FIFTH EDITION

Fluid and Electrolyte Balance

Nursing Considerations

Norma M. Metheny, PhD, RN, FAAN

Professor and Dorothy A. Votsmier Endowed Chair
Saint Louis University School of Nursing
St. Louis, Missouri

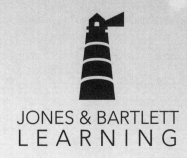

JONES & BARTLETT
LEARNING

World Headquarters
Jones & Bartlett Learning
40 Tall Pine Drive
Sudbury, MA 01776
978-443-5000
info@jblearning.com
www.jblearning.com

Jones & Bartlett Learning Canada
6339 Ormindale Way
Mississauga, Ontario L5V 1J2
Canada

Jones & Bartlett Learning International
Barb House, Barb Mews
London W6 7PA
United Kingdom

Jones & Bartlett Learning books and products are available through most bookstores and online booksellers. To contact Jones & Bartlett Learning directly, call 800-832-0034, fax 978-443-8000, or visit our website, www.jblearning.com.

Substantial discounts on bulk quantities of Jones & Bartlett Learning publications are available to corporations, professional associations, and other qualified organizations. For details and specific discount information, contact the special sales department at Jones & Bartlett Learning via the above contact information or send an email to specialsales@jblearning.com.

The author, editor, and publisher have made every effort to provide accurate information. However, they are not responsible for errors, omissions, or for any outcomes related to the use of the contents of this book and take no responsibility for the use of the products and procedures described. Treatments and side effects described in this book may not be applicable to all people; likewise, some people may require a dose or experience a side effect that is not described herein. Drugs and medical devices are discussed that may have limited availability controlled by the Food and Drug Administration (FDA) for use only in a research study or clinical trial. Research, clinical practice, and government regulations often change the accepted standard in this field. When consideration is being given to use of any drug in the clinical setting, the health care provider or reader is responsible for determining FDA status of the drug, reading the package insert, and reviewing prescribing information for the most up-to-date recommendations on dose, precautions, and contraindications, and determining the appropriate usage for the product. This is especially important in the case of drugs that are new or seldom used.

Production Credits
Publisher: Kevin Sullivan
Acquisitions Editor: Amy Sibley
Editorial Assistant: Rachel Shuster
Production Assistant: Sara Fowles
Marketing Manager: Meagan Norlund
V.P., Manufacturing and Inventory Control: Therese Connell
Composition: Auburn Associates, Inc.
Cover Design: Kristin E. Parker
Cover Image: © Ed Isaacs/Dreamstime.com
Printing and Binding: Malloy, Inc.
Cover Printing: Malloy, Inc.

Library of Congress Cataloging-in-Publication Data
Metheny, Norma Milligan.
Fluids and electrolytes balance : nursing considerations / Norma Metheny. —5th ed.
     p. ; cm.
   Rev. ed. of: Fluid and electrolyte balance / Norma M. Metheny. 4th ed.
   c2000.
   Includes bibliographical references and index.
  ISBN 978-0-7637-8164-4 (pbk.)
  1. Body fluid disorders. 2. Body fluid disorders—Nursing. 3. Water-electrolyte imbalances. 4. Water-electrolyte imbalances—Nursing.
I. Metheny, Norma Milligan. Fluid and electrolyte balance. II. Title.
  [DNLM: 1. Water-Electrolyte Imbalance—Nurses' Instruction.
  2.   Water-Electrolyte Balance—Nurses' Instruction. WD 220 M592f 2011]
  RC630.F556 2011 (2012)
  616.3'992—dc22
                                                                2010021081

6048
Printed in the United States of America
15   14   13   12   11   10 9 8 7 6 5 4 3 2

Contents

Preface

The fifth edition of *Fluid and Electrolyte Balance: Nursing Considerations* continues in the tradition established by the prior editions of this textbook. It provides current and comprehensive information related to the nursing care of patients with fluid, electrolyte, and acid–base imbalances in a readable and user-friendly manner. Because concepts of fluid and electrolyte balance apply to a broad spectrum of patient problems, the book's scope is wide. While written simply, in an effort to promote ease of understanding for students, it contains enough information to stimulate the interest of advanced practitioners.

The most current research findings related to conditions affecting fluid and electrolyte balance are integrated throughout the text. The book retains its strong focus on understanding the pathophysiology of fluid and electrolyte imbalances as a basis for providing care to patients with these conditions. Additional case studies are included in this edition to emphasize important information pertinent to patients with fluid and electrolyte imbalances.

Contributors

Contributor (Fifth Edition)

Linda Haycraft, RN, MSN(R), CPNT
Assistant Professor
Saint Louis University School of Nursing
St. Louis, Missouri

Recognition of Former Contributors (Fourth Edition)

Dr. Charold L. Baer
Professor Emerita
Oregon Health and Sciences University
Portland, Oregon

Joan Clark, RN, MSN, BC, ANP
St. Louis Hematology/Oncology Specialists
St. Louis, Missouri

Susan L. Cole, APN, RN
Cape Girardeau, Missouri

Mary Ellen Grohar-Murray, RN, PhD
Professor of Nursing
Saint Louis University
St. Louis, Missouri

Marilyn Hackenthal, RN, MSN
Former Professor of Nursing
Lewis and Clark Community College
Alton, Illinois

J. Keith Hampton, MSN, APRN, ACNS-BC
Professional Practice and Nursing Standards Coordinator
University of Missouri Health Care
Columbia, Missouri

Dorothy C. James, RN, PhD
Center of Nursing Excellence
St. John's Mercy Medical Center
St. Louis, Missouri

Kathryn L. Neunaber, ANP, BA, NP
Washington University School of Medicine
St. Louis, Missouri

Catherine C. Powers, MSN, RN, ACNS-BC
Clinical Nurse Specialist, Heart and Vascular Program
Barnes-Jewish Hospital
St. Louis, Missouri

Sherry Beth Robinson, RNCS, PhD
Southern Illinois University
Springfield, Illinois

Patsy L. Ruchala, RN, DNSc
Director, Orvis School of Nursing
University of Nevada
Reno, Nevada

Lynn Schallom, RN, MSN, CCRN, CCNS
Evidence Based Practice Critical Care CNS
Barnes-Jewish Hospital
St. Louis, Missouri

Deirdre M. Schweiss, MSN, RN, CPNP
Associate Professor of Nursing
Saint Louis University
St. Louis, Missouri

UNIT I

Basic Concepts

Chapter 1

Fundamental Concepts and Definitions

BODY FLUIDS AND THEIR DISTRIBUTION

Body fluid is either *intracellular* (within the cells) or *extracellular* (outside the cells). Extracellular fluid (ECF) is further subdivided into intravascular fluid (plasma) and interstitial fluid (fluid lying between the cells, or tissue fluid). The ECF interfaces with the outside world and is modified by it, but the intracellular fluid (ICF) remains stable. Constantly moving throughout the body, the ECF contains the ions and nutrients needed to maintain cell life.[1] In addition to carrying nutrients to the cells, the ECF carries wastes away from the cells by means of the capillary bed. The peripheral circulation includes approximately 10 billion capillaries with a total surface area estimated to be close to one-eighth the surface area of a football field.[2]

Water accounts for approximately 60% of the body weight of a normal adult male. Approximately two-thirds of the total body water (TBW) is inside the cells; the remaining one-third is outside the cells (in the interstitial space or plasma space). For example, a lean male weighing 70 kilograms (kg) may have 42 liters (L) of body fluid (60% of 70 kg). Of that 42 L, approximately 28 L is found in the intracellular space, 10.5 L in the interstitial space, and 3.5 L in the plasma.[3] In an adult, the average blood volume represents 7% of body weight and contains both extracellular fluid (in the form of plasma) and cellular fluid (the fluid within the red blood cells).[4]

Women have less body water than men because they have proportionately more fat (a tissue characterized by low water content). After 40 years of age, mean values for TBW in percentage of body weight decrease for both men and women; however, the sex differentiation remains. After 60 years of age, the percentage may decrease to 52% in men and 46% in women (even less in obese persons). The reduction in body fluid is explained by the fact that aging brings a decrease in lean body mass in favor of fat. Obese individuals have considerably less body fluid than persons of lean build, regardless of gender.

A premature infant's body is approximately 90% water; the newborn infant's body is 70% to 80% water. In addition to having proportionately more body fluid than adults, infants have relatively more fluid in the extracellular compartment, a condition that predisposes them to developing fluid volume deficit more readily than adults (**Figure 1-1**). As infants become older, their total body fluid percentage decreases—a change that occurs most rapidly during the first 6 months of life. By the end of the second year of life, the total body fluid approaches the adult percentage of 60% (36% cellular and 24% extracellular). At puberty, the adult body composition is attained and, for the first time, there is a sex differentiation in fluid content. **Table 1-1** lists general variations in total body fluid with age.

Microscopically, one might visualize the body fluids as shown in **Figure 1-2**. Also, part of the ECF consists of transcellular fluids, primarily representing secretions from epithelial cells and sometimes having ionic compositions different from the plasma and interstitial fluids. Examples of transcellular fluid include cerebrospinal fluid (CSF), secretions in the gastrointestinal (GI) tract, and fluid found in the peritoneal and pleural cavities. Collectively, these fluids account for 1 to 2 L of body fluid.[5]

BODY ELECTROLYTES AND THEIR DISTRIBUTION

Body fluid consists primarily of water and electrolytes. An *electrolyte* is a substance that develops an electrical charge when dissolved in water. Examples of electrolytes include sodium, potassium, calcium, chloride, and bicarbonate.

(a) Adult

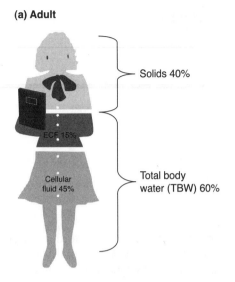

Solids 40%

ECF 15%

Cellular fluid 45%

Total body water (TBW) 60%

Figure 1-1a Fluid and solid components of body weight in adult

(b) Newborn

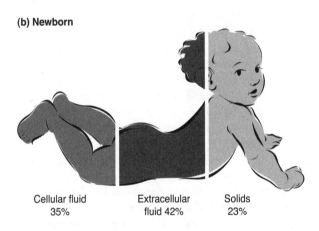

Cellular fluid 35%   Extracellular fluid 42%   Solids 23%

Figure1-1b Fluid and solid components of body weight in newborn

Table 1-1 Approximate Values of Total Body Fluid as a Percentage of Body Weight in Relation to Age and Gender

Age	Approximate Total Body Fluid (Percentage of Body Weight)
Premature infant	90%
Full-term newborn	70–80%
1 year	64%
Puberty to 39 years	Men: 60% Women: 52%
40–60 years	Men: 55% Women: 47%
> 60 years	Men: 52% Women: 46%

As indicated earlier, the bulk of body fluid is located within the intracellular fluid (ICF) of the body's approximately 100 trillion cells.[6] The electrolyte content of ICF differs significantly from that of ECF. **Table 1-2** lists the electrolytes in plasma (ECF); **Table 1-3** lists the electrolytes in ICF. Because special techniques are required to measure the concentration of electrolytes in the ICF, it is customary to measure the electrolytes in the ECF—namely, in the plasma. Plasma electrolyte concentrations are used in assessing and managing patients with electrolyte imbalances. Some tests are performed on serum (the portion of plasma left after clotting); for practical purposes, the terms *serum electrolytes* and *plasma electrolytes* are used interchangeably.

The major electrolytes in the ECF are sodium (Na^+) and chloride (Cl^-), with a great preponderance of sodium ions (142 mEq/L) compared with other cations. Sodium ions are restricted primarily to the ECF and are of primary importance in regulating body fluid volume. Retention of sodium is associated with fluid retention; in contrast, loss of sodium is usually associated with decreased fluid volume. The major electrolytes in the ICF are potassium, phosphate, and magnesium. Release of the large stores of intracellular potassium through cellular trauma can be extremely dangerous because the ECF can tolerate only small potassium concentrations (about 5 mEq/L).

The body expends a great deal of energy maintaining the extracellular preponderance of sodium and the intracellular preponderance of potassium. It does so by means of cell membrane pumps, which exchange sodium and potassium ions. (See the discussion of the sodium–potassium pump later in this chapter.)

Those elements that develop a positive charge in water are called *cations*—for example, sodium (Na^+), potassium (K^+), calcium (Ca^{++}), and magnesium (Mg^{++}). Electrolytes that develop negative charges when dissolved in water are called *anions*—for example, chloride (Cl^-), and bicarbonate (HCO_3^-). In all body fluids, anions and cations are always present in equal amounts because positive and negative changes must be equal. In fact, all solutions (whether biological or nonbiological) are electrically neutral; this condition is sometimes called the law of *electroneutrality*.

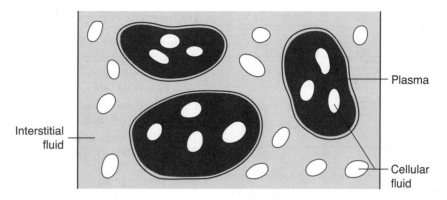

Figure1-2 Microscopic visualization of body fluid distribution

Table 1-2 Plasma Electrolytes

Electrolytes	Concentration (mEq/L)
Cations	
Sodium (Na⁺)	142
Potassium (K⁺)	5
Calcium (Ca⁺⁺)	5
Magnesium (Mg⁺⁺)	2
Total cations	**154**
Anions	
Chloride (Cl⁻)	103
Bicarbonate (HCO₃⁻)	26
Phosphate (HPO₄⁻⁻)	2
Sulfate (SO₄⁻⁻)	1
Organic acids	5
Proteinate	17
Total anions	**154**

UNITS OF MEASURE FOR ELECTROLYTES

Concentrations of solutes can be expressed in several ways—for example, milligrams per deciliter (mg/dL), milliequivalents per liter (mEq/L), or millimoles per liter (mmol/L). Because all of these units may be used in clinical settings, a brief review of their meanings is appropriate.

Milligrams per 100 mL (100 mL = 1 dL) expresses the weight of the solute per unit volume. In contrast, a *milliequivalent* of an ion is its atomic weight expressed in milligrams divided by the valence. The latter measure is most favored in the United States for expressing the small concentrations of electrolytes in body fluids because it emphasizes the principle that ions combine on a milliequivalent for milliequivalent basis, not millimole for millimole or milligram for milligram. Also, the important concept of *electroneutrality* is clarified when using milliequivalents because milliequivalents of cations and anions exist in equal numbers in the body fluids (**Figure 1-3**). This obligatory relationship is not evident if the ionic concentrations are measured in millimoles per liter or in milligrams per deciliter. Because electrolytes in body fluids are active chemicals (anions and cations) that unite in varying combinations, it is considered more logical to express their concentration as a measure of chemical activity rather than as a measure of weight.

Countries using the Système Internationale (SI) units express electrolyte content in body fluids in *millimoles*. To understand millimoles, it is necessary to review the definition of a mole. One *mole* (mol) of a substance is defined as

Table 1-3 Approximation of Major Electrolyte Concentrations in Intracellular Fluid

Electrolytes	Concentration (mEq/L)
Cations	
Potassium (K⁺)	150
Magnesium (Mg⁺⁺)	40
Sodium (Na⁺)	10
Total cations	**200**
Anions	
Phosphates and sulfates	150
Bicarbonate (HCO₃⁻)	10
Proteinate	40
Total anions	**200**

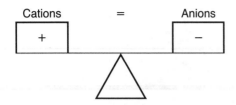

Figure1-3 Number of cations equals number of anions

the molecular (or atomic) weight of that substance in grams (g). For example, a mole of sodium is equivalent to 23 g (the atomic weight of sodium is 23). A millimole is one-thousandth of a mole, or the molecular or atomic weight expressed in milligrams. Thus a millimole of sodium is equivalent to 23 mg. Univalent elements, such as sodium (Na^+) and potassium (K^+), have identical numbers for milliequivalents and millimoles; that is, 140 mEq of Na^+ = 140 mmol of Na^+ and 5 mEq of K^+ = 5 mmol of K^+. However, different numbers are required for electrolytes that are not univalent. To convert from units of millimoles per liter to milliequivalents per liter, use the following formula:

mEq/L = mmol/L × valence

For example, because the valence of calcium is 2, l mmol of calcium = 2 mEq of calcium (**Figure 1-4**). Although the milliequivalent is not an SI unit, it is so widely used and conceptually useful that it is likely to persist for some time.

MOVEMENT OF BODY FLUIDS AND ELECTROLYTES ACROSS COMPARTMENTS

As described earlier, body fluids are constantly moving to carry nutrients to the cells as well as to carry wastes away from the cells. A number of mechanisms are in place to facilitate fluid and electrolyte movement within the body.

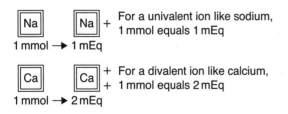

Figure1-4 Millimoles versus milliequivalents for univalent and divalent ions

Hydrostatic Pressure and Oncotic Pressure

Normal movement of fluids through the capillary wall into the tissues depends on two forces: *hydrostatic pressure* (exerted by pumping of the heart) and *oncotic pressure* (exerted by nondiffusible plasma proteins, primarily albumin). Oncotic pressure is defined as the osmotic pressure generated by large solutes (such as albumin) and is sometimes called colloid osmotic pressure. At the arterial end of the capillary, fluids are filtered through its wall by a hydrostatic pressure that exceeds the oncotic pressure exerted by plasma proteins. In contrast, because oncotic pressure is greater than hydrostatic pressure in the venous end of the capillary, fluids reenter the capillary here (**Figure 1-5**).

Osmosis

When two different solutions are separated by a membrane impermeable to the dissolved substances, a shift of water occurs through the membrane from the region of low solute concentration to the region of high solute concentration until the solutions are of equal concentrations (**Figure 1-6**). The magnitude of this force depends on the number of particles dissolved in the solutions, not on their weights.

Osmolality Versus Osmolarity

The number of dissolved particles in a unit of water determines the solution's concentration and can be expressed as either osmolality or osmolarity. *Osmolality* refers to the number of milliosmoles per kilogram of water (mOsm/kg), while *osmolarity* refers to the number of milliosmoles per liter of solution (mOsm/L).[7] The total volume in osmolality is 1 L of water plus the relatively small volume occupied by the solute. In contrast, the total volume in osmolarity is less than 1 L by an amount equal to the solute volume. Because body fluids have a very low solute content, the difference between osmolality and osmolarity is negligible. Therefore, the terms are often used interchangeably in practice settings.

Whether described as osmolality or osmolarity, the concentrations of solutes are important in determining fluid movement between the body's physiologic compartments. In the ECF, the primarily determinant of osmolality is sodium. In the ICF, potassium salts and organic phosphate esters largely determine the effective osmolality.[8] See Chapter 10 for information about the osmolarity of common intravenous fluids.

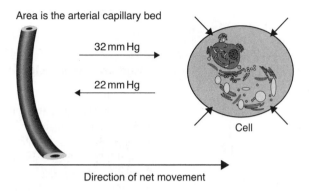

Figure1-5a Delivery of water, electrolytes, and other nutrients to cells

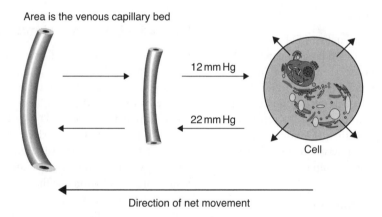

Figure1-5b Transport of urea, CO_2, and other wastes away from cells

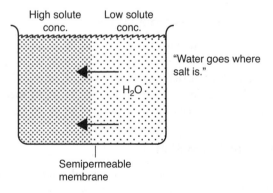

Figure1-6 Osmosis

Tonicity

The term *tonicity* is sometimes used instead of osmolarity or osmolality. Solutions may be termed isotonic, hypotonic, or hypertonic. *Isotonic* solutions have the same effective osmolality as body fluids (normal range is 280–295 mOsm/kg). Examples of near-isotonic parenteral fluids include 0.9% sodium chloride (308 mOsm/L) and lactated Ringer's solution (273 mOsm/L). In contrast, a *hypotonic* solution has a lower osmolarity than body fluids; an example of a hypotonic parenteral fluid is 0.45% sodium chloride (154 mOsm/L). Finally, an example of a *hypertonic* parenteral fluid is 3% sodium chloride (1027 mOsm/L).

Diffusion

The continued movement of molecules among each other in liquids, or in gases, is called *diffusion*. An example of diffusion is the exchange of oxygen and carbon dioxide (CO_2) between the alveoli and capillaries.

Filtration

Filtration is the transfer of water and dissolved substances from a region of high pressure to a region of low pressure; the force behind it is hydrostatic pressure. An example of filtration is the passage of water and electrolytes from the arterial capillary bed to the interstitial fluid. In this instance, the hydrostatic pressure is furnished by the pumping action of the heart.

Sodium–Potassium Pump

Sodium concentration is greater in the ECF than in the ICF; therefore, there is a tendency for sodium to enter the cells by diffusion. This tendency is offset by the workings of the sodium–potassium pump, which is located in the cell membrane; in the presence of adenosine triphosphate (ATP), this pump actively moves sodium from the cell into the ECF. Conversely, potassium is the predominant cation in the ICF; the high intracellular potassium concentration is maintained by pumping potassium into the cell.

Active Transport of Calcium and Hydrogen Ions

The calcium pump is another primary active transport mechanism; it acts to maintain the very low concentrations of calcium inside the cells at a concentration approximately 10,000 times less than that in the ECF.[9] Active transport of hydrogen ions occurs in the gastric glands as well as in the kidneys' distal tubules and cortical collecting ducts.[10]

ROUTES OF GAINS AND LOSSES

Water and electrolytes are gained in various ways. In healthy humans, fluids are gained by drinking and eating (much of solid food is actually fluid). In illness, fluids may be gained by the parenteral route (intravenously or subcutaneously) or by means of an enteral feeding tube in the stomach or intestine. Organs of fluid loss include the lungs, skin, GI tract, and kidneys. When fluid balance is critical, *all routes of gain* and *all routes of loss* must be recorded and the volumes compared. For critically ill patients, even small gains of fluid (such as that provided by humidifiers) must be considered.

Fluid Loss from Kidneys

Although losses from the lungs, skin, and GI tract are determined by changing environmental events, losses from the kidney can be regulated by homeostatic organs. As such, the kidneys play a crucial role in the regulation of ECF volume in healthy and disease states.

The usual volume of urine output in the adult is between 1 and 2 L/day. A general rule of thumb is approximately 1 mL of urine per 1 kilogram of body weight per hour (1 mL/kg/hr), with a range of 0.5 to 2 mL/kg/hr. Table 2-1 on page 19 shows that in a healthy adult, the average 24-hour intake and output of water are approximately equal.

Fluid Loss from Gastrointestinal Tract

Each day, the healthy small intestine absorbs both fluids that are ingested and fluids that are secreted into the GI tract. Thus, although in adults approximately 6 L of fluid circulates through the GI system every 24 hours (called the "GI circulation"), only 100 to 200 mL is lost through the GI tract each day. Obviously, very large losses can be incurred from the GI tract if abnormal conditions occur (such as diarrhea, fistulas, or vomiting). Diarrheal fluid losses tend to be isotonic with the ECF; however, diarrheal losses from the terminal part of the large intestine are hypotonic and reflect losses of free water. Not only does vomiting cause fluid loss by the ejection of ingested and secreted fluids in the stomach and upper small intestine, but it is also usually associated with nausea that further limits oral intake of fluid.

Water Vapor Loss from Lungs

The lungs normally eliminate water vapor (*insensible loss*) at a rate of 300 to 400 mL/day.[11] The rate of loss is much greater with increased respiratory rate, depth, or both. Losses from the lungs depend on external factors, such as humidity and oxygen concentration.

Fluid Loss from Skin

Visible water and electrolyte loss through the skin occurs by sweating (*sensible perspiration*). Sweat is a hypotonic fluid containing several solutes—chiefly sodium, chloride, and potassium. Actual sweat losses vary according to environmental temperature, from 0 to 1000 mL or more per hour. Significant sweat losses occur if the patient's body temperature exceeds 38.3°C (101°F).

Continuous water loss by evaporation (approximately 600 mL/day) occurs through the skin as *insensible perspiration*, a nonvisible form of water loss. The presence of fever greatly increases insensible water loss through the lungs and the skin. Loss of the natural skin barrier in major burns also increases water loss by this route.

HOMEOSTATIC MECHANISMS

The body is equipped with homeostatic mechanisms to keep the composition and volume of body fluid within narrow limits of normal. Major organs involved include the kidneys, lungs, heart, adrenal glands, parathyroid glands, and the pituitary gland. See **Table 1-4**.

Kidneys

The kidneys are vital to the regulation of fluid and electrolyte balance. They normally filter 180 L of plasma per day in a normal adult, while excreting only 1.8 L of urine. They act both autonomously and in response to blood-borne messengers, such as aldosterone and *antidiuretic hormone* (ADH).

The kidneys have the following major functions in fluid balance homeostasis:

- *Regulation of electrolyte concentrations in the ECF by selective retention and excretion.* The kidney can modify the quantity of solutes and water excreted in the urine according to the intake of these substances. For example, experimental studies have shown that many people can maintain normal plasma sodium concentrations when sodium intake is as much as 10 times normal or as low as one-tenth of normal.[12]
- *Regulation of acid–base balance.* The kidneys contribute to acid–base balance by excreting acids (such as sulfuric acid and phosphoric acid) that are generated by the metabolism of proteins.
- *Excretion of metabolic wastes (primarily acids) and toxic substances.* Urine contains high concentrations of urea (allowing metabolic end products to be excreted, rather than accumulating in the body).

Obviously, renal failure results in multiple fluid and electrolyte problems (see Chapter 17).

Heart and Atrial Natriuretic Factor

Plasma must reach the kidneys in sufficient volume to permit regulation of water and electrolytes. The pumping action of the heart provides circulation of blood through the kidneys under sufficient pressure for urine to form; of course, renal perfusion makes renal function possible. A hormone

---

Table 1-4 Summary of Homeostatic Hormones and Their Effects on Fluid and Electrolyte Balance

Hormone	Origin	Effects
Aldosterone	Adrenal cortex	Increases renal retention of sodium and subsequent expansion of ECF; also causes renal excretion of potassium.
Antidiuretic hormone (ADH), same as arginine vasopressin (AVP)	Hypothalamus, stored in posterior pituitary gland	Causes renal retention of water with subsequent dilution of serum sodium concentration. Sometimes called the "water-conserving hormone."
Atrial natriuretic factor (ANF)	Right atrium of heart	Causes diuresis of sodium and water, thereby decreasing intravascular volume.
Calcitonin	Thyroid gland	Reduces plasma calcium concentration (action opposite that of parathyroid hormone).
Cortisol	Adrenal cortex	Increases renal retention of sodium and subsequent expansion of ECF; also causes renal excretion of potassium. Cortisol's action is much less intense than that of aldosterone.
Oxytocin	Hypothalamus	Has primary effects on the uterus and lactation, but also possesses significant ADH activity. At high doses, oxytocin can produce ADH effects (water retention with subsequent dilution of serum sodium concentration).
Parathyroid hormone (PTH)	Parathyroid glands, located on four corners of thyroid gland	Increases plasma calcium concentration by stimulating release of calcium from bone, increasing renal retention of calcium, and increasing gastrointestinal absorption of calcium.

known as *atrial natriuretic factor* (ANF) or atrial natriuretic peptide (ANP) is released in the right atrium. The primary stimulus for release of ANF is atrial distention, which is associated with an increased blood volume that stretches the right atrium. This hormone acts by a variety of mechanisms to cause a diuresis of sodium and water, thereby decreasing the intravascular volume. ANF increases sodium excretion partly by suppressing renin and aldosterone release and partly by exerting a direct inhibitory effect on sodium reabsorption by the kidney.[13] In addition, ANF is a vasodilator, acting to lower the systemic blood pressure.[14]

Lungs and Acid–Base Balance

The lungs are also vital in maintaining homeostasis. Alveolar ventilation is responsible for the daily elimination of about 13,000 mEq H^+, as opposed to only 40 to 80 mEq H^+ excreted daily by the kidneys.

Under the control of the medulla, the lungs act promptly to correct metabolic acid–base disturbances by regulating the amount of carbon dioxide (CO_2) in the ECF. (Recall that when CO_2 is dissolved in water, carbonic acid is formed.) For example, to compensate for metabolic alkalosis, the lungs hypoventilate to retain CO_2; the increased acidity helps correct excess alkalinity of body fluids. Just the opposite occurs with metabolic acidosis: The lungs hyperventilate to remove CO_2, which helps decrease the excess acidity of body fluids. Pulmonary dysfunction can produce a rapid change (matter of seconds) in acid–base balance. Hypoventilation causes respiratory acidosis; hyperventilation causes respiratory alkalosis. When the lungs are at fault, the kidneys must compensate for the pH disturbances. Acid–base regulation is discussed in depth in Chapter 9.

The lungs also remove approximately 300 mL of water daily through exhalation (insensible water loss) in the healthy adult. Abnormal conditions, such as hyperventilation or continuous coughing, increase this loss. Conversely, mechanical ventilation with excessive moisture decreases the loss.

Pituitary Mechanism and Antidiuretic Hormone

Specialized cells located in the hypothalamus manufacture ADH, which is stored in the posterior lobe of the pituitary gland and released as needed. ADH is also known as *arginine vasopressin* (AVP) and vasopressin; the terms are used interchangeably.[15] ADH makes the body retain water; therefore, it is sometimes called the "water-conserving" hormone. The kidney is the target organ of ADH; as such, the amount of water retained or excreted by the kidneys is partially regulated by ADH, which attaches to specialized receptor sites in the collecting and distal renal tubules.[16] When ADH secretion increases, urine volume decreases because of renal retention of water. The opposite occurs when ADH production is low—that is, output of dilute urine is increased.

Minor changes in body fluid osmolality occur during normal living and lead to minor physiological changes in ADH production. A rising plasma osmolality, such as occurs with salt intake, increases ADH production and, therefore, water retention. For example, a 2% elevation in plasma osmolality leads to a two- to three-fold increase in ADH levels (thus causing water to be conserved by the kidney and urine volume to decrease).[17] Conversely, a falling plasma osmolality, such as occurs with water intake, decreases ADH production and enhances renal water excretion (**Figure 1-7**). Therefore, plasma osmolality and ADH are in constant interaction. In the presence of a falling

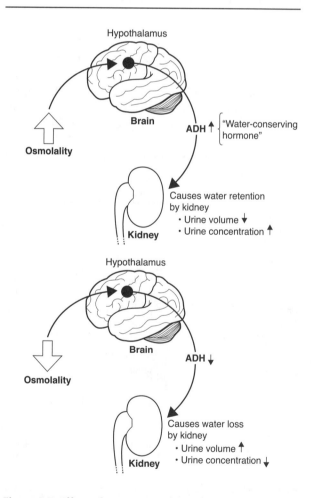

Figure1-7 Effect of serum osmolality on ADH release and urine output

blood volume, ADH secretion and subsequent water retention are stimulated. ADH is rapidly released in response to physiological stimuli and begins to act within minutes; it is rapidly metabolized in the liver and kidney (its half-life in the circulation is only 15 to 20 minutes).[18]

ADH is a potent vasoconstrictor. For example, in the presence of shock, formation of this hormone is increased, causing constriction of peripheral vessels as well as increased water retention by the kidneys.[19] However, the role of ADH in maintaining blood pressure is minor when compared to the effects of the renin–angiotensin and sympathetic nervous systems.[20] In recognition of this role, ADH is gaining acceptance in the treatment of distributive or vasodilatory shock.[21]

Syndrome of inappropriate antidiuretic hormone secretion (SIADH) and *diabetes insipidus* (DI) are disorders of water balance caused by ADH disturbances at opposite ends of a continuum. In SIADH, excessive ADH secretion causes water retention. The opposite happens in DI, which is characterized by large dilute urine volumes due to inadequate amounts of ADH. These pathological states are discussed further in Chapters 4 and 19.

Oxytocin is another hormone that is synthesized in the hypothalamus and has a chemical structure very similar to ADH. While its primary effects are on the uterus and lactation, it also possesses significant ADH activity.[22] At high doses, oxytocin can produce ADH effects.[23] See Chapter 23 for a discussion of the relationship between oxytocin administration and fluid balance.

Adrenal Glands and Aldosterone

The primary adrenocortical hormone that influences fluid balance is *aldosterone*, a mineralocorticoid secreted by the outer zone of the adrenal cortex. This hormone acts chiefly on the distal tubules of the kidney to cause sodium retention and expansion of the ECF, along with renal excretion of potassium. Conditions that can stimulate aldosterone secretion include a decrease in the plasma sodium concentration or an increase in the plasma potassium concentration. However, the primary regulator of aldosterone secretion appears to be angiotension II, which is produced by the renin-angiotensin system. A decreased blood volume or flow activates this system and increases aldosterone secretion (**Figure 1-8**). The opposite happens when a state of volume overexpansion exists.

Cortisol, another adrenocortical hormone, has only a fraction of the mineralocorticoid potency of aldosterone. However, secretion of cortisol in large quantities can produce sodium and fluid retention and potassium deficit.

Parathyroid Glands and Parathyroid Hormone

Most persons have four parathyroid glands (**Figure 1-9**). These pea-sized glands, which are embedded in the corners of the thyroid gland, regulate calcium and phosphate balance by means of *parathyroid hormone* (PTH). PTH release is, in turn, regulated by the serum calcium concentration. In other words, PTH production is stimulated by hypocalcemia

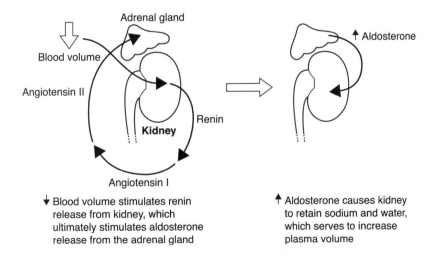

Figure1-8 Effect of hypovolemia on the renin-angiotensin-aldosterone system

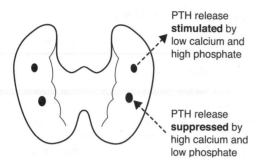

Figure 1-9 Effect of serum calcium and phosphorus on PTH release

and is suppressed by hypercalcemia. PTH production during hypocalcemia helps to correct the low plasma calcium concentration by stimulating release of calcium from the bone into the ECF. PTH also promotes renal conversion of vitamin D to *calcitriol* (1,25-dihydroxyvitamin D_3). Calcitriol is the most active form of vitamin D and causes increased absorption of calcium from the GI tract as well as release of calcium from bone; it also increases renal absorption of calcium. Vitamin D is synthesized in skin following exposure to light and is also absorbed from ingested food.[24]

Another hormone that bears consideration in the regulation of calcium is *calcitonin*, a substance secreted by the thyroid gland. The action of calcitonin on calcium is opposite to that of PTH; that is, it reduces plasma calcium concentration. Calcitonin is sometimes administered to help control hypercalcemia when other more prominent treatments are ineffective.

A reciprocal relationship exists between extracellular calcium and phosphate levels, in that an elevation of one usually causes a depression of the other (**Figure 1-10**). Thus a high extracellular phosphate concentration (common in renal failure) causes a secondary depression of extracellular calcium; as a result, PTH release is stimulated. This explains

why patients with chronic renal failure have reduced bone calcium concentrations.

SUMMARY

The concepts introduced in this chapter are expanded upon in the specific chapters on fluid, electrolyte, and acid–base balance as well is in the chapters dealing with clinical situations associated with fluid and electrolyte problems.

NOTES

1. Guyton, A. C., & Hall, J. E. (2006). *Textbook of medical physiology* (11th ed.). Philadelphia: W. B. Saunders, p. 3.
2. Guyton & Hall, note 1, p. 181.
3. Cooper, D. H., Krainik, A. J., Lubner, S. J., & Reno, H. E. (2007). *The Washington manual of medical therapeutics* (32nd ed.). Philadelphia: Lippincott Williams & Wilkins, p. 54.
4. Guyton & Hall, note 1, p. 293.
5. Guyton & Hall, note 1, p. 292.
6. Guyton & Hall, note 1, p. 3.
7. Hahn, R. F., Prough, D. S., & Svensen, C. H. (2007). *Perioperative fluid therapy*. London: Informa Healthcare USA, p. 247.
8. Cooper et al., note 3, p. 59.
9. Guyton & Hall, note 1, p. 54.
10. Guyton & Hall, note 1, p. 54.
11. Guyton & Hall, note 1, p. 292.
12. Guyton & Hall, note 1, p. 308.
13. Feehally, J., Floege, J., & Johnson, R. J. (2007). *Comprehensive clinical nephrology* (3rd ed.). Philadelphia: Mosby Elsevier, p. 24.
14. Rose, B. D., & Post, T. W. (2001). *Clinical physiology of acid–base and electrolyte disorders* (5th ed.). New York: McGraw-Hill, p. 187.
15. Brunton, L., Parker, K., Blumenthal, D., & Buxton, I. (2008). *Goodman and Gilman's manual of pharmacology and therapeutics*. New York: McGraw-Hill, p. 505.
16. Garner, D. G., & Shoback, D. (2007). *Greenspan's basic and clinical endocrinology* (8th ed.). New York: McGraw-Hill Medical, p. 890.
17. Brunton et al., note 15, p. 499.
18. Rose & Post, note 14, p. 168.
19. Guyton & Hall, note 1, p. 281.
20. Rose & Post, note 14, p. 172.
21. McPhee, S., Papadakis, M. A., & Tierney, L. M. (2008). *2008 current medical diagnosis and treatment*. New York: McGraw-Hill Lange, p. 420.
22. Rose & Post, note 14, p. 709.
23. Brunton et al., note 15, p. 978.
24. Cooper et al., note 3, p. 78.

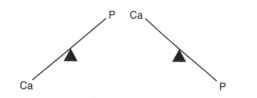

Figure 1-10 Reciprocal relationship between calcium and phosphorus

Chapter 2

Nursing Assessment

Nursing assessment of fluid and electrolyte balance requires a review of the patient's history and laboratory data as well as careful clinical observation. In summary, the nurse must know what to look for, where and how often to look, and when to expect certain changes as a result of interventions.

HISTORY

The following questions should be considered in the nursing history:

1. Is a disease process or injury state present that can disrupt fluid and electrolyte balance? If so, which types of imbalances usually result from this condition? (For example, a patient with end-stage renal disease would be at increased risk for hyperkalemia, hyperphosphatemia, hypocalcemia, and metabolic acidosis.)
2. Is the patient receiving any medication or treatment that might disrupt fluid and electrolyte balance? If so, how might this therapy upset fluid balance? (For example, a patient receiving a potassium-conserving diuretic would be at increased risk for hyperkalemia.)
3. Is there an abnormal loss of body fluids and, if so, from which source? Which types of imbalances are usually associated with the loss of these fluids? (For example, a patient with severe vomiting would be at increased risk for hypokalemia and metabolic alkalosis.)
4. Have any dietary restrictions been imposed? If so, how might fluid balance be affected?
5. Has the patient taken adequate amounts of water and other nutrients orally or by some other route? If not, how long has the inadequate intake been present?

6. How does the total intake of fluids compare with the total output of fluid? (For example, does the fluid intake greatly exceed output?)

CLINICAL ASSESSMENT

After the history described in the preceding section has been reviewed, the nurse should be able to identify potential problems related to fluid and electrolyte imbalances. At this point, a thorough nursing assessment is indicated. Of course, nursing assessment is not a one-time procedure, but rather must be performed at regular intervals to detect changes. The assessments described in this section are also included in subsequent chapters as they pertain to specific imbalances and age groups.

Facial Appearance and Sunken Eyes

An individual with a severe *fluid volume deficit* (FVD) has a pinched facial expression. A significant FVD causes decreased intraocular pressure; thus the eyes appear sunken and feel soft to the touch. Sunken eyes are a valid indicator of FVD in both infants and elderly patients.

Moisture in Oral Cavity

A dry mouth may be the result of FVD or of mouth breathing. If it is due to FVD, all of the oral tissues will be dry. In contrast, if the dryness is due to mouth breathing, the areas where the gums and cheek membranes meet will remain moist. Dry, sticky mucous membranes are noted with sodium excess (hypernatremia).

Thirst

Thirst is a subjective sensory symptom that has been defined as an awareness of the desire to drink. When plasma osmolality increases, water is pulled from the cells in the thirst center and thirst is stimulated. The value of thirst is, of course, that it stimulates fluid intake and helps to dilute extracellular fluids and return osmolality toward normal.

In general, any factor that causes intracellular dehydration will cause a sensation of thirst; examples of metabolic problems that can stimulate thirst include hypernatremia, hypercalcemia, hyperglycemia, and fever. For example, a 2 mEq/L elevation of the serum sodium above normal can stimulate thirst.[1] The sense of thirst is so protective of the normal serum sodium level that hypernatremia virtually never occurs unless thirst is impaired or rendered ineffective because of unconsciousness or inaccessibility of water. Thirst is diminished in the elderly; see Chapter 25 for a discussion of decreased thirst associated with aging. Obviously, patients with a decreased level of consciousness are not fully cognizant of thirst. A decreased blood volume caused by hemorrhage can stimulate thirst even though there is no change in plasma osmolality.[2] Dryness of the mouth causes the desire to drink (not to relieve thirst, but instead to relieve mouth dryness).

Skin Turgor

In a healthy person, pinched skin will immediately fall back to its normal position when released. This elastic property, referred to as turgor, partially depends on the interstitial fluid volume. In an individual with FVD, the skin flattens more slowly after the pinch is released and may remain elevated for several seconds. (See **Figure 2-1.**)

Although the purpose of the skin turgor test is to measure interstitial fluid volume, it also measures skin elasticity. Because persons older than 55 to 60 years of age have decreased skin elasticity, skin turgor is more difficult to assess in these individuals. Probably the best site to assess skin turgor in elderly people is over the forehead or sternum. For children, skin turgor is often assessed over the abdominal area and on the medial aspects of the thighs.

In children, skin turgor begins to diminish after 3% to 5% of the body weight is lost. Obese infants with FVD, however, may have deceptively normal skin turgor. Also, infants with hypernatremia may have firm skin that feels thick (thus disguising a water deficit in the child).

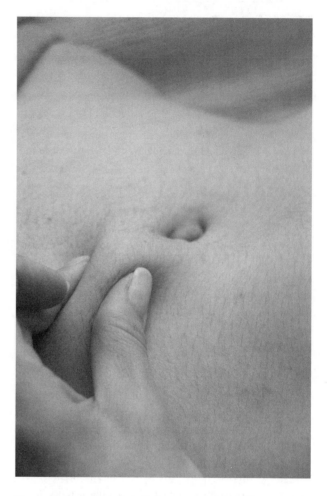

Figure 2-1 Tissue turgor © Stowman L Stines/ShutterStock, Inc.

Tongue Turgor

In a person with FVD, the tongue is smaller and has additional longitudinal furrows, again reflecting loss of interstitial fluid. Fortunately, tongue turgor is not affected appreciably by age; thus it is a useful assessment for all age groups.

Capillary Refill

Capillary refill time is commonly used to assess fluid status in children. It is tested by applying pressure to a fingernail for 5 seconds, releasing the pressure, and noting how rapidly the normal color returns. Color will return in less than 1 to 2 seconds in a healthy person. In addition to reduced peripheral perfusion (due to fluid deficit), a delayed capillary refill could indicate constriction of the peripheral vessels, decreased cardiac output, or anemia. Nurses should be aware that capillary refill assessment is less reliable in cigarette smokers than in nonsmokers. While some authors question the usefulness of capillary refill time in adults,[3, 4] investigators have reported that a capillary refill time greater than 4.5 seconds following initial resuscitation in a group of critically ill adult patients was related to worsening organ failure.[5]

Tearing

Tearing is decreased in patients with FVD. For example, in a study reported in 2003, 132 parents were asked to record symptoms of dehydration present in their children upon admittance to a pediatric emergency department.[6] Parental report of a normal tearing state was correlated with a reduced likelihood of significant dehydration, while decreased tears and a sunken fontanelle were associated with dehydration severe enough to require hospital admission.

Edema

Edema is defined as an excessive accumulation of interstitial fluid (the body fluid that bathes the cells). Edema usually does not become clinically apparent until the interstitial volume has increased by at least 2.5 to 3 L.[7] Causes of edema include the following conditions:

- Increased capillary permeability, which allows fluid to leak into the interstitium (as in burns or localized trauma)
- Increased capillary hydraulic pressure, which forces fluid into the interstitium (as in heart failure or venous obstruction)
- Decreased plasma oncotic pressure associated with hypoalbuminemia, which fosters the transfer of fluid into the interstitium
- Lymphatic obstruction, which permits local edema (as in node enlargement of malignancy)

Edema formation may be either localized (as in thrombophlebitis) or generalized (as in heart failure and nephrotic syndrome). *Dependent edema* is defined as an excess of interstitial fluid accumulating predominantly in the lower extremities of ambulatory patients and in the pre-

sacral region of bedridden patients. *Generalized edema* is spread throughout the body, with interstitial fluid typically accumulating in the periorbital and scrotal regions because of the relatively lower tissue hydrostatic pressure in these regions. Edema related to salt retention generally consists of pitting, which can be manifested by pressing a finger into soft tissue, preferably over a bone (**Figure 2-2**). After the pressure is removed, the "pit" gradually disappears.

The description of peripheral edema is often subjective. For example, it is sometimes estimated by using plus signs (ranging from 1+ to 4+). Measuring an extremity or body part with a millimeter tape, in the same area each day, is a more objective assessment method. Little or no peripheral edema is noted with only water retention (as occurs in excessive secretion of antidiuretic hormone [ADH]).

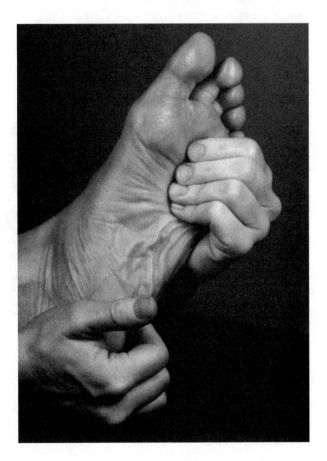

Figure 2-2 Pitting edema © Al Wekelo/Dreamstime.com

Pulmonary Edema

Pulmonary edema results from excessive shifting of fluid from the vascular space into the pulmonary interstitium and air spaces. Cardiogenic pulmonary edema occurs when the pulmonary capillary pressure exceeds the forces that normally maintain fluid within the vascular space; these forces include serum oncotic pressure and interstitial hydrostatic pressure. Accumulation of extravascular lung water affects pulmonary functioning and gas exchange, causing dyspnea, anxiety, expectoration of pink frothy fluid, and use of accessory respiratory muscles.

Neuromuscular Irritability

Assessment for neuromuscular irritability is especially important when calcium and magnesium deficits are suspected. Common assessments include checking for Chvostek's sign and Trousseau's sign as well as testing of deep-tendon reflexes.

Chvostek's Sign

To test Chvostek's sign, the facial nerve is tapped approximately 2 cm anterior to the earlobe. A positive response consists of a unilateral twitching of the facial muscles, including the eyelid and lips. Chvostek's sign is indicative of either hypocalcemia or hypomagnesemia, although it is not specific for these conditions. For example, approximately 25% of normal individuals have a mildly positive Chvostek's sign.[8]

Trousseau's Sign

To test for Trousseau's sign, a blood pressure cuff is inflated approximately 20 mm Hg above systolic pressure for 3 minutes.[9] A positive reaction is the development of a hand cramp (**Figure 2-3**). The hand cramp is characterized by the thumb and fifth finger coming together while the second and fourth fingers are extended. Although Trousseau's sign is more specific for hypocalcemia than is Chvostek's sign, approximately 1% to 4% of normal individuals have a positive Trousseau's sign.[10]

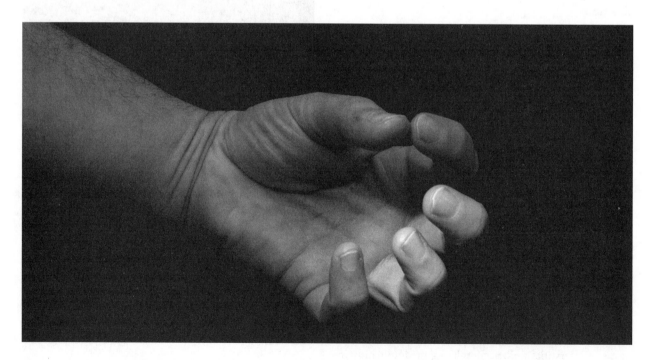

Figure 2-3 Carpopedal spasm © Kodo34/Dreamstime.com

Deep-Tendon Reflexes

The common deep-tendon reflexes include the biceps, triceps, brachioradialis, patellar, and Achilles reflexes. A deep-tendon reflex is elicited by briskly tapping a partially stretched tendon with a rubber percussion hammer. The response in the prospective muscle is a sudden contraction. Deep-tendon reflexes may be hyperactive in the presence of hypocalcemia, hypomagnesemia, and alkalosis. They may be hypoactive in the presence of hypercalcemia, hypermagnesemia, and acidosis. Of course, many factors other than electrolyte disturbances can produce abnormalities in deep-tendon reflexes. As with other signs, deep-tendon reflexes should be evaluated in light of other clinical signs, patient history, and laboratory data.

Body Temperature

Elevation in body temperature in a hypernatremic patient may occur due to excessive water loss. The elevated body temperature is probably related to lack of available fluid for sweating. Also, dehydration probably has a direct effect on the hypothalamus (the heat-regulating portion of the brain).

In a cool room, a patient with an isotonic fluid volume deficit may be slightly hypothermic (probably related to the decreased basal metabolic rate associated with FVD). After partial correction of the FVD, the temperature generally increases to an appropriate level.

Changes in body temperature do not merely reflect fluid balance problems. In fact, fever can *cause* fluid balance problems if not promptly recognized and treated. Fever leads to an increase in metabolic rate and, as a result, in formed metabolic wastes, which require fluid to make a solution for their renal excretion; therefore, fluid loss is increased. Fever also causes hyperpnea, an increase in breathing rate, resulting in extra water vapor loss through the lungs. Because fever increases loss of body fluids, temperature elevations must be detected early and appropriate interventions taken. A 10% increase in need for water is associated with every degree of body temperature above 37°C.[11]

Pulse

Tachycardia is one of the earliest signs of decreased vascular volume associated with FVD. In addition, the pulse feels less full when FVD is present. Conversely, the pulse may feel bounding when fluid volume excess is present.

Respirations

Deep, rapid respirations may be a compensatory mechanism for metabolic acidosis; alternatively, they can be the primary problem that causes respiratory alkalosis. Slow, shallow respirations may be a compensatory mechanism for metabolic alkalosis; alternatively, they may be the primary problem that causes respiratory acidosis.

Weakness or paralysis of respiratory muscles is likely in severe hypokalemia or hyperkalemia and in severe hypermagnesemia (the respiratory center may be paralyzed at a serum magnesium level of 10–15 mEq/L). Moist rales, in the absence of cardiopulmonary disease, indicates fluid volume excess.

Blood Pressure

Blood pressure represents the force exerted on blood vessels by circulating blood. It can be measured directly with an indwelling arterial catheter or indirectly by means of a blood pressure cuff and sphygmomanometer. In most situations, the indirect method is used. Accurate readings mandate selection of a blood pressure cuff that is appropriate to the patient's size. For example, the width of the cuff's inflatable bladder should be approximately 40% of the upper arm circumference in the average adult).[12] A too-narrow cuff will lead to falsely high readings while a too-wide cuff on a small arm will lead to falsely low readings.

In an adult older than 18 years of age, normal systolic pressure is less than 120 mm Hg and normal diastolic pressure is less than 80 mm Hg.[13] Hypotension is generally defined as a systolic pressure less than 90 mm Hg.[14] However, it is important to recognize that a seemingly normal systolic blood pressure (such as 120 mm Hg) is actually low in a patient who is usually hypertensive.[15]

Pulse Pressure

Pulse pressure is defined as the arithmetic difference between systolic blood pressure and diastolic blood pressure. A pulse pressure less than 30 mm Hg is common in patients with hypovolemia. In a hypovolemic patient, a narrow pulse pressure indicates a decreasing cardiac output (falling systolic blood pressure) and an increasing peripheral vascular resistance (increased diastolic blood pressure). The latter represents an attempt by the body to maintain the falling blood pressure through vasoconstriction. An example of a low pulse pressure is seen in a patient with a systolic blood pressure of 102 mm Hg and a diastolic blood pressure of 86 mm Hg; in this instance, the pulse pressure is 16 mm Hg. Monitoring changes in pulse pressure is helpful when assessing response to fluid volume replacement.

Mean Arterial Pressure

Mean arterial pressure (MAP) is the preferred method to evaluate unstable patients.[16] A mean arterial pressure of 60 mm Hg is needed to perfuse the coronary arteries, brain, and kidneys (usual range is 70–110 mm Hg). Mean arterial pressure can be calculated by the following equation: MAP = [(2 × diastolic) + systolic]/3.

For example, if the diastolic pressure is 80 mm Hg and the systolic pressure is 120 mm Hg, the MAP would be approximately 93 mm Hg. Diastole counts twice as much as systole because two thirds of the cardiac cycle is spent in diastole.

Orthostatic Blood Pressure

One method for detecting volume depletion involves measuring the blood pressure and pulse rate with the patient lying flat and then in a standing position. Standing from a supine position causes an abrupt drop in venous return, for which sympathetically mediated cardiovascular adjustments normally compensate. In the healthy individual, cardiac return is maintained by increased peripheral resistance and a slight increase in heart rate; systolic pressure falls only slightly, and diastolic pressure may actually rise a few millimeters of mercury. In contrast, a fall in systolic pressure greater than 20 mm Hg, especially when accompanied by light-headedness and tachycardia, may suggest orthostatic hypotension due to intravascular volume deficit.[17] According to some authors, to be specific for hypovolemia, an increase in pulse rate must be greater than 20 to 30 beats per minute when changing from a supine to a standing position.[18, 19] Of course, conditions associated with autonomic neuropathy (such as diabetes) can also produce these kinds of orthostatic blood pressure and pulse changes, as can sympatholytic antihypertensive medications.

Central Venous Pressure

Central venous pressure (CVP) refers to the pressure in the right atrium or vena cava; it provides information about blood volume, the effectiveness of the heart's pumping action, and vascular tone. When CVP is measured with a water manometer, pressure in the right atrium is usually 0 to 4 cm of water and pressure in the vena cava is approximately 4 to 11 cm of water. When CVP is measured with a transducer system, the normal range is 0 to 7 mm Hg. A below-normal CVP may indicate decreased blood volume, vasodilatation, or a condition that reduces venous return to the heart. Conversely, an above-normal CVP may indicate excessive blood volume, vasoconstriction, or heart failure. More important than absolute values are the upward or downward trends; these trends are determined by taking frequent readings (often every 30–60 minutes).

It is always important to evaluate CVP in reference to other available clinical data, such as blood pressure, fluid intake, and urinary output. For example, a rise in CVP paralleling a rise in systolic blood pressure in a previously hypotensive patient indicates adequate fluid volume replacement. Conversely, a low CVP persisting after fluid volume replacement may be a sign of continued occult bleeding.

In patients with normal cardiac function and relatively normal pulmonary function, the CVP remains an acceptable guide to blood volume.

Pulmonary Artery Pressure

In critically ill patients, CVP monitoring may not be sufficient as an assessment technique. In these patients, it may be necessary to use more invasive hemodynamic monitoring, such as a pulmonary artery catheter, to evaluate clinical status and fluid infusion rates. The pulmonary artery catheter provides direct measurements from the right atrium, right ventricle, pulmonary arteries, and pulmonary capillary wedge pressure. This device is helpful in assessing fluid balance status in patients with confusing clinical pictures, especially those for whom errors in fluid management and drug therapy have major consequences.

URINE VOLUME AND CONCENTRATION

Urine Volume

The normal urinary output in an adult is approximately 1 mL/kg body weight/hr, with boundaries of 0.5 to 2 mL/kg/hr. **Table 2-1** shows that the usual urine volume in adults is approximately 1,500 mL/day (range 1000 to 2000 mL/day). This is equivalent to 40 to 80 mL/hr in the typical adult. Urine volume in children is less and is dependent on age and weight. (See Chapter 24.)

Table 2-1 Average Intake and Output in an Adult for a 24-Hour Period

Intake		*Output*	
Oral liquids	1300 mL	Urine	1500 mL
Water in food	1000 mL	Stool	200 mL
Water produced by metabolism	300 mL	Insensible:	
		Lungs	300 mL
		Skin	600 mL
Total	2600 mL	Total	2600 mL

During periods of stress, the 24-hour urine volume in the adult may diminish to 750 to 1200 mL/day (or 30–50 mL/hr). Urine volume is somewhat less during periods of stress because of increased production of stress hormones (aldosterone and ADH). A low urine volume suggests fluid volume deficit, and a high urine volume suggests fluid volume excess (provided the kidneys are normal and able to respond to an increased fluid volume).

A number of factors can alter urine volume:

- *Amount of fluid intake.* In healthy individuals, a large fluid intake produces a large urine volume. Conversely, a small fluid intake results in a small urine output. Healthy adult kidneys can reduce urine output to approximately 500 mL of concentrated urine when fluid intake is markedly reduced.
- *Losses from skin, lungs, and gastrointestinal tract.* Urine volume is decreased when large fluid losses from the skin, lungs, and gastrointestinal (GI) tract occur.
- *Amount of waste products for excretion.* Urine volume is increased in conditions with high solute loads, such as diabetes mellitus, high-protein tube feedings, thyrotoxicosis, and fever.
- *Renal concentrating ability.* Urine volume is decreased when the kidneys cannot concentrate urine normally; this condition is common in elderly patients. See Chapter 25.
- *Blood volume.* Urine volume is low when the patient is hypovolemic; conversely, urine volume is high when hypervolemia is present (provided the kidneys are functioning normally).
- *Hormonal influences.* Conditions in which aldosterone and ADH production are increased are associated with reduced urine output, because these hormones cause

retention of sodium and water. The absence of effective ADH results in large losses of urine, a condition referred to as neurogenic diabetes insipidus.

Urine Concentration: Specific Gravity and Osmolality

The kidneys continuously vary the concentration of electrolytes and other substances excreted in urine to help maintain homeostasis. Measures of the kidney's ability to perform this important activity are urine specific gravity (SG) and urine osmolality. Urine SG can be measured by clinicians with a reagent strip, urinometer, or a refractometer. Urine osmolality is a laboratory test.

The urine SG test indicates the relative proportion of dissolved solids to the total volume of solution; the urine osmolality test indicates the number of particles per unit of solution. Whereas large molecules (such as glucose, albumin, and radiocontrast dyes) do not interfere with osmolality test results, they do interfere with the accuracy of the urine SG test when it is performed with a urinometer or refractometer (but not a reagent strip). Thus, when measuring urine concentration in a patient with glucosuria or proteinuria, it is preferable to use a SG reagent strip or the osmolality test.

The urinary SG test is used in most clinical settings and compares the density of urine with that of distilled water (1.000). Because urine contains electrolytes and other substances (such as sodium chloride, sulfate, phosphate, and urea), its SG is greater than 1.000 (range 1.003 to 1.035). A random urine specimen with a SG of 1.023 or higher indicates normal renal concentrating ability. A healthy adult with a normal fluid intake will produce a urine with an osmolality of in the range of 500 to 850 mOsm/kg. If the person is dehydrated, the osmolality may be as high as 1400 mOsm/kg; conversely, it may be as low as 40 mOsm/kg if water overload is present.

The significance of urine SG and osmolality readings has to be evaluated in relation to the patient's clinical status. For example, both urinary SG and osmolality are elevated when FVD is present, as the healthy kidney seeks to retain needed fluid and, therefore, excretes solutes in a small concentrated urine volume. After a period of dehydration, it is reasonable to expect the urine osmolality to be approximately 3 times higher than the plasma osmolality. A very low SG is seen in patients with neurogenic diabetes insipidus, a condition in which the individual excretes large volumes of water due to the absence of ADH. A fixed low urine SG at about 1.010 is a serious condition referred to as *isosthenuria;* it indicates that the diseased kidney has lost its ability to vary the concentration of urine and essentially excretes the urinary filtrate unchanged.

FLUID INTAKE/OUTPUT MEASUREMENT

Many serious fluid balance problems can be averted by maintaining a careful vigil on the patient's intake and output (I & O) and recording the volumes accurately on the patient's medical record. A recognized standard of care is initiating I & O records on any patient with a disease or condition that places her or him at risk for fluid deficit or overload.[20]

In litigation situations, it is common practice for expert nurse witnesses to evaluate the accuracy and completeness of I & O records, especially in cases where fluid and electrolyte problems are present. Not only is it important to evaluate I & O for each shift, but it is also important to compare differences (gains or losses) over a period of several days. Several case studies are reported in Chapter 4 that demonstrate adverse outcomes from situations in which caregivers did not heed the warnings inherent in vast differences in fluid intake and output.

Critically ill patients may require an hourly summary of fluid gains and losses. However, most patients require summaries for 8- or 12-hour shifts (whatever is employed at the involved institution). It is important to evaluate I & O records according to each shift as well as over a period of several subsequent days to obtain a full picture of the patient's fluid volume status.

Positive Versus Negative Fluid Balance

Although a healthy individual has similar fluid intake and output volumes (Table 2-1), patients who are ill may have either a *positive fluid balance* (intake exceeding output) or a *negative fluid balance* (output exceeding intake). During treatment, it is sometimes necessary to induce a positive fluid balance, or even a negative fluid balance, depending on the patient's clinical status.

For example, a positive fluid balance is desirable for a short period of time when a severely fluid-volume-depleted patient is receiving aggressive fluid replacement therapy to correct the condition. In contrast, a positive fluid balance is *not* desirable when a patient in renal failure consumes more fluids than can be excreted by the diseased kidneys. Similarly, a negative fluid balance may be desirable during the short period of time in which intravenous diuretics are administered to a patient with heart failure who is experiencing pulmonary edema. A negative fluid balance may be dangerous, however, when a patient with severe vomiting and diarrheal fluid losses is not receiving fluid replacement therapy.

Factors to Consider When Measuring Fluid Intake and Output

The following factors should be considered when measuring I & O:

- Measure and record the volume of *all* fluids taken into the body:
  ○ Oral liquids. (Provide caregivers with a list of the volume of fluid contained in glasses and bowls used in the facility.)
  ○ Foods that are liquid at room temperature.
  ○ Ice chips. (Record as half the volume of water; for example, 100 mL of ice chips is equivalent to 50 mL of water.)
  ○ Intravenous fluid. (Consider small bags of solutions used to administer intravenous medications in addition to the large bags of primary intravenous solutions.)
  ○ Subcutaneous fluids. (Use of subcutaneous fluids is increasing, especially in long-term care settings where it may be difficult to gain intravenous access. See Chapter 10.)
  ○ Formula and water administered through GI feeding tubes.
  ○ Fluids used to flush enteral feeding tubes (should be recorded as intake).
  ○ Fluids used to flush nasogastric drainage tubes (should be recorded as intake; fluid withdrawn from the tubes should be recorded as output).
  ○ Enema solutions.
- Measure and record all fluids eliminated from the body. If not possible to directly measure the lost fluid with a calibrated device, attempt to estimate the volume as closely as possible.
  ○ Urine.
  ○ Vomitus.
  ○ Liquid stool.

- ∘ Drainage from gastric suction tubes.
- ∘ Drainage from chest tubes.
- ∘ Fluid recovered from closed wound drainage tubes.
- Estimate fluid loss from sources that cannot be directly measured.
    - ∘ For example, is sweating mild or profuse? Is sweating so severe that it requires linen changes?
    - ∘ Is the patient hyperventilating? If so, this could result in considerable loss of water vapor. Recall that in normal situations approximately 300 mL of water vapor is lost via this route.
    - ∘ Is there drainage from large wounds? If so, attempt to estimate the amount of drainage on dressings.
- Educate all personnel involved with I & O measurement about the importance of accurate measurements to the patient's welfare.
- Educate the patient and family about the need for I & O measurements; enlist their help in assuring accurate measurements. Provide the patient and family with a list of common conversions between household measures and the metric system (**Table 2-2**).

BODY WEIGHT MEASUREMENT

Weighing patients with potential or actual fluid balance problems daily is of great clinical importance for the following reasons:

- Accurate body weight measurements are usually easier to obtain than are accurate I & O measurements.

Table 2-2 Conversion from Common Household Measures to the Metric System

Household Measure	Metric Equivalent
One teaspoon	5 mL
One tablespoon	15 mL
One fluid ounce	30 mL
One cup (8 ounces)	240 mL
One pint (16 ounces)	480 ml (approximately one-half liter [0.5 L])
One quart (32 ounces)	960 mL (approximately one liter [1 L])
One pound	454 mg (approximately one-half kilogram [0.5 kg])
2.2 pounds	1 kg (1000 mg)

- Rapid variations in weight, when measured correctly, reflect changes in body fluid volume in most patients.

A rapid body weight loss or gain of 1 kg (2.2 lb) is approximately equivalent to the loss or gain of 1 L of fluid (or expressed another way, a loss or gain of 500 mL of fluid is equivalent to a loss or gain of 1 lb). While direct fluid gains and losses from the body are reflected in body weight changes, patients who have experienced a fluid shift from the bloodstream to injured tissues (such as may occur in burns or trauma) will weigh the same as before the fluid shift occurred. In this unique situation, body weight is *not* helpful in assessing fluid volume status.

Body weight as an index of fluid balance is based on the assumption that the patient's dry weight remains relatively stable. Over a short period (hour-to-hour), this assumption is valid, and changes in body weight reflect changes in body fluid volume rather than tissue mass changes. To assess these small hourly changes, it is necessary to use extremely accurate metabolic scales, which are not available on most patient care units.

Body weight loss will occur when the total fluid intake is less than the total fluid output. In children, a rapid loss of 5% or less of total body weight indicates mild FVD, whereas a 6% to 10% loss represents moderate FVD and a rapid loss of greater than 10% represents severe FVD. Conversely, a rapid gain in body weight will occur when the total fluid intake is greater than the total fluid output.

Long-term (day-to-day) body weight variations reflect changes in tissue mass as well as body fluid volume. Thus factors affecting tissue mass (e.g., caloric intake and metabolic status) must also be evaluated. It is generally assumed that a relative deficit of 3400 calories is needed to lose 1 lb of tissue mass; this deficit can be the result of inadequate caloric intake, increased metabolic rate, or both.

The following practices should be followed when weighing patients:

1. Use the same scale each time, because variations among scales may be significant. Measure weight in the morning before breakfast and after voiding.
2. Be sure the patient is wearing the same or similar clothing each time and that the clothing is dry.
3. If the patient is unable to stand for weighing on a small portable scale or a stand-on scale, use a sling-type scale. Wheelchair and under-bed scales are also commercially available.

Of course, accurate body weights can be obtained only when the scales used for the weighing procedure are accurate. Unfortunately, a small but significant percentage of scales in clinical use are inaccurate and imprecise to a clinically important degree because of breakage and loss of calibration. To minimize inaccuracies in weight measurements, medical institutions should test the accuracy of their clinical scales periodically.

EVALUATION OF LABORATORY DATA

Data from laboratory tests provide the nurse with valuable information about the patient's fluid and electrolyte status. Specimens must be collected properly to obtain valid results, and all findings must be evaluated in light of the patient's history and clinical status. Treatment for an abnormality reported on an improperly performed laboratory test can be quite serious. When in doubt, it is wise to confirm a grossly abnormal test result.

Obtaining Blood Specimens

Avoid Excessive Blood Sample Volume

Phlebotomy for blood samples contributes to anemia, especially when tests are performed frequently using more blood than actually required for the analysis. For example, acquired iron-deficiency anemia has been found in more than 50% of critically ill patients within the first two weeks of their hospitalization.[21] According to one source, phlebotomy may account for greater blood loss than pathologic bleeding in ICU patients.[22] The amount of blood (25 to 40 mL) withdrawn daily from critically ill patients is about three times the amount taken from patients on general wards.[23] All too often, the volume of blood collected for laboratory tests exceeds the volume required, resulting in a sizable amount of blood being wasted.[24] Laboratories need to make a concerted effort to use smaller collection tubes whenever possible to reduce unnecessary blood loss through this practice.[25]

Prevention of Hemolysis of Specimen

Regardless of whether blood is drawn from a peripheral line or from a central line, it is important to prevent hemolysis of the blood sample because it can lead to erroneous test results. *Hemolysis* is defined as the breakage of red blood cells, which causes hemoglobin to enter the plasma and produces a pink to red tinge in the plasma when the blood is centrifuged. Because potassium, phosphate, and magnesium are major cellular ions, rupture of red blood cells results in spillage of these electrolytes into the plasma, causing falsely high serum levels. Hemolyzed specimens are a frequent occurrence in clinical laboratories, with a prevalence as high as 3.3% of all routine samples, nearly five times higher than other causes for unsuitable blood specimens.[26]

Hemolysis of blood specimens may result from any of the following causes:

- Delay in transporting the specimen to the laboratory for testing.
- Use of a syringe with excessive suction applied to the plunger.[27] (Hemolysis is less likely when blood is collected in evacuated tubes than when collected with syringes.)
- Drawing blood through a small needle or catheter, which may rupture the red blood cells as they pass through the needle/catheter.
- Vigorously shaking the tube to mix the blood with anticoagulant.[28]

Obtaining Peripheral Venous Blood Samples

Two general principles should be kept in mind when obtaining venous blood samples:

- *Avoid drawing blood samples from a site above an infusing IV line.* Specimens for serum biochemical and hematologic profiles should be drawn from the opposite arm or *below* the IV.[29]
- *Avoid having the patient repeatedly clench and unclench the fist when blood is being drawn for potassium measurement.* Prolonged use of a tourniquet with fist exercises before venipuncture may cause a spurious elevation in potassium concentrations of as much as 1 mEq/L.[30]

To evaluate the effect of exercise on potassium levels, one investigator put a tourniquet on both of his arms; his right hand was relaxed during the procedure while his left hand was repeatedly clenched and unclenched for 15 seconds, continuing as the blood was drawn from both arms. The concentration of potassium in blood obtained from the left (pumping) arm was 1.04 mEq/L higher than in blood obtained from the right arm at the same time.[31]

Obtaining Specimens from Central Venous and Arterial Devices

Central venous access devices are used frequently in intensive care settings to collect blood samples. Although this practice eliminates the need for numerous peripheral venipunctures, it can present a problem when blood specimens drawn from the catheters are contaminated by constituents in recently administered intravenous fluids. For example, one study showed that even small amounts of lactated Ringer's solution in catheters used for blood sampling caused falsely elevated serum lactate results; the investigators emphasized that when blood specimens are drawn from indwelling lines, all IV solutions need to first be cleared from the line.[32] The appropriate volumes to be discarded should be established by each laboratory.

The arterial catheter is also a convenient source of blood specimens in the critically ill patient. It is especially helpful for obtaining samples for arterial blood gases in patients with acute metabolic problems and in patients in respiratory failure.[33] Although most blood samples from arterial catheters are obtained reliably, several sources for error exist. The most common is dilution or contamination of the sampled blood with flush fluid. For example, introduction of heparin into the blood sample can cause faulty activated partial thromboplastin time results. Moreover, if sodium citrate is used as a flush solution and is inadvertently mixed with the blood sample, hypocalcemia and a low pH might be reported in the laboratory analysis.[34]

There is a tendency to do more blood draws when a central line is in place, as opposed to when the blood must be drawn from a peripheral line. For example, in a study of 977 critically ill children, blood draws were 2.3 to 4 times more frequent when the children had an arterial line or a central venous catheter than when they had peripheral venous lines alone.[35] A common dilemma in hospital settings relates to performing sufficient blood draws to monitor the patient's clinical status without causing or contributing to anemia; this concern is especially evident in pediatric settings. For this reason, hospital laboratories have specific protocols for blood tests and recommend withdrawing the minimal amount of blood needed to perform each test.

Obtaining Urine Specimens

Single Specimen

For a single urine specimen, the first voided morning specimen is ideal because of its greater concentration. Nevertheless, a fresh specimen collected at any time is reliable for most purposes. To avoid false readings, the specimen must be collected in a clean container. Ideally, the urine specimen should be delivered to the laboratory and analyzed within one hour after collection.[36]

24-Hour Specimen

A 24-hour urine specimen is often indicated in the measurement of urinary excretion of electrolytes. The urine collection container should be obtained from the laboratory and contain the needed preservative for the specified test. Failure to save all urine during the period negates the accuracy of tests performed on the specimen; thus it is important to enlist the patient's help in saving all urine to add to the collection container. Specific directions provided by the laboratory for the test need to be following precisely. Start and stop times need to be recorded, and the urine container should be refrigerated unless otherwise noted.

INTERPRETING LABORATORY TESTS USED TO MEASURE FLUID AND ELECTROLYTE BALANCE

Blood tests used to assess fluid and electrolyte status are listed in **Table 2-3**, and urine tests used for the same purpose are listed in **Table 2-4**. The usual reference ranges for the tests and significance of variations are also included in these tables. Commonly used units of measures are reported, with SI units appearing in parentheses.

Laboratory reports in the chart should be reviewed at regular intervals to note the patient's current status and to detect trends in the data. Because normal ranges for laboratory tests vary slightly from institution to institution, it is necessary to evaluate results according to the standards listed by the laboratory performing the tests. Laboratory tests used to diagnose specific fluid and electrolyte problems are discussed in greater depth in Chapters 3 through 9.

Table 2-3 Blood Tests Used to Evaluate Fluid and Electrolyte Status

Test	Usual Reference Range	Comments
Serum potassium	3.5–5.0 mEq/L (3.5–5.0 mmol/L)	• A falsely elevated level (pseudohyperkalemia) can occur when the blood sample is allowed to sit at room temperature and hemolyze (causing release of cellular K into the bloodstream). A falsely high K level can also occur when a tourniquet is applied for a prolonged period and the hand is repeatedly clenched and unclenched. (See Chapter 5 for further discussion of this problem.)
		• Serum K concentration is often increased when acidosis is present because this condition causes K to shift from the cells to the plasma. Conversely, plasma K concentration is often decreased when alkalosis is present because this condition causes K to shift into the cells. (See Chapter 9 for further discussion of cellular K shifts associated with pH balance.)
Serum sodium	135–145 mEq/L (135–145 mmol/L)	• An osmotic pull of water from cells when hyperglycemia is present can dilute the plasma sodium concentration. The serum Na may fall by 1.5–2.4 mEq/L for every 100 mg/dL rise in the plasma glucose level.[37, 38]
		• Although this condition is sometimes called "pseudohyponatremia," it is actually true hyponatremia because the plasma sodium concentration is diluted by fluid pulled from the cells.[39]
		• See Chapter 4 for further discussion of hyponatremia.
Total serum calcium	8.9–10.3 mg/dL (2.23–2.57 mmol/L)	• Total Ca is measured in most clinical settings to evaluate Ca status.
		• This test measures a combination of ionized Ca and the amount of Ca bound to anions, predominantly albumin.
		• To evaluate the effective calcium level, the clinician must first know the serum albumin level to apply the following rule: A fall in serum albumin of 1 g/dL decreases plasma Ca by approximately 0.8 mg/dL.
		• Alkalosis lowers the ionized calcium level.
		• Acidosis increases the ionized calcium level.
		• See Chapter 6 for further discussion of the relationship between albumin and calcium, and pH and calcium.
Ionized calcium	4.6–5.1 mg/dL (1.15–1.27 mmol/L)	• Measurement of ionized Ca is favored in seriously ill patients because it is the ionized fraction of Ca that is physiologically active and clinically important.
		• See Chapter 6 for further discussion of ionized Ca measurement.
Serum magnesium	1.3–2.1 mEq/L (0.65–1.1 mmol/L)	• Hemolysis of the blood sample invalidates the results by releasing Mg from the red blood cells into the serum. (Recall that Mg, like K, is primarily an intracellular ion.)
Serum phosphate	2.5–4.5 mg/dL (0.81–1.45 mmol/L)	• Hemolysis of the sample invalidates the results by releasing phosphate from the red blood cells into the serum. (Recall that phosphate, like K and Mg, is primarily an intracellular ion.)
		• Phosphate levels are normally higher in children than in adults. (See Chapter 24 for variations in phosphate according to age.)
Serum chloride	97–110 mEq/L (97–110 mmol/L)	• A lower than normal concentration indicates hypochloremia (commonly associated with hypokalemia and metabolic alkalosis).
		• A higher than normal concentration indicates hyperchloremia, a form of metabolic acidosis (often seen with excessive administration of isotonic saline).

Table 2-3 *(continued)*

Carbon dioxide content	22–31 mEq/L (22–31 mmol/L)	• Primarily a measure of bicarbonate in venous blood. It is low when metabolic acidosis is present and is high when metabolic alkalosis is present. • CO content should not be confused with the partial pressure of carbon dioxide ($PaCO_2$) obtained during arterial blood gas analysis.
Serum osmolality	280–295 mOsm/kg	• Can be measured by laboratory or calculated by the following equation: 2(Na) + G/18 + BUN/2.8. • Becomes elevated when Na, glucose, or blood urea nitrogen levels are above normal.
Anion gap (AG)	12 ± 2 mEq/L	• Useful in ascertaining the cause of metabolic acidosis. (See Chapter 9 for further discussion of significance of high and normal AG levels.) • Calculated by the following equation: AG = Na − (Cl + HCO_3).
Serum creatinine	0.6–1.5 mg/dL (53–133 mcmol/L)	• More specific indicator of renal function than is blood urea nitrogen. • See Chapter 17 for information regarding interpretation of serum creatinine levels
Blood urea nitrogen (BUN)	10–20 mg/dL	• Elevated when fluid volume depletion is present because of reduction in renal blood flow (results in reduced clearance of urea in urine). • High protein intake or bleeding into the GI tract can also elevate BUN. • BUN is lowered in the presence of fluid volume overload.

BUN/creatinine (Cr) ratio	Highly variable; normal values can range between 10:1 and 20:1	• Concurrent measurement of serum BUN and creatinine is helpful in identifying fluid volume deficit
		• Fluid volume contraction causes renal retention of BUN and thus leads to serum BUN:Cr ratio > 20:1.[40]
		  • For example, if BUN is 40 mg/dL and Cr is 1 mg/dL, the BUN:Cr ratio is 40:1 and is an indication of fluid volume deficit.
		• Intrinsic renal failure is likely when *both* the serum Cr and BUN levels rise while maintaining a ratio of less than 20:1.
		  • For example, if BUN is 63 mg/dL and Cr is 3.5 mg/dL, the BUN:Cr ratio is 18:1 and is an indication of intrinsic renal failure.

Hematocrit	Male: 44–52% Female: 39–47%	• Represents the percentage of red blood cells per unit volume of plasma. • Elevated in fluid volume deficit (because red blood cells are contained in a relatively smaller plasma volume). • Decreased in fluid volume excess (because the red blood cells are contained in a relatively larger plasma volume). • Changes are interpretable in terms of fluid balance only when no changes in the red blood cell mass have occurred (such as bleeding or hemolysis).
Fasting blood glucose	65–110 mg/dL (3.58–6.05 mmol/L)	• Markedly elevated glucose level causes an osmotic diuresis and resultant fluid volume deficit.
Albumin	3.6–5.0 g/dL (35–48 g/L)	• Decreased serum albumin level lowers the colloidal osmotic pull in the intravenous space and allows fluids to shift to the tissues (causing edema). • Important to know albumin level when evaluating total calcium values.
Plasma lactate	0.6–1.7 mmol/L (0.6–1.7 mmol/L)	• Lactic acidosis considered to be present if the plasma lactate level > 4–5 mmol/L. • Most cases of lactic acidosis are due to marked tissue hypoperfusion.

Table 2-4 Urine Tests Used to Evaluate Fluid and Electrolyte Status

Test	Usual Reference Range	Comments
Urinary pH	4.6–8.0 (average is 6.0)	• Urine pH fluctuates throughout the day. • The specimen should be examined soon after collection because urine that is left standing too long becomes alkaline due to bacterial-induced splitting of urea into ammonia. • Urine pH is increased with use of alkalinating agents, such as sodium bicarbonate or potassium citrate. • Urine pH is decreased with use of acidifying agents, such as ascorbic acid and sodium acid phosphate.
Urine specific gravity (SG)	Varies from 1.003 to 1.035 1.016–1.022 (with normal fluid intake)	• SG depends on state of hydration • Varies with fluid intake and the solute load to be excreted by the kidneys. • Elevated in FVD, as a normal kidney seeks to retain needed fluid and excrete solutes in as little fluid as possible. • SG fixed at 1.010, regardless of fluid intake, signals significant renal disease.[41]
Urine osmolality	50–1400 mOsm/kg	• In a normal person, the urine osmolality is greater than 1.2 times that of serum osmolality. Following a period of dehydration, the urine osmolality should be about 3 times higher than the serum osmolality.
Urinary sodium	No fixed normal values; kidneys vary the rate of excretion to match dietary intake	• Urinary Na levels must be evaluated in light of the total clinical picture. • Urine Na < 25 mEq/L in hypovolemic states, reflecting renal conservation of sodium to maintain blood volume. • Urine Na > 40 mEq/L in SIADH, diuretic therapy, and adrenal insufficiency.[42]
Urinary potassium	Kidneys vary the rate of excretion to match dietary intake and endogenous production of potassium	• Used to assess cause of hypokalemia. • Low value suggests nonrenal K loss (usually from GI tract) or diuretic use (if urine was collected after the diuretic effect has worn off).[43]

NOTES

1. Guyton, A. C., & Hall, J. E. (2006). *Textbook of medical physiology* (11th ed.). Philadelphia: W. B. Saunders, p. 162.

2. Guyton & Hall, note 1, p. 361.

3. Anderson, B., Kelly, A. M., & Kerr, D. (2008). Impact of patient and environmental factors on capillary refill time in adults. *American Journal of Emergency Medicine, 26*(1), 62–65.

4. Lewin, J., & Maconochie, I. (2008). Capillary refill time in adults. *Emergency Medicine Journal, 25*, 325–326.

5. Lima, A., Jansen, T. C., van Bommel, J. I., & Bakker, J. (2009). The prognostic value of the subjective assessment of peripheral perfusion in critically ill patients. *Critical Care Medicine, 37*(3), 934–938.

6. Porter, S. C., Fleisher, G. R., Kohane, I. S., & Mandl, K. D. (2003). The value of parental report for diagnosis and management of dehydration in the emergency department. *Annals of Emergency Medicine, 41*(2), 196–205.

7. Rose, B. D., & Post, T. W. (2001). *Clinical physiology of acid–base and electrolyte disorders* (5th ed.). New York: McGraw-Hill, p. 479.

8. Garner, D. G., & Shoback, D. (2007).: *Greenspan's basic and clinical endocrinology* (8th ed.). New York: McGraw-Hill Medical, p. 311.

9. Garner & Shoback, note 8, p. 311.

10. Garner & Shoback, note 8, p. 311.

11. Pestana, C. (2000). *Fluids and electrolytes in the surgical patient* (5th ed.). Philadelphia: Lippincott Williams & Wilkins, p. 26.

12. Bickley, L. S., & Szilagyi, P. G. (2009). *Bates' guide to physical examination and history taking* (10th ed.). Philadelphia: Wolters Kluwer/Lippincott Williams & Wilkins, p. 116.

13. Bickley & Szilagyi, note 12, p. 115.

14. Fink, M. P., Abraham, E., Vincent, J. L., & Kochanek, P. M. (2005). *Textbook of critical care* (5th ed.). Philadelphia: Elsevier Saunders, p. 736.

15. Rose & Post, note 7, p. 423.

16. Hardin, S., & Kaplow, R. (2010). *Cardiac surgery essentials for critical care nursing.* Sudbury, MA: Jones and Bartlett, p. 150.

17. Bickley & Szilagyi, note 12, p. 119.

18. Feehally, J., Floege, J., & Johnson, R. J. (2007). *Comprehensive clinical nephrology* (3rd ed.). Philadelphia: Mosby, p. 84.

19. Bongard, F. S., Sue, D. Y., & Vintch, J. R. (2008). *Current diagnosis and critical care* (3rd ed.). New York: McGraw-Hill/Lange, p. 16.

20. Alford, D. M. (2003). The clinical record: Recognizing its value in litigation. *Geriatric Nursing, 24*(4), 228–230.

21. von Ahsen, N., Muller, C., Serke, S., Frei, U., & Eckardt, K. U. (1999). Important role of nondiagnostic blood loss and blunted erythropoeitic response in the anemia of medical intensive care patients. *Critical Care Medicine, 27*(12), 2630–2639.

22. von Ahsen et al., note 21.

23. Vincent, J. L., Baron, J. F., Reinhart, K., Gattinoni, L., Thijs, L., Webb, A., et al. (2002). Anemia and blood transfusion in critically ill patients. *Journal of the American Medical Association, 288*(12), 1499–1507.

24. Dale, J. C., & Ruby, S. G. (2003). Specimen collection volumes for laboratory tests. *Archives of Pathology and Laboratory Medicine, 127*(2), 162–168.

25. Smoller, B. R., Kruskall, M. S., & Horowitz, G. L. (1989). Reducing adult phlebotomy blood loss with the use of pediatric-sized blood collection tubes. *American Journal of Clinical Pathology, 91*(6), 701–703.

26. Lippi, G., Blanckaert, N., Bonini, P., Green, S., Kitchen, S., Palicka, V., et al. (2008). Haemolysis: An overview of the leading cause of unsuitable specimens in clinical laboratories. *Clinical Chemistry & Laboratory Medicine, 46*(6), 764–772.

27. Baer, D. M., Ernst, D. J., Willeford, S. I., & Gambino, R. (2006, November). Investigating elevated potassium values. *Medical Laboratory Observer, 38*(11), 26.

28. Baer et al., note 27, p. 24.

29. Watson, K., I'Kell, R., & Joyce, J. (1983). Data regarding blood drawing sites in patients receiving intravenous fluids. *American Journal of Clinical Pathology, 79,* 119.

30. McPherson, R. A., & Pincus, M. R. (2007). *Henry's clinical diagnosis and management by laboratory methods* (21st ed.). Philadelphia: Saunders, p. 158.

31. Baer et al., note 27, p. 30.

32. Jackson, E.V Jr., Wise, J., Sigal, B., Miller, J., Bernstein, W., Kassel, D., et al. (1997). Effects of crystalloid solutions on circulating lactate concentrations: Part I. Implications for the proper handling of blood specimens obtained from critically ill patients. *Critical Care Medicine, 25*(22), 1840.

33. Parrillo, J. E., & Dellinger, R. P. (2008). *Critical care: Principles of diagnosis and management in the adult* (3rd ed.). St. Louis: Mosby Elsevier, p. 54.

34. Fink et al., note 14, p. 1798.

35. Bateman, S. T., Lacroix, J., Boven, K., Forbes, P., Barton, R., Thomas, N.J., et al. (2008). Anemia, blood loss and blood transfusions in North American children in the intensive care unit. *American Journal of Respiratory and Critical Care Medicine, 178,* 26–33, p. 28.

36. McPherson & Pincus, note 30, p. 27.

37. McPherson & Pincus, note 30, p. 160.

38. Kollef, M. H., Bedient, T. J., Isakow, W., & Witt, C. A. (2008). *The Washington manual of critical care.* Philadelphia: Wolters Kluwer/Lippincott Williams & Wilkins, p. 155.

39. McPhee, S. T., & Papadakis, M. A. (2008). *2008 Current medical diagnosis & treatment.* New York: McGraw-Hill, p. 758.

40. Feehally et al., note 18, p. 84.

41. McPherson & Pincus, note 30, p. 396.

42. Chung, H. M., Kluge, R., & Schrier, R. L. (1987). Clinical assessment of extracellular fluid volume in hyponatremia. *American Journal of Medicine, 83,* 905.

43. Rose & Post, note 7, p. 863.

UNIT II

Overview of Fluid and Electrolyte Problems: Nursing Considerations

Chapter 3

Fluid Volume Imbalances

Fluid volume imbalances are common in all age groups and types of settings. Although they sometimes occur alone, fluid volume imbalances may also be coupled with one or more electrolyte problems. In this chapter, fluid volume imbalances are primarily discussed in their "pure" form (without the presence of other disturbances). Specific variations in fluid volume imbalances associated with age extremes are also discussed in Chapters 24 and 25. In Chapters 13 through 23, fluid volume imbalances are discussed in relation to specific clinical situations.

ISOTONIC FLUID VOLUME DEFICIT

Fluid volume deficit (FVD) results when water and electrolytes are lost in an isotonic fashion (**Figure 3-1**). This condition should not be confused with *dehydration,* which refers primarily to a loss of water (resulting in hypernatremia). Unless concurrent electrolyte imbalances are present, serum electrolyte levels remain essentially unchanged in isotonic fluid volume deficit.

Causes

Causes and clinical signs of FVD are summarized in **Table 3-1.** This imbalance is almost always due to loss of body fluids and occurs more rapidly when coupled with decreased intake for any reason. It is possible to develop FVD solely on the basis of inadequate intake, provided the decreased intake is prolonged.

Losses of Gastrointestinal Fluids

In adults, approximately 8 L of fluid enters the small intestine daily, consisting primarily of salivary, gastric, biliary, pancreatic, and small intestinal secretions.[1] Most of these secretions are reabsorbed in the ileum and proximal colon, leaving only 100 to 200 mL of relatively electrolyte-free fluid to be excreted daily in the stool.[2] When any abnormal route of loss is present, such as vomiting, diarrhea, gastrointestinal (GI) suction, fistulas, or drainage tubes, it becomes evident how large losses can occur (resulting in FVD). Fluids trapped in the GI tract (as in intestinal obstruction) are physiologically outside the body (third-space effect). Indeed, any condition that interferes with the absorption of fluids from the GI tract can cause serious FVD.

Polyuria

The polyuria associated with hyperosmolar syndromes can lead to profound FVD. This situation is common in patients with hyperglycemia (as in diabetic ketoacidosis) and in patients receiving concentrated tube feedings. To excrete the excess solute load, the kidneys must also excrete a large urine volume. In the absence of an adequate exogenous source of water, fluid will be "pulled in" from the plasma, from the tissue space, and even from the cells to promote urinary excretion, thereby depleting the extracellular fluid spaces.

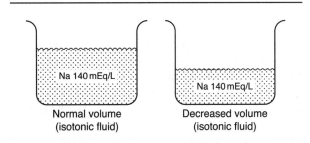

Figure 3-1 Fluid volume deficit

Table 3-1 Summary of Causes and Clinical Signs of Fluid Volume Deficit

Causes	Clinical Signs
Loss of water and electrolytes, as in the following conditions:	• Weight loss over short period (except in third-space fluid losses)
• Vomiting	∘ 2% (mild deficit, such as a 2.4-lb loss in a 120-lb person)
• Diarrhea	∘ 5% (moderate deficit, such as a 6-lb loss in a 120-lb person)
• Excessive laxative use	∘ 8% (severe deficit, such as a 10-lb loss or more in a 120-lb person)
• Fistulas	• Decreased skin and tongue turgor
• GI suction	• Dry mucous membranes
• Polyuria	• Urine output < 30 mL/hr in adult
• Fever	• Postural hypotension (systolic pressure drops by more than 20 mm Hg
• Excessive sweating	when the patient moves from lying to standing or sitting position)
• Third-space fluid shifts	• Weak, rapid pulse
	• Slow capillary refill time
Decreased intake, as in the following conditions:	• Decreased body temperature, unless infection is present
• Anorexia	• Central venous pressure < 4 cm water in vena cava
• Nausea	• BUN elevated out of proportion to serum creatinine
• Inability to gain access to fluids	• Urinary specific gravity elevated
• Depression	• Marked oliguria, late
	• Altered sensorium
	• Cold extremities, late

Fever

An elevated body temperature can cause FVD if extra fluids are not supplied. For example, fever causes hyperventilation and increased insensible water vapor loss from the lungs. Fever also increases the metabolic rate and, therefore, increases production of waste products; as a result, urine volume is increased to allow for the renal elimination of these wastes. Fluid requirements increase by 10% to 12.5% for each 1°C increase in body temperature above 37°C.[3, 4] Put another way, water losses in an adult generally increase by 100 to 150 mL per day for each degree of body temperature above 37°C.[5]

Sweating

Sweat is a hypotonic fluid containing primarily water, salt (sodium chloride), and potassium. Sweat can vary in volume from 0 to 1000 mL/hr or more. Thus a person might potentially become volume depleted from severe perspiration in the absence of adequate fluid replacement. Frequently, a sodium imbalance is superimposed on the volume depletion (either hyponatremia if excessive water is ingested, or hypernatremia if no liquids are consumed).

Decreased Intake

A number of circumstances can interfere with normal fluid intake, including anorexia, nausea, and fatigue. Patients who are unable to swallow because of neurological impairment frequently have at least some degree of FVD. Others predisposed to this condition include patients who are reluctant to swallow because of oral or pharyngeal pain or those who are unable to gain access to fluids because of decreased mobility. In some cases, depression may be so severe as to interfere with normal fluid intake.

Clinical Signs

Clinical signs of FVD are summarized in **Table 3-1**. Fluid volume deficit can develop slowly or with great rapidity, and can be mild, moderate, or severe, depending on the degree of fluid loss.

Weight Loss

Rapid weight loss reflects a loss of body fluid because fluctuations in body mass do not occur quickly. For example, it is generally assumed that it takes a caloric deficit of approximately 3400 kcal to lose 1 lb (0.45 kg) of actual weight. Theoretically, a typical adult on bedrest with a normal metabolism would have to take in zero calories to achieve a "real" weight loss of 1 lb in 2 days (assuming basal caloric needs are approximately 1800 calories per day). In reality, because 500 mL of fluid weighs about 1 lb, it is easy to lose this amount of weight very quickly during direct loss of body fluids (as in diarrhea or vomiting). Indeed, it is possible to lose much larger amounts of weight in a short period of time.

Decreased Skin and Tongue Turgor

In most healthy persons, pinched skin will immediately fall back to its original position when released. This elastic property, called "turgor," is partially dependent on interstitial fluid volume. In a person with FVD, the skin may remain slightly elevated for many seconds after being pinched, indicating a deficit of fluid in the interstitial compartment (one segment of extracellular fluid [ECF]). Because tissue turgor also reflects the degree of skin elasticity, it is less valid as a sign of FVD in patients older than 55 to 60 years (because skin elasticity decreases with age). Although reduced skin turgor is an important finding, turgor might potentially appear normal in obese individuals or anyone with only a mild fluid deficit.

In a person with FVD, the tongue is smaller and has additional longitudinal furrows, again reflecting loss of interstitial fluid. Fortunately, tongue turgor is not affected appreciably by age; as a consequence, it is a useful assessment for all age groups. In a study of 55 emergency room patients, ranging in age from 61 to 98 years, tongue dryness and increased longitudinal tongue furrows were found to be good indicators of FVD (as were dry oral mucous membranes, sunken eyes, confusion, speech difficulty, and upper-body muscle weakness).[6]

Decreased Moisture in Oral Cavity

A dry mouth may be due to FVD or to mouth breathing. If due to FVD, all of the oral tissues will be dry. In contrast, if the dryness is due to mouth breathing, the areas where the gums and cheek membranes meet will remain moist. If the serum sodium is elevated concurrently with FVD, the mucous membranes may feel dry and sticky.

Decreased Urinary Output

Decreased urinary output reflects inadequate perfusion of the kidney. A urine volume less than 30mL/hr in an adult is

cause for concern. Persistent oliguria in a severely volume-depleted patient can result in renal damage (a condition referred to as "acute tubular necrosis," discussed later in this chapter).

Increased Urinary Specific Gravity

Elevation of urinary specific gravity (SG) reflects fluid conservation by the kidneys (a compensatory response to a reduced fluid intake). Urinary SG can range from 1.003 to 1.035 (with 1.003 being very dilute and 1.035 being very concentrated). Thus a healthy renal response to FVD would be a reduced urine volume with an elevated urinary SG, indicating reduced water in the urine.

Elevated Blood Urea Nitrogen/Creatinine Ratio

Measurement of blood urea nitrogen (BUN) and creatinine concentrations is quite helpful in the diagnosis of FVD. Fluid volume contraction causes increases tubular reabsorption of urea, leading to an increased serum BUN concentration (but not an appreciably increased serum creatinine concentration). In other words, when FVD leads to a reduced glomerular filtration rate, the blood urea nitrogen (BUN) level rises slowly out of proportion to the serum creatinine. In this situation, the BUN:creatinine (Cr) ratio is usually greater than 20:1.

Changes in Vital Signs

Body temperature may be subnormal due to decreased metabolism, unless infection is present. In contrast, body temperature may be elevated in patients with water deficit (hypernatremia), also referred to as dehydration.

Postural hypotension and increased pulse rate are signs of hypovolemia (a condition present in FVD). On changing from a lying to an upright position, a drop in systolic pressure greater than 20 mm Hg and an increase in the pulse rate suggest intravascular volume deficit. The blood pressure should be assessed immediately after the patient assumes the erect position and again 2 to 3 minutes later (if indicated) to determine whether the pressure drop is sustained. Postural hypotension with dizziness strongly suggests hypovolemia in the absence of autonomic neuropathy or use of medications that are associated with postural hypotension (such as sympatholytic drugs for hypertension).[7] As fluid volume depletion worsens, blood pressure becomes low in all positions due to loss of compensatory mechanisms.

As always, the patient's baseline blood pressure should be used to assess the degree of blood pressure drop (not the commonly accepted "normal" value of 120/80 mm Hg). Notably, blood pressure measured by a sphygmomanometer may reflect a lower pressure than is found if arterial pressure is being simultaneously measured with an intra-arterial catheter (because peripheral vasoconstriction leads to decreased intensity of Korotkoff sounds). Tachycardia occurs as the heart pumps faster to compensate for the decreased plasma volume.

Changes in Central Venous Pressure

Direct measurement of central venous pressure (CVP), which is frequently performed in acutely ill patients, will reveal a reading less than normal in those persons with FVD (provided cardiopulmonary function is not impaired). Sometimes the jugular veins are observed to detect changes in CVP because, in the presence of hypovolemia, filling of these veins is visibly decreased.

Decreased Capillary Refill

Measuring the time required for capillaries to fill after compression of the nail bed is helpful in assessing the degree of fluid depletion. A study of this phenomenon done in 30 healthy infants (2 to 24 months of age) indicated that normal capillary refill time was 0.81 ± 0.31 seconds.[8] In a study of 32 infants with diarrhea, capillary refill time was compared with laboratory indicators of FVD. The investigators found the following results:

- A refill time less than 1.5 seconds suggests either a normal volume or a deficit of less than 50 mL/kg.
- A refill time of 1.5 to 3.0 seconds suggests a deficit between 50 and 100 mL/kg.
- A refill time of more than 3.0 seconds suggests a deficit greater than 100 mL/kg.

Another group of investigators studied an outpatient sample of 102 children younger than the age of 4 years. They found that increased capillary refill time was a good indicator of fluid depletion in these pediatric patients (as was decreased skin turgor and increased thirst).[9]

Other Changes

Altered sensorium is the result of decreased cerebral perfusion, secondary to decreased blood volume. Cold extremities reflect peripheral vasoconstriction, a mechanism that increases the central blood volume and thus perfusion of more vital organs (such as the brain and heart). The hematocrit is elevated above baseline due to loss of intravascular fluid (and subsequent concentration of the formed ele-

ments of blood). A relative increase in serum albumin concentration also occurs due to hemoconcentration.[10]

Treatment

Fluid Replacement

The kidneys require substantial blood flow to maintain their metabolism; therefore, sustained hypovolemia may result in acute tubular necrosis.[11] For this reason, prompt treatment of FVD is imperative to prevent renal damage. In planning fluid replacement for the patient with FVD, it is necessary to consider usual maintenance fluid volume requirements and other factors (such as fever) that can influence fluid needs. Chapter 10 discusses formulas used to determine both maintenance and replacement fluid requirements. When the deficit is not severe, the oral route is preferred for replacement, provided the patient is able to drink. In contrast, when fluid losses are acute, the intravenous (IV) route or the intraosseous route is required. In subacute settings, fluids may also be administered subcutaneously (hypodermoclysis). See Chapters 24 and 25.

Isotonic electrolyte solutions (such as lactated Ringer's solution or 0.9% NaCl [normal saline]) are frequently used to treat the hypotensive patient with FVD because these fluids expand plasma volume. As soon as the patient becomes normotensive, a hypotonic electrolyte solution (such as 0.45% NaCl) may be used to provide both electrolytes and free water for renal excretion of metabolic wastes. These and other fluids are discussed in Chapter 10.

Fluid Challenge Test

If the patient with severe FVD is oliguric, it is necessary to determine whether the depressed renal function is the result of reduced renal blood flow secondary to FVD (prerenal azotemia) or, more seriously, the result of acute tubular necrosis (ATN) due to prolonged FVD. The therapeutic test used in the latter situation is the "fluid challenge test." Although the amount of fluid to be given must be determined on an individual basis, in adults this volume typically ranges between 500 and 1000 mL of normal saline (0.9% NaCl) infused over a period of 30 to 60 minutes.[12] During this period, the urine output and cardiopulmonary status should be carefully monitored. Whenever monitoring urine output, it is imperative to ensure that the urinary catheter is not occluded. If urine output does not increase with fluid challenges, invasive hemodynamic monitoring may be required to exclude cardiac causes of decreased cardiac output.[13]

Key Clinical Points for Isotonic Fluid Volume Deficit

- Measure and evaluate intake and output (I & O) at least at 8-hour intervals; sometimes hourly measurements are critical. For a valid evaluation of the patient's fluid balance status, it is also necessary to compare the total I & O measurements for several consecutive days. (See Case Study 3-3.)
- Monitor body weight daily. Remember that an acute weight loss of 1 lb represents a fluid loss of approximately 500 mL.
- Monitor for postural hypotension (i.e., a drop in the systolic blood pressure reading greater than 20 mm Hg) when the patient is quickly moved from a lying to a sitting position.
- Monitor concentration of urine. In a volume-depleted patient with healthy kidneys, the urinary SG will be more than 1.020 (indicating a healthy renal response by conserving water and salt while excreting metabolic wastes in as little fluid as possible). Urine with a high SG due to FVD will have a dark yellow color.
- Monitor the BUN/Cr ratio. In a patient with FVD and healthy kidneys, the BUN:Cr ratio will be higher than 20:1. (See Table 2-2.)
- Consult with the physician for intravenous or tube feeding directives if the patient is unable to consume fluids by mouth. This intervention is important to prevent renal damage related to prolonged FVD.
- When oral fluids are tolerated, select fluids that will replace needed electrolytes. For example, select fluids containing sodium and potassium for a patient who has a FVD due to vomiting. **Table 3-2** lists the electrolyte content of commonly available beverages, **Table 3-3** lists the electrolyte content of common foods, and **Table 3-4** lists the potassium content of common food additives and condiments. See Table 13-1 for a summary of the electrolyte content of selected body fluids.
- Be familiar with the usual types of intravenous fluids used to treat FVD (review the treatment section earlier in this chapter and see Chapter 10).
- Understand the principles underlying the fluid challenge test and the parameters for nursing assessment (see the treatment section earlier in this chapter).
- Monitor the response to fluid intake. If therapy is providing adequate fluids, the following will be observed:
  - Increased urinary volume toward 40 to 60 mL/hr in adults
  - If previously hypotensive, increased blood pressure toward normal
  - Return of pulse rate to baseline
  - Improved sensorium and sense of vitality
  - Improved skin and tongue turgor
  - Decreased dryness of oral mucosa
  - Increased CVP toward normal
  - Normal, or no worse, breath sounds
  - Decreased urinary SG as urinary volume increases

THIRD-SPACING OF BODY FLUIDS

Third-spacing of body fluids is a unique situation leading to decreased intravascular volume and largely presents with the same characteristics as FVD. Because this condition is

---

Table 3-2 Sodium and Potassium Content of Selected Beverages

Beverage	Sodium (mg)	Potassium (mg)
Carbonated cola, 12 fl oz	26	7
Coffee (brewed from grounds with tap water, 6 fl oz)	4	87
Cranberry juice cocktail, bottled, 8 fl oz	5	35
Milk, 1%, 1 cup	107	366
Orange juice, canned, unsweetened, 1 cup	10	458
Prune juice, canned, 1 cup	10	707
Tea, brewed with tap water, 6 fl oz	5	68
Tomato juice, canned, with added salt, 1 cup	654	556
Vegetable juice cocktail, canned, 1 cup	653	467

Source: Information from USDA National Nutrient Database for Standard Reference, Release 21. United States Department of Agriculture Research Service, 2008.

Table 3-3 Sodium and Potassium Content of Selected Foods

Food	Sodium (mg)	Potassium (mg)
Apple, raw, one	1	148
Apricots, dried, 10 halves	4	407
Bacon, cooked, 3 slices	439	107
Baked beans, canned plain, 1 cup	871	569
Banana, raw, one	1	422
Beans, white canned, 1 cup	13	1189
Beef broth or bouillon, prepared with equal volume water, 1 cup	636	154
Bologna, 2 slices	417	179
Bread, rye, 1 slice	211	53
Broccoli, raw, 1 cup	29	278
Cantaloupe, raw, 1 cup	26	427
Cheddar cheese, 1 oz	176	28
Cottage cheese, creamed, 1 cup	764	218
Crackers, whole wheat, 4 crackers	105	48
Egg, whole scrambled, 1 large	171	84
Fish, salmon pink, canned with solids and bone, 3 oz	471	277
Fish, tuna salad, 1 cup	824	365
Gelatin dessert, dry mix prepared with water, ½ cup	101	1
Honeydew melon, raw, 1 cup	31	388
Nuts, almonds, 24 nuts	0	200
Nuts, pecans, 20 halves	0	116
Orange, raw, one	0	237
Potato, whole, baked, one	20	1081
Strawberries, raw, 1 cup	2	254
Tomato, red ripe, one	6	292
Watermelon, raw, 1 cup	2	170
Yogurt, plain, low-fat, 8 oz	159	531

Source: Information from USDA National Nutrient Database for Standard Reference, Release 21. United States Department of Agriculture. Agricultural Research Service, 2008

more difficult to diagnose than direct loss of body fluids, it is discussed separately here. In addition, third-space fluid losses are discussed in the clinical chapters dealing with specific conditions associated with this phenomenon.

Pathophysiology

Third-spacing refers to a shift of fluid from the vascular space into a portion of the body from which it is not easily exchanged with the rest of the ECF. This sequestration of fluid results from altered capillary permeability secondary to injury, ischemia, or inflammation. The trapped fluid, although still technically within the body, is essentially unavailable for functional use. Termed *nonfunctional* because it is not able to participate in the normal functions of the ECF compartment, the third-spaced fluid might just as well have been lost externally. Fluid can be sequestered from the intravascular space in body spaces (such as the pleural, peritoneal, pericardial, or joint cavities) or it may become trapped in the bowel by obstruction or in the interstitial space as edema after burns or other trauma. Furthermore, it can be trapped in inflamed tissues, as in peritonitis, pancreatitis, or fasciitis.

Table 3-4 Sodium Content of Common Food Additives and Condiments

Additive	Sodium Content (mg)
Table salt, 1 teaspoon	2325
Baking powder, 1 teaspoon	363–488
Baking soda, 1 teaspoon	1259
Yellow mustard, 1 teaspoon	57
Catsup, 1 tablespoon	167

Source: Information from USDA National Nutrient Database for Standard Reference, Release 21. United States Department of Agriculture, Agricultural Research Service. 2008.

The following points are major considerations in differentiating the FVD associated with third-spacing from that associated with fluid lost through vomiting or diarrhea:

- Third-space fluid losses cannot be directly observed and measured. In contrast, it is possible to measure fluid lost from vomiting, diarrhea, fistulas, and other causes.
- Body weight does not change when third-space fluid shifts occur (because the fluid is trapped within the body). In contrast, when direct losses of fluid are incurred by the body, the weight diminishes in proportion to the amount of lost fluid.

Phases of Third-Space Fluid Shifts and Clinical Signs

Third-space fluid shifts occur in two phases. The first involves a shift of fluid from the intravascular space into a nonfunctional fluid space. Clinical manifestations expected with a significant shift of fluid are essentially those of FVD because, although the fluid is in the body, it is functionally unavailable for use. During this period, expect to see the following signs and symptoms:

- Tachycardia and hypotension (effective blood volume is reduced as the fluid shifts out of the vascular space)
- Urine volume less than 30 mL/hr in the adult (decreased plasma volume causes a fall in renal perfusion and, therefore, less urine formation)
- High urinary SG and osmolality (renal attempt to conserve needed water)

- Elevated hematocrit (red blood cells become suspended in a smaller plasma volume as the fluid shifts out of the intravascular space)
- Postural hypotension
- Low CVP
- Poor skin and tongue turgor

As with any cause of hypovolemia associated with reduced renal blood flow, it is important to correct the reduced plasma volume before renal perfusion becomes compromised to the extent that acute tubular necrosis occurs.

After a variable number of days, the fluid shifts back to the vascular space and may impose a temporary hypervolemia. Resolution of the third-spacing phenomenon is slower than the accumulation of this fluid. In some cases, the shift of fluid back to the intravascular space occurs within 48 to 72 hours. In other cases, it may not occur for 10 days or longer. For example, fluid shifts from major burns or peritonitis are generally reversed within 2 to 3 days, whereas those associated with septic shock may not occur until the underlying cause of the sepsis is addressed. As the extra fluid in the tissues or body spaces shifts back into the intravascular compartment, it is excreted through the kidneys. Excessive fluid administration during the period when fluid is shifting back into the bloodstream may cause circulatory overload, especially in patients with cardiac or renal failure.

Assessment is primarily directed at detecting hypervolemia before serious effects occur. For example, observe for polyuria (hourly urine volume may be as high as 200 mL as the excess fluid is excreted), distended neck veins (a sign of fluid overload), moist lung sounds, shortness of breath, elevated CVP, and elevated systolic blood pressure.

Examples of Conditions Associated with Third-Spacing of Body Fluids

Hip Fracture

A patient with a fractured hip may lose 1500 to 2000 mL of blood into the tissues surrounding the injury site.[14] The third-spaced fluid will eventually be reabsorbed (over a period of days or weeks). Until this fluid restoration occurs, however, the deficit can cause an acute reduction in the vascular volume if it is not replaced.

Surgical Procedures

Following surgery, the amount of fluid "third-spaced" at the surgical site depends on the extent and nature of the surgical undertaking. For example, minor operative procedures (e.g., appendectomy) are associated with considerably less fluid sequestration than are major operative procedures (e.g., an extensive colon resection). After abdominal surgery, particularly pelvic surgery, fluid accumulates in the peritoneum, bowel wall, and other traumatized tissues. In the surgical patient, it is difficult to assess fluid loss due to sequestration into the interstitial compartment. Such unrecognized deficits of ECF during the early postoperative period are manifested primarily as circulatory instability.

Burns

Altered capillary permeability of burned tissue results in an exudation of plasma at the burn site. Fluid flux also increases across capillaries in nonburned tissue, apparently as a result of hypoproteinemia rather than an alteration in capillary permeability. Formation of edema occurs primarily in the first 24 hours after the burn occurs, with the greatest losses being observed during the first 8 to 12 hours in mild to moderate burn injuries and during the first 12 to 24 hours with extensive burn injuries.

Intestinal Obstruction

In acute intestinal obstruction, fluid volumes of as much as 6 L or more can accumulate within the lumen and wall of the gut. (See Chapter 13 for a more in-depth discussion of intestinal obstruction.)

Inflammation of Intra-abdominal Organs

Important third-space fluid losses can occur into the peritoneum, the bowel wall, and other tissues in the presence of inflammatory lesions of the intra-abdominal organs. The extent of these losses may not be fully appreciated unless one considers that the total area of the peritoneum is approximately the same as that of the skin.[15]

Sepsis

Sepsis produces a generalized capillary leak that leads to a decrease in the functional ECF volume (while generating interstitial edema). As sepsis persists, protein malnutrition produces hypoproteinemia, which in turn may increase the formation of edema. Other toxic insults to the capillary endothelium (such as may occur secondary to snakebites or after the administration of certain drugs, such as interleukin-2) may result in the "capillary leak" syndrome. In these situations, edema forms at the expense of the intravascular volume.

Pancreatitis

In pancreatitis, inflammation and auto-digestion by pancreatic enzymes lead to peripancreatic edema as well as fluid loss into the retro-peritoneal tissue; a dramatic decrease in plasma volume causes systemic hypovolemia. Clinical signs of this type of fluid loss include hypotension, tachycardia, oliguria, and increased hematocrit due to hemoconcentration. When hemorrhagic pancreatitis occurs, the third-space fluid shift is accompanied by direct blood loss; in this situation, the hematocrit level will likely drop rather than become elevated. See Chapter 20 for an in-depth discussion of fluid and electrolyte problems associated with pancreatitis.

Ascites

The major difference between the fluid shifts described previously in this section and that associated with cirrhotic ascites is the rate of fluid accumulation. In patients with cirrhosis, ascites usually develops slowly, allowing time for renal conservation of sodium and water to replenish the effective circulating blood volume.[16] As a result, patients with cirrhosis typically present with symptoms of edema instead of hypovolemia. An exception could occur if rapid fluid removal by paracentesis results in a rapid shift of fluid from the vascular space to the peritoneum (producing hypovolemia). When a large volume of ascitic fluid is removed by paracentesis, some authorities recommend the simultaneous intravenous infusion of salt-poor albumin (such as 10 g per 1 L of ascitic fluid removed) to prevent rapid contraction of the intravascular space by fluid shifting.[17] See Chapter 21 for a more detailed discussion of cirrhosis with ascites.

Fluid Replacement in Third-Space Fluid Shifts

Treatment of third-spacing is directed at correcting the cause of the third-space shift of body fluids. As is the case with any cause of FVD, the reduced plasma volume must be corrected before renal damage occurs.

Although the choice of a replacement fluid depends on the existence of concurrent electrolyte abnormalities, most third-space losses are properly replaced with a balanced salt solution such as lactated Ringer's solution or isotonic saline (0.9% sodium chloride). Attempts to correct the fluid deficit with hypotonic solutions (such as 5% dextrose in water or half-strength saline) may result in clinically significant hyponatremia. Any deficits in red blood cell concentration may require correction by the administration of packed cells to maintain the optimal oxygen-carrying capacity of the blood. Large quantities of replacement fluids are often needed to maintain an effective circulating volume. Plasma or plasma substitutes may also be considered for use in addition to replacement electrolyte solutions for patients who have suffered protein loss (e.g., in burns or peritonitis).

Fluid replacement therapy must be tailored to the patient's response. For example, during the first phase, when fluid has shifted from the intravascular space, the aim of fluid therapy is to stabilize blood pressure and pulse and maintain an adequate urine volume (usually 30–50 mL/hr) in an adult.

FLUID VOLUME EXCESS

Fluid volume excess (FVE) is the result of the abnormal retention of water and sodium in about the same proportions in which they normally exist in the ECF (**Figure 3-2**). It always occurs secondary to an increase in the total body sodium content, which in turn leads to an increase in total body water. Because, in most situations, the body maintains isotonic retention of both substances, the serum sodium concentration remains essentially normal.

Causes

Causes and clinical signs of FVE are summarized in **Table 3-5**. This kind of imbalance may be caused by simple overloading with fluids or by diminished function of the home-

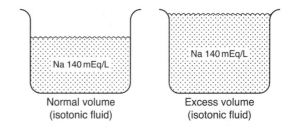

Figure 3-2 Fluid volume excess

ostatic mechanisms responsible for regulating fluid balance. Etiological factors can include the following conditions:

- Compromised regulatory mechanisms, as in congestive heart failure, renal failure, cirrhosis of the liver, and steroid excess.
- Overzealous administration of sodium-containing fluids, particularly in patients with impaired regulatory mechanisms. The commonly used isotonic fluids— 0.9% NaCl and lactated Ringer's solution—contain considerable amounts of sodium and, if used to excess, can easily exceed the tolerance of patients with impaired regulatory mechanisms. Note that 0.9% NaCl contains 154 mEq/L sodium and that lactated Ringer's solution contains 130 mEq/L sodium.
- Excessive ingestion of sodium chloride or other sodium salts in the diet. Table 3-4 identifies the sodium

Table 3-5 Summary of Causes and Clinical Signs of Fluid Volume Excess

Causes	Clinical Signs
Compromised regulatory mechanisms: • Renal failure • Congestive heart failure • Cirrhosis of liver • Cushing's syndrome	• Weight gain over a short period: ○ 2% (mild excess, such as 2.4 lb in a 120-lb person) ○ 5% (moderate excess, such as 6 lb in a 120-lb person) ○ 8% (severe excess, such as 10 lb or more in a 120-lb person) • Peripheral edema (excess of fluid in interstitial space) • Distended veins • Central venous pressure > 11 cm H$_2$O in the vena cava • Moist rales in lungs • Polyuria (if renal function is normal) • Ascites, pleural effusion (when fluid volume excess is severe, fluid transudates into body cavities) • Decreased blood urea nitrogen (due to dilution) • Bounding, full pulse • Pulmonary edema, if severe

content of compounds used to improve the texture or flavor of food or to extend freshness. Other "hidden" gains of sodium may result from the use of proprietary drugs such as sodium-containing antacids and hypertonic sodium phosphate enemas.

Clinical Signs

The clinical signs of FVE are linked to an excess of fluid in the extracellular compartment and are summarized in Table 3-5. Pitting edema is depicted in Figure 2-2.

Treatment

When reversal of the primary problem is impossible, symptomatic treatment often consists of the administration of diuretics and restriction of sodium and fluids. In some conditions, only one of these therapies is necessary. Sodium-restricted diets and diuretic administration are discussed in this section, along with the effect of bedrest on mobilization of edematous fluid.

Sodium-Restricted Diets

Sodium content in foods may be expressed as grams of salt, milligrams of sodium, or milliequivalents of sodium. To understand conversions of grams of salt to grams of sodium, recall that sodium represents about 40% of the weight of table salt (sodium chloride). Therefore, 1 g of sodium chloride is equivalent to 0.4 g of sodium. To convert milligrams of sodium to milliequivalents of sodium, divide the number of milligrams by 23 (the atomic weight of sodium); for example, 1000 mg sodium is equivalent to approximately 43 mEq sodium.

The typical American diet includes roughly 10 to 12 g salt (NaCl) per day (or 4 to 4.8 g sodium). About one-third comes from the salt shaker, one-third from processed foods, and one-third from the food itself. Recall that processed foods often have hidden sources of sodium in the form of preservatives (such as monosodium glutamate, baking powder, baking soda, brine, and disodium phosphate). Tables 3-1 and 3-2 list the sodium and potassium content of some common beverages and foods; Table 3-3 summarizes the sodium content of common food additives. These figures clearly indicate how plentiful sodium is in the average diet.

Sodium-restricted diets are commonly prescribed for patients with fluid excess problems, such as occur with congestive heart failure, hepatic failure with ascites, renal failure, and hypertension. Some patients do well with only mildly restricted diets, whereas others require severe restrictions. A mildly sodium-restricted diet requires only light salting of food (roughly half the usual amount) in cooking and at the table, no addition of salt to foods that are already seasoned (such as canned foods and foods ready to cook or eat), and avoidance of foods that are high in sodium. Examples of such foods include salty snack foods, olives, pickles, and luncheon meats.

Patients should be made aware that most canned and "ready-to-eat'" foods have added salt and, therefore, should be used only as their specific diets allow. Foods that may be consumed freely include most fresh vegetables and fruits and unprocessed cereals. Cooking from scratch is usually the best way to prepare low-sodium food, and several excellent cookbooks are available for this purpose. Low-sodium baking powder can be found in the dietetic section of many grocery stores, and low-sodium milk, milk products, and bakery goods are available in most large cities. Patients on sodium-restricted diets should also consider the sodium content in over-the-counter drugs. For example, one Alka-Seltzer tablet (without aspirin) contains nearly 450 mg of sodium.

Because a substantial portion of sodium is ingested in the form of seasoning, use of substitute seasonings plays a major role in cutting sodium intake. Lemon juice, onion, and garlic are excellent substitute flavoring agents. Most salt substitutes contain potassium chloride and should be used cautiously by those individuals taking potassium-conserving diuretics and by those patients who have renal impairment. Salt substitutes containing ammonium chloride can be harmful to patients with liver damage. (Salt substitutes are discussed further in Chapter 5.)

Diuretics

Diuretics are commonly used drugs that promote increased urine flow (**Table 3-6**). More specifically, they act by inhibiting salt and water reabsorption by the renal tubules. By inducing a negative fluid balance, these medications are useful in the treatment of conditions associated with fluid volume excess.

For the most part, diuretics can be grouped into three major classes:

- Loop diuretics (such as furosemide, bumetanide, and ethacrynic acid), which act in the thick ascending loop of Henle
- Thiazide-type diuretics (such as chlorothiazide and hydrochlorothiazide), which act in the distal tubule and connecting segment

Table 3-6 Summary of Commonly Used Diuretics

Drug	Comments
Thiazides (examples): • Chlorothiazide (Diuril) • Hydrochlorothiazide (HCTZ)	• Cause loss of sodium, chloride, and potassium. • Decrease urinary calcium excretion, and sometimes result in a slightly elevated serum calcium level. • Act by inhibiting sodium reabsorption in the distal tubule and, to a lesser extent, the inner medullary collecting duct.
Loop diuretics (examples): • Furosemide (Lasix) • Bumetanide (Bumex)	• Cause loss of sodium, chloride, and potassium. • Act primarily in the thick segment of the medullary and cortical ascending limbs of the loop of Henle. • Potassium supplements or extra dietary potassium may be necessary when these agents are used routinely. • Increase urinary calcium excretion.
Potassium-conserving diuretics (examples): • Spironolactone (Aldactone) • Triamterene (Dyrenium) • Amiloride (Midamor)	• Conserve potassium while promoting loss of sodium. • Spironolactone inhibits action of aldosterone. (Recall that the hormone aldosterone causes sodium retention and potassium excretion.) • These drugs reduce potassium excretion and may lead to hyperkalemia; thus potassium supplements are contraindicated, as are salt substitutes containing potassium. • Often combined with thiazides for effective diuresis. In this case, the hypokalemic tendency of the thiazides may offset the hyperkalemic tendency of triamterene and spironolactone (examples of such combinations are Dyazide and Aldactazide).

• Potassium-sparing diuretics (such as amiloride, spironolactone, and triamterene), which act in the cortical collecting tube

Examples of other diuretics include acetazolamide, a carbonic anhydrase inhibitor, and mannitol, a non-reabsorbable polysaccharide that acts as an osmotic diuretic. To achieve excretion of excess fluid, either a single diuretic (such as a thiazide) or a combination of agents may be selected (such a thiazide and spironolactone). The latter combination is particularly helpful in that the two drugs have different sites of action, which enables this dual-agent therapy to provide more effective control of fluid volume excess.

Diuretics may be given orally or parenterally, depending on the drug and the status of the patient. For example, patients with advanced congestive heart failure may have difficulty in absorbing orally administered furosemide (due to decreased intestinal perfusion and perhaps intestinal mucosal edema). In this situation, removal of edema with intravenous furosemide therapy and stabilization of cardiac function may partially correct this absorptive effect, thereby allowing oral therapy to be reinstituted.

Diuretics can have undesirable side effects, such as extracellular FVD, hyponatremia, alterations in potassium excretion, magnesium wasting, alterations in calcium excretion, and acid–base disturbances.

Extracellular Fluid Volume Depletion. Depletion of the ECF volume is a common complication of diuretic use, especially when the potent loop-acting diuretics are used. Some patients have a relatively large initial response to diuretics and develop true volume depletion. This complication is most likely to occur in patients who are concurrently losing fluids from other routes (e.g., vomiting or diarrhea) or who are unable to consume sufficient amounts of salt and water.

Hyponatremia. Hyponatremia is seen relatively often in patients taking diuretics. Hyponatremia associated with diuretic use is typically due to a thiazide-type diuretic (as opposed to a loop diuretic). Indeed, hydrochlorothiazide may cause rapidly developing and severe hyponatremia in some patients.[18]

Hypokalemia. Urinary potassium losses are increased by the thiazide and loop diuretics, often leading to the development of hypokalemia (generally defined as a serum potassium concentration less than 3.5 mEq/L). Because potassium homeostasis is essential for normal myocardial function, low serum potassium may cause fatal arrhythmias. Other problems associated with hypokalemia may include defects in renal concentrating ability, sluggish insulin release (leading to carbohydrate intolerance), and predisposition to rhabdomyolysis (due to decreased striated muscle blood flow). Electrocardiographic changes may occur even when the plasma potassium concentration is near the low end of the normal range.[19] Studies have shown that cardiac patients with serum potassium less than 4 mEq/L have worse outcomes than do those with potassium levels greater than 4 mEq/L.[20] Therefore, an attempt is made to keep the plasma potassium level in the mid-to-high normal range (such as 4 mEq/L or greater) in patients with cardiac conditions to minimize their risk for arrhythmias.

Hyperkalemia. The potassium-conserving diuretics (e.g., spironolactone, amiloride, and triamterene) reduce potassium secretion and, as a result, can cause hyperkalemia. To prevent this problem, these drugs should be used with great caution (if at all) in patients with impaired renal function or in those treated with a potassium supplement or an angiotensin-converting enzyme (ACE) inhibitor (which also decreases potassium secretion).

Magnesium Wasting. Magnesium depletion can be induced by the chronic administration of loop and thiazide diuretics. Compared to loop diuretics, the thiazides have little acute effect on magnesium handling; nonetheless, they can be associated with chronic magnesium depletion (perhaps because of the effect of hypokalemia).[21] Atrial and ventricular arrhythmias can occur in patients with hypomagnesemia, especially those who are treated with digoxin.[22]

Alterations in Calcium Excretion. Thiazide diuretics interfere with urinary calcium excretion with both short- and long-term use. Thus long-term thiazide administration may lead to overt hypercalcemia. Use of amiloride also decreases calcium excretion. Conversely, bumetanide, furosemide, and ethacrynic acid all increase urinary calcium excretion and, therefore, are useful in the treatment of acute hypercalcemic conditions.

Metabolic Acid–Base Disturbances. Hypokalemia secondary to usage of thiazide and loop diuretics is often accompa-nied by metabolic alkalosis. In contrast, the potassium-sparing diuretics can result in both hyperkalemia and metabolic acidosis.

Bedrest

Bedrest alone can induce diuresis, particularly in patients with heart failure. The mobilization of edematous fluid when a person is in the supine position probably increases the effective blood volume, thereby improving renal perfusion. Metabolic requirements of peripheral tissues are usually decreased by bedrest, so that less demand is placed on the weakened myocardium of patients with congestive heart failure. This action can transfer as much as 400 to 500 mL of interstitial fluid into the central circulation over a few days.[23] Bedrest increases the glomerular filtration rate and enhances renal response to diuretics.

Summary of Clinical Considerations for Fluid Volume Excess

1. Assess for the presence, or worsening, of fluid volume excess:
   - Monitor I & O and evaluate the patient at regular intervals for excessive fluid retention.
   - Monitor changes in body weight; be alert for acute weight gain.
   - Assess breath sounds at regular intervals for rales.
   - Monitor the degree of peripheral edema; look for edema in most dependent parts of body (feet and ankles in ambulatory patients, sacral region in bedridden patients). Check for pitting edema (see Figure 2-2) and measure the extent of edema with millimeter tape.
   - Monitor the degree of distention of the peripheral veins.
   - Monitor laboratory values (look for low BUN and hematocrit; however, realize that abnormalities in these values may be caused by other conditions, such as low protein intake and anemia).
2. Encourage adherence to sodium-restricted diet, if prescribed. Assist the dietitian in diet instruction. Review the section on sodium-restricted diets provided earlier in this chapter.
3. Instruct patients requiring sodium restriction to avoid over-the-counter drugs without first checking with the healthcare adviser.
4. When fluid retention persists despite adherence to dietary sodium intake, consider hidden sources of sodium, such as water supply or use of water softeners.

5. When indicated, encourage the patient to take rest periods. Lying down favors diuresis of edematous fluid.

6. Monitor the patient's response to diuretics and parenteral fluids.

7. Teach self-monitoring of weight and I & O measurements to patients with chronic fluid retention (such as those with congestive heart failure, renal disease, or cirrhosis of liver).

8. If dyspnea and orthopnea are present, position the patient in semi-Fowler's position to favor lung expansion.

9. Turn and reposition the patient frequently; be aware that edematous tissue is more prone to skin breakdown than is normal tissue.

CASE STUDIES

Case Study 3-1

An 80-year-old man developed fluid volume deficit as a result of overzealous diuretic use. After a 13-lb weight loss over 4 days, the CVP dropped to 1 cm water. Skin turgor over the sternum and medial aspect of the thigh was poor (when the patient's skin was pinched, it remained elevated for 6 seconds). Urine output was low, at 20 mL/hr, and the BUN was greatly elevated, at 80 mg/dL (normal, 10–20 mg/dL). Boxy temperature was 36.3°C (97.4°F), pulse was 96 and weak in volume, and blood pressure was 140/90 mm Hg supine and 122/84 mm Hg in a sitting position.

Commentary. This patient had lost 6 L of fluid in a relatively short period; his CVP was far below the normal level of 4 to 11 cm H$_2$O. His BUN was elevated, and his urine volume was low, particularly for an elderly person. These factors, plus positional hypotension and increased pulse rate, were indicative of FVD. Note that the body temperature was not elevated, probably reflecting the slowed metabolic rate associated with FVD not complicated by infection.

Case Study 3-2

A 35-year-old woman developed FVD after 4 days of severe diarrhea and poor intake. She weighed 119 lb on admission (her pre-illness weight was 128 lb). Her BUN was 40 mg/dL and serum creatinine was 1.3 mg/dL. Skin turgor was poor and urine output was 15 mL/hr (SG 1.030). Blood pressure was 120/80 mm Hg recumbent and fell to 98/60 mm Hg when erect. Pulse was 110, weak, and regular.

Commentary. This patient lost 7% of her body weight in 4 days; her BUN was twice the normal level, whereas her serum creatinine was normal. Postural hypotension, poor turgor, and oliguria all point to FVD.

Case Study 3-3

A 16-year-old uninsured girl in the first trimester of pregnancy developed nausea and frequent bouts of gagging and vomiting. She was unable to eat but drank small quantities of tea and ginger ale over a 3-day period. Her mother cared for her and measured her fluid intake and output. Because the patient's condition did not improve, her mother took her to the emergency department of a nearby hospital on day 4. She received intravenous fluids and medication for nausea and was subsequently discharged.

	Intake	Output
Day 1	700 ml	900 ml (urine) 350 ml (vomitus)
Day 2	500 ml	850 ml (urine) 200 ml (vomitus)
Day 3	300 ml	750 ml (urine) 250 ml (vomitus)
24-hour total	1500 ml	3300 ml

*Note the negative fluid balance of 1800 ml (3300 ml–1500 ml)

Commentary. As noted in the I & O chart, the patient lost more fluid than she took in on each of the 3 days (negative fluid balance ranging between 550 mL and 700 mL for each day). By observing the I & O record over the 72-hour period, it was clear that the patient was sorely in need of fluid replacement. Obviously, treatment should have been sought before day 4.

NOTES

1. Brunicardi, F. C., Andersen, D. K., Billiar, T. R., Dunn, D. L., Hunter, J.G., & Pollock, R. E. (2005). *Schwartz's principles of surgery.* (8th ed.). New York: McGraw-Hill Medical Publishing Division, p. 1021.

2. Rose, B. D., & Post, T. W. (2001). *Clinical physiology of acid–base and electrolyte disorders* (5th ed.). New York: McGraw-Hill, p. 416.

3. Pestana, C. (2000). *Fluids and electrolytes in the surgical patient* (5th ed.). Philadelphia: Lippincott Williams & Wilkins, p. 26.

4. Matarese, L. E., & Gottschlich, M. M. (2003). *Contemporary nutrition support practice: A clinical guide* (2nd ed.). Philadelphia: Saunders, p. 125.

5. Kollef, M. H., Bedient, T. J., Isakow, W., & Witt, C. A. (2008). *The Washington manual of critical care*. Philadelphia: Lippincott Williams & Wilkins, p. 157.

6. Gross, C. R., Lindquist, R. D., Wooley, A. C., Granieri, R., Allard, K., & Webster, B. (1992). Clinical indications of dehydration severity in elderly patients. *Journal of Emergency Medicine, 10,* 267, 274.

7. Rose & Post, note 2, p. 420.

8. Saavedra, J., Harris, G., Song, L., & Finberg, L. (1991). Capillary refilling in the assessment of dehydration. *American Journal of Diseases of Children, 145,* 296.

9. MacKenzie, A., Barnes, G., & Shann, F. (1992). Clinical signs of dehydration in children. *Lancet, 2,* 504.

10. Feehally, J., Floege, J., & Johnson, R. J. (2007). *Comprehensive clinical nephrology* (3rd ed.). Philadelphia: Mosby, p. 84.

11. Bongard, F. S., Sue, D. Y., & Vintch, J. R. (2008). *Current diagnosis and treatment, critical care* (3rd ed.). New York: McGraw-Hill Medical Publishing, p. 225.

12. Cooper, D. H., Krainik, A. J., Lubner, S. J., & Reno, H. E. (2007). *The Washington manual of medical therapeutics* (32nd ed.). Philadelphia: Lippincott Williams & Wilkins, p. 322.

13. Marik, P.E. (2001). *Handbook of evidence-based critical care*. New York: Springer, p. 110.

14. Rose & Post, note 2, p. 419.

15. Fink, M. P., Abraham, E., Vincent, J. L., & Kochanek, P. M. *Textbook of critical care* (5th ed.). Philadelphia: Elsevier Saunders, p. 1034.

16. Rose & Post, note 2, p. 419.

17. Bongard et al., note 11, p. 719.

18. Brunton, L., Parker, K., Blumenthal, D., & Buxton, I. (2008). *Goodman and Gilman's manual of pharmacology and therapeutics.* New York: McGraw-Hill, p. 546.

19. Bongard et al., note 11, p. 37.

20. Ahmed, A., Zannad, F., Love, T. E., Tallai, J., Gheorghiade, M., Ekundavo, O. J., & Pitt, B. (2007). A propensity matched study of the association of low serum potassium levels and mortality in chronic heart failure. *European Heart Journal, 28*(11), 334–343.

21. Rose & Post, note 2, p. 461.

22. Cooper et al., note 12, p. 90.

23. Ring-Larsen, H., Henriksen, J. H., Wilken, C., Clausen, J., Pals, H., & Christensen, N. J. (1986). Diuretic treatment in decompensated cirrhosis and congestive heart failure: Effect of posture. *British Medical Journal: Clinical Research Edition, 292,* 1351.

Chapter 4

Sodium Imbalances

SODIUM BALANCE

Sodium imbalances have multiple causes and are common occurrences in both acute and chronic care settings. They are among the most difficult imbalances to understand because of their intricate relationship with water balance and the variety of mechanisms that can disrupt sodium homeostasis. Before discussion of the types of sodium imbalances, it is helpful to briefly review some basic facts about sodium.

Distribution

More than 95% of the body's physiologically active sodium is found in the extracellular fluid (ECF); in contrast, the intracellular concentration of sodium is small. The sodium–potassium adenosine triphosphate (ATP) pump works to maintain this asymmetrical distribution of sodium. Sodium is, by far, the most plentiful electrolyte in the ECF, with a concentration ranging from 135 to 145 mEq/L.

Role in Water Distribution

The fact that sodium does not easily cross the cell wall membrane, in addition to being the dominant electrolyte in terms of quantity, accounts for its primary role in controlling water distribution as well as ECF volume. In general, a loss or gain of sodium is accompanied by a loss or gain of water.

Effect on Cells

Extracellular sodium concentration has a profound effect on body cells. A low serum sodium level (*hyponatremia*) results in a diluted ECF and allows water to be drawn into the cells. Conversely, a high serum sodium level (*hypernatremia*) results in a concentrated ECF and allows water to be pulled out of cells. (See **Figure 4-1**.)

Dietary Sodium

The typical American diet provides 4 to 5 g of sodium per day (approximately 10 to 12 g of sodium chloride); Chapter 3 describes dietary sources of sodium. Tables 3-2 and 3-3 list the sodium content in selected beverages and foods. The amount of sodium provided in commonly used IV fluids is described in **Table 4-1**.

A healthy person can maintain sodium balance over a wide range of intake because the normal kidney can conserve or excrete sodium as needed. A sodium intake of 1.5 g per day is probably adequate for healthy individuals who are not losing sodium through extensive exercise and sweating.[1]

HYPONATREMIA

Definition

Hyponatremia is probably the most frequent electrolyte disorder in hospitalized patients. It refers to a serum sodium level that is below normal (135 mEq/L).[2] A low serum concentration does not necessarily mean that the total body sodium is less than normal. Hyponatremia is a complex imbalance with many causes, most of which can be classified as involving either excessive water gain (dilutional hyponatremia) or excessive sodium loss (depletional hyponatremia).

| Hypernatremia | Hyponatremia |

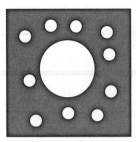 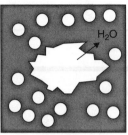 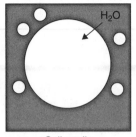

Normal cell size; Normal serum Na concentration | Cell shrinks as H$_2$O is pulled out of cell | Cell swells as H$_2$O is pulled into cell

Figure 4-1 Effect of serum sodium level on cells

Table 4-1 Approximate Sodium Content of Selected Parenteral Fluids

Parenteral Fluid	Sodium (mEq/L)
0.9% NaCl ("isotonic saline")	154
0.45% NaCl (half-strength saline)	77
0.33% NaCl	56
0.22% NaCl	38
0.11% NaCl	19
3% NaCl	513
5% NaCl	855
Lactated Ringer's solution	130

Incidence

Approximately 2.5% of hospitalized patients have hyponatremia; the incidence is much higher (15%) in critical care settings.[3, 4] The mortality rate in hospitalized patients with hyponatremia is approximately 30% to 40%, reflecting the severity of the underlying disease process (not the hyponatremia itself).[5]

Pathophysiology

Acute hyponatremia is arbitrarily defined as having developed in less than 48 hours, whereas *chronic hyponatremia* is defined as being present for greater than 48 hours. Hyponatremia may occur as a result of any of the following conditions:

- Loss of sodium, as through the kidney, gastrointestinal (GI) tract, or skin.
- Gain of water, as in high antidiuretic hormone (ADH) secretion and excessive water intake.
- Edematous states (such as severe heart failure, cirrhosis, and severe nephrotic syndrome).
- Shift of water from the cell to the ECF, as may occur in hyperglycemia. For example, the serum sodium concentration may fall by 1.5 to 2.4 mEq/L for each 100 mg/dL increase in glucose concentration above normal.[6, 7] In this situation, the plasma sodium concentration is diluted by water withdrawn from the cells.[8]

Hyponatremia can range from mild to severe. When severe, it is often a marker of serious underlying disease. In addition, severe hyponatremia can itself cause major neurological damage and death. As illustrated in **Figure 4-2**, hyponatremia can be superimposed on a normal fluid volume, a fluid volume deficit (FVD), or a fluid volume excess (FVE).

Cellular Swelling and Hyponatremic Encephalopathy

As noted in Figure 4-1, a decrease in the serum sodium concentration causes a shift of water from the ECF to the intracellular space, resulting in cellular edema. Unlike other tissues in the body, the brain's capacity to expand is limited by the barrier posed by the bony cranium. Increased intracranial pressure resulting from brain edema may lead to

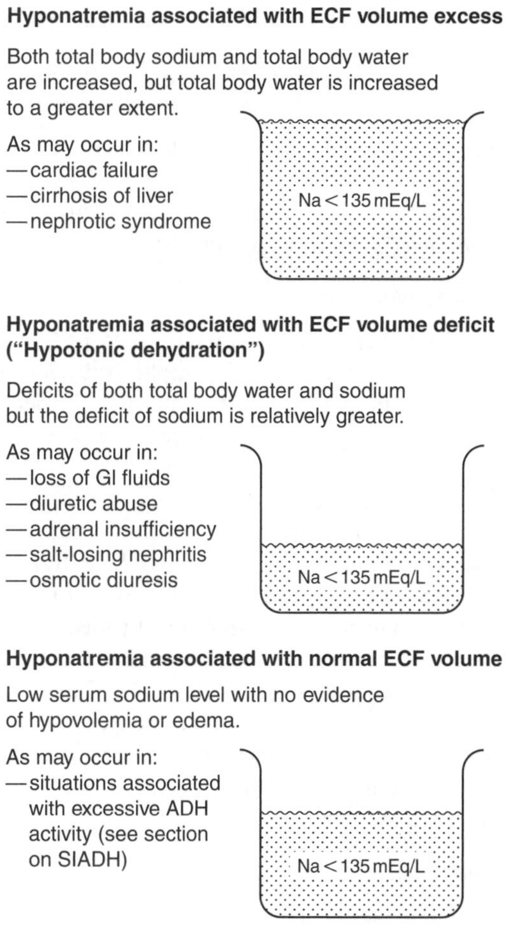

Hyponatremia associated with ECF volume excess

Both total body sodium and total body water are increased, but total body water is increased to a greater extent.

As may occur in:
—cardiac failure
—cirrhosis of liver
—nephrotic syndrome

Na < 135 mEq/L

Hyponatremia associated with ECF volume deficit ("Hypotonic dehydration")

Deficits of both total body water and sodium but the deficit of sodium is relatively greater.

As may occur in:
—loss of GI fluids
—diuretic abuse
—adrenal insufficiency
—salt-losing nephritis
—osmotic diuresis

Na < 135 mEq/L

Hyponatremia associated with normal ECF volume

Low serum sodium level with no evidence of hypovolemia or edema.

As may occur in:
—situations associated with excessive ADH activity (see section on SIADH)

Na < 135 mEq/L

Figure 4-2 (A) Hyponatremia associated with ECF volume excess; (B) Hyponatremia associated with ECF volume deficit; (C) Hyponatremia associated with normal ECF volume

herniation and death or irreversible brain damage if brain adaptation fails. In this condition, which is called *hyponatremic encephalopathy*, cerebral edema compresses the respiratory center and causes hypoxemia. To prevent this catastrophic event, the brain responds to swelling by attempting to remove sodium from the cells via the Na-KPase system (in so doing, the osmotic pull of water into the cells can be reduced).[9]

The individuals most susceptible to death or permanent brain damage from hyponatremia are prepubescent children and menstruant-age women, primarily because they lack adequate adaptive mechanisms to deal with brain swelling.[10]

In children, discrepancy between skull size and brain size is an important factor in the genesis of brain damage. In adults, estrogen has been shown to impair brain adaptation, decreasing both cerebral blood flow and oxygen utilization.

Causes of Hyponatremia

Causes of hyponatremia are listed in **Table 4-2** and are briefly described here.

Gastrointestinal Fluid Losses

Gastric fluid loss by vomiting or gastric suction can predispose an individual to hyponatremia by the direct loss of sodium. As a rule, hyponatremia from gastric fluid loss is not severe unless there is a concurrent excess intake of water. Vomiting is associated with increased production of ADH and, therefore, predisposes the person to water retention; however, this effect is generally not significant if the patient does not receive a large quantity of water (either by mouth of intravenously). A case was reported in which a young, previously healthy woman with severe vomiting and diarrhea associated with gastroenteritis drank copious amounts of water, causing her serum sodium concentration to drop to 106 mEq/L; this unfortunate scenario led to her death.[11] In the hospital setting, the erroneous administration of excessive electrolyte-free solutions (such as 5% dextrose in water) can seriously dilute the serum sodium concentration.

Loss of intestinal fluid by diarrhea can result in an isotonic FVD (an equal loss of water and sodium, resulting in decreased fluid volume but a normal serum sodium concentration). At times, sodium loss in diarrhea can exceed water loss, resulting in hyponatremia. At other times, water loss through diarrhea can exceed sodium loss, leading to hypernatremia.

Excessive Release of Antidiuretic Hormone

Syndrome of inappropriate antidiuretic hormone secretion (SIADH) produces a special kind of hyponatremia that is associated with excessive water retention. In conditions producing SIADH, either too much ADH is released or the individual exhibits an intensified renal response to the hormone. Release of ADH is termed *inappropriate* because in normal situations a low serum sodium level would suppress ADH activity. Many of the causes of hyponatremia listed in the remainder of this section are related to SIADH.

Table 4-2 Summary of Causes Hyponatremia

Loss of Sodium
- Use of diuretics
- Loss of GI fluids
- Adrenal insufficiency
- Osmotic diuresis
- Salt-losing nephritis

Gains of Water
- Excessive intravenous administration of D_5W or other hypotonic fluids
- Psychogenic polydipsia
- Excessive water administration with isotonic of hypotonic tube feedings
- Excessive water intake during heavy exercise (exercise-associated hyponatremia)

Disease States or Conditions Associated with SIADH
- Oat-cell carcinoma of lung
- Carcinoma of the duodenum or pancreas
- Head trauma
- Stroke
- Pulmonary disorders (tuberculosis, pneumonia, asthma, respiratory failure)
- Early postoperative period when ADH levels are elevated above normal

Drugs Associated with Hyponatremia
- Thiazide diuretics
- Tricyclic antidepressants
- SSRIs (e.g., citalopram, escitalopram, fluoxetine, paroxetine, sertraline)
- Antineoplastic agents (e.g., cyclopramide, vincristine, cisplatin)
- Carbamazepine
- Oxytocin
- Desmopressin acetate (DDAVP)
- Chlorpropamide
- Ecstasy (3,4-methylenedioxymethnylamphetamine)

GI = gastrointestinal; SIADH = syndrome of inappropriate antidiuretic hormone secretion; ADH = antidiuretic hormone; SSRI = selective serotonin reuptake inhibitors.

Adrenal Insufficiency

Hyponatremia is a common complication of adrenal insufficiency and is due to the effect of aldosterone deficiency. Recall that a reduced aldosterone level causes increased renal loss of sodium.

Sweating

Sweat is a hypotonic fluid with a sodium concentration of about 30 to 65 mEq/L.[12] Although sweat production is low in the basal state, it may occur at a rate as high as 1500 mL/hr in subjects exercising in a dry, hot climate.[13]

Salt-Losing Nephritis

A variety of kidney diseases can result in renal salt wasting. Among these are chronic interstitial nephropathy, medullary cystic disease, and polycystic kidney disease. The degree of renal sodium wasting can range from mild to severe.

Diuretics

Diuretic-induced severe hyponatremia is primarily a complication of thiazide-type drugs (not loop diuretics).[14] Thiazide-induced hyponatremia is more common in women than in men.[15, 16] In a study of 64 patients admitted to hospitals for treatment of hyponatremia, thiazides were either the only cause or a major contributing factor in more than half of the cases.[17] In yet another study, thiazides were found to be responsible for 94% of the 129 cases of diuretic-induced severe hyponatremia reported in the literature between 1962 and 1990.[18]

Antidepressants

Hyponatremia may be induced by antidepressants (such as tricyclic antidepressants and selective serotonin reuptake inhibitors [SSRIs]). Use of these agents should be considered as a possible cause of hyponatremia in patients of all ages, although the risk appears to be greater in the elderly. As many as 12% of older adults taking SSRIs may present with clinical symptoms.[19] In a study reported by Bouman et al., 4 of 32 elderly patients taking SSRIs developed symptomatic hyponatremia due to SIADH.[20] Examples of SSRIs include citalopram (Celexa), escitalopram (Lexapro), fluoxetine (Prozac), fluvoxamine (Luvox), paroxetine (Paxil), and sertraline (Zoloft).[21]

Risk factors for antidepressant-induced hyponatremia include low body weight, old age, female sex, use of other medications that can cause hyponatremia (such as diuretics), and a previous history of hyponatremia.[22] Hyponatremia associated with antidepressant use usually occurs within the first few weeks of treatment.[23] Because symptoms of hyponatremia can mimic depression or psychosis, it is important for providers to be aware of the potential for this imbalance and to periodically monitor patients' serum electrolytes. Some authors recommend checking serum sodium levels in older adults at least once during the first month of use of antidepressants.[24] If hyponatremia is found, the medication should be discontinued until the imbalance is corrected.[25]

Antineoplastic Agents

Cyclophosphamide (Cytoxan) is an antineoplastic alkylating agent that can increase renal sensitivity to ADH and perhaps stimulate its release when given IV in high doses. Given that a high fluid intake is generally prescribed to lessen the possibility of hemorrhagic cystitis associated with cyclophosphamide, severe hyponatremia can result from this combination. Use of isotonic saline rather than water to maintain a high urine output can minimize the risk of this complication.[26]

Vincristine is another antineoplastic drug that can cause hyponatremia, apparently by exerting a neurotoxic effect on the hypothalamus, leading to an increased release of ADH. A recent retrospective study of a pharmaceutical company's global safety database found the reported rate of SIADH with vincristine was very low (1.3 cases per 100,000 patients).[27] The data suggested that Asian patients may be at increased risk for hyponatremia associated with vincristine use.

Cisplatin is a widely used agent in cancer treatment and can lead to hyponatremia in 4% to 10% of cases due to salt wasting.[28] Most of these cases are attributable to the sodium-losing nephropathy of SIADH.[29]

Carbamazepine

Carbamazepine, which is prescribed as an anticonvulsant, is a well-established cause of ADH release (which, of course, favors water retention). Hyponatremia associated with carbamazepine use is particularly common in psychiatric patients with polydipsia. As many as 20% of patients receiving carbamazepine may develop a serum sodium concentration of less than 135 mEq/L.[30] Several factors have been reported to increase the risk of hyponatremia associated with carbamazepine use: age greater than 40 years, concurrent use of medications associated with hyponatremia, psychiatric condition, psychogenic polydipsia, and female gender.[31] Overall, hyponatremia is a prevalent and potentially dangerous problem in patients with psychiatric conditions.

Nonsteroidal Anti-inflammatory Drugs

The nonsteroidal anti-inflammatory drugs (NSAIDs) decrease renal water excretion because decreased synthesis of prostaglandins potentiates the action of ADH on the kidney. Despite this effect, hyponatremia due solely to these agents is rare.[32] Instead, NSAIDS tend to exacerbate the tendency toward hyponatremia in patients with other risk factors for hyponatremia.

Oxytocin in Pregnancy

Oxytocin, like vasopressin (ADH), is synthesized in the hypothalamus and released by the pituitary gland. Although its primary effects relate to uterine function and milk production, this hormone also possesses significant antidiuretic activity. Administration of oxytocin to induce labor, therefore, can cause hyponatremia if improperly used. The intravenous administration of oxytocin in dextrose and water to stimulate labor has resulted in water retention, severe hyponatremia, and seizures in both the mother and the fetus.[33] The relationship between oxytocin and hyponatremia is discussed in Chapter 23.

Desmopressin Acetate to Treat Nocturnal Enuresis

Children. Intranasal desmopressin acetate (DDAVP) has been used extensively to treat nocturnal enuresis ("bedwetting"), a condition that affects millions of children in the United States. This drug causes decreased urine formation and thus presumably reduces urination (and the potential for enuresis). Although the medication has proved safe and effective for many who are affected by enuresis, it has the potential to cause serious hyponatremia.[34] As such, it is important to follow basic rules when DDAVP is used, such as prescribing the smallest effective dose and limiting fluid intake prior to bedtime.

A report of five enuretic children on desmopressin who suffered from hyponatremic encephalopathy demonstrates the need for appropriate water restriction when this agent is prescribed.[35] Despite the appearance of warning symptoms of hyponatremia (including headache and vomiting), the children continued to drink too much fluid, and medical attention was not sought early. These five case reports emphasize the need to educate parents about fluid restriction and symptoms of dilutional hyponatremia. Some question the use of DDAVP to treat enuresis in children, particularly because the condition usually resolves spontaneously with age.[36]

Adults. The problem of DDAVP-associated hyponatremia during the treatment of nocturnal enuresis is not limited to children. For example, a 29-year-old woman with a long history of nocturnal enuresis developed severe symptomatic hyponatremia shortly after beginning intranasal DDAVP use.[37] Monitoring electrolytes periodically may help prevent hyponatremia and its potentially serious sequelae. It is recommended that DDAVP medication be used no longer than 3 months without stopping for 1 week for full reassessment.[38] DDAVP therapy should be temporarily interrupted during acute illness, febrile episodes, and conditions associated with increased water intake.[39]

It is very important to educate patients and their families about how DDAVP works and how they can minimize the possibility of adverse events. Extreme caution is needed in patients with cognitive impairment who cannot control their fluid intake themselves.[40] Fluid intake should be limited 1 hour before and 8 hours after the dose.[41] Hyponatremia related to DDAVP use has also been reported in elderly patients.[42, 43]

Ecstasy (MDMA)

Use of 3,4-methylenedioxymethnylamphetamine (MDMA) —the "club drug" called "Ecstasy"—can enhance the release of ADH from the hypothalamus and cause hyponatremia, which can in turn cause severe neurological symptoms.[44] It appears that young, menstruant-age women are at particularly high risk for the development of severe, symptomatic hyponatremia after using Ecstasy.[45] Hyponatremia-related death from MDMA is due to a "perfect storm" of increased secretion of ADH, polydipsia, and recommendations to drink copiously at parties where Ecstasy is used.[46]

Postoperative Hyponatremia

In a study of 1088 postoperative patients, Chung et al. reported a 4.4% incidence of hyponatremia (serum Na < 130 mEq/L) within 1 week after surgery.[47] Predisposing factors included a temporary increase in vasopressin (ADH) release after anesthesia and the stress of surgery. Pain enhances the release of vasopressin by direct stimulation of the hypothalamus. Nausea, which is frequently present in postoperative patients, can increase vasopressin release by as much as 1000-fold; the nausea does not have to be associated with vomiting. Because of the tendency for hyponatremia in newly postoperative patients, the administration of electrolyte-free solutions during the first 2 to 4 postoperative days should be avoided. In fact, because elevated plasma levels of vasopressin are a nearly universal occurrence in the first few postoperative days, some authors state that it may be important to avoid the use of any hypotonic IV solution in the immediate postoperative period.[48]

Increased Risk in Menstruant-Age Women Undergoing Surgical Procedures. Deaths have occurred in young women who underwent relatively simple surgical procedures (such as hysterectomy or cholecystectomy) and then received excessive volumes of hypotonic fluids postoperatively. Postoperative hyponatremia is a more serious problem in menstruant-age women than in postmenopausal women or men. One report indicated that although women and men are equally likely to develop hyponatremia and hyponatremic encephalopathy after surgery, menstruant-age women are approximately 25 times more likely to die or have permanent brain damage (compared with either men or postmenopausal women) if this condition develops.[49]

The significantly higher mortality from postoperative hyponatremia in menstruant-age women may be due, at least in part, to physical factors (such as estrogen) that affect the ability of the brain to adapt to hyponatremia. In a study of 40 young women with hyponatremic encephalopathy, all experienced nausea and vomiting, 34 had headache, and some had other symptoms, including weakness, slurred speech, lethargy, confusion, disorientation, bizarre behavior, urinary incontinence, dyspnea, and decorticate posturing.[50] Of the 40 women, 36 sustained an abrupt respiratory arrest postoperatively; at the time of respiratory arrest, the mean plasma sodium level was 113 mEq/L (range, 91–128 mEq/L). Although early symptoms are somewhat nonspecific, the diagnosis can be easily established by measuring the plasma sodium level with virtually no risk to the patient and at minimal cost.[51]

Direct absorption of hypotonic irrigating fluid through the veins during endometrial ablation or transurethral prostatectomy can cause serous hyponatremia. See Chapter 14 for a more extensive discussion of these procedures.

Central Nervous System Disorders

Among the central nervous system (CNS) conditions that may be associated with hyponatremia are head trauma, neoplasms, and infectious disorders. Sometimes the hyponatremia is due to SIADH; at other times it may be due to cerebral salt wasting (CSW) discussed in detail in Chapter 19).

Malignant Tumors and SIADH

An oat-cell carcinoma of the lung can cause SIADH. Other malignancies associated with this syndrome include carcinomas of the duodenum and pancreas, Hodgkin's disease, leukemia, and lymphoma. In some instances, malignant cells from patients with SIADH have been shown to synthesize and release a substance similar to native ADH ("ectopic ADH production"). Chapter 22 discusses SIADH in oncology patients in more detail.

Compulsive Water Drinking

Primary polydipsia is often present in psychiatric illness and with the prescription of antipsychotic medications that cause a dry mouth.[52] This excessive water intake can occasionally cause severe symptomatic hyponatremia, a syndrome also referred to as "compulsive water drinking" or "self-induced water intoxication." The syndrome of psychosis, intermittent hyponatremia, and polydipsia is a potentially life-threatening problem. Primary polydipsia affects as many as 7% of patients with schizophrenia.[53] Dilutional hyponatremia is thought to occur when the rapid ingestion of voluminous quantities of water exceeds the excretory capacity of normally functioning kidneys. Patients who smoke may be more likely to be symptomatic because nicotine contributes to transient release of vasopressin. A study of a group of psychiatric patients with hyponatremia found that heavy smoking was a contributing factor to development of this condition.[54]

Pulmonary Disorders Associated with SIADH

Pulmonary disorders associated with hyponatremia include pneumonia, acute asthma, tuberculosis, acute respiratory failure, pneumothorax, and empyema. The causes are not entirely clear, although increased production of antidiuretic hormone has been suggested. For example, mechanical ventilation, especially when combined with positive expiratory pressure, stimulates ADH release by impeding venous return, thereby decreasing cardiac output. Acute hypoxia and hypercapnia also stimulate ADH secretion.[55] Bioassays from tuberculous lung tissue have demonstrated ADH activity.

Acquired Immunodeficiency Syndrome

Hyponatremia is very common in patients with acquired immunodeficiency syndrome (AIDS).[56] For example, Vitting et al. reported that 56% of the patients with AIDS followed prospectively in their study were hyponatremic (mean serum sodium level, 125 ± 4 mEq/L).[57] In another study, Agarwal et al. found that about 35% of 103 patients with AIDS admitted for opportunistic infections had serum sodium levels lower than or equal to 130 mEq/L.[58] In a study of 86 children infected with human immunodeficiency virus-1 (HIV-1), the incidence of hyponatremia was approximately 25%.[59] Conditions that may play a role in hyponatremia in this setting include *Pneumocystis carinii*

pneumonia, malignancies, and CNS disease.[60] Hyponatremic states are also aggravated by the excessive use of hypotonic fluids.

Endurance Exercise Hyponatremia

Hyponatremia can occur after endurance exercise (such as in marathons and triathlon events).[61] In fact, as many as 10% of ultradistance athletes experience serum sodium levels less than 135 mEq/L; however, symptoms usually do not appear until this level is less than 125 mEq/L.[62] Most often exercise-induced hyponatremia is due to excess free water intake, which fails to replace sodium losses incurred from sweating.[63] Some authorities recommend that marathon organizers provide a mechanism whereby medical personnel can measure serum sodium concentrations on site and be able to administer a 100 mL bolus of 3% sodium chloride when appropriate prior to transferring the symptomatic athlete to an acute care facility.[64]

Clinical Signs of Hyponatremia

Clinical signs of hyponatremia vary, but generally depend on the following factors:

- Magnitude of the serum sodium decrease. In general, the lower the serum sodium level, the more likely symptoms are to be severe (**Table 4-3**).
- *Speed of development (acute versus chronic).* The neurologic symptoms of acute hyponatremia are likely due to cerebral edema, secondary to the entry of water into brain cells.[65] In contrast, patients with chronic hyponatremia have time for cerebral adaptation to occur, resulting in return of brain volume toward normal and abatement of neurological symptoms.[66] Two patients having similar low serum sodium values may exhibit vastly different symptoms if hyponatremia developed slowly in one and quickly in the other. In acute hyponatremia, symptoms develop at a higher rate than they do when hyponatremia is chronic.
- *Cause of hyponatremia (gain of water or loss of sodium).* Acute water overloading is more likely to cause severe symptoms than is the chronic loss of sodium.
- *Age and gender differences.* Menstruant-age women seem to be at substantially greater risk for irreversible brain damage than are men or postmenopausal women.[67] Sex hormones may be responsible for this difference, because no gender difference is noted in terms of the risk of symptomatic hyponatremia in prepubertal children.[68] Young women account for most

Table 4-3 Summary of Facts Regarding Clinical Manifestations of Hyponatremia

Clinical Manifestations of Hyponatremia
- Nausea and vomiting
- Abdominal cramping
- Lethargy
- Headache
- Seizures
- Respiratory arrest
- Coma

Severity of Symptoms
- Hyponatremia due to water overload ("dilutional hyponatremia") is generally associated with more severe symptoms than is hyponatremia due to sodium loss.
- Rapidly developing hyponatremia is more likely to be associated with severe symptoms than is slowly developing hyponatremia.
- Patients are usually asymptomatic when the serum sodium concentration is greater than 125 mEq/L (although occasional patients may be symptomatic at higher levels).
- Women of child-bearing age are especially susceptible to adverse effects of hyponatremia (presumably because of the effect of female hormones on the ability of the brain to adapt to osmotic changes). Respiratory arrest has occurred in young women with serum sodium levels of 125 mEq/L or greater after acute water overloading in the early postoperative period.

Volume Status
- Hyponatremia due to water overload increases body weight but does not cause appreciable edema because approximately two-thirds of the retained water is located inside the cells.
- Hyponatremia due to sodium loss is generally associated with ECF volume depletion and symptoms of weakness and postural dizziness.

Laboratory Data
- Hyponatremia due to sodium loss from a non-renal route (such as the GI tract) is associated with a low urinary sodium level (e.g., less than 15 mEq/L), indicating renal conservation of needed sodium.
- Hyponatremia due to SIADH is generally associated with a urinary sodium level greater than 20 mEq/L.

ECF = extracellular fluid; SIADH = syndrome of inappropriate antidiuretic hormone secretion.

of the reported cases of fatalities secondary to hyponatremia, presumably because their brains are less able to adapt to the effects of hyponatremia than are those of men or postmenopausal women.

- *Early versus late symptoms.* Early manifestations of hyponatremia include those involving the gastrointestinal system, such as nausea and abdominal cramps. However, most of the major manifestations of clinical hyponatremia are of a neurologic nature and are related to brain cellular swelling. In general, patients with acute decreases in serum sodium levels have a higher mortality rate than do those with more slowly developing hyponatremia. Brain edema associated with hyponatremia can lead to devastating clinical entities, such as pulmonary edema, central diabetes insipidus, cerebral infarction, cortical blindness, persistent vegetative state, respiratory arrest, and coma.

Treatment of Hyponatremia

Basic principles to consider in the treatment of hyponatremia are (1) raising the plasma sodium concentration at a safe rate and (2) treating the underlying cause. Major considerations include the cause of the hyponatremia and the severity of the imbalance.

Sodium Replacement if Hyponatremia Is Due to Sodium Loss

Sodium can be replaced orally if the patient is able to consume sodium-rich fluids and foods. More commonly, in acutely ill patients, sodium is replaced in the form of sodium-containing intravenous fluids, such as isotonic saline (0.9% sodium chloride) or lactated Ringer's solution.

Water Restriction if Chronic Hyponatremia Is Due to Water Overload

In normovolemic patients with chronic asymptomatic hyponatremia, water restriction is generally recommended. Water restriction to less than 1000 to 1500 mL/day is usually successful in reversing hyponatremia between 125 and 135 mEq/L in patients who are water overloaded and asymptomatic.[69] Of course, this approach includes restricting *all* fluids (not just electrolyte-free water).[70]

Hypertonic Saline and Furosemide if Hyponatremia Causes Neurologic Symptoms

The most potent combination therapy for treating symptomatic hyponatremia is the cautious administration of a small volume of hypertonic saline (often 3% NaCl) and a loop diuretic (usually furosemide).[71] (See Table 4-1 for the sodium content of some parenteral fluids.). Furosemide given in conjunction with hypertonic saline induces a loss of sodium and water while the hypertonic saline solution replaces sodium, resulting in a net gain of body sodium. The recommended speed and method of treatment of hyponatremia depend on the magnitude of symptoms, their duration, and the status of the ECF volume (**Table 4-4**).

Complication of Too-Rapid Correction of Hyponatremia: Central Pontine Myelinolysis

The goal of therapy in symptomatic hyponatremia is to reduce brain water and increase the plasma sodium level only to the point necessary to maintain normal respiration and keep the patient alert and free of seizures and, at the same time, prevent central pontine myelinolysis (CPM). CPM is a condition thought to result from shrinkage of neurons away from their myelin sheaths, due to water shifts associated with rapid correction of hyponatremia. The greatest risk for CPM occurs when the hyponatremia is corrected by more than 12 mEq/L in a 24-hour period.[76] Actually, the total amount of correction during a 24-hour period appears to be more important than the rate of correction; that is, an initial rapid rate of correction that is tapered off after several hours for a total rise of less than 12 mEq/L over 24 hours may carry less risk than does a steady rate of decline that exceeds 12 mEq/L in a 24-hour period.[77]

Relatively rapid correction is indicated in patients with symptomatic hyponatremia who are experiencing seizures or other acute neurological symptoms.[78, 79] In this setting, the plasma sodium may be raised at an initial rate of 1.5 to 2.0 mEq/L/hr hour for the first 3 to 4 hours because the risk of persistent severe hyponatremia is greater than the possible danger of CPM from too-rapid correction.[80, 81] Even then, however, the total increase probably should not exceed 10 to 12 mEq/L over the first 24 hours.[82] Some authors prefer an

---

Table 4-4 Considerations in Administering Hypertonic Saline Solutions (3% and 5% NaCl)

- Hypertonic saline should be administered to patients only in intensive care settings where close monitoring of response to the fluid can be observed.
- A volumetric pump is needed to provide the precise desired flow rate. Even then, it is important to recognize that pumps may fail; thus the volume of fluid remaining in the infusion bag should be monitored.
- Frequent monitoring of plasma sodium concentrations is needed to determine if the desired rate of sodium correction is being achieved.
- During the administration of hypertonic saline, it is important to monitor for fluid volume overload, especially in patients with underlying cardiopulmonary problems.
- It is important to monitor neurological signs; worsening of these signs could signal the appearance of central pontine myelinolysis (CPM). The greatest risk for CPM occurs when the hyponatremia is corrected by more than 12 mEq/L in a 24-hour period.[72]
- The desired rate of plasma sodium elevation depends on how long the hyponatremia has been present; generally, the rate of correction is faster when hyponatremia is acute (present less than 48 hours) than when it is chronic (present for more than 48 hours). Although there is not firm agreement on precise amounts, the following recommendations are reasonable:
  ○ In acute hyponatremia, the plasma sodium may be raised at an initial rate of 1.5–2.0 mEq/L/hr for the first 3–4 hours because the risk of persistent severe hyponatremia is greater than the possible danger of CPM from too rapid correction.[73]
  ○ Even then, the total increase probably should not be greater than 10–12 mEq/L over the first 24 hours.[74]
  ○ In chronic hyponatremia, sodium replacement can be achieved more slowly, such as a gradual correction of less than 10 mEq/L in 24 hours.[75]

increase of no more than 10 mEq/L over the first 24 hours (to allow a margin of error from the 12 mEq/L thought to be the maximal allowed amount of elevation) and an increase of less than 18 mEq/L over the first 48 hours.[83] The patients at highest risk for developing CPM are those with preexisting hypokalemia, malnutrition, alcoholism, female gender, and advanced age.[84, 85] Symptoms of CPM include dysarthria, dysphagia, behavioral disturbances, ataxia, quadriplegia, and coma.[86]

The rate of sodium level correction is slower in asymptomatic hyponatremia patients. For example, the plasma sodium concentration in these individuals should be raised at a maximal rate of less than 0.5 mEq/L/hr (and, more importantly, should be less than 10 mEq/L in the first day and less than 18 mEq/L over the first two days).[87] Other authors recommend that chronic hyponatremia be corrected no faster than 8 mEq/L in the first 24 hours.[88] Patients with liver disease and hypokalemia may require an even slower rate of correction (closer to 6 mEq/L per day) because of their increased risk for developing CPM.[89] Active correction of hyponatremia is stopped when the patient's symptoms are abolished, or the total magnitude of the correction has been achieved.[90]

Arginine Vasopressin Receptor Antagonists

When a patient has dilutional hyponatremia due to excessive ADH activity (as in congestive heart failure), drugs known as arginine vasopressin (AVP) receptor antagonists may be prescribed. The AVP receptor antagonists—conivaptan, tolvaptan, lixivaptan, and satavaptan—are a relatively new class of agents that have been shown to normalize serum concentration by causing water diuresis.[91] Studies have indicated that these agents can be advantageous in treating SIADH, heart failure, and liver failure.[92] Hyponatremia is a frequent complication of advanced cirrhosis and is associated with increased morbidity and mortality; further, it represents a risk factor for complications after liver transplant.[93] While short-term treatment with an AVP receptor antagonist can produce a marked increase in free water excretion and subsequent improvement in hyponatremia, the long-term efficacy of these drugs in improving serum sodium concentration remains under investigation.[94] Chapter 16 discusses how vasopressin receptor antagonists are used to treat heart failure and Chapter 21 describes their use in treating cirrhosis.

Clinical Considerations for Hyponatremia

1. Identify patients at risk for hyponatremia. As noted in Table 4-2, many common conditions can lower the serum sodium concentration.

2. Being aware of patients at risk for hyponatremia is crucial to monitoring for the occurrence of subtle early changes associated with this imbalance. A profound hyponatremia can be fatal if not detected early and treated appropriately.

3. Review medications that the patient is taking, noting those that predispose him or her to hyponatremia (see Table 4-2).

4. Monitor fluid losses and gains for all patients at risk for hyponatremia. Look for loss of sodium-containing fluids (such as GI secretions or sweat), particularly in conjunction with a low-sodium diet or excessive water intake either orally or IV.

5. Monitor daily weights, noting acute weight gains (reflecting excessive fluid retention).

6. Monitor laboratory data, looking for serum sodium levels lower than normal.

7. Monitor for presence of GI symptoms, such as anorexia, nausea, vomiting, and abdominal cramping, as they may be early signs of hyponatremia. These symptoms must be evaluated in relation to other findings, such as fluid gains and losses, amount of sodium intake, and laboratory data.

8. Monitor for CNS changes, such as lethargy, confusion, muscular twitching, convulsions, and coma. Be aware that more severe neurological signs are associated with very low sodium levels that have fallen rapidly due to water overloading.

9. For patients who are able to consume a normal diet, encourage foods and fluids with a high sodium content. See Tables 3-2 and 3-3 for examples of beverages and foods high in sodium content. For example, a cup of beef broth/bouillon contains approximately 636 mg of sodium and a cup of canned tomato juice contains approximately 654 mg of sodium (each equivalent to roughly 28 mEq of sodium).

10. When administering sodium-containing IV fluids to patients with cardiovascular disease, monitor them especially closely for signs of circulatory overload, including moist rales in the lungs. The greater the sodium concentration, the greater the risk.

11. Avoid giving large water supplements to patients who are receiving isotonic tube feedings, particularly if routes of abnormal sodium loss are present or if water is being retained abnormally (as in SIADH); see Chapter 12.

12. Be aware of the clinical signs of SIADH and know how to monitor for this condition. See **Tables 4-5** and **4-6**.

13. Use extreme caution when administering hypertonic saline solutions (3% or 5% NaCl). Be aware that these fluids can be lethal if infused carelessly. See Table 4-4.

HYPONATREMIA CASE STUDIES

Case Study 4-1

A 50-year-old man was started on hydrochlorothiazide and a low-sodium diet for the treatment of hypertension. After 2 weeks, he began to complain of weakness, abdominal cramping, leg cramps, and postural dizziness. On examination, he was found to have decreased skin turgor and flat neck veins in the supine position. Laboratory data included Na 118 mEq/L, K 2.2 mEq/L, Cl 66 mEq/L, and plasma osmolality 240 mOsm/kg.

Commentary. This patient was obviously hyponatremic, as indicated by the low plasma sodium level and osmolality. In this instance, the hyponatremia was accompanied by decreased skin turgor and flat neck veins. In addition, the plasma potassium and chloride levels were quite low. Thiazide diuretics promote both sodium and potassium excretion and predispose patients to hypochloremic alkalosis (metabolic alkalosis). Sodium loss, coupled with a low sodium intake, caused the hyponatremia in this case.

Case Study 4-2

A 58-year-old man with a history of inoperable oat-cell carcinoma of the lung was admitted to the hospital; according to his family, he had a 2-week history of progressive lethargy. Laboratory data included plasma Na 105 mEq/L, urinary Na 76 mEq/L, Cl 72 mEq/L, and urinary osmolality 800 mOsm/kg.

Commentary. The history of an oat-cell lung tumor strongly suggests the presence of ectopic ADH production. Lethargy is a prominent symptom of hyponatremia due to water excess. Laboratory data revealed an extremely low plasma sodium level. In contrast, note the relatively high urinary sodium level, indicating the kidneys' inability to retain sodium even though severe hyponatremia is present.

Case Study 4-3

Following an automobile accident, a 30-year-old woman was admitted to the emergency department of a small suburban hospital. She had sustained facial fractures and a possible head injury (evidenced by temporary loss of consciousness at

Table 4-5 Summary of Clinical Manifestations of SIADH

Water Retention

- Intake of fluid greatly exceeds urinary output (as evidenced by I & O records)
- Acute weight gain (reflecting water retention)
- No significant peripheral edema (because water is primarily retained inside the cells, not in the interstitial space)
- Signs of cerebral edema (see neurological symptoms below)

Gastrointestinal Symptoms

- Anorexia
- Nausea
- Vomiting
- Abdominal cramps

Neurological Symptoms

- Lethargy
- Headache
- Pupillary changes
- Seizures
- Respiratory arrest

Laboratory Findings Reflecting Overhydration

- Below normal plasma sodium concentration
- Below normal plasma osmolality
- Below normal BUN

Urinary Signs

- Urinary sodium > 20 mEq/L (as opposed to that seen when hyponatremia is primarily due to sodium loss)
- Urinary specific gravity > 1.012
- Urine osmolality is usually higher than plasma osmolality (urine contains important amounts of sodium; also, plasma is diluted with water)

SIADH = syndrome of inappropriate antidiuretic hormone secretions; I & O = intake and output; BUN = blood urea nitrogen; SG = specific gravity.

the accident scene). During the first 3 days of her hospitalization, she received an average of 4 L of fluid daily (despite persistent low urinary output). The patient became increasingly lethargic and complained of headache and nausea. On the fourth day, she had a grand mal seizure and was noted to have papilledema and Babinski's sign. At that time, her serum sodium level was 110 mEq/L. Despite intensive treatment, she died within a week. On autopsy, her brain was found to be swollen, and she weighed 10 lb more than when admitted (despite almost no caloric intake during her hospitalization).

Table 4-6 Nursing Assessment for SIADH

Identify patients at risk (such as those with excessive production of ADH by tumor, those with temporary excessive release of ADH following surgery, or those receiving drugs that potentiate ADH activity (see Table 4-2).

Maintain accurate I & O records.
• Look for fluid intake greatly exceeding output; I & O should be totaled and the overall picture observed for several consecutive days.

Maintain daily body weight records.
• Look for a sudden weight gain (recall that 1 L of fluid weighs approximately 2.2 lb).
• Although there will be an acute weight gain, do not expect to detect significant peripheral edema because most of the excess fluid will be retained inside the cells (not in the interstitial space)

Monitor serum sodium concentrations.
• Recognize the effect of rapidity of onset, degree of decrease, and gender on the probability for adverse effects of hyponatremia.
• Be especially alert for a sharp decline in the serum sodium concentration over a short period of time.

Observe for gastrointestinal symptoms, which usually occur early.
• Be alert for anorexia, nausea, vomiting, and abdominal cramping.

Observe the neurological status carefully.
• Be particularly alert for lethargy and headache; these symptoms occur relatively early. Later neurological symptoms include seizures and coma.

ADH = antidiuretic hormone.

Commentary. Patients with head injuries (especially when facial injuries are also present) are at risk for SIADH and should be monitored closely for its development. Care should be taken to avoid fluid overloading in patients with head injuries (see Chapter 19). Note that this patient did not have any concurrent injuries that necessitated large fluid volume replacement. Her weight on autopsy was greater than her weight on admission because water was abnormally retained in cells throughout her body. No peripheral edema was present because the excess water was retained intracellularly, not in the interstitial space. This patient's death could have been prevented had her care-givers looked at the I & O record and paid attention to the obvious warning signs of SIADH. For example, despite a fluid intake of 4000 mL/day, she excreted less than 600 mL on most days. Nurses' notes made frequent mention of the presence of lethargy, nausea, abdominal cramping, and headache.

Case Study 4-4

A 23-year-old healthy woman (the mother of two children) underwent an elective vaginal hysterectomy. Postoperatively, this 110-lb woman received 5% dextrose in 0.45% NaCl at a rate of 175 mL/hr for approximately 20 hours, even though her urinary output was less than 500 mL each shift. No abnormal routes of fluid loss were present. On the evening after the surgery, she complained of nausea and headache. In the early morning of the first postoperative day, she was combative and disoriented. Two hours later, blood work revealed a serum sodium level of 126 mEq/L (no baseline sodium level was available because preoperative values were not obtained). Thirty minutes later, she was unresponsive to verbal stimuli; at this time, her serum sodium level was 122 mEq/L. Despite resuscitative efforts, she progressed on a downhill course and subsequently died several weeks later without regaining consciousness.

Commentary. Cerebral edema was apparent on autopsy. This patient suffered hyponatremic encephalopathy, resulting in respiratory arrest and her subsequent death. (See the discussion of postoperative hyponatremia in menstruant-age women in this chapter.) The cause of the hyponatremia was the excessive administration of hypotonic fluid during a period when her ability to excrete fluid was limited (due to the effects of increased ADH activity in the postoperative period). Recall that ADH activity is increased for the first 2 to 4 postoperative days due to the stress of surgery as well as the presence of pain and nausea. The I & O record for the day of surgery showed a disproportionately large fluid intake/output ratio for all three shifts.

Time (Shift)	IV Intake (mL)	Urine Output (mL)
7–3	2900	675
3–11	950	600
11–7	1150	500
Total	5000	1775

In fact, from the time of her return from surgery to the catastrophic neurological event, this patient received approximately 5 L of hypotonic fluid and excreted less than 2 L of urine. The excess hypotonic fluid caused her serum sodium level to drop quickly, accounting for the severe neurological symptoms despite a serum sodium level of more than 120 mEq/L. This patient's death could have been easily prevented by the administration of an isotonic fluid (or at least by avoiding the greatly excessive rate of the hypotonic electrolyte fluid). Had her symptoms been recognized earlier and the appropriate treatment instituted, this condition could likely have been safely reversed.

Case Study 4-5

An 88-year-old woman, who had started taking an antidepressant (escitalopram) two weeks earlier, developed confusion and weakness and had difficulty caring for herself.[95] When she was admitted to an acute care facility, her serum sodium concentration was found to be 124 mEq/L. The patient was placed on fluid restriction and treated with intravenous normal saline. Additional laboratory studies showed that she had SIADH. A decision was made to discontinue the antidepressant. Upon doing so, the patient's serum sodium level rose to the normal level over the next two days. In addition, her clinical status improved to baseline.

Commentary. Escitalopram (Lexapro) is a SSRI drug whose use can lead to hyponatremia, especially in elderly individuals. As this case demonstrates, simply discontinuing the drug is usually sufficient to allow the serum sodium level to return to normal. A review of the patient's history revealed that she was also taking a thiazide diuretic, another drug that can lead to hyponatremia. The combination of two sodium-lowering drugs intensified this patient's chance of developing hyponatremia.

Case Study 4-6

A case was reported in which a 50-year-old woman visited the emergency room with symptoms of nausea and fatigue.[96] She had drunk 4000 mL of water over a 3-hour period because she feared having a urinary tract infection. Her serum sodium concentration was 126 mEq/L and her plasma osmolality was low (248 mOsm/kg). Further, her circulating vasopressin level was inappropriately high. (The expected ADH level when serum osmolality is less than 290 mOsm/kg is less than 2 pg/mL.[97]) The patient was treated

with saline, and her serum sodium concentration returned to normal by the third day of hospitalization.

Commentary. This patient was diagnosed with water intoxication (dilutional hyponatremia) secondary to the large intake of fluid (4000 mL) over a short period of time (3 hours). It was speculated that the relatively high serum vasopressin level was due to nausea; nausea is a recognized cause of increased vasopressin release.[98] This patient may have been spared from more severe effects of hyponatremia because of her age (50 years). Recall that older (postmenopausal) women are less susceptible to adverse brain changes secondary to hyponatremia.

Case Study 4-7

A case was reported in which a 75-year-old woman was admitted to the ER with confusion and a history of hypertension and depression.[99] A CT scan of the head showed mild atrophy. At the time of admission, her serum sodium concentration was 133 mEq/L. Among the medications she was taking were amiodipine (antihypertensive), hydrochlorothiazide (diuretic), aplrazolam (antianxiety agent), and esomeprazole (proton pump inhibitor). On day 7 of her admission, she was prescribed escitalopram (Lexapro, a SSRI). Five days later, her serum sodium level had decreased to 116 mEq/L. Because escitalopram was considered to be causative of the hyponatremia, it was discontinued. The patient's serum sodium concentration slowly increased to 139 mEq/L over a period of 5 days.

Commentary. This case is an example of hyponatremia occurring in a patient receiving multiple drugs (escitalopram, hydrochlorothiazide, and esomeprazole) that can lower the serum sodium concentration. The fact that her serum sodium was below normal at the time of her admission should have raised a red flag about adding escitalopram to her medication regimen.

Case Study 4-8

A 28-year-old previously healthy mother of two children was admitted to the hospital for a "tummy tuck" and abdominal hysterectomy. Her body weight was 110 lb; no baseline electrolyte values were available prior to surgery. The intravenous fluid order following transfer from the recovery room to the general unit was 2000 mL of 5% dextrose in water. This volume of fluid was administered over a

5-hour period (5 P.M. to 10 P.M.) the evening of the operative day. At 8:30 P.M., the patient complained of nausea; at 10:15 P.M., she was found unresponsive and cyanotic. Shortly afterward, she was pronounced dead.

Commentary. The rapid administration of 2 L of sodium-free fluid, combined with the high ADH level associated with surgery, undoubtedly caused the patient to develop hyponatremia. Further, the hyponatremia developed very quickly (making matters worse than had it occurred over a period of days). These facts, coupled with the patient's gender and young age, predisposed her to hyponatremic encephalopathy. The lesson to be learned from this tragic case is that sodium-free fluid is contraindicated as a postoperative fluid, especially in young women. See Chapter 14 for a more detailed discussion of intravenous fluids in postoperative patients.

Case Study 4-9

A 25-year-old, 97-lb woman was admitted to an acute care facility for an open cholecystectomy. The serum sodium level on the day prior to surgery was 147 mEq/L (upper limit of normal for the reporting laboratory). The surgical procedure was well tolerated. Postoperative orders called for 5% dextrose in water with added KCl (20 mEq/L) at a rate of 125 mL/hr. The fluid order was implemented at 1 P.M. At 8:30 P.M., the evening nurse noticed that the patient had not voided, but did not have a distended bladder. The patient complained of nausea and was given hydroxyzine (Vistaril) 25 mg; at 1 A.M. the next day, the patient remained nauseated and the drug was administered again. By 6 A.M., the patient began vomiting; she was still unable to void but her bladder was not distended. The physician was notified and blood was collected for stat electrolytes. At 8 A.M., the patient complained of a severe headache and the nausea persisted. At 10 A.M., the laboratory reported that the serum sodium level was 123 mEq/L. At that time, the fluid order was changed from D5W to 0.9% sodium chloride at a rate of 125 mL/hr.

Later in the day, the patient was found unresponsive, with clear fluid flowing from her mouth. She became cyanotic and was transferred to an intensive care unit, where she was placed on life support. A CT scan showed diffuse cerebral edema with herniation (consistent with hyponatremic encephalopathy). The patient developed central diabetes insipidus over the next two days and was subsequently removed from life support at the request of the family.

Commentary. Upon review of the patient's I & O record from the end of surgery until the time of respiratory arrest, it was found that she received 3640 mL of fluid and excreted only 1255 mL (fluid gain of 2385 mL). In other words, her fluid intake was approximately 2.7 times greater than her fluid output. This red flag should have alerted the caregivers that something was wrong. Recall that ADH is greatly increased in the immediate postoperative period; thus the kidneys are unable to excrete a large fluid load. Making matters worse, the bulk of the fluid this patient received was sodium free (causing rapid dilution of her serum sodium concentration).

Note that this patient's serum sodium level dropped from a high normal level (147 mEq/L) on the day prior to surgery to 123 mEq/L on the first postoperative day. The rapidity of the development of hyponatremia is a major factor in determining how the body can react to the imbalance. Because the patient was female and of menstruant age, her brain had difficulty adjusting to the cerebral edema associated with her hyponatremia. This patient's tragic death could have been prevented had the proper postoperative fluid orders been implemented.

HYPERNATREMIA

Definition

Hypernatremia refers to a greater-than-normal serum sodium level (> 145 mEq/L). This condition occurs in as many as 2% of general hospital patients and in as many as 15% of critically ill patients.[100] It is also more common in institutionalized elderly patients.[101] In nonhospitalized patients, hypernatremia is primarily a condition seen in the elderly; however, hospital-acquired hypernatremia occurs in patients of all ages. In adults, a serum sodium concentration greater than 160 mEq/L is associated with a high mortality rate. Nevertheless, hypernatremia in adults usually occurs in the setting of serious disease and this high mortality likely reflects the seriousness of the underlying problem.[102] Arguing against this conclusion, other authors point out that hypernatremia alone carries significant morbidity.[103]

Pathophysiology

Hypernatremia is caused by water deficit or, less often, an excessive gain of sodium. This type of imbalance is especially prevalent among elderly individuals. Chapter 25 (Table 25-1) summarizes the differences between precipitating causes of simple FVD and hypernatremia associated with FVD in elderly individuals.

Normally, the body defends itself against the development of hypernatremia by both increasing the release of ADH and stimulating thirst through the osmoreceptors in the hypothalamus. Thus, when the serum sodium level begins to increase, the resultant retention of water and increased water intake lower the sodium concentration. Naturally, failure of these responses can lead to hypernatremia. Hypernatremia is almost never seen in an alert patient with a normal thirst mechanism and access to water. Because of blunted thirst perception in elderly persons, however, these individuals may fail to experience thirst during times of extensive fluid loss. (See Chapter 25.)

As noted in Figure 4-1, hypernatremia favors the shrinkage of cells as fluid is pulled out into the hypertonic ECF. It is this cellular dehydration in the brain that produces its contraction and is largely responsible for the neurological symptoms of hypernatremia. Contraction of the brain may, in turn, cause mechanical traction on delicate cerebral vessels and produce vascular trauma. For example, it can rupture bridging veins, thereby causing subdural, subarachnoid, or intra-parenchymal hemorrhage. This problem appears to be more prevalent in infants and small children.[104]

The cerebral shrinking caused by hypernatremia is transient, however. When hypernatremia is present for more than a few hours, brain cells begin to adapt to the extracellular hyperosmolality by raising the amount of intracellular solutes, thereby minimizing its water loss. With increased intracellular solute, water movement back into the brain is initiated and the brain volume moves toward normal. This adaptation accounts for the relative absence of symptoms in patients with slow-developing high serum sodium levels. Conversely, severe hypernatremia that develops over a period of less than 24 hours is often fatal.

Causes of Hypernatremia

Causes of hypernatremia are listed in **Table 4-7** and are briefly described in this section. In general, the etiology of hypernatremia is quite different in children and in adults. For example, in infants, the most common cause is watery diarrhea, whereas in the elderly population, it is infirmity with inability to obtain sufficient free-water intake.[105]

Water Deprivation

Hypernatremia may occur in any patient with a diminished mental status in whom the ability to perceive and respond to thirst is impaired.[106] In adults, hypernatremia is most often seen in patients who are 65 years of age or older. Not

Hypernatremia associated with a near normal ECF volume

Loss of water causes elevation of serum sodium level; does not lead to volume contraction unless water losses are massive.

As may occur in:
—increased insensible water loss (as in hyperventilation)

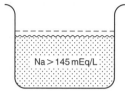

Hypernatremia associated with ECF volume deficit ("Hypertonic dehydration")

Losses of both sodium and water but relatively greater loss of water.

As may occur in:
—profuse sweating
—diarrhea, particularly in children
—aged individuals with poor water intake (recall that the aged kidney loses part of its ability to concentrate urine and thus cannot conserve water as it should)

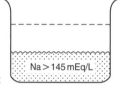

Hypernatremia associated with fluid volume excess

Gains of both sodium and water, but relatively greater gain of sodium.

As may occur:
—administration of hypertonic sodium solutions or substances (such as sodium bicarbonate in cardiac arrest)

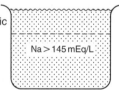

Figure 4-3 (A) Hypernatremia associated with a near normal ECF volume; (B) Hypernatremia associated with ECF volume deficit; (C) Hypernatremia associated with fluid volume excess

only are older persons at increased risk for illness and diminished mental status, but increasing age is also associated with decreased thirst and decreased ability of the kidneys to conserve water in times of need. Infants, because they are unable to ask for water, are also at increased risk.

Breastfeeding-Associated Hypernatremia

Hypernatremic dehydration requiring hospitalization is sometimes observed in breastfed neonates.[107] It may be

Table 4-7 Causes of Hypernatremia

- Deprivation of water, most commonly in unconscious or debilitated patients who are unable to perceive or respond to thirst (such as the elderly stroke patient)
- Deprivation of water in infants, very young children, or mentally impaired individuals who are unable to communicate their thirst
- Breastfed infants when maternal milk is high in sodium content or when inadequate lactation is present
- Hypertonic tube feedings without adequate water supplements (see Chapter 12)
- Greatly increased insensible water loss (as in hyperventilation or in extensive denuding effects of uncovered second- or third-degree burns)
- Watery diarrhea
- Ingestion of salt in unusual amounts (as in faulty preparation of oral electrolyte-replacement solutions)
- Excessive parenteral administration of sodium-containing fluids
- Diabetes insipidus if the patient does not experience, or cannot respond to, thirst; or if fluids are excessively restricted.
- Heatstroke
- Near drowning in sea water (which has a Na concentration in the range of 300 to 500 mEq/L)

related to high sodium content in maternal milk or to inadequate lactation. An increased incidence is found in primiparous women and in those discharged from the hospital within 48 hours after birth. Hypernatremic dehydration in neonates due to inadequate breastfeeding is a life-threatening disorder and can damage the neonate's central nervous system. Follow-up of infants for weight loss and other signs of inadequate breastfeeding is important for this reason.[108] Breastfeeding-associated hypernatremia is discussed in detail in Chapter 24.

Watery Diarrhea

Hypernatremia can result from watery diarrhea in children, especially when their intake of water is diminished by nausea. Other causes of hypernatremia in children include fever (with its increased insensible water loss) and excessive sodium administration in poorly prepared electrolyte-replacement solutions.

Insensible Water Loss

A typical adult with a normal body temperature will lose approximately 1000 mL of water per day through respira-

tion and evaporation from the skin (insensible water loss). When any condition is present that increases this insensible water loss (such as fever, hyperventilation, pulmonary infections, tracheostomy, exposure to hot environmental temperatures, or massive burns), hypernatremia may result.

Excessive Sodium Intake

The oral ingestion or intravenous infusion of too much salt can induce hypernatremia. Acute or fatal hypernatremia due to excessive sodium intake has been reported following improperly prepared oral electrolyte solutions (addition of too much NaCl or $NaHCO_3$). Fatalities have resulted from the administration of 5% NaCl solution instead of the intended 5% dextrose in 0.9% NaCl solution because parenteral fluid containers were not checked carefully. Other causes of hypernatremia include excessive administration of $NaHCO_3$ during cardiac arrest or in the treatment of lactic acidosis. Elevated serum sodium levels can even occur from the administration of an isotonic NaCl solution (0.9% NaCl) if the patient's fluid deficit is primarily water.

Ingestion of sea water (which has a sodium concentration in the range of 300 to 500 mEq/L) can lead to severe hypernatremia.[109] In one reported case, a 35-year-old fisherman developed severe hypernatremia (sodium level of 175 mEq/L) following near drowning at sea during a hurricane. The patient eventually recovered after treatment with oxygen and intravenous fluids that slowly returned his serum sodium concentration to a normal range.[110]

Diabetes Insipidus

Diabetes insipidus (DI) is a disorder of water balance that is associated either with a lack of ADH or resistance of the kidney to ADH, leading to water diuresis. Hypernatremia will result if insufficient water is replaced. The two types of DI are central and nephrogenic.

Central DI (CDI) is caused by a relative lack of ADH and is sometimes called vasopressin-sensitive DI because it responds favorably to ADH administration. It is also referred to as neurogenic diabetes insipidus. This form of DI may occur after head trauma (particularly in cases involving fractures at the base of the skull or surgical procedures near the pituitary) or as a result of infection, primary tumor, or metastatic tumor. It may also be idiopathic: Approximately 50% of the patients with CDI have no known underlying pathology. See Chapter 19 for a discussion of the treatment of CDI.

Nephrogenic DI (NDI) is caused by failure of the kidney to respond to ADH, rather than by a deficit of the hormone.

This condition is sometimes referred to as vasopressin-resistant DI because the administration of vasopressin does not relieve the disorder. It may occur as a rare genetic disorder or may be acquired. Acquired NDI is much more common and may result from electrolyte disorders (such as hypokalemia or hypercalcemia) or use of lithium. Fortunately, NDI caused by hypercalcemia and hypokalemia is usually reversible after correction of the imbalance. Drugs that may induce NDI include demeclocycline and lithium.

The most prevalent signs of DI are polyuria and polydipsia. Depending on the severity of the disease, the degree of polyuria in DI can range from 3 to 20 L in 24 hours. In complete CDI and NDI, the urinary specific gravity and osmolality are quite low (less than 1.010 and 300 mOsm/L, respectively). In partial CDI and NDI, the urinary specific gravity and osmolality are somewhat higher (1.010–1.023 and 300–800 mOsm/L, respectively), because the patient has some remaining ability to concentrate urine.

As a rule, the patient with an intact thirst mechanism will drink sufficient fluids to maintain sodium balance (i.e., an essentially normal serum sodium and serum osmolality). Unfortunately, the frequency of urination and drinking often interferes with other activities when the condition is severe. If the patient is not able to perceive or respond to thirst or if parenteral fluid replacement is inadequate, polyuria will lead to severe dehydration (hypernatremia and hyperosmolality of plasma) along with weight loss, tachycardia, and even shock.

Clinical Signs of Hypernatremia

Symptoms of hypernatremia are dependent on the degree and rate of rise in the serum sodium concentration.[111] **Table 4-8** summarizes the clinical signs of hypernatremia. Severe neurological damage tends to occur with acute elevations in sodium greater than 158 mEq/L, but patients with chronic hypernatremia may be only mildly symptomatic with serum sodium concentrations ranging between 170 and 180 mEq/L.[112]

When the patient is awake, thirst is the usual early sign of developing hypernatremia (provided the thirst mechanism is intact). It should be noted that thirst, by stimulating water intake, normally protects against hypernatremia. Thus hypernatremia generally occurs in individuals who are either unable to perceive or unable to respond to thirst (e.g., elderly adults, infants, or anyone with an altered mental status).

Table 4-8 Clinical Signs of Hypernatremia

- Thirst
- Elevated body temperature
- Dry and sticky mucous membranes
- Restlessness and weakness in moderate hypernatremia
- Disorientation, delusions, and hallucinations in severe hypernatremia; alternatively, the patient may be lethargic when undisturbed and irritable and hyperreactive when stimulated
- Lethargy, stupor, or coma (The level of consciousness depends not only on actual sodium levels, but also on the rate of development of hypernatremia. For example, a patient may have a serum sodium level of 170 mEq/L and remain conscious if the imbalance developed slowly.)
- Muscle irritability and convulsions
- Signs of irritability and high-pitched cry in infants

Laboratory Data

- Serum sodium > 145mEq/L
- Serum osmolality > 295 mOsm/kg
- Urinary specific gravity > 1.015 as the kidneys attempt to conserve needed water, provided water loss is from a route *other* than the kidney (e.g., GI tract, skin, or lungs)
- Urinary specific gravity will be very low if the physiological defect involves water loss from the kidney (as occurs in complete diabetes insipidus)

As in hyponatremia, the primary manifestations of hypernatremia are neurological in nature. The earliest signs are lethargy, weakness, and irritability. These symptoms can progress to twitching, seizures, coma and death if the hypernatremia is severe. Although convulsions may occur with an acute, rapid increase in plasma sodium by 15 to 20 mEq/L within 24 hours or less, they are more typically observed with a sodium concentration greater than 160 mEq/L. Presumably these symptoms are the consequence of cellular dehydration (resulting from pulling of fluid from the cells into the hyperosmotic ECF). If hypernatremia is severe, permanent brain damage can occur, especially in children. Brain damage is apparently due to subarachnoid hemorrhages that result from tearing of vessels during brain contraction. Because of rupture of cerebral vessels, a lumbar puncture may reveal blood in the cerebrospinal fluid. Symptoms in infants often include marked irritability and a high-pitched cry, with a depressed sensorium ranging from lethargy to frank coma. In adults, the symptoms of hypernatremia are often difficult to separate from those of the underlying pathology, which is often of a catastrophic nature.

As is the case with hyponatremia, the rapidity of onset is an important determinant of the severity of symptoms as well as the eventual outcome of hypernatremia. A high plasma sodium level that evolves over days to weeks is associated with minimal to mild neurological symptoms because the CNS cells have time to adapt to hyperosmolar changes.

If the hypernatremia is accompanied by FVD, other symptoms such as postural hypotension may occur. Other physical signs of water deficit include dry, hot skin with decreased sweating; thick, rubbery-feeling skin; and fever of CNS origin. Hypernatremia is the only state in which dry, sticky mucous membranes are characteristic.

Hypernatremic states are associated with increased risk for thrombosis.[113] For example, reports have cited aortic and cerebral venous thrombosis as well as peripheral venous thrombosis in children with hypernatremia.[114,115]

Treatment of Hypernatremia

Hypernatremia is treated either by the addition of water or by the removal of sodium, depending on the cause of the imbalance. If water loss is the cause, water needs to be added; if sodium excess is the cause, sodium needs to be removed.

Too rapid correction of hypernatremia can result in cerebral edema, seizures, permanent neurological damage, and death, for the following reasons. Hypernatremia initially pulls water from brain cells and produces brain contraction; however, after a few hours the brain begins to adapt by increasing the intracellular solute level. Rapid lowering of the plasma sodium can render the plasma relatively hypoosmotic to the brain cells and allow water to be pulled into the cells, producing cerebral edema. (Note that the blood–brain barrier prevents the intracellular solutes from being diluted at the same rate as the solute in the plasma.) Thus, rapid correction of hypernatremia can cause cerebral edema, seizures, and permanent neurological damage.

The maximal recommended rate of correction of the serum sodium is 0.5 mEq/L/hr (or 12 mEq/L in 24 hours) in symptomatic patients.[116] Other sources recommend limiting the total decrease in sodium over a 24-hour period to 10 mEq to allow for a margin of error.[117]

The safest route for administering water is by mouth or by nasogastric tube. Alternatively, hypotonic saline solutions or 5% dextrose in water may be cautiously given intravenously.

If the hypernatremic patient is also hypovolemic, a solution of 0.9% sodium chloride (osmolality 308 mOsm/L) may be given to expand the plasma volume while still lowering the plasma sodium concentration. Once the hypovolemia is corrected, switching to a more dilute sodium fluid (such as a 0.45% NaCl or 0.22% NaCl) may be done to further gradually dilute the plasma sodium concentration.

Treatment of Diabetes Insipidus

The standard treatment for patients with complete central (neurogenic) diabetes insipidus is ADH replacement by means of vasopressin administration. Vasopressin may be administered in different forms—orally, parenterally, or nasal spray—depending on the clinical situation. Until the polyuria of CDI is controlled by vasopressin therapy, careful attention must be paid to replacement of fluid, particularly if the patient has a decreased level of consciousness or other disturbances interfering with the perception of thirst or the ability to drink. A potential complication of vasopressin therapy is excessive retention of water, resulting in hyponatremia. Fortunately, hyponatremia is uncommon if minimal effective doses are used.[118]

Paradoxically, thiazide diuretic agents are sometimes used to decrease the polyuria associated with both central and nephrogenic diabetes insipidus.[119] It is thought that thiazides act by decreasing the number of sodium ions that reach the distal tubules of the kidneys.

Clinical Considerations for Hypernatremia

1. Identify patients at risk for hypernatremia (review Table 4-7).
2. Monitor fluid losses and gains. Look for abnormal losses of water or low water intake, and for large gains of sodium such as may occur with prescription drugs having high sodium content. Monitor for symptoms of hypernatremia (see Table 4-8), evaluating them in relation to other factors in the patient's history.
3. Monitor serum sodium levels as frequently as indicated.
4. Prevent hypernatremia in debilitated patients who are unable to perceive or respond to thirst by offering them fluids at regular intervals. If fluid intake remains inadequate, consult with the physician to plan an alternate route for intake, either by tube feedings or by the parenteral route.
5. If tube feedings are used, give sufficient water to keep the serum sodium and the blood urea nitrogen (BUN) levels within normal limits (see Chapter 12).
6. Monitor the patient's response to corrective parenteral fluids by reviewing serial sodium levels and observing any changes in neurological signs. With gradual

decrease in the serum sodium level, the neurological signs should improve, not worsen. Be aware that the serum sodium level should be decreased gradually.

7. For patients with DI:
   a. Recognize the clinical manifestations of DI (**Table 4-9**).
   b. Ensure that the alert patient with DI and an intact thirst mechanism is allowed to drink at will. Also ensure that this individual is near a bathroom, because frequent voiding is anticipated until the condition is brought under control.
   c. Ensure that the patient with a decreased level of consciousness or other disability interfering with drinking is given adequate fluid. If the patient is unable to take fluids orally, consult with the physician to obtain parenteral fluid orders.
   d. Be aware that a potential complication of vasopressin administration is water intoxication (excessive retention of water causing a low serum sodium level). This consideration is particularly important because it is difficult to regulate vasopressin dosage in patients with rapidly fluctuating clinical state.

HYPERNATREMIA CASE STUDIES

Case Study 4-10

A 70-year-old, previously healthy woman suffered a stroke that rendered her partially paralyzed and unable to swallow normally. With assistance, she was able to consume fluids and nutrients without significant aspiration. The patient expressed a desire to be rehabilitated and tried to cooperate fully in her care. After treatment in an acute care facility, she was transferred to a skilled nursing facility for rehabilitation. While there, she did not receive adequate fluid or nutrients and lost more than 7 lb; her serum sodium level increased from normal to 160 mEq/L, and she developed a sacral decubitus ulcer. From the skilled nursing home, she was transferred to a long-term care facility, where the care was even worse. At no time while in either facility was the patient offered a feeding tube to assist in fluid and nutrient intake.

When the patient's neurological status deteriorated, her family insisted that she be re-admitted to the acute care facility. At that time, the following laboratory values were obtained: serum Na 168 mEq/L, hematocrit 60%, BUN 60 mg/dL, and creatinine 2 mg/dL (BUN:Cr ratio = 30:1). While in the acute care facility she was treated with 0.9%

Table 4-9 Clinical Manifestations of Diabetes Insipidus

Excessive urinary output regardless of fluid intake:

- Urinary output usually ranges between 3 and 20 L per 24 hours (depending on the severity of the pathologic process)
- Urinary output often exceeds 200 mL/hr
- Complete DI: urinary specific gravity is less than 1.010 and urinary osmolality is less than 300 mOsm/L
- Partial DI: urinary specific gravity may be in the range of 1.010–1.023 and urinary osmolality may be in the range of 300–800 mOsm/L
- Kidneys are unable to concentrate urine by fluid restriction (a common test for this disorder)

Intense thirst in the alert patient, resulting in an intake that corresponds to the urinary volume

Serum osmolality and sodium levels greater than normal if water intake does not match urinary losses (severe hypovolemia may occur with inadequate fluid intake)

NaCl and later 0.45% NaCl until her serum sodium concentration dropped to 149 mEq/L over a period of 3 days. A feeding tube was placed and isotonic feedings were started. Despite correct management in the acute care facility, the patient developed multiple clots and died.

Commentary. There was no excuse for the failure to provide adequate fluid and nutrients to this patient, who wished to receive all needed therapeutic interventions. Another disturbing feature of this case is the use of a standard form that included a series of nursing diagnoses. One of the diagnoses was entitled "potential for inadequate fluid and nutrient intake due to swallowing deficit"; others were "potential for skin breakdown due to incontinence" and "potential for electrolyte imbalances." All of these diagnoses were checked off each day, indicating that the staff was aware of the potential problems. The nursing diagnosis "potential for electrolyte imbalances" was checked off when the patient already had a severe imbalance (hypernatremia). Even so, the staff did not act on the nursing diagnoses by providing fluid and nutrients. It is likely that the patient could have taken adequate fluids by mouth with proper feeding techniques; certainly, fluids and nutrients could have been provided by a feeding tube if she was unable to take adequate fluids orally.

This patient's death was clearly related to hypernatremia, a condition associated with a high mortality rate. Her hypernatremia could have been avoided had the staff provided adequate fluids.

Case Study 4-11

An 80-year-old woman living in a nursing home had a stroke and developed aphasia and hemiplegia. Because of her neurological deficits, she required a great deal of assistance to eat and drink. Because of lack of attention from the staff, she ingested insufficient water and developed a serum sodium concentration of 188 mEq/L.

Commentary. A serum sodium concentration greater than 150 mEq/L is virtually never seen in an alert patient with a normal thirst mechanism and access to water. This hypernatremic patient represents a common problem—namely, decreased awareness and inability to drink. One researcher has stated that hypernatremic dehydration constitutes a "sentinel health event" in patients without documented rapid free-water loss. A sentinel health event is defined as an illness or death that should be preventable, given adequate care, or at least should cause those caring for the patient to ask why the event occurred. In the absence of free-water loss, hypernatremic dehydration probably indicates fluid deprivation (a form of neglect).

Case Study 4-12

A 60-year-old woman with a serum sodium level of 185 mEq/L was transferred from a nursing home to an acute care facility. Aggressive IV therapy with large volumes of 5% dextrose in water was instituted, and her serum sodium dropped to 145 mEq/L in 5 hours. She became unresponsive; a lumbar puncture revealed an opening pressure of 32 cm H_2O (normal is 10–20 cm H_2O).

Commentary. This patient had been hypernatremic for some time, allowing her brain to adapt to the hyperosmolal state by increasing brain osmolality. (In hypernatremia, brain volume initially declines and then begins to adapt toward normal within several hours.) Once this cerebral adaptation has occurred, any rapid lowering of the serum sodium level creates an osmotic gradient, allowing water to move into the brain, increasing brain size, and causing cerebral edema. This outcome is precisely what happened in this case: Had the serum sodium been decreased gradually, the cerebral edema would not have occurred.

Case Study 4-13

Over a 16-hour period, a young child was inadvertently given 800 mL of 5% NaCl solution (containing 855 mEq/L of sodium). The prescribed fluid was 5% dextrose in 0.9% sodium chloride. The patient developed lethargy, convulsions, and coma before the error was discovered. Despite resuscitative efforts, the child died.

Commentary. Instead of the prescribed fluid, this child received a grossly hypertonic sodium solution causing fatal brain damage. This terrible event would never have occurred had the fluid been checked properly before being administered.

Case Study 4-14

A 55-year-old comatose woman with a basal skull fracture was transferred to a medical center from a small suburban hospital. Her urine output was 200 mL/hr and her serum sodium level was 170 mEq/L. The low urine osmolality (80 mOsm/kg) reflected the large water content of the patient's urine. A diagnosis of central diabetes insipidus (CDI) was made and vasopressin was administered. After 3 days of this treatment, her serum sodium level had fallen to 130 mEq/L.

Commentary. This patient was not hydrated adequately at the onset, which caused her to develop hypernatremia. The staff should have been alert for CDI because of the nature of the injury (basal skull fracture). Excessive use of vasopressin caused the development of hyponatremia.

Case Study 4-15

A physician prescribed 20 mL of 0.9% NaCl to be administered over 30 minutes to a hypotensive newborn.[120] Instead of a vial of 0.9% NaCl, the nurse inadvertently obtained a vial of 14.6% NaCl. (Unfortunately, the vial's label did not clearly warn that the solution was highly concentrated and required dilution.) Two doses were administered from the vial and the infant developed apnea and required intubation. Blood was drawn and showed a serum sodium level of 195 mEq/L.

Commentary. The greatly elevated serum sodium level resulted in severe, permanent brain damage, requiring that the child be institutionalized. An important lesson to learn from the tragic event reported here is the need to carefully check all vials before administering any solution.

Also see Case Studies 14-3, 14-4, 19-1, 19-2, 19-3, 19-4, and 25-1 for a discussion of other patients with sodium imbalances.

NOTES

1. Nix, S. (2009). *Williams' basic nutrition and diet therapy* (13th ed.). St. Louis: Mosby Elsevier, p. 132.
2. Schrier, R. W., & Bansal, S. (2008). Diagnosis and management of hyponatremia in acute illness. *Current Opinion in Critical Care, 14*(6), 627–634.
3. Bongard, F. S., Sue, D. Y., & Vintch, J. R. (2008). *Current diagnosis and treatment, critical care* (3rd ed.). New York: McGraw-Hill/Lange, p. 24.
4. Kolleff, M. H., Bedient, T. J., Isakow, W., & Witt, C. A. (2008). *The Washington manual of critical care.* Philadelphia: Lippincott Williams & Wilkins, p. 153.
5. Kolleff et al., note 4, p. 153.
6. McPhee, S. J., Papadakis, M. S., & Tierney, L. M. (2008). *2008 current medical diagnosis and treatment.* New York: McGraw-Hill, p. 732.
7. Kolleff et al., note 4, p. 155.
8. McPherson, R. A., & Pincus, M. R. (2007). *Henry's clinical diagnosis and management by laboratory methods* (21st ed.). Philadelphia: Saunders, p. 149.
9. Ayus, J. C., Achinger, S. G., & Arieff, A. (2008). Brain cell volume regulation in hyponatremia: Role of sex, age, vasopressin, and hypoxia. *American Journal of Physiology: Renal Physiology, 295*(3), F619–F624.
10. Ayus et al., note 9.
11. Sjoblom, E., Hojer, J., Ludwigs, S., & Pirskanen, R. (1997). Fatal hyponatremic brain edema due to common gastroenteritis with accidental water intoxication. *Intensive Care Medicine, 23,* 348–350.
12. Rose, B. D., & Post, T. W. (2001). *Clinical physiology of acid–base and electrolyte disorders* (5th ed.). New York: McGraw-Hill, p. 286.
13. Rose & Post, note 12, p. 286.
14. Rose & Post, note 12, p. 702.
15. Bongard et al., note 3, p. 25.
16. Hoorn, E. J., & Zietse, R. (2008). Hyponatremia revisited: Translating physiology to practice. *Nephron Physiology, 108,* 46–59.
17. Sterns, R. H. (1987). Severe symptomatic hyponatremia, treatment and outcome: A study of 64 cases. *Annals of Internal Medicine, 107,* 656–664.
18. Sonnenblick, M., Friedlander, Y., & Rosin, A. J. (1993). Diuretic-induced severe hyponatremia: Review and analysis of 129 reported patients. *Chest, 103,* 601–606.
19. Fabian, T. J., Amico, J. A., Kroboth, P. D., Mulsant, B. H., Corey, S. E., Begley, A. E., et al. (2004). Paroxetine-induced hyponatremia in older adults: A 12-week prospective study. *Archives of Internal Medicine, 164,* 327–332.
20. Bouman, W., & Pinner, G. (1998). Incidence of selective serotonic reuptake inhibitor (SSRI) induced hyponatremia due to the syndrome of inappropriate antidiuretic hormone (SIADH) secretion in the elderly. *International Journal of Geriatric Psychiatry, 13,* 12–15.
21. Bowen, P. D. (2009). Use of selective serotonin reuptake inhibitors in the treatment of depression in older adults: Identifying and managing potential risk for hyponatremia. *Geriatric Nursing, 30*(2), 85–89.
22. Mago, R., Mahajan, R., & Thase, M. E. (2008). Medically serious adverse effects of newer antidepressants. *Current Psychiatry Reports, 10*(3), 249–257.
23. Mago et al., note 22.
24. Mago et al., note 22.
25. Sharma, H., & Pompei, P. (1996). Antidepressant-induced hyponatremia in the aged. Avoidance and management strategies. *Drugs & Aging, 8*(6), 430–5.
26. Rose & Post, note 12, p. 707.
27. Hammond, I. W., Ferguson, J. A., Kwong, K., Muniz, E., & Delisle, F. (2002). Hyponatremia and syndrome of inappropriate anti-diuretic hormone reported with the use of Vincristine: An over-representation of Asians? *Pharmacoepidemiology & Drug Safety, 11*(3), 229–234.
28. Peyrade, F., Taillan, B., Lebrun, C., Bendini, J. C., Passeron, C., & Dujardin, P. (1997). Hyponatremia during treatment with cisplatin. *La Presse Medicale, 26,* 1523–1525.
29. Iywe, A. V., Krasnow, S. H., Dufour, D. R., & Arcenas, A. S. (2003). Sodium-wasting nephropathy caused by cisplatin in a patient with small-cell lung cancer. *Clinical Lung Cancer, 5*(3), 187–189.
30. Kuz, G. M., & Manssourian, A. (2005). Carbamazepine-induced hyponatremia: Assessment of risk factors. *Annals of Pharmacotherapy, 39*(11), 1943–1946.
31. Kuz & Manssourian, note 30.
32. Rose & Post, note 12, p. 708.
33. Rose & Post, note 12, p. 709.
34. Donoghue, M. B, Latimer, M. E., Pillsbury, H. L., & Hertzog, J. H. (1998). Hyponatremic seizure in a child using desmopressin for nocturnal enuresis. *Archives of Pediatric and Adolescent Medicine, 152,* 290–292
35. Ecoffey, M., Merz, A., Egil, D., & Panchard, M. (2006). Role of prescribing doctor in hyponatremic seizures of enuretic children on desmopressin. *Archives de Pediatrie, 13*(3), 262–265.
36. Bloom, D. A. (1993). The American experience with desmopressin. *Clinical Pediatrics,* special issue, 28–31.
37. Bernstein, S. A, & Williford, S. (1997). Intranasal desmopressin-associated hyponatremia: A case report and literature review. *Journal of Family Practice, 44*(2), 203–208.
38. Toumba, M., & Stanhope, R. (2006). Morbidity and mortality associated with vasopressin analogue treatment. *Journal of Pediatric Endocrinology, 19*(3), 197–201.
39. Toumba & Stanhope, note 38.
40. Toumba & Stanhope, note 38.
41. Toumba & Stanhope, note 38.
42. Johnson, T. M., Miller, M., Tang, T., Pillion, D. J., & Ouslander, J. G. (2006). Oral DDAVP for nighttime urinary incontinence in characterized nursing home residents: A pilot study. *Journal of the American Medical Directors Association, 7,* 6–11.

43. Weatherall, M. (2004). The risk of hyponatremia in older adults using desmopressin for nocturia: A systematic review and meta-analysis. *Neurology & Urodynamics, 23,* 302–305.

44. McPhee et al., note 6, p. 761.

45. Budisavljevic, M. N., Stewart, L., Sahn, S. A., & Ploth, D. W. (2003). Hyponatremia associated with 3,4-methylene-dioxymethylamphetamine ("Ecstasy") abuse. *American Journal of the Medical Sciences, 326*(2), 89–93.

46. Campbell, G. A., & Rosner, M. H. (2008). The agony of ecstasy: MDMA (3,4-methylenedioxymethamphetamine) and the kidney. *Clinical Journal of the American Society of Nephrology, 3*(6), 1852–1860.

47. Chung, H. M., Kluge, R., Schrier, R. W., & Anderson, R. J. (1986). Postoperative hyponatremia. A prospective study. *Archives of Internal Medicine, 146,* 333–336

48. Ayus, J. C., Wheeler, J. M, & Arieff, A. I. (1992). Postoperative hyponatremic encephalopathy in menstruant women. *Annals of Internal Medicine, 117,* 891–897.

49. Ayus et al., note 48, p. 893.

50. Ayus et al., note 48, p. 893.

51. Ayus et al., note 48, p. 893.

52. Bagshaw, S. M., Townsend, D. R., & McDermid, R. C. (2009). Disorders of sodium and water balance in hospitalized patients. *Canadian Journal of Anesthesia, 56,* 151–167.

53. Rose & Post, note 12, p. 711.

54. Ellinas, P. A., Rosner, F., & Jaume, J. C. (1993). Symptomatic hyponatremia associated with psychoses, medications, and smoking. *Journal of the National Medical Association, 85,* 135–141.

55. Brown, R. G. (1993). Disorders of water and sodium balance. *Postgraduate Medicine, 93,* 227.

56. Glassock, R. J, Cohen, A. H., Danovitch, G., & Parsa, K. P. (1990). Human immunodeficiency virus (HIV) and the kidney. *Annals of Internal Medicine, 12,* 35–49.

57. Vitting, K. E., Gardenswartz, M. H., Zabetakis P. M., Tapper, M. L., Gleim, G. W., Agrawal, M., et al. (1990). Frequency of hyponatremia and nonosmolar vasopressin release in the acquired immunodeficiency syndrome. *Journal of the American Medical Association, 263,* 973–978.

58. Agarwal, A., Soni, A., & Ciechanowsky, M., (1989). Hyponatremia in patients with the acquired immunodeficiency syndrome. *Nephron, 53,* 317–21.

59. Tolaymat, A., al-Mousily, F., Sleasman, J., Paryani, S., & Nelberger, R. (1995). Hyponatremia in pediatric patients with HIV-1 infection. *Southern Medical Journal, 88,* 1039–1042.

60. Rose & Post, note 12, p. 707.

61. McPhee et al., note 6, p. 761.

62. O'Connor, R. E. (2006). Exercise-induced hyponatremia: Causes, risks, prevention, and management. *Cleveland Clinic Journal of Medicine, 73(3),* S13–S18.

63. O'Connor, note 62.

64. Moritz, M. L. & Ayus, J. C. (2008). Exercise-associated hyponatremia: Why are athletes still dying? *Clinical Journal of Sports Medicine, 18*(5), 379–381.

65. Marik, P. E.(2001). *Handbook of evidence-based critical care.* New York: Springer, p. 253.

66. Marik, note 65, p. 253.

67. Rose & Post, note 12, p. 719.

68. Arieff, A. I., Ayus, J. C, & Fraser, C. L. (1992). Hyponatremia and death or permanent brain damage in healthy children. *British Medical Journal, 304,* 1218–1222.

69. Bongard et al., note 3, p. 28.

70. Bongard et al., note 3, p. 28.

71. Bongard et al., note 3, p. 28.

72. Cooper, D. H., Krainik, A. J., Lubner, S. J., & Reno, H. E. (2007). *The Washington manual of medical therapeutics* (32nd ed.). Philadelphia: Lippincott Williams & Wilkins.

73. Marik, note 65, p. 253.

74. Marik, note 65, p. 253.

75. Marcucci, L., Martinez, E. A., Haut, E. R., Slonim, A. D., & Suarez, J. I. (2007). *Avoiding common ICU errors.* Philadelphia: Wolters Kluwer/Lippincott Williams & Wilkins, p. 422.

76. Sterns, R. H., Riggs, J. E., & Schochet, S. S. (1986). Osmotic demyelination syndrome following correction of hyponatremia. *New England Journal of Medicine, 314,* 1535–1542.

77. Cooper et al., note 72, p. 63

78. Marik, note 65, p. 253.

79. Cooper et al., note 72.

80. Marik, note 65, p. 253.

81. Cooper et al., note 72, p. 63.

82. Marik, note 65, p. 253.

83. Cooper et al., note 72, p. 64.

84. Kolleff et al., note 4, p. 157.

85. Parrillo, J. E., & Dellinger, R. P. (2008). *Critical care: Principles of diagnosis and management in the adult* (3rd ed.). Philadelphia: Mosby Elsevier, p. 1222.

86. Parrillo & Dellinger, note 85, p. 1222.

87. Marik, note 65, p. 253.

88. Reilly, R. F., & Perazella, M. A. (2007). *Acid–base, fluids and electrolytes.* New York: McGraw-Hill Medical, p. 82.

89. Reilly & Perazella, note 88, p. 83.

90. Gardner, D. G., & Shoback, D. (2007). *Greenspan's basic and clinical endocrinology* (8th ed.). New York: McGraw-Hill Medical, p. 168.

91. Ghali, J. K. (2008). Mechanisms, risks, and new treatment options for hyponatremia. *Cardiology, 111*(3), 147–157.

92. Hoorn, E. J., & Zietse, R. (2008). Hyponatremia revisited: Translating physiology to practice. *Nephron Physiology, 108,* 46–59

93. Gines, P., & Guevara, M. (2008). Hyponatremia in cirrhosis: Pathogenesis, clinical significance, and management. *Hepatology, 48*(3), 1002–1010.

94. Gines & Guevara, note 93.

95. Bowen, note 21.

96. Hiramatsu, R., Takeshita, A., Taguchi, M., & Takeuchi, Y. (2007). Symptomatic hyponatremia after voluntary excessive water

ingestion in a patient without psychiatric problem. *Endocrine Journal, 54*(4), 643–645.

97. Gardner & Shoback, note 90, p. 934.

98. Stern, R. M. (2002). The psychophysiology of nausea. *Acta Biologica Hungarica, 53*(4), 589–599

99. Covyeou, J. A., & Jackson, C. W. (2007). Hyponatremia associated with escitalopram. *New England Journal of Medicine, 356*(1), 94–95.

100. Fink, M. P., Abraham, E., Vincent, J. L., & Kochanek, P. M. (2005). *Textbook of critical care* (5th ed.). Philadelphia: Elsevier Saunders, p. 63.

101. Gardner & Shoback, note 90, p. 86.

102. Feehally, J., Floege, J., & Johnson, R. J. (2007). *Comprehensive clinical nephrology* (3rd ed.). Philadelphia: Mosby Elsevier, p. 109.

103. Fink et al., note 100, p. 63.

104. Parrillo & Dellinger, note 85, p. 1223.

105. Bagshaw et al., note 52.

106. Rose & Post, note 12, p. 746.

107. Moritz, M. L., Manole, M. D., Bogten, D. L., & Ayus, J. C. (2005). Breastfeeding-associated hypernatremia: Are we missing the diagnosis? *Pediatrics, 116*(3), 343–347.

108. Unal, S., Arhan, E., Kara, N., Unca, N., & Aliefendioglu, D. (2008). Breast-feeding associated hypernatremia: Retrospective analysis of 169 term newborns. *Pediatrics International, 50*(1), 29–34.

109. Ellis, R. J. (1997). Severe hypernatremia from sea water ingestion during near-drowning in a hurricane. *Western Journal of Medicine, 167*(6), 430–433.

110. Ellis, note 109.

111. Marcucci et al., note 75, p. 422.

112. Kastin, A., Lipsett, M., Ommaya, A., & Moser, J. M. (1965). Asymptomatic hypernatremia: Physiological and clinical study. *American Journal of Medicine, 38,* 306–315.

113. Grant, P. J., Tate, G. M., Hughes, J. R., Davies, J. A., & Prentice, C. R. (1985). Does hypernatremia promote thrombosis? *Thrombosis Research, 40*(3), 393–399.

114. Iglesias, F. C, Chimenti, C. P., Vazques, L. P., Camacho, P., Guerrero, S. M., & Blanco, B. D. (2006). Aortic and cerebral thrombosis caused by hypernatremic dehydration in an exclusively breast-fed infant. *Anales de Pediatria, 65*(4), 381–383.

115. Bergada, I., Aversa, L., & Heinrich, J. J. (2004). Peripheral venous thrombosis in children and adolescents with adipsic hypernatremia secondary to hypothalamic tumors. *Hormone Research, 61(3)* 108–110.

116. Marik, note 65, p. 254.

117. Cooper et al., note 72, p. 65.

118. McPhee et al., note 6, p. 954.

119. McPhee et al., note 6, p. 954.

120. Cohen, M. R. Sodium chloride vial concentration above 0.9% should make you nervous. *Intravenous Nurses Society Newsline.* 1994; 15:8, 10.

Chapter 5

Potassium Imbalances

Disturbances in potassium balance are common in all age groups and in a variety of patient care settings. Before discussing hypokalemia and hyperkalemia, it is helpful to review some pertinent factors about potassium balance.

POTASSIUM BALANCE

The typical adult has a total body potassium content of between 3000 and 4000 mEq, 98% of which is situated inside the cells. The remaining 2% is found in the extracellular fluid (ECF); this portion is important in neuromuscular function. Potassium plays a major role in the transmission of nerve impulses, muscle contraction, tissue synthesis, carbohydrate metabolism, and maintenance of intracellular acid–base balance and tonicity. Changes in the electrocardiogram (ECG) associated with serum potassium variations are illustrated in **Figure 5-1.**

Aldosterone, a hormone secreted by the adrenal cortex, is crucial in the regulation of potassium. The target organ of aldosterone is the kidney, where sodium and potassium retention and excretion are regulated. Approximately 80% of the potassium excreted daily from the body is removed by way of the kidneys. The other 20% is lost through the bowel (15%) and sweat glands (5%).[1]

The typical American diet contains approximately 3 g (80 mEq) of potassium per day; a high-potassium diet may contain 4.5 to 7 g (120–180 mEq) per day.[2] Because potassium is plentiful in the normal diet, poor dietary intake rarely causes hypokalemia; however, this factor contributes to other causes of hypokalemia. For patients who are unable to eat, potassium must be replaced daily, either enterally or parenterally; an intake of 40 to 60 mEq/day suffices in the adult if no abnormal losses are occurring.

HYPOKALEMIA

The normal potassium range in the bloodstream, as reported by most laboratories, is between 3.5 and 5.0 mEq/L. *Hypokalemia* refers to a below-normal potassium concentration. When defined as a plasma potassium less than 3.5 mEq/L, hypokalemia is found in more than 20% of hospitalized patients.[3] Mild hypokalemia is arbitrarily defined as ranging between 3.0 and 3.4 mEq/L; this degree of potassium depletion is usually well tolerated in the absence of digitalis therapy or severe hepatic disease. Moderate hypokalemia is arbitrarily said to range between 2.5 and 3.0 mEq/L, whereas severe hypokalemia is generally defined as a plasma level less than 2.5 mEq/L.[4]

Hypokalemia usually indicates a real deficit of total potassium stores. In some cases, however, it may occur in patients having normal potassium stores when alkalosis is present (because alkalosis causes a temporary shift of serum potassium into the cells). Hypokalemia is a common disturbance with a number of etiologies. Frequently, a combination of factors is present at one time to predispose the person to developing hypokalemia.

Causes

Gastrointestinal Losses

Relatively large amounts of potassium are present in intestinal fluids; for example, diarrheal fluid may contain as much as 80 to 90 mEq/L.[5, 6] Given this fact, potassium deficit occurs frequently with diarrhea and recent ileostomy. Hypokalemia is especially likely to occur in individuals with a high-output villous adenoma (a type of polyp in the colon).[7]

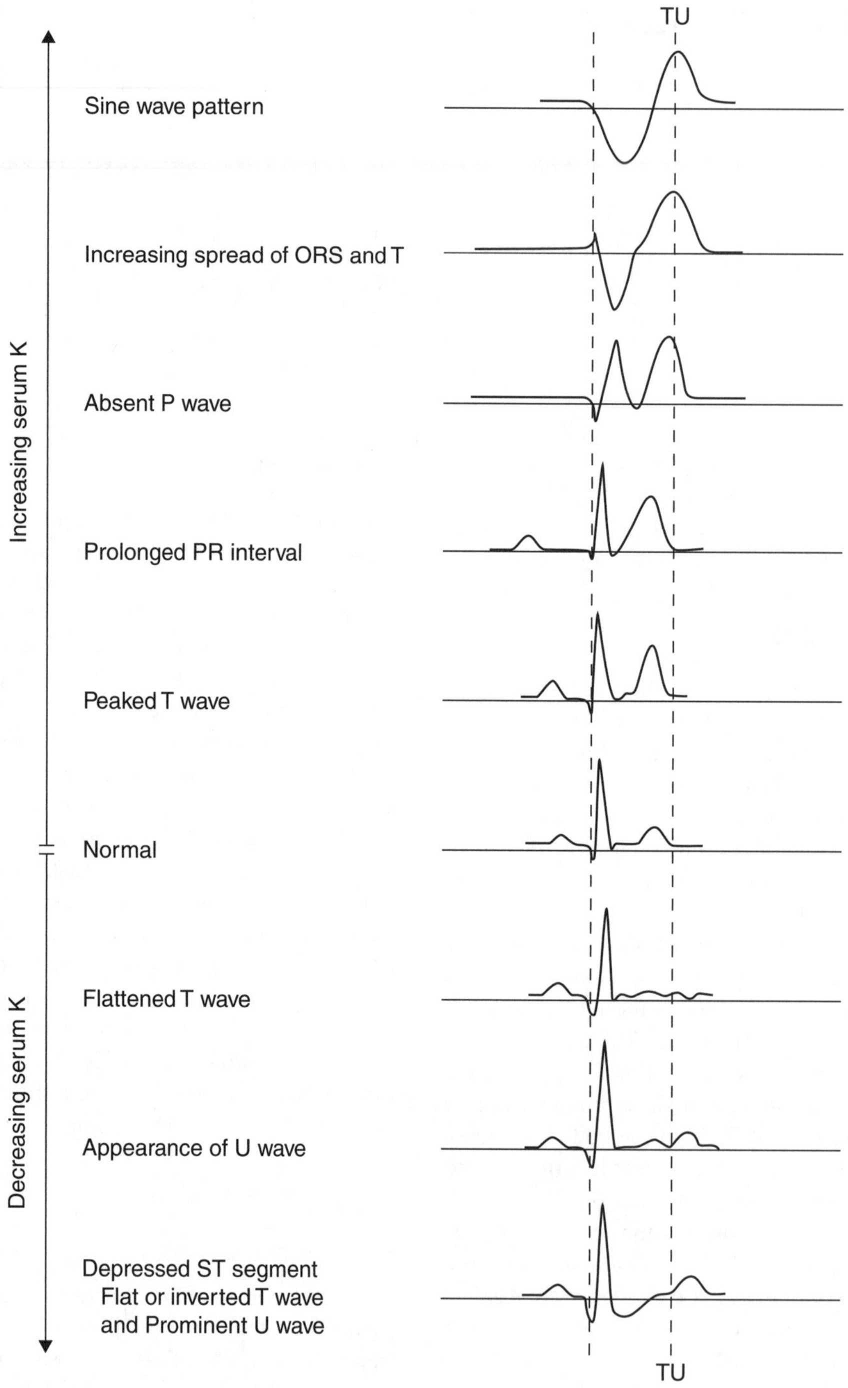

Figure 5-1 ECG manifestations of hypokalemia and hyperkalemia
Source: Zull, DN. Disorders of potassium metabolism. *Emerg Med Clin N Am* 1989/Vol. 7 Issue 4 pages 771–794. Copyright Elsevier.

Vomiting and gastric suction frequently lead to hypokalemia, partly because of actual potassium loss in gastric fluid, but largely because of increased renal potassium loss associated with metabolic alkalosis. Recall that loss of acidic gastric fluid causes metabolic alkalosis, after which the kidneys attempt to conserve hydrogen ions to correct the pH disturbances. In this process, potassium ions are lost in greater amounts.

Medications

Table 5-1 identifies medications associated with hypokalemia. Potassium-losing diuretics (such as the thiazides and furosemide) are among the most frequent causes of hypokalemia, particularly when given in high doses to patients with poor potassium intake. As many as 50% of patients receiving potassium-losing diuretics may develop hypokalemia.[18] Another way in which diuretics increase the likelihood of hypokalemia is by stimulating production of aldosterone (following intravascular volume contraction from diuresis).

As indicated in Table 5-1, the plasma potassium concentration can fall after the administration of a beta-adrenergic agonist (such as albuterol or dobutamine) to treat asthma or heart failure.[19] Ritodrine and terbutaline (inhibitors of uterine contraction) can also cause the plasma potassium level to drop to as low as 2.5 mEq/L after 4 to 6 hours of their intravenous administration.[20]

Insulin promotes the entry of potassium into skeletal muscle and hepatic cells; thus patients with persistent insulin hypersecretion may experience hypokalemia. Later in the chapter, insulin administration is discussed as a therapeutic measure for the temporary relief of life-threatening hyperkalemia. Catecholamines also promote potassium entry into the cells. Therefore, transient hypokalemia can be induced when epinephrine release is enhanced by the stress of an acute illness (such as in an episode of coronary ischemia).

Chronic ingestion of licorice (as candy, certain chewing tobaccos, cough mixtures, and herbal medicines) can produce hypokalemia because licorice contains glycyrrhizic acid, a substance that has mineralocorticoid activity (which

Table 5-1 Medications Associated with Hypokalemia

Medication	Comments
Potassium-losing diuretics (e.g., hydrochlorothiazide, furosemide)	Diuretic therapy is the most common cause of hypokalemia. Both the thiazide and loop diuretics favor renal potassium wasting. A low plasma potassium level has been found in 10% to 40% of patients treated with thiazide diuretics.[8] The degree of potassium loss is largely dose dependent. When low-dose thiazides (e.g., 12.5 to 25 mg of hydrochlorothiazide) are given, the risk for hypokalemia is decreased.[9] If larger doses are needed, it may be necessary to combine the thiazide diuretic with a potassium-sparing diuretic.
B_2-adrenergic agonists (e.g., albuterol, ritodrine, terbutaline)	Nebulized albuterol (standard dose) can reduce the serum potassium by 0.2 to 0.4 mEq/L; a second dose within one hour can reduce it by almost 1 mEq/L.[10] Inhibitors of uterine contraction (ritodrine and terbutaline) can reduce the serum potassium to as low as 2.5 mEq/L after 4 to 6 hours of intravenous administration.[11] These drugs cause a transient shift of potassium from the plasma into the cells.[12]
Amphotericin B	Amphotericin B causes renal potassium wasting through inhibition of hydrogen ions secretion by the renal collecting-duct cells as well as by inducing magnesium depletion.[13] Hypokalemia occurs in as many as half of patients treated with amphotericin B.[14] When this agent is used, it is recommended that its use be discontinued as soon as possible.[15]
Aminoglycosides (e.g., gentamicin, tobramycin)	Renal tubular damage due to aminoglycosides, such as gentamicin, can lead to hypokalemia combined with hypocalcemia, hypomagnesemia, and alkalosis.
Cisplatin	Cisplatin commonly causes hypomagnesemia and hypokalemia by increasing renal magnesium and potassium losses.
Cathartics	Cathartics stimulate emptying of the bowel, thereby causing loss of potassium. The small bowel secretions contain as much as 80 mEq potassium per liter.
Glucocorticoids	Glucocorticoids increase potassium excretion through their effect on the renal filtration rate and distal sodium delivery.[16] When given over a long period of time, these drugs reduce serum potassium only slightly (0.2–0.4 mEq/L).[17]

favors potassium loss). For example, one report described a 55-year-old woman who developed a serum potassium concentration of 2.0 mEq/L after habitually consuming more than 2 pounds of licorice candy per week.[21]

Adrenal Conditions

Excessive aldosterone production enhances renal potassium wasting and, therefore, commonly leads to hypokalemia. For example, a case was reported in which a 55-year-old man with primary hyperaldosteronism (caused by an adrenal adenoma) developed severe weakness and a serum potassium concentration of 1.4 mEq/L.[22] Far more common than primary hyperaldosteronism is secondary hyperaldosteronism, a condition that occurs in patients with cirrhosis, nephrotic syndrome, and congestive heart failure. High serum glucocorticoid levels associated with the administration of large doses of steroids can also cause potassium loss.

Hypomagnesemia

Hypomagnesemia is observed in as many as 40% of patients with hypokalemia. In some cases, the underlying abnormality causes both imbalances.[23] At other times, hypomagnesemia contributes to the development of hypokalemia. When this is the case, correction of the hypokalemia requires the concurrent restoration of magnesium balance. Magnesium depletion should be suspected when hypokalemia does not respond to replacement.[24]

Alkalosis

Recall that potassium is constantly shifting in and out of cells according to the body's needs, under the influence of the Na/K ATPase pump. In alkalosis, hydrogen ions shift out of the cells to help correct the pH defect; potassium ions from the ECF then move into the cells to maintain electroneutrality. (See Chapter 9 for a more thorough discussion of the effects of alkalemia on plasma potassium concentration.)

Refeeding Syndrome

Vigorous feeding of chronically malnourished patients can lead to serious hypokalemia if inadequate potassium is supplied. The feeding causes an acute increase in insulin, which in turn stimulates cellular uptake of potassium for the synthesis of glycogen and lean body tissue.[25] Other electrolytes that shift into the cells during the refeeding syndrome are magnesium and phosphate. See Chapter 12 for a more detailed discussion of this condition.

Barbiturate Coma Therapy

A recent case report outlined a sequential occurrence of life-threatening hypokalemia and rebound hyperkalemia following barbiturate coma therapy.[26] In this case, a 53-year-old man underwent barbiturate coma therapy following traumatic subarachnoid hemorrhage and subdural hematoma. Ten hours after the start of thiopental administration, the patient developed profound hypokalemia (1.0 mEq/L) accompanied by severe bradycardia and cardiac arrest. When the thiopental infusion was stopped suddenly, the patient's potassium level increased to 8.9 mEq/L, necessitating emergency management with calcium gluconate and a glucose/regular insulin infusion. A similar case was reported in a 14-year-old boy who was treated with a thiopental infusion for management of increased intracranial pressure following a severe head injury.[27] Throughout the infusion, the patient had persistent hypokalemia; upon cessation of the infusion, he developed a dysrhythmia associated with a serum potassium level of 7.0 mEq/L. In both cases, potassium had been administered to correct the hypokalemia experienced during the coma.

Hypokalemic Periodic Paralysis

Hypokalemic periodic paralysis is a rare disorder that is characterized by intermittent muscle weakness following an intracellular influx of potassium. It may be familial (through an autosomal dominant inheritance pattern) or acquired (associated with thyrotoxicosis); it is predominantly seen in men.[28] Muscle weakness may be so pronounced that the patient is temporarily paralyzed. Without intervention, the paralytic attacks may last for 7 to 14 days.

Sweat Losses

Potassium deficit from heavy perspiration is most likely to occur in persons who are acclimated to heat. This condition occurs because the sweat glands in acclimated individuals excrete more potassium than do the sweat glands of persons who are not acclimated to heat stress. The mechanism involved is presumably an aldosterone-related effect to conserve sodium (the primary electrolyte in sweat). Sweat losses exceeding 10 L/day have been reported in individuals exercising in a hot climate.

Poor Intake

Patients who are unable or unwilling to eat a normal diet for a prolonged period are prone to developing hypokalemia. However, strict fasting usually induces only a moderate depletion of total body potassium if normal homeostatic mechanisms are present. In most cases, poor intake is coupled with other problems, which may collectively increase the risk of hypokalemia. For example, in addition to poor intake, individuals with anorexia nervosa frequently abuse diuretics and laxatives and induce vomiting to maintain a low body weight. Likewise, alcoholics frequently have other factors predisposing them to hypokalemia, such as vomiting, diarrhea, and magnesium deficiency.

Clinical Signs

While hypokalemia is usually well tolerated in otherwise healthy people, it can be life-threatening when severe (possibly culminating in cardiac or respiratory arrest). In patients with cardiovascular disease, even mild or moderate hypokalemia increases the risk of morbidity and mortality.[29]

Clinical signs are usually not present until the potassium level falls below 3.0 mEq/L. Symptoms may appear sooner in patients who are receiving digitalis (which predisposes them to dysrhythmias) and patients with hepatic failure (who are more prone to hepatic encephalopathy because of increased ammonia production). Hypokalemia is rarely suspected on the basis of clinical presentation alone; the diagnosis is usually made by measurement of the serum potassium level.[30]

Cardiovascular Effects

Arrhythmias. The major cardiac effects of hypokalemia are abnormalities of electrophysiology and contractility. Most important is the potential for a variety of atrial and ventricular arrhythmias, particularly in patients with ischemic myocardial disease and those receiving digitalis preparations. Because hypokalemia is associated with increased binding of digitalis to Na/K ATPase, cardiac sensitivity to digitalis preparations is heightened by hypokalemia. As mentioned earlier, hypokalemia and hypomagnesemia often occur together; the most serious consequence of this combination of imbalances is increased cardiac irritability and risk for arrhythmias.

In patients without underlying heart disease, abnormalities in cardiac conduction are unusual, even when the serum potassium concentration is less than 3 mEq/L.[31] Some physicians advocate maintaining plasma potassium concentrations above 4.0 mEq/L in patients with heart disease.[32]

Hypertension. Potassium has an antihypertensive effect; the apparent mechanisms for this effect are enhanced sodium excretion, direct vasodilation, and lower cardiovascular reactivity to norepinephrine or angiotensin II.[33] Many clinical studies support the blood pressure-lowering effects of potassium supplementation. For example, significant reductions in systolic blood pressure were demonstrated in a study of 55 hypertensive patients who were treated with potassium chloride supplementation (64 mEq/day) for four weeks as compared with placebo.[34]

Considerable variation in dietary potassium intake is noted, depending on individual preferences. African Americans tend to consume less dietary potassium, which may lead to a state of physiological potassium deficiency and contribute to the higher incidence of hypertension in this population.[35] Maintenance of adequate dietary potassium intake shows promise for the prevention and treatment of hypertension.

Muscular Effects

Skeletal Muscle Weakness. Muscle weakness does not usually become noticeable until the plasma potassium concentration is less than 2.5 mEq/L; the lower extremities usually show involvement first (particularly the quadriceps).[36] Later, in severe cases, the muscles of the trunk and upper extremities are affected, with respiratory failure occurring eventually if the condition is not corrected.

Smooth Muscle Weakness. Moderate hypokalemia, which is characterized by serum potassium concentrations in the range of 2.5 to 3.0 mEq/L, may cause constipation (from disturbed smooth-muscle function). Other symptoms of hypokalemia, such as anorexia, nausea, vomiting, prolonged gastric emptying, gaseous distention, and paralytic ileus, are due to weakness of the smooth muscles of the GI tract and impairment of the response to parasympathetic stimulation.

Rhabdomyolysis. Hypokalemia predisposes individuals to reduced skeletal muscle blood flow, which in turn can lead to rhabdomyolysis (disintegration of striated muscle fibers with excretion of myoglobin in the urine). The effects of the muscle ischemia are exacerbated by exercising because hypokalemia blocks the vasodilation that normally occurs during exercise. Rhabdomyolysis is usually seen only when the plasma potassium level is less than 2.5 mEq/L.[37] For example, rhabdomyolysis was diagnosed in a 93-year-old hypertensive woman with severe hypokalemia (1.3 mEq/L) secondary to the long-term use of licorice-containing herbal medicines.[38]

Impaired Urine-Concentrating Ability

Prolonged potassium depletion can interfere with renal concentrating ability. This, in turn, results in dilute urine, polyuria, nocturia, and polydipsia (nephrogenic diabetes insipidus). These symptoms are not uncommon when chronic hypokalemia is present. The reduced ability to concentrate urine is the result of a decreased renal responsiveness to antidiuretic hormone (ADH). The polyuria associated with hypokalemia is usually mild, as the urine output usually remains less than 3 L/day.[39] Fortunately, the problem is usually reversible with correction of the hypokalemia.

Elevated Plasma Glucose

Hypokalemia predisposes patients to hyperglycemia by impairing both insulin release and end-organ sensitivity to insulin.[40] In a six-year study of 84,380 women, high potassium intake was associated with a lower risk of developing type 2 diabetes.[41] In contrast, thiazide diuretics are associated with an increased risk of diabetes, possibly through a hypokalemic connection. To determine whether thiazide-induced diabetes is mediated by changes in potassium, a group of investigators analyzed data from 3790 nondiabetic subjects.[42] These researchers found that a decreased serum potassium level was independently associated with higher risk for diabetes and concluded that potassium supplementation might prevent thiazide-induced diabetes.

Treatment

Shifting of potassium in and out of the cells makes it difficult to precisely identify the amount of potassium needed to correct a potassium deficit merely by assessing plasma potassium levels. Although the degree of body potassium depletion does not correlate well with the plasma potassium concentration, it has been estimated that a decrease of 1 mEq/L may represent a total body potassium deficit of 200 to 400 mEq.[43] As with other imbalances, the aim of treatment in hypokalemia is to prevent life-threatening outcomes (not to totally correct the imbalance in a short period of time). Indeed, the administered potassium needs time to equilibrate with cellular stores; it may take days to totally correct the entire body potassium deficit.

Dietary Potassium Intake

For patients at risk for hypokalemia, a diet with ample potassium content should be provided. Usual maintenance requirements for potassium are 40 to 60 mEq/day (unless abnormal routes of potassium loss are present). **Table 5-2** lists some foods with high potassium content. However, once hypokalemia has developed, especially when it coincides with metabolic alkalosis, dietary potassium intake may be ineffective replacement. This is because potassium in most foods is complexed to anions (such as citrate) that metabolize into bicarbonate. Therefore, patients with significant hypokalemia associated with metabolic alkalosis should be given potassium chloride (KCl).[44]

Oral Potassium Supplements

When dietary intake is inadequate, an oral potassium supplement may be prescribed. In some cases, a potassium-containing salt substitute may be sufficient to provide extra

---

Table 5-2 Examples of High-Potassium Foods and Beverages

Food	Potassium
Apricots, dried, 10 halves	407 mg (10 mEq)
Baked beans, 1 cup	569 mg (15 mEq)
Bananas, raw, 1 medium	422 mg (11 mEq)
Broccoli, boiled, 1 cup	437 mg (11 mEq)
Dates, Deglet Noor, 1 cup	1168 mg (30 mEq)
French fries, large (fast food)	930 mg (24 mEq)
Grapefruit juice, canned, 1 cup	405 mg (10 mEq)
Halibut, Atlantic or Pacific, cooked, ½ fillet	916 mg (23 mEq)
Honeydew melon, 1 cup	388 mg (10 mEq)
Lima beans, boiled, 1 cup	955 mg (24 mEq)
Milk, 1% fat, 1 cup	366 mg (9 mEq)
Nuts, almonds, 24 nuts	200 mg (5 mEq)
Orange, 1 medium	237 mg (6 mEq)
Orange juice, canned, 1 cup	458 mg (12 mEq)
Potato, baked, flesh and skin, one	1081 mg (28 mEq)
Plums, dried (prunes), five	307 mg (8 mEq)
Raisins, dried, seedless, 1 cup	1086 mg (28 mEq)
Taco, large (fast food), one	729 mg (19 mEq)
Tomato, red, raw, 1	292 mg (7 mEq)
Tomato soup with 2% milk, 1 cup	466 mg (12 mEq)
Vegetable juice cocktail, 1 cup	467 mg (12 mEq)
Watermelon, 1 wedge	320 mg (8 mEq)
Yogurt, plain, low-fat, 8 oz	443 mg (11 mEq)

Source: Information from USDA National Nutrient Database for Standard Reference, Release 21. United States Department of Agriculture, Agricultural Research Service. (2008).

potassium. See **Table 5-3** for examples of the wide variance in potassium content in salt substitutes and seasoning agents. Oral potassium replacement is favored because it allows the plasma potassium concentration to rise slowly and equilibrate with the potassium concentration within the cells. Also, larger doses may be given by the oral route than by the intravenous route.[45] Although oral replacement is safer than intravenous replacement, it is not without risk. Because KCl is efficiently absorbed through the GI tract, it is possible to cause hyperkalemia with oral supplements.[46]

Intravenous Potassium Replacement

When dietary potassium intake is inadequate, and when oral potassium supplements are not feasible, the intravenous (IV) route becomes necessary for replacement. The IV route is mandatory for patients with severe hypokalemia (i.e., potassium level of less than 2.5 mEq/L). **Table 5-4** summarizes information regarding the safe intravenous administration of potassium.

Table 5-3 Potassium Content of Some Salt Substitutes and Seasoning Agents

Preparation	Potassium (mg/teaspoon)	Potassium (mEq/teaspoon)
Nu-Salt	3180	82
AlsoSalt	1424	37
Mrs. Dash, salt-free, original	40	1

Although potassium chloride (KCl) is typically used to compensate for potassium deficits, other potassium salts are also available, such as potassium acetate and potassium phosphate. Potassium acetate can be used to treat patients with hypokalemia associated with metabolic acidosis (as in renal tubular acidosis and potassium-losing nephritis); the acetate is metabolized to bicarbonate and helps correct the acidosis. Potassium phosphate may be used when the patient has deficits of both potassium and phosphate.

Table 5-4 Considerations in Administering Potassium Intravenously

Dilute Potassium Solutions Prior to Administration
Concentrated potassium solutions from ampoules should *never* be directly administered into a vein.

Maximal Concentration of Potassium Solutions According to Delivery Site
- *Peripheral vein:* The most frequently recommended maximal concentration of KCl in a peripheral vein is 40 mEq/L. [47]
- *Central vein:* The maximal recommended concentration in a central vein is 100 mEq/L.[48]

Rate of Administration
In usual situations, potassium is administered at a rate not exceeding 10 mEq/hr.
- Infusion rate should not exceed 20 mEq/hr unless malignant ventricular arrhythmia or paralysis is present.[49]

Protocols for Safe Administration of Potassium
Protocols for the safe administration of potassium solutions in specific institutions and agencies should be jointly written by pharmacists, nurses, and physicians. General precautions include the following measures:
- Specify limits for the concentration of potassium to be used in peripheral and central veins (see the recommendations earlier in this table).
- Limit the amount of potassium available in a single container for peripheral and venous delivery (such as 40 mEq/L for peripheral veins and 10 mEq/100 mL for central veins) to minimize the possibility of accidental over-infusion.
- Use an infusion pump to control the flow rate, and carefully monitor the rate to be sure that the pump is working properly.
- Check urine volume; a urine output greater than 30 mL/hr in an adult is recommended to avoid producing transient hyperkalemia. If potassium replacement is needed in an oliguric patient, the amount must be reduced according to the level of renal function.
- Check the infusion site frequently for extravasation. KCl inadvertently administered into subcutaneous tissue produces pain and tissue injury and needs to be detected early.
- Preparation of potassium solutions for intravenous use should be performed in the pharmacy.
- The concentrated forms of KCl solution should not be stored in patient care areas; if they are, they should be kept in a separate locked cabinet and clearly marked as "Must be diluted before administration."

Possibility for Errors in Administering Intravenous Potassium. From 1996 to 1998, the Accreditation Committee of JCAHO's Board of Commissioners reported that medication errors involving the administrating of potassium chloride (KCl) was a serious problem.[50] For example, during these two years, the Joint Commission reviewed 10 patient deaths stemming from misadministration of KCl; in 8 of the cases, the error involved direct infusion of concentrated KCl. A contributing factor in all 10 cases was the availability of concentrated KCl on the nursing units. In 6 of 8 cases, KCl was mistaken for other medications (due to similarities in packaging and labeling). Among the medications confused with KCl were heparin, furosemide (Lasix), and sodium chloride. Because of these problems, JCAHO (now known as The Joint Commission) suggested that healthcare organizations eliminate the availability of concentrated KCl outside of the pharmacy, unless safeguards are in place. Some institutions remain reluctant to remove KCl from patient care areas for fear that the medication will not be immediately available in emergency situations. If potassium chloride is kept on the units, it has been recommended that it be stored in a locked cupboard, separate from all other solutions.[51] Further, it is recommended that the medication be clearly marked, indicating that it must be diluted before administration.

To help reduce medication errors involving KCl, a multidisciplinary group of investigators developed a mandatory request form for physicians ordering intravenous KCl.[52] Before the form was implemented, the incidence of post-infusion elevations of serum potassium in the involved institution was 7.7% (103/1341). After implementation of the form, the incidence of post-infusion elevations of serum potassium was 0% (0/150). Among the 16 items included on the form are the patient's weight in kilograms, laboratory potassium and creatinine values before infusion, and other sources of potassium.

Pain at Infusion Site of KCl. Administration of KCl in a peripheral vein at a concentration greater than 40 mEq/L is often associated with discomfort; the discomfort increases as the concentration of KCl increases. Pain at the infusion site is more likely if the patient already has phlebitis (due to prolonged cannulation of the site or previous infusions of irritating medications at the site).

In a double-blind study of 28 subjects, researchers evaluated the effectiveness of a pretreatment IV bolus of 3 mL lignocaine (versus a placebo bolus dose of 3 mL of 0.9% NaCl) at the infusion site in alleviating pain associated with the administration of concentrated KCl solutions (20 mEq/100 mL) over a 2-hour period.[53] They concluded that pain at the IV site was reduced in the group whose members received the lignocaine bolus dose.

In an earlier study, the effect of lidocaine in alleviating pain caused by intravenous KCl administration was evaluated in six healthy volunteers.[54] Each subject received KCl in a concentration of 200 mEq/L (10 mEq KCl in 50 mL D_5W) in both arms. One of the infusions had 10 mg lidocaine added (although the subjects were not told which infusion contained the lidocaine). The solutions were infused over 1 hour and each person was asked to rate the degree of pain in each arm on a 7-point scale (1 = mild, 7 = severe). Pain was less in the arm with the lidocaine (mean = 3.17) than in the arm without lidocaine (mean = 6.17). It is worth noting, however, that the pain was reported as at least moderate in the group receiving the lidocaine.

A report from the Institute of Safe Medication Practices (ISMP) described a case in which a physician prescribed three sequential IV potassium chloride infusions of 40 mEq in 250-mL bags for a patient with severe hypokalemia.[55] Each of the bags was to infuse over a period of 4 hours. During infusion of the first bag, the patient complained of burning pain at the infusion site. The physician then prescribed 25 mg of lidocaine to be added to each of the subsequent bags to relieve venous discomfort. Unfortunately, an error was made by the nurse who added the lidocaine to the bags; 250 mg was added to each bag (rather than the prescribed 25 mg to each bag). Thus the patient received 500 mg of lidocaine during the course of the next two infusions. Fortunately, because the patient had a pacemaker, adverse effects attributable to the infusions were suppressed.

In another report, regular insulin was erroneously added to a potassium infusion instead of lidocaine; multiple bags were prepared in this manner, resulting in recurrent hypoglycemia before the error was detected.[56] A question was raised by the authors: "Do the benefits of adding lidocaine to KCl infusions outweigh the risks?"[57] Whenever an extra step is added to a process, the risk for error increases. It is also possible that adding lidocaine could mask infection or vein injury that presents as phlebitis. Evidence that lidocaine can produce significant pain reduction with KCl infusions is limited, given the small sample sizes and different protocols used in the studies to test its efficacy for this purpose.

Clinical Considerations

1. Take measures to prevent hypokalemia when possible. Prevention may take the form of encouraging extra potassium intake for at-risk patients (when the diet allows). Some foods high in potassium are listed in Table 5-2. Of course, one must always consider dietary restrictions imposed by other conditions (e.g., diabetes mellitus or obesity).

2. Monitor for hypokalemia in at-risk patients (**Table 5-5**). Because hypokalemia can be life-threatening, it is important to detect this condition early.

3. Assess patients receiving digitalis who are at risk for hypokalemia especially closely for symptoms of digitalis toxicity because hypokalemia potentiates the action of digitalis. Be aware that the physician usually prefers to keep the serum potassium level in the high normal range (> 4.0 mEq/L) in patients receiving digitalis.

4. When hypokalemia is due to abuse of laxatives or diuretics, education of the patient may help alleviate the problem. Part of the nursing history and assessment should be directed at identifying problems amenable to prevention through education.

5. Educate patients regarding the use of salt substitutes, keeping the following facts in mind:
   • Salt substitutes may contain 60 mEq or more of potassium per teaspoon.
   • As with any potassium-containing substance, there is a danger of hyperkalemia with excessive use, particularly if renal function is impaired.
   • Although salt substitutes are often viewed as helpful for those taking potassium-losing diuretics (such as furosemide or thiazides), they can be dangerous for patients taking potassium-conserving diuretics (such as spironolactone, tramterene, and amiloride) and angiotensin-converting enzyme (ACE) inhibitors.

Table 5-5 Summary of Hypokalemia

Causes	*Clinical Signs*
Gastrointestinal Loss	*Skeletal Muscle*
Diarrhea	Fatigue
Laxative abuse	Weakness (initially most prominent in legs, especially the quadriceps, and then extending to the arms; involvement of respiratory muscles soon follows)
Villous adenoma	
Prolonged gastric suction	Cramps
	Rhabdomyolysis
Nonpharmacologic Renal Loss	
Hyperaldosteronism	*Cardiovascular System*
Osmotic diuresis	Increased sensitivity to digitalis
	ST-segment depression
Drugs	Flattened T waves
See drugs listed in Table 5-1	Ventricular arrhythmias
	Cardiac arrest
Shift into Cells	
Alkalosis	*Gastrointestinal System*
Excessive insulin administration	Decreased bowel motility (intestinal ileus)
Hyperalimentation	
	Renal System
Poor Intake	Impaired urinary concentrating ability when hypokalemia is prolonged, causing dilute urine, polyuria, nocturia, and polydipsia
Anorexia nervosa	
Alcoholism	Increased ammonia production and H^+ excretion
Debilitation	
	Lab Data
	Serum potassium < 3.5 mEq/L
	Often associated with alkalosis

6. Be thoroughly familiar with considerations involved with administering potassium intravenously. See Table 5-4.

HYPOKALEMIA CASE STUDIES

Case Study 5-1

A 40-year-old woman was admitted to the hospital with complaints of progressive muscle weakness. She had been taking a thiazide diuretic for several weeks and had recently developed vomiting and diarrhea. Postural hypotension was present (110/70 mm Hg when supine and 90/60 mm Hg when upright). Skin turgor was reduced. Laboratory data included the following: plasma K 2 mEq/L, HCO₃ 40 mEq/L (normal approximately 24 mEq/), Cl 70 mEq/L. (normal approximately 100 mEq/L).

Commentary. This patient had increased losses of potassium from the GI tract as well as in her urine. Her major presenting symptom—diffuse progressive muscle weakness—is common in hypokalemia. In addition to hypokalemia, signs of fluid volume deficit were present (i.e., reduced skin turgor and postural hypotension). Although postural hypotension is usually thought of as being a symptom of fluid volume deficit, it can also be a sign of hypokalemia. On questioning, it was found that the patient was taking a friend's diuretic to induce weight loss. Note the presence of hypochloremic alkalosis, evidenced by the below-normal chloride level and greatly elevated bicarbonate level.

Case Study 5-2

A 65-year-old man with a draining intestinal fistula was receiving a total parenteral nutrition (TPN) solution at the rate of 120 mL/hr. The total potassium intake was 100 mEq/day. On a routine ECG, flattened T waves, ST-segment depression, and arrhythmias were detected. A blood sample was then drawn that revealed a plasma potassium level of 2.5 mEq/L. The rate of TPN infusion was tapered promptly, the serum glucose levels were monitored closely, and an IV infusion of KCl was initiated in a peripheral vein at the rate of 10 mEq/hr. After alleviation of the signs of hypokalemia, the TPN infusion was slowly reinstated, with adequate potassium being added to the solution.

Commentary. Potassium requirements in patients who are receiving TPN vary. Most often the potassium need is higher than normal because, during nutritional repletion, potassium will be deposited in the newly synthesized cells, causing serum levels to fall abruptly if potassium is not supplied in sufficient amounts. This patient's needs were even greater than usual because intestinal fistulas result in significant potassium loss.

Case Study 5-3

A case was reported in which a 21-year-old hypertensive woman at 31 weeks of gestation was admitted to labor and delivery with a 2-week history of progressive fatigue and weakness.[58] In the 2 days prior to admission, she had difficulty ambulating and could not climb stairs without assistance. Laboratory analysis showed a serum potassium level of 1.7 mEq/L, a bicarbonate level of 32.3 mEq/L, and an arterial pH of 7.53 (evidence of severe hypokalemia and metabolic alkalosis). The patient also showed signs of rhabdomyolysis (breakdown of striated muscle, evidenced by an elevated creatine phosphokinase). Upon inquiry into the patient's history, it was found that she was consuming 1 box (454 g) of pure baking soda (sodium bicarbonate) per day. The baking soda was discontinued and the patient improved significantly; the weakness and hypertension quickly resolved and her electrolytes and creatine phosphokinase levels returned to normal over the course of 1 week. She went on to deliver a normal fetus at 39 weeks gestation.

Commentary. The patient's eating disorder (pica) caused her to consume large quantities of baking soda (sodium bicarbonate), which led to metabolic alkalosis and subsequently to hypokalemia. Elevations in serum pH cause an influx of potassium into the cells as hydrogen ions are released to help balance the elevated serum bicarbonate levels. The hypertension was likely due to the high sodium load in sodium bicarbonate. In the United States, pica is most commonly seen in pregnant women and children as well as among persons of lower socioeconomic status.[59] Women who are most at risk during pregnancy are patients who are African American, have a family history of pica, and live in rural areas.[60]

Case Study 5-4

A case was reported in which a 77-year-old grandmother was admitted with nausea and vomiting after babysitting her infant grandchild who was infected with rotavirus.[61] The vomiting persisted for 3 days and the patient was able to consume only scant amounts of water, ginger ale, and crackers, even several days after the vomiting ceased. Upon examination in the emergency department, the patient had tachycardia, orthostatic hypotension, and poor skin turgor. Laboratory results included an elevated hematocrit (48%), consistent with mild volume depletion. The serum potassium was 3.5 mEq/L, and the magnesium and phosphorus levels were within normal range. While in the hospital, the patient was treated with 10% dextrose in 0.9% sodium chloride intravenously and started on a full liquid diet with premeal antiemetics to reduce prandial nausea. Serum chemistries on hospital day 2 showed a potassium level of 2.5 mEq/L in addition to below-normal magnesium and phosphorus levels.

Commentary. The patient was diagnosed with refeeding syndrome resulting from intravenous dextrose solution and oral feedings after a week of minimal oral intake. Infusions of potassium phosphate and magnesium sulfate were administered along with oral potassium phosphate supplements and the electrolyte levels normalized over the next 2 days.

Case Study 5-5

A case was reported in which a 15-year-old girl presented to her pediatrician with complaints of muscle weakness and dizziness.[62] Her weight was in the 75th percentile for her age and her height was in the 15th percentile for her age. Upon the discovery of hypotension, she was transferred to the emergency department, where laboratory studies provided the following data: serum Na 135 mEq/L, serum K 2.1 mEq/L, serum Cl 91 mEq/L, serum CO_2 content 33 mEq/L. At that time, the patient was given 2 L of normal saline intravenously and discharged to home with instructions to take oral potassium chloride supplements for several days. Two days later, the patient returned to her pediatrician with complaints of persistent weakness and intermittent hypotension. The patient reported nocturia (routinely getting up one to two times during the night to void). It was found that her father took furosemide, receiving a 90-day supply at a time. Furosemide was identified in the teenager's urine; upon repeated questioning, the patient admitted to taking one to two tablets of her father's furosemide at night every 3 to 4 days so that the missing pills would not be noticed. She did this in an attempt to lose weight; she hoped to pursue a dancing career after finishing high school.

Commentary. CO_2 content in venous blood reflects the serum bicarbonate concentration; in this case, it showed metabolic alkalosis secondary to the hypokalemia caused by the unauthorized ingestion of furosemide (a potassium-losing diuretic). The most common cause for these imbalances in children is vomiting; however, there was no evidence of vomiting in this patient. Reviewing the patient's social history was important in identifying furosemide abuse.

Case Study 5-6

A case was reported in which a 19-year-old girl with cerebral palsy developed a postoperative wound infection following spinal fusion for scoliosis.[63] She was treated with intravenous gentamicin. The antibiotic was continued for 20 days; the patient also received intravenous hyperalimentation. On day 17 of therapy, the patient was found to have hypokalemia (2.7 mEq/L), hypomagnesemia (1 mg/dL), and metabolic alkalosis (serum bicarbonate 33 mEq/L). The serum creatinine and blood urea nitrogen levels remained within normal range and the gentamicin trough level was maintained within the therapeutic range. Supplemental potassium and magnesium were given, and the electrolyte abnormalities resolved 5 days after gentamicin was discontinued.

Commentary. Elevations of serum creatinine and BUN concentrations are not uncommon in patients receiving gentamicin therapy; fortunately, this was not a problem in this patient. However, she did experience hypokalemic metabolic alkalosis and hypomagnesemia, secondary to increased renal loss of potassium and magnesium associated with the use of gentamycin.

Case Study 5-7

For the past 6 months, a 65-year-old man had received diuretics to manage his hypertension. During a visit to his physician, he reported that he was more thirsty than usual and frequently had to get up at night to urinate (nocturia). Laboratory analysis found his serum potassium to be 2.4 mEq/L. The patient was hospitalized for evaluation; it was found that he could concentrate his urine to only 300 mOsm/kg on fluid restriction (instead of the expected 1200–1400 mOsm/kg in normal renal function). After correction of the hypokalemia, his renal concentrating ability and urine volume eventually returned to normal.

Commentary. This patient had acquired nephrogenic diabetes insipidus (NDI) due to hypokalemia. Many patients with potassium depletion complain of polyuria associated with reduced renal concentrating ability (due to poor responsiveness of the kidneys to ADH in patients with sustained hypokalemia). This resistance to ADH may be due to an interference with the generation and action of cyclic adenosine monophosphate. Although the NDI associated with hypokalemia is usually reversible, recall that more severe changes are possible with prolonged hypokalemia. The serum sodium level was not elevated in this case because the patient managed to drink sufficient fluids to match the increase output of dilute urine.

HYPERKALEMIA

Hyperkalemia refers to a greater than normal serum potassium concentration. It seldom occurs in patients with normal renal function. In fact, fewer than 1% of healthy adults develop hyperkalemia, attesting to the potent mechanisms that can increase renal excretion of potassium when necessary.[64] According to researchers, the incidence of hyperkalemia is twice as high in hospitalized adults older than 60 years of age than in younger hospitalized adults.[65] Like hypokalemia, hyperkalemia is often due to iatrogenic (treatment-induced) causes. Although less common than hypokalemia, it is often more dangerous because cardiac arrest is more frequently associated with high serum potassium levels.

Causes

Some of the causes of hyperkalemia are simple and straightforward, such as direct gain of potassium exceeding the kidney's excretory rate. Others are related to shifts of potassium out of the cells into the plasma, or to decreased production of aldosterone, which causes potassium retention. A number of commonly used drugs produce potassium-elevating effects, particularly when patients have preexisting abnormalities in potassium metabolism.

Pseudohyperkalemia

Hemolyzed Blood Specimen. A number of causes of factitious ("pseudo") hyperkalemia exist. The most common cause is a hemolyzed blood sample (a condition in which potassium leaks from the ruptured erythrocytes into the plasma). The laboratory can detect this condition by noting a pink tinge to the plasma (caused by release of hemoglobin by the damaged red blood cells). Other causes of pseudohyperkalemia include marked leukocytosis or thrombocytosis, drawing blood above a site where potassium is infusing, and obtaining a sample from an extremity in which repeated clenching and unclenching of the fist has been performed. Pseudohyperkalemia should be suspected when there is no apparent cause for elevated plasma potassium and there are no changes in muscle strength or on ECG tracings.

Fist Clenching. Although the effect of fist clenching has been recognized for many years, it continues to be a problem. Don et al. reported a case in which a man was admitted for evaluation of hyperkalemia.[66] Blood drawn from this individual in an outpatient setting (using a tourniquet with repeated fist clenching and unclenching) had a serum potassium concentration of 6.9 mEq/L. In the hospital, blood drawn from an indwelling catheter (without use of a tourniquet and fist clenching) had a normal value of 4.1 mEq/L. (The concentration increased to 5.1 mEq/L within 1 minute after application of a tourniquet and repeated fist clenching.) The researchers concluded that it is advisable to avoid fist clenching altogether when obtaining samples for potassium testing and to rely on venous stasis alone, if needed, as an aid in performing phlebotomy.

A more recent report indicated that finger flexing during venipuncture can cause pseudohyperkalemia.[67] Investigators compared plasma potassium readings from 500 consecutive blood draws when squeeze balls were used during venipuncture to 500 consecutive readings obtained after use of squeeze balls was stopped. The incidence of above-normal potassium levels decreased from 10.5% when squeeze balls were used to 2.6% when they were not used.

Pseudohyperkalemia is an important problem. For example, it can mask a real illness where hypokalemia is actually present.[68] Conversely, a falsely elevated potassium value in a presurgical work-up can delay surgery unnecessarily; worse yet, instituting treatment for a "high" potassium level that is factitious can be disastrous.[69] Some clinicians favor withholding treatment for elevated serum potassium levels in stable patients until a confirmatory ECG can be obtained.

Although absence of ECG evidence for hyperkalemia is usually consistent with a factitious reading, it does not necessarily preclude the presence of hyperkalemia. That is, although ECG abnormalities are typically present, they may be absent in nearly half of patients with elevated serum potassium levels. Moderate levels of hyperkalemia are more difficult to detect by ECG than are severe potassium elevations. A study of 220 ECGs performed on patients at risk for hyperkalemia indicated that ECG interpretations made by two physicians were not especially good predictors of hyperkalemia; this finding prompted the researchers to caution that it is prudent to delay treatment for hyperkalemia in stable patients until confirmatory serum values can be obtained to confirm the presence of hyperkalemia.[70]

The best evidence of hyperkalemia is a correctly repeated laboratory assay that confirms the original report; the evidence is strengthened by an ECG report that also indicates the presence of hyperkalemia.

Renal Failure

A major cause of hyperkalemia is decreased renal excretion of potassium. This relationship is understandable when one considers that the kidney is the major route of potassium excretion. Significant hyperkalemia, therefore, is commonly seen in patients with untreated renal failure, particularly when potassium is being liberated from cells during infectious processes or when exogenous sources of potassium are excessive (as in diet or medications).

Hypoaldosteronism

A deficiency of adrenal steroids causes sodium loss and potassium retention; thus hypoaldosteronism and Addison's disease predispose patients to hyperkalemia. Hyporeninemic hypoaldosteronism (type IV renal tubular acidosis) is also a renal cause of hyperkalemia. This condition is usually seen in elderly persons with mild renal insufficiency, many of whom have diabetes as well.

Drugs That Predispose Patients to Hyperkalemia

Table 5-6 summarizes the drugs that predispose patients to hyperkalemia. Potassium-conserving diuretics, such as spironolactone (Aldactone), triamterene (Dyrenium), and amiloride (Midamor), are commonly implicated as causes

Table 5-6 Summary of Medications Associated with Hyperkalemia

Medication	Comments
ACE inhibitors: captopril (Capoten), enalapril (Vasotec), ramipril (Altace), benazepril (Lotensin)	Mean increase in plasma potassium concentration after ACE inhibitors is less than 0.3 to 0.4 mEq/L if renal function is normal; clinically important hyperkalemia is possible if the patient is taking potassium supplements or has renal disease.[71]
Beta-adrenergic receptor blockers: atenolol (Tenormin), propranolol (Inderal), metoprolol (Lopressor)	Usually associated with only minimal elevation of plasma potassium concentration (e.g., less than 0.5 mEq/L). More likely to elevate plasma potassium concentration if administered to patients with renal disease.[72]
Aldosterone antagonists: spironolactone (Aldactone), eplerenone (Inspra)	Predispose patients to hyperkalemia by impairing renal excretion of potassium. Probability of hyperkalemia is high if patient is also taking ACE inhibitors.[73]
Other potassium-sparing diuretics: amiloride, triamterene	Predispose patients to hyperkalemia by impairing renal excretion of potassium. Probability of hyperkalemia high if patient has renal disease.
Heparin	Hyperkalemia occurs in approximately 7% of patients receiving long-term heparin therapy. Typically the hyperkalemia is moderate and rarely is life-threatening.[74]
Nonsteroidal anti-inflammatory drugs (NSAIDs): aspirin, ibuprofen (Advil, Motrin), naproxen	In patients with normal renal function, mean plasma potassium elevation is approximately 0.2 mEq/L. In patients with chronic renal disease, elevation of plasma potassium can exceed 1 mEq/L.[75]
Trimetoprim (contained in Bactrim)	Potassium levels rise progressively over 4 to 5 days in patients receiving standard or high-dose trimetoprim, especially if chronic renal disease is present; more than 50% of inpatients on this drug have potassium levels exceeding 5.0 mEq/L; 20% have levels greater than 5.5 mEq/L.[76]
Cyclosporin	Can cause hyperkalemia in patients with organ transplants.
Drospirenone and ethinyl estradiol: Yasmin, Yas	Drospirenone in these products has a mineralocorticoid effect, equivalent to spironolactone 25 mg.[77]
Nutritionals and herbal supplements	Examples of herbs with high potassium content include Noni juice, alfalfa, dandelion, horsetail, and nettle.[78]
Digitalis overdose	Can cause hyperkalemia through inhibition of the Na/K ATPase pump, allowing for a shift of intracellular potassium to the plasma.

of hyperkalemia—particularly when there is renal dysfunction, potassium supplementation, or concomitant use of other drugs predisposing patients to potassium retention. Serious and even fatal complications have been associated with use of these drugs.[79]

Beta-adrenergic blockers (such as propranolol) increase the risk of hyperkalemia by interfering with the entry of potassium into the cells. The increase in plasma potassium concentration is usually modest (0.2–0.5 mEq/L) and is corrected upon discontinuation of the drug.[80] Dangerous hyperkalemia is rarely due to beta blockers alone,[81] but these agents can exacerbate hyperkalemia in patients with other risk factors. Digoxin has produced fatal hyperkalemia when taken in large amounts.[82] Although digitalis toxicity is aggravated by hypokalemia, severe digitalis intoxication poisons the Na/K ATPase pump, resulting in potassium release from the cells and hyperkalemia.

Captopril (an ACE inhibitor) is one of the drugs most frequently implicated in producing hyperkalemia.[83] Significant hyperkalemia has been reported in association with captopril in patients with renal insufficiency, presumably due to the inhibitory effect of the drug on aldosterone secretion.[84]

Cyclosporin can cause hyperkalemia through a combination of mechanisms. For example, it can decrease potassium excretion, decrease prostaglandin production, and lower plasma renin and aldosterone levels. Cyclosporin-induced hyperkalemia does not seem to be related either to dosage or duration of therapy.[85]

Heparin administration blocks a step in aldosterone synthesis, and can conceivably be associated with hyperkalemia. While not usually a cause of this condition in itself, it can contribute to hyperkalemia caused by other sources.

Trimethoprim-sulfamethoxazole can cause hyperkalemia, especially when renal insufficiency is present; the mechanism appears to be its amiloride-like action.[86] In one study, hyperkalemia occurred in 20% to 53% of patients with AIDS while they were receiving high doses of trimethoprim in combination with sulfamethoxazole or dapsone for the treatment of *Pneumocystis carinii* pneumonia.[87]

Nonsteroidal anti-inflammatory drugs (NSAIDs), when taken by patients with renal insufficiency, predispose users to hyperkalemia. The hyperkalemia appears to be related to reduced plasma and urinary aldosterone levels.[88] (See Table 5-6.)

Drosirenone is contained in some birth control pills. For example, Yasmin contains 3 mg of drosperinone and is comparable to a 25-mg dose of spironolactone in terms of predisposing to hyperkalemia.[89] Thus recommendations from the manufacturer are that the drug not be used in patients with conditions that predispose them to developing hyperkalemia (i.e., renal or adrenal insufficiency). Similarly, recommendations are that women receiving daily, long-term pharmacologic treatment for chronic conditions with medications that can increase the serum potassium concentration (e.g., ACE inhibitors, potassium-sparing diuretics, aldosterone antagonists, heparin, NSAIDs) have these levels monitored during the first treatment cycle with drosperinone. Although product labeling for the oral contraceptive (Yasmin) recommends potassium monitoring in the first month of use for women concurrently receiving medications that could increase serum potassium levels, there is evidence of limited compliance with this recommendation by prescribing physicians.[90] Among barriers to compliance with potassium testing identified in a recent study were selective physician acceptance of the recommendations and failure of some healthcare plans to pay for the testing. A recent study compared the incidence of hyperkalemia in more than 22,000 patients receiving drospirenone to that observed in more than 44,000 patients receiving other oral contraceptives and found no significant difference.[91]

High Potassium Intake

Although sustained hyperkalemia is rarely observed after potassium ingestion in individuals with normal renal function, it can occur with massive oral potassium ingestion or by rapid IV potassium administration. A case was reported in which a young physician took potassium in the form of a potassium-containing salt substitute to ward off hypokalemia after diuretic use and a bout of diarrhea.[92] On admission to a hospital, her plasma potassium concentration was 8.4 mEq/L. An ECG revealed signs of severe hyperkalemia (peaked T waves, absent P wave, and a broadened QRS complex). She experienced cardiorespiratory arrest and was resuscitated. After treatment, the hyperkalemia resolved; however, post-hypoxic brain damage occurred. Although excessive potassium intake by the oral route is less dangerous than the IV route (because GI absorption may be limited by either vomiting or diarrhea from the large potassium load), the previously described case illustrates that care is required with potassium administration in all situations. Cases have been reported in which both intentional and accidental oral potassium overdoses have resulted in fatalities.[93, 94]

Although potassium-containing salt substitutes are often recommended for patients requiring sodium restriction, they are contraindicated for patients on potassium-restricted diets or those with renal disease who have diminished capacity to excrete potassium. As shown in Table 5-3, the potassium content in most salt substitutes is quite high.

Because it is possible to exceed the renal tolerance of any patient with rapid IV potassium administration, extreme caution is required when administering potassium solutions. (See Table 5-4.) In addition, blood transfusions can be a source of excessive potassium administration. The serum concentration of potassium increases as storage time of blood increases; therefore, aged blood should not be given as transfusions to patients with impaired renal function (see Chapter 10).

In a patient with renal failure, the potassium content in tube feedings may be sufficient to cause hyperkalemia, as may intravenous hyperalimentation solutions containing usually recommended potassium concentrations. See Chapter 12.

Tissue Injury

Recall that cellular fluid has a very high potassium concentration (approximately 150 mEq/L). Thus it is understandable that elevated plasma potassium concentrations are noted following extensive tissue trauma (as in crush injuries or burns), when potassium leaks out of the cells into the plasma. For example, in a study of 372 patients who sustained crush injuries during a major earthquake, investigators found that hyperkalemia was a major cause of early deaths.[95] Similarly, hyperkalemia can occur during lysis of malignant cells after chemotherapy or radiation therapy, especially in patients with lymphomas, leukemia, and meyloma. See the discussion of tumor lysis syndrome in Chapter 22.

Acidosis

Potassium leaks out of the cells in acidosis, as hydrogen ions enter the cells to help correct the acidic extracellular pH. However, evidence suggests that the extent of potassium shifting from the cells that occurs in acidosis is greatly influenced by the cause of the acidosis. More extensive shifting is associated with metabolic acidosis due to the accumulation of non-organic acids (as occurs in diarrhea and renal failure) than in metabolic acidosis due to organic acids (such as lactic acidosis or ketoacidosis). Respiratory acidosis has less effect on potassium shifting than does metabolic acidosis. (Chapter 9 provides a more thorough discussion of this topic.)

Clinical Signs

Hyperkalemia can cause a variety of problems, most of which are related to the effects of potassium on cellular membrane potential (**Table 5-7**). By far, the most prominent is the effect of hyperkalemia on the myocardium.

Cardiac Effects

As the plasma potassium concentration is increased, disturbances in cardiac conduction occur. (See Figure 5-1.) The earliest changes, which often appear when the serum potassium level exceeds 6 mEq/L, are peaked narrow T waves and a shortened QT interval. If the serum potassium level continues to rise, the PR interval becomes prolonged and is followed by disappearance of the P waves. Finally, there is decomposition and prolongation of the QRS complex. Ventricular arrhythmias and cardiac arrest may occur at any point in this progression.

Hyperkalemia slows the heart rate, may cause atrioventricular block, and prolongs depolarization.[96] Factors exaggerating ECG changes of hyperkalemia include low serum sodium and calcium levels, acidosis, and a high serum magnesium concentration. These changes are counteracted by an increased serum calcium level, explaining why calcium infusion is used an emergency treatment for serious hyperkalemia.

In profound hyperkalemia, the heart becomes dilated and flaccid due to decreased strength of contraction (related to a decreased number of active muscle units). Detrimental myocardial effects of hyperkalemia are more pronounced when the serum potassium level becomes elevated rapidly.

Neuromuscular Effects

Skeletal muscles are particularly sensitive to hyperkalemia, resulting in muscle weakness and even paralysis related to a depolarization block in muscle. Typically, muscle weakness does not occur until the plasma potassium concentration is more than 8 mEq/L.[97] Muscle weakness and paralysis usually affect the large muscles of the legs first, followed by the trunk and upper extremity muscles. Cardiac muscle is also weakened by hyperkalemia; the ultimate cause of death may be cardiac failure in diastole.

Gastrointestinal Changes

Gastrointestinal symptoms, such as nausea, intermittent intestinal colic, and diarrhea, can occur in hyperkalemic patients.[98] These changes have been attributed to hyperactivity of smooth muscle.

Table 5-7 Summary of Hyperkalemia

Causes	Clinical Signs
Pseudohyperkalemia	*Neuromuscular Effects*
• Prolonged tight application of tourniquet; fist clenching and unclenching immediately before or during blood drawing	• Vague muscular weakness
• Hemolysis of blood sample	• Flaccid muscle paralysis (first noticed in legs, later in arms and trunk; respiratory muscles and muscles supplied by cranial nerves are usually spared)
• Leukocytosis	• Paresthesias of face, tongue, feet, and hands
• Thrombocytosis	
	Cardiovascular System
Decreased Potassium Excretion	• Tall, peaked T waves
• Oliguric renal failure	• Widened QRS complex progressing to sine waves
• Potassium-conserving diuretics	• Ventricular arrhythmias
• Hypoaldosteronism	• Cardiac arrest
High Potassium Intake	*Gastrointestinal System*
• Excessive use of oral potassium supplements	• Nausea
• Excessive use of salt substitutes	• Intermittent intestinal colic or diarrhea
• Rapid IV potassium administration	
• Rapid transfusion of aged blood	*Laboratory Data*
	• Serum potassium > 5.0 mEq/L
Shift of Potassium Out of Cells	• Often associated with acidosis
• Acidosis	
• Tissue damage, as in crush injuries	
• Malignant cell lysis after chemotherapy	
Drugs	
See Table 5-6.	

Treatment

Restriction of Potassium Intake and Drugs Potentiating Hyperkalemia

In non-acute situations, adequate treatment may be limited to restriction of dietary potassium and discontinuance of agents predisposing to hyperkalemia (including potassium-sparing diuretics, potassium supplements, and potassium-containing salt substitutes). Other drugs that predispose patients to hyperkalemia are listed in Table 5-6. Low-potassium foods are listed in **Table 5-8.**

Methods to Promote Potassium Excretion

Sodium Polystyrene Sulfonate. Sodium polystyrene sulfonate is a cation-exchange resin that can be given orally or rectally to remove potassium from the body by exchanging sodium for potassium in the intestinal tract. Each gram of

resin may bind 1 mEq of potassium and release 1 to 2 mEq of sodium; because of the released sodium, use of this resin is limited in patients with congestive heart failure.[99] The onset of action of the resin is relatively slow; therefore, it is typically administered to treat mild to moderate cases of hyperkalemia. If used to treat severe hyperkalemia, it is given in conjunction with more rapid-acting treatments to lower serum potassium levels. When given orally, the resin is usually administered with an osmotic agent (such as sorbitol) to prevent constipation. If the oral route cannot be used, the drug can be given by enema and retained for a period of at least 30 to 60 minutes. Each enema can lower the plasma potassium concentration by as much as 0.5 to 1.0 mEq/L.[100]

Dialysis. Dialysis can remove potassium effectively but is reserved for patients in whom more conservative methods do not suffice. Although peritoneal dialysis can be started relatively quickly, it is not as effective as hemodialysis in

Table 5-8 Examples of Low-Potassium Foods and Beverages

Food	Potassium (mg)
Butter, 1 tablespoon	3 (< 1 mEq)
Cake, angel food, 1 piece	26 (< 1 mEq)
Candy, vanilla fudge, 1 piece	8 (< 1 mEq)
Candy, hard, 1 piece	0 (0 mEq)
Carbonated beverage, cola, 12 fl oz	7 (< 1 mEq)
Carrot, baby, raw, 1 medium	24 (< 1 mEq)
Cheese, low fat, cheddar or Colby, 1 oz	19 (<1 mEq)
Cookie, butter, 1 cookie	6 (<1 mEq)
Crackers, cheese, regular, 10 crackers	15 (<1 mEq)
Cream, heavy whipping, 1 tablespoon	15 (<1 mEq)
Gelatin dessert, dry mix, prepared with water, ½ cup	1 (< 1 mE1)
Grape drink, canned, 8 fl oz	30 (<1 mEq)
Honey, 1 tablespoon	11 (<1 mEq)
Jams and preserves, 1 tablespoon	15 (<1 mEq)
Margarine, 1 teaspoon	1 (<1 mEq)
Mustard, 1 teaspoon	7 (<1 mEq)
Radish, raw, one	10 (<1 mEq)
Rolls, hamburger or hotdog plain, one	40 (1 mEq)
Salad dressing, French, 1 tablespoon	3 (<1 mEq)
Snacks, Kellogg's Rice Krispies Treat, 1 bar	9 (<1 mEq)
Sugars, brown sugar, 1 teaspoon	4 (<1 mEq)

Source: USDA National Nutrient Database for Standard Reference, Release 21. United States Department of Agriculture, Agricultural Research Service, 2008.

removing potassium from the body. That is, the rate of potassium removal is many times faster with hemodialysis than with peritoneal dialysis. A major limitation of hemodialysis is the time needed to prepare the patient for the procedure.

Emergency Measures

Rationales for the use of medications to treat severe hyperkalemia emergently are summarized in **Table 5-9.**

Clinical Considerations

1. Be aware of patients at risk for hyperkalemia and monitor for its occurrence. Because hyperkalemia is life-threatening, it is imperative to detect this condition early.

2. Take measures to prevent hyperkalemia when possible by following guidelines for administering potassium safely. (See Table 5-4.)
3. Avoid administration of potassium-conserving diuretics, potassium supplements, or salt substitutes to patients with poor renal function.
4. Caution patients to use salt substitutes with a high potassium content sparingly if they are taking other supplementary forms of potassium or are taking potassium-conserving diuretics (e.g., spironolactone, triamterene, amiloride).
5. Caution hyperkalemic patients to avoid foods high in potassium content. (See Table 5-2.)
6. To avoid false reports of hyperkalemia, take the following precautions:
   - Avoid prolonged use of a tourniquet while drawing blood samples.
   - Do not allow the patient to exercise the extremity immediately before drawing a blood sample.
   - Avoid drawing a blood specimen from a site above an infusion of potassium solution (or any solution, for that matter). See the section on obtaining blood samples in Chapter 2.
   - Take the blood sample to the laboratory as soon as possible (serum must be separated from cells within 1 hour after collection).

HYPERKALEMIA CASE STUDIES

Case Study 5-8

A 60-year-old man visited his family physician complaining of chronic tiredness and increased skin pigmentation. On examination, his blood pressure was low (98/60 mm Hg). Blood tests revealed a plasma potassium level of 6.8 mEq/L and a plasma sodium level of 132 mEq/L. The blood urea nitrogen (BUN) was 20 mg/dL and the serum creatinine was 1.2 mg/dL.

Commentary. This patient was diagnosed as having adrenal insufficiency. Recall that aldosterone regulates sodium and potassium balance by causing sodium retention and potassium excretion. Thus a deficit of aldosterone results in potassium retention and elevation of the plasma potassium level. Note that this patient had normal renal function, as evidenced by the BUN and creatinine levels. Increased skin pigmentation is common in adrenal insufficiency.

Table 5-9 Drugs Used in Emergency Treatment of Hyperkalemia

Medication	Comments
Calcium gluconate or calcium chloride	The IV administration of calcium immediately antagonizes the effects of hyperkalemia on the myocardial conduction system and on myocardial repolarization.
	Onset of action is immediate; effect lasts approximately 30 to 60 minutes.[101]
	Calcium does *not* lower plasma potassium concentration.
	If using $CaCl_2$, infuse in a central vein to avoid the possibility of extravasation and tissue necrosis.
	Calcium should be used only when absolutely necessary in patients taking digitalis because hypercalcemia potentiates the toxic effects of digitalis on the myocardium.
Regular insulin and glucose	Intravenous insulin stimulates potassium uptake by the cells, thereby reducing the plasma potassium concentration.
	Onset of action is about 15 minutes; effect lasts approximately 6 to 8 hours.[102]
	It is not necessary to administer glucose with the insulin if the patient's glucose level is significantly elevated.
Albuterol	Temporarily forces plasma potassium into cells.
	Can be given by nebulized inhalation or by IV drip.
	Onset of action is approximately 10 to 30 minutes; effect lasts approximately 3 to 6 hours.[103]
	Risks for arrhythmias suggest that this form of therapy be used only when conventional therapy has failed or fluid overload is a concern.[104]
Sodium bicarbonate	Most effective in patients with metabolic acidosis.
	Short-term bicarbonate infusion apparently does not cause a shift of potassium into the cells.[105]
	Possible problems associated with this treatment include expansion of the ECF and precipitation of congestive heart failure in patients with cardiac disease, as well as precipitation of tetany in patients with preexisting hypocalcemia.
Loop diuretics	Increases renal excretion of potassium.
	Onset of action is approximately 30 to 60 minutes; effects last approximately 4 to 6 hours.[106]
	Loop diuretics are of limited value in patients with severely impaired glomerular filtration rates.

Case Study 5-9

A 30-year-old man with chronic renal failure developed vomiting and diarrhea. Because he became very weak, his family brought him to the emergency room. In addition to severe muscle weakness, the patient had decreased skin turgor. An ECG revealed tall, peaked T waves and widening of the QRS complex. Blood tests revealed a plasma potassium level of 9.4 mEq/L and a creatinine level of 2.9 mg/dL.

Commentary. Due to fluid volume depletion after the bout of vomiting and diarrhea, this patient developed decreased renal perfusion and a reduced ability to excrete potassium. Because of the life-threatening situation (evidenced by the high plasma potassium level and the ECG changes), he was treated with calcium gluconate and sodium bicarbonate. A dextrose and saline solution was administered to achieve volume replacement. After volume was restored to normal, kidney perfusion improved and the patient was again able to excrete potassium. Remember that patients with chronic renal failure can become seriously ill when fluid volume is depleted.

Case Study 5-10

A 65-year-old woman in renal failure was admitted to the emergency room complaining of abdominal cramping and numbness in her extremities. Laboratory data revealed a BUN of 96 mg/dL and a creatinine of 3.9 mg/dL. The serum potassium was 8.6 mEq/L. She was given a retention enema of Kayexalate (sodium polystyrene sulfonate) in 20% sorbitol. She received 50 mL of 50% dextrose and 10 units of regular insulin IV. An infusion of 5% dextrose and 0.45% NaCl containing two ampules of sodium bicarbonate was started at a rate of 25 mL/hr. By the next day, the patient's serum potassium level was reduced to 5.0 mEq/L.

Commentary. Kayexalate is an ion-exchange resin that causes sodium to be exchanged for potassium in the intestine, resulting in potassium excretion by this route. Hypertonic dextrose and insulin favor cellular uptake of potassium. Sustained sodium bicarbonate administration, by alkalinizing the plasma, contributed to the shift of potassium into the cells.

Case Study 5-11

A 75-year-old man with a history of coronary artery disease and myocardial infarction presented at cardiac rehabilitation with complaints of malaise, fatigue, agitation, dyspnea on exertion, and nausea with one episode of vomiting.[107] His medications included torsemide 60 mg once daily, spironolactone 25 mg once daily, Lanoxin 0.25 mg once daily and, enalapril 10 mg once daily., He was immediately admitted to the hospital, where he was noted to have dry mucous membranes, sunken eyes, and a blood pressure of 112/64 mm Hg. The following laboratory results were obtained: Na 139 mEq/L, K 6.4 mEq/L, Cl 100 mEq/L, BUN 74 mg/dL, Cr 2.8 mg/dL. The patient was treated with 10% calcium gluconate IV and 30 g Kayexalate by mouth. Two hours after the Kayexalate was administered, his potassium level had decreased to 5.4 mEq/L. It was assumed that the acute renal failure was due to overdiuresis and possible nephrotoxic effects of enalapril (an ACE inhibitor). The patient was taken off spironolactone (a potassium-sparing diuretic) and was slowly rehydrated with 0.9% NaCl (50 mL/hr) to correct the fluid volume depletion. The enalapril was discontinued and hydralazine was titrated up to 100 mg every 6 hours on discharge. On the day of discharge, the patient's BUN was 45 mg/dL and the serum creatinine was 1.8 mg/dL.

Commentary. Hyperkalemia is a relatively common imbalance in the elderly, and it is often related to prescribed medications (such as potassium-sparing diuretics and ACE inhibitors, as present in this case).

Case Study 5-12

A case was reported in which a 72-year-old man with congestive heart failure and other major comorbidities was admitted to the hospital with a complaint of weakness.[108] Within 36 hours of admission, he had an acute myocardial infarction and later developed cellulites of the foot. Later, he developed edema of the lower extremities and scrotum, which did not respond well to oral furosemide. Thus, furosemide was prescribed intravenously to reduce the patient's edema. Minutes after the injection was administered, the patient experienced a full cardiopulmonary arrest. Resuscitation was not instituted per previous request of the patient.

Commentary. An investigation was undertaken by the hospital, the homicide squad of the local police department, and the county coroner. During the investigation, a nurse confessed to injecting 40 mEq of potassium chloride IV instead of 40 mg of furosemide.

Case Study 5-13

A case was reported in which an 81-year-old man with atherosclerotic coronary artery disease and chronic renal failure was admitted to the hospital for treatment of cellulitis of both upper extremities.[109] A central line was placed for the administration of antibiotics. The physician ordered twice-daily heparin flushes to all three central line ports. After a routine flush by a nurse, the patient yelled and threw back his head; the nurses said that his face turned pale and his "eyes rolled." Ventricular fibrillation was shown on telemetry monitoring. Within minutes, the patient progressed to full cardiopulmonary arrest. Resuscitation was not started in accordance with the patient's previously documented request.

Commentary. An investigation showed that the port of the central line had been irrigated with 6 mL (4.4 mEq/mL) of potassium phosphate instead of the intended 5 mL of heparin.

Case Study 5-14

A case was reported in which a 10-month-old female infant was admitted to the hospital for surgical repair of a congenital ventricular septal defect.[110] The surgery was performed without complication, and the initial postoperative period was uneventful. Approximately 12 hours after the surgery, the patient experienced seizure activity and head twitching; her eyes rolled back. Peaked T waves and widening of the QRS complex were demonstrated by telemetry. About 20 minutes after the onset of symptoms, the serum potassium level was found to be 10 mEq/L and the patient became progressively hypotensive. Sodium bicarbonate, glucose, calcium, and Kayexalate were administered. Defibrillation was then attempted and resulted in a slow atrial fibrillation with no ventricular activity. Potassium levels were determined 65 and 95 minutes after the onset of symptoms and found to be 11.2 mEq/L and 12.4 mEq/L, respectively. The infant died more than an hour and a half after the onset of symptoms.

Commentary. No anatomic cause of death was identified on autopsy. Although an extensive investigation was undertaken, the source of the apparent exogenous potassium remains unknown. Cause of death was attributed to hyperkalemia from an unknown exogenous source.

Case Study 5-15

A case was reported in which a 6-month-old female infant was admitted to the hospital for surgical repair of aortic stenosis.[111] The surgery was performed without incident, but the patient developed complete heart block and required an external pacemaker and use of a ventilator. Blood chemistry on the third postoperative day showed a potassium value of 2.9 mEq/L. The attending physician prescribed potassium chloride to be given intravenously over a two-hour period. During the infusion, the patient developed cardiac arrest. During the attempted resuscitation, the serum potassium level was found to be 9.3 mEq/L. Evident on telemetry monitoring were changes consistent with hyperkalemia (peaked T waves and ST elevation). Although resuscitative efforts were attempted over a one-hour period, the infant died.

Commentary. The intravenous fluid was secured by risk management personnel, and analysis of the remaining fluid showed that the pharmacy had prepared an incorrectly mixed, concentration form of potassium chloride. Although the hospital followed the correct protocol and had the potassium solution prepared in the pharmacy, the pharmacist made a grave error in preparing the mixture.

Case Study 5-16

A case was reported in which a 23-year-old woman whose legs were crushed for almost 7 hours during an underground rail disaster was admitted to the hospital.[112] Her legs were found to be swollen and bruised; fractures were present. Bladder catheterization produced a small amount of brown urine, and laboratory analysis revealed a serum potassium concentration of 8.8 mEq/L. Early treatment consisted of an insulin and glucose infusion and peritoneal dialysis (followed by hemodialysis on day 2). Lower limb fasciotomies were performed bilaterally; in the ninth week after the injury, her right leg was disarticulated at the hip. A series of complications occurred that ultimately led to her death in week 13 without ever having regained consciousness.

Commentary. The extremely high serum potassium level was due to release of cellular potassium into the extracellular space following the massive crush injuries to the patient's legs. The brown urine was due to discoloration of urine with myoglobin, a substance released from the injured striated muscles (rhabdomyolysis).

Also see Case Studies 22-2 and 25-2 for a discussion of other patients with potassium problems.

NOTES

1. Mandal, A. K. (1997). Hypokalemia and hyperkalemia. *Medical Clinics of North America, 81,* 611–639.

2. McPhee, S. J., Papadakis, M. S., & Tierney, L. M. (2008). *2008 current medical diagnosis and treatment.* New York: McGraw-Hill, p. 1079.

3. Gennari, F. J. (1998). Hypokalemia. *New England Journal of Medicine, 339,* 451–458.

4. Bloomfield, R. L., Wilson, D. J., & Buckalew, V. W. (1986). The incidence of diuretic-induced hypokalemia in two distinct clinic settings. *Journal of Clinical Hypertension, 2,* 331–338.

5. McPhee et al., note 2, p. 765.

6. Gennari, note 3.

7. Zull, D. N. (1989). Disorders of potassium metabolism. Emergency *Medical Clinics of North America, 7,* 771–794.

8. Gennari, note 3.

9. McPhee et al., note 2, p. 383.

10. Gennari, note 3.

11. Gennari, note 3.

12. Reilly, R. F., & Perazella, M. A. (2007). *Acid–base, fluids and electrolytes.* New York: McGraw-Hill, p. 149.

13. Gennari, note 3.

14. Rose, B. D., & Post, T. W. (2001). *Clinical physiology of acid–base and electrolyte disorders* (5th ed.). New York: McGraw-Hill, p. 854.

15. Fink, M. P., Abraham, E., Vincent, J. L., & Kochanek, P. M. (2005). *Textbook of critical care* (5th ed.). Philadelphia: Elsevier Saunders, p. 1109.

16. Gennari, note 3.

17. Gennari, note 3.

18. Bloomfield et al., note 4.

19. Rose & Post, note 14, p. 840.

20. Braden, G. L., von Oeyen, P. T., Germain, M. J., Watson, D. J., & Haag, B. L. (1997). Ritodrine and terbutaline induced hypokalemia in preterm labor: Mechanisms and consequences. *Kidney International, 51*, 1867–1875.

21. Chataway, S. J., Mumford, C. J., & Ironside, J. W. (1997). Self-induced myopathy. *Postgraduate Medical Journal, 73*, 593–594.

22. Goto, A., Takanashi, Y., Kismimoto, M., Minowada, S., Albe, H., Hasuo, K., et al. (2009). Primary aldosteronism associated with severe rhabdomyolysis due to profound hypokalemia. *Internal Medicine, 48*(4), 219–223.

23. Rose & Post, note 14, p. 855.

24. McPhee et al., note 2, p. 765.

25. Matarese, L. E., & Gottschlich, M. (2003). *Contemporary nutrition support practice: A clinical guide* (2nd ed.). Philadelphia: Saunders, p. 455.

26. Jung, J. Y., Lee, C., Ro, H. Kim, H. S., Joo, K. W., Kim, Y., et al. (2009). Sequential occurrence of life-threatening hypokalemia and rebound hyperkalemia associated with barbiturate coma therapy. *Clinical Nephrology, 71*(3), 333–337.

27. Neil, M. J., & Dale, M. C. (2009). Hypokalemia with severe rebound hyperkalemia after therapeutic barbiturate coma. *Anesthesia & Analgesia, 108*(6), 1867–1868.

28. Anderson, K. M. (1998). Hypokalemic periodic paralysis: A case study. *American Journal of Critical Care, 7*, 236–239.

29. Gennari, note 3.

30. Gennari, note 3, p. 452.

31. Gennari, note 3, p. 451.

32. Rose & Post, note 14, p. 845.

33. Barri, Y. M, & Wingo, C. S. (1997). The effects of potassium depletion and supplementation on blood pressure: A clinical review. *American Journal Medical Science, 314*, 37–40.

34. Khanna, A., & White, W. B. (2009). The management of hyperkalemia in patients with cardiovascular disease. *American Journal of Medicine, 122*(3), 215–221.

35. Zemel, P., Gualdoni, S., & Sowers, J. R. (1988). Racial differences in mineral intake in ambulatory normotensives and hypertensives. *American Journal of Hypertension, 1*, 146S–148S.

36. Braden et al., note 20.

37. Rose & Post, note 14, p. 860.

38. Yasue, H., Itoh, T., Mizuno, Y., & Harada, E. (2007). Severe hypokalemia, rhabdomyolysis, muscle paralysis, and respiratory impairment in a hypertensive patient taking herbal medicines containing licorice. *Internal Medicine, 46*(9), 575–578.

39. Rose & Post, note 14, p. 860.

40. Barri & Wingo, note 33.

41. Colditz, G. A., Manson, J. E., Stampfer, M. J., Rosner, B. Willett, W. C., & Speizer, F. E. (1992). Diet and risk of clinical diabetes in women. *American Journal of Clinical Nutrition, 55*, 1018–1023.

42. Shafi, T., Appel, L. J., Miller, E. R., Klag, M. J., & Parekh, R. S. (2008). Changes in serum potassium mediate thiazide-induced diabetes. *Hypertension, 52*, 1022–1029.

43. Zull, note 7, p. 785.

44. Zull, note 7, p. 785.

45. Cooper, D. H., Krainik, A. J., Lubner, S. J., & Reno, H. E. (2007). *The Washington manual of medical therapeutics* (32nd ed.). Philadelphia: Lippincott Williams & Wilkins, p. 73.

46. Hultgren, H. N., Swenson, R., & Wettach, G. (1975). Abstract. Cardiac arrest due to oral potassium administration. *American Journal of Medicine, 58*, 139–142.

47. Kollef, M. H., Bedient, T. J., Isakow, W., & Witt, C. A. (2008). *The Washington manual of critical care*. Philadelphia: Lippincott Williams & Wilkins, p. 161.

48. Kollef et al., note 47, p. 161.

49. Kollef et al., note 47, p. 161.

50. Anonymous. Patient safety alert: Medication error prevention: potassium chloride. (2001). *International Journal for Quality in Health Care, 13*(2), 155.

51. Cohen, M. R. (1997). ISMP medication error report analysis: Still more errors with potassium chloride injection concentrate. *Hospital Pharmacy, 32*, 998.

52. White, J. R., Veltri, M. A., & Fackler, J. C. (2005). Preventing adverse events in the pediatric intensive care unit: Prospectively targeting factors that lead to intravenous potassium chloride order errors. *Pediatric Critical Care Medicine, 6*(1), 25–32.

53. Lim, E. T., Khoo, S. T., & Tweed, W. A. (1992). Efficacy of lignocaine in alleviating potassium chloride infusion pain. *Anesthesia and Intensive Care, 20*, 196–198.

54. Morrill G. B., & Katz, M. D. (1988). The use of lidocaine to reduce the pain induced by potassium chloride infusion. *Journal of Intravenous Nursing, 11*, 105–108.

55. Institute for Safe Medication Practices. (2004, February 12). ISMP medication safety alert: Safety issues with adding lidocaine to IV potassium infusions.

56. Institute for Safe Medication Practices, note 55.

57. Institute for Safe Medication Practices, note 55.

58. Grotegut, C. A., Dandolu, V., Katari, S., Whiteman, V. E., Geifman-Holtzman, O., & Teitelman, M. (2006). Baking soda pica: A case of hypokalemic metabolic alkalosis and rhabdomyolysis in pregnancy. *Obstetrics & Gynecology, 107*(2), 484–485.

59. Rose, E. A., Porcerelli, J. H., & Neale, A. V. (2000). Pica: Common but commonly missed. *Journal of the American Board of Family Practice, 13*, 353–358.

60. Horner, R. D., Lackey, C. J., Kolasa, K. S., & Warren, K. (1991). Pica practices of pregnant women. *Journal of the American Dietetic Association, 91*, 34–38.

61. Marinella, M. A. (2003). The refeeding syndrome and hypophosphatemia. *Nutrition Reviews, 61*(9), 320–323.

62. Seifert, M. E., & Rasoulpour, M. (2009). Hypokalemia and nocturia in a 15 year-old girl. *Clinical Pediatrics, 48*(3), 317–319.

63. Shetty, A. K., Rogers, N. L., Mannick, E. E., & Aviles, D. H. (2000). Syndrome of hypokalemic metabolic alkalosis and

hypomagnesemia associated with gentamicin therapy: Case reports. *Clinical Pediatrics, 39,* 529–533.

64. Feehally, J., Floege, J., & Johnson, R. J. (2007). *Comprehensive clinical nephrology* (3rd ed.). Philadelphia: Mosby Elsevier, p. 117.

65. Kleinfeld, M., & Corcoran, A. J. (1990). Hypertension in the elderly. *Comprehensive Therapy, 16,* 49–53.

66. Don, B. R., Sebastian A, Cheitlin, M., Christiansen, M., & Schambelan, M. (1990). Pseudohyperkalemia caused by fist clenching during phlebotomy. *New England Journal of Medicine, 322,* 1290–1292.

67. Gambino, R., Sanfilippo, M., & Lazcano, L. (2009). Pseudohyperkalemia from finger flexion during venipuncture masks true hypokalemia [letter]. *Annals of Clinical Biochemistry, 46*(2), 177.

68. Baer, D. M., Ernst, D. J., & Willeford, S. I. (2006). Investigating elevated potassium values. *Medical Laboratory Observer,* 38:24.

69. Baer et al., note 68.

70. Wrenn, K. D., Slovis, D. M., & Slovis, B. S. (1991). The ability of physicians to predict hyperkalemia from the ECG. *Annals of Emergency Medicine, 20,* 1229–1232.

71. Khanna & White, note 34.

72. Rose & Post, note 14, p. 845.

73. Khanna & White, note 34.

74. Feehally et al., note 64, p. 119.

75. Khanna & White, note 34.

76. McPhee et al., note 2, p. 767.

77. Eng, P. M., Seeger, J. D., Loughlin, J., Oh, K., & Walker, A. M. (2007). Serum potassium monitoring for users of ethinyl estradiol/drospirenone taking medications predisposing to hyperkalemia: Physician compliance and survey of knowledge and attitudes. *Contraception, 75,* 101–107.

78. Hollander-Rodriguese, J. C., & Calvert, J. F. (2006). Hyperkalemia. *American Family Physician, 73*(2), 283–290.

79. Schwartz, A. B., & Cannon-Babb, M. (1989). Hyperkalemia due to drugs in diabetic patients. *American Family Practice, 39,* 225–231

80. Schwartz & Cannon-Babb, note 79.

81. Zull, note 7.

82. Schwartz & Cannon-Babb, note 79.

83. Rimmer, J. M, Horn, J. F, & Gennari, F. J. (1987). Hyperkalemia as a complication of drug therapy. *Archives of Internal Medicine, 147,* 867–869.

84. Rimmer et al., note 83.

85. Schwartz & Cannon-Babb, note 79.

86. Beck, L. H. (1998). Changes in renal function with aging. *Clinical Geriatric Medicine, 14,* 199–209.

87. Medina, I., Mills, J., Leoung, G., Hopewell, P. C., Lee, B., Modin, G., et al. (1990). Oral therapy for *Pneumocystis carinii* pneumonia in the acquired immunodeficiency syndrome: A controlled trial of trimethoprim sulfamethoxazole versus trimethoprim-dapsone. *New England Journal of Medicine, 323,* 776–782.

88. Schwartz & Cannon-Babb, note 79.

89. Eng et al., note 89.

90. Eng et al., note 77.

91. Loughlin, J., Seeger, J. D., Eng, P. M., Foegh, M., Clifford, C. R., Cutone, J., et al (2008). Risk of hyperkalemia in women taking ethinylestradiol/drospirenone and other oral contraceptives. *Contraception, 78*(5), 377–383.

92. Shim van der Loeff, H. J., Strack van Schijndel, S., & Thijs, L. G. (1988). Cardiac arrest due to oral potassium intake. *Intensive Care Medicine, 15,* 58–59.

93. Illingsworth, R. N, & Proudfoot, A. T. (1980). Rapid poisoning with slow-release potassium. *British Medical Journal, 281,* 485–486.

94. Wetli, C. V, & Davis, J. H. (1978). Fatal hyperkalemia from accidental overdose of potassium chloride. *Journal of the American Medical Association, 240,* 1139.

95. Oda, J., Tanaka, H., Yashioka, T., Iwai, A., Yamamura, H., Ishikawa, K., et al. (1997). Analysis of 372 patients with crush syndrome caused by the Hanshin-Awaji earthquake. *Journal of Trauma: Injury Infection & Critical Care, 42*(3), 470–475.

96. Rimmer et al., note 83, p. 869.

97. Rose & Post, note 14, p. 909.

98. Rimmer et al., note 83, p. 869.

99. Rose & Post, note 14, p. 917.

100. Rose & Post, note 14, p. 917.

101. Kollef et al., note 47, p. 164.

102. Kollef et al., note 47, p. 164.

103. Kollef et al., note 47, p. 164.

104. Bongard, F. S., Sue, D. Y., & Vintch, J. R. (2008). *Current diagnosis and treatment, critical care* (3rd ed.). New York: McGraw-Hill/Lange, p. 42.

105. Weisberg, L. S. (2008). Management of severe hyperkalemia. *Critical Care Medicine, 36*(12), 3246–3251.

106. Kollef et al., note 47, p. 164.

107. Weber, L. (1998). Iatrogen induced hyperkalemia in an elderly male: A case study. Unpublished paper. Saint Louis University School of Nursing.

108. Wetherton, A. R., Corey, T. S., Buchino, J. J., & Burrows, A. M. (2003). Fatal intravenous injection of potassium in hospitalized patients. *American Journal of Forensic Medicine and Pathology, 24*(2), 128–131.

109. Wetherton et al., note 108.

110. Wetherton et al., note 108.

111. Wetherton et al., note 108.

112. Selig, M. (1978). Crush syndrome. *Australian Family Physician, 7*(1), 32–33.

Chapter 6

Calcium Imbalances

Because many factors affect calcium regulation, there are a multitude of causes of disturbed calcium balance. For this reason, both hypocalcemia and hypercalcemia are relatively common imbalances. To facilitate understanding of calcium disturbances, it is helpful to review factors that affect calcium balance.

CALCIUM BALANCE

Distribution and Function

Calcium is the body's most abundant divalent cation.[1] More than 99% of the body's calcium is concentrated in the skeletal system, and approximately 1% is rapidly exchangeable with blood calcium (the remainder is more stable and exchanged only slowly). The small amount of calcium located outside the bone circulates in the serum, partly bound to protein and partly ionized. Calcium has a major role in transmission of nerve impulses. It helps regulate muscle contraction and relaxation, including normal heartbeat. Calcium has a vital role in the cardiac action potential and is essential for cardiac pacemaker automaticity. This ion is also involved in blood clotting and hormone secretion. Recommended adequate intake for calcium for both men and women aged 19 to 50 years is 1000 mg/day; some experts recommend increasing this amount to 1200 mg/day for those persons older than 50 years.[2]

Evidence suggests that calcium and vitamin D play important roles in the primary prevention of colorectal neoplasia.[3] It appears that calcium binds bile acids in the bowel lumen, inhibiting bile-induced mucosal damage.[4] Calcium is closely tied to magnesium and phosphorus regulation.[5]

Measurement of Calcium in Blood

The test most frequently performed in clinical settings to measure serum calcium is total calcium, with results normally ranging from 8.9 to 10.3 mg/dL (roughly equivalent to 2.23 to 2.57 mmol/L). The total calcium in serum is the sum of the ionized (47%) and non-ionized (53%) calcium components. In the non-ionized portion, calcium is primarily bound to albumin (and, to a lesser extent, to other anions such as citrate and phosphate). When serum albumin levels and pH are within normal ranges, readings from total calcium are generally useful. In contrast, when the serum albumin level is abnormal, corrections must be made in the reported total serum calcium levels. In noncritically ill patients, it is estimated that a 1.0 g/dL decrease in the serum albumin is accompanied by a 0.8 mg/dL decrease in the total calcium. The following is a convenient formula sometimes used to calculate the "corrected" calcium level when hypoalbuminemia is present:

$$\text{Corrected calcium (mg/dL)} = \text{measured serum calcium} + 0.8 \times (4.0 - \text{measured serum albumin g/dL})$$

For example, if the patient's serum albumin level is below normal by 1 g/dL (e.g., 3.0 g/dL rather than 4.0 g/dL), a measured total serum calcium concentration of 8.0 mg/dL should be adjusted upward to 8.8 mg/dL. In this situation, the ionized calcium level would be estimated at approximately half of the adjusted value. The direct relationship between albumin and total calcium often leads clinicians to ignore a low total serum calcium level in the presence of a similarly low serum albumin level.

The ionized calcium level in the bloodstream is affected by plasma pH. For example, when the arterial pH increases (alkalosis), more calcium becomes bound to protein. Although the total serum calcium remains unchanged, the ionized portion decreases. Therefore, symptoms of hypocalcemia often occur when alkalosis is present (despite a normal total calcium level). Acidosis (low pH) has the opposite effect; that is, less calcium is bound to protein and, therefore, more exists in the ionized form. Signs of hypocalcemia will develop only rarely in the presence of acidosis, even when the total serum calcium level is lower than normal.

Direct measurement of ionized calcium by the laboratory is highly desirable, especially in critically ill patients. Recall that the ionized calcium concentration is the physiologically active and clinically important component.[6] Whole blood, heparinized plasma, or serum may be used for the measurement of calcium ionization.[7] Instructions from the laboratory that is performing the analysis need to be carefully followed to assure accurate results. The normal value for urinary calcium is dependent on dietary calcium intake. Urine specimens collected for calcium analysis need to be appropriately acidified to prevent calcium salt precipitation.[8]

Regulation

Many biochemical and hormonal factors act to maintain a normal calcium balance. Among the most important are parathyroid hormone (PTH), calcitonin, and calcitriol (an active metabolite of vitamin D). PTH promotes transfer of calcium from the bone to the plasma, thereby raising the plasma calcium level. The bones and teeth are ready sources for replenishment of low plasma calcium levels. PTH also augments the intestinal absorption of calcium and enhances the net renal calcium reabsorption. Calcium is absorbed primarily in the duodenum and jejunum.[9]

Calcitonin (which is produced in the thyroid as well as several other tissues) is a physiological antagonist of PTH. Calcitonin secretion is directly stimulated by a high serum calcium concentration. At high levels, calcitonin inhibits bone resorption; the resultant reduced flux of calcium from bone causes a reduction in the serum calcium level.

Calcitriol (1,25-dihydroxyvitamin D) is a hormone that increases the extracellular calcium concentration by three main actions: promotion of calcium absorption from the intestine, enhancement of bone resorption of calcium, and stimulation of renal tubular reabsorption of calcium. Calcitriol has a synergistic effect with parathyroid hormone on bone resorption.

Osteoporosis

Osteoporosis is associated with prolonged low intake of calcium. It is characterized by loss of bone mass, which in turn causes bones to become porous, brittle, and susceptible to fracture. In the United States, osteoporosis is estimated to cause 1.5 million fractures annually, primarily of the hip and spine.[10] Although serum calcium levels are usually normal in individuals with osteoporosis, total body calcium stores are greatly diminished. Bone loss begins at an earlier age in women than in men and is accelerated by menopause. However, men also develop a negative calcium balance in later years, at which point they may become vulnerable to osteoporosis. A dual process is involved in osteoporosis: increased bone resorption and inadequate bone formation. Menopause leads to rapid bone loss in women because estrogen deficiency reduces calcium absorption and increases excretion; as a result, bone loss far outpaces bone deposition.

Risk of developing serious bone problems is greater in postmenopausal, physically inactive women who are elderly, thin and small-framed, and smokers, and in those who have a diet deficient in calcium.[11] Inactivity predisposes to bone loss by reducing the efficiency of calcium use. Conversely, regular physical exercise (such as running, walking, or bicycling) slows the rate of bone loss and improves calcium balance. Considering the magnitude of the problems associated with osteoporosis, prevention is the only cost-effective approach. Also important in the prevention of osteoporosis is elimination of bone toxins (such as cigarettes and heavy alcohol ingestion). Hypogonadal women who take estrogen have a reduced risk of developing osteoporosis; thus it is one factor to consider when deciding whether to take estrogen (hormone replacement therapy [HRT]).[12] It appears that low doses of estrogen are adequate to prevent postmenopausal osteoporosis; however, once osteoporosis has developed, it is not an effective treatment.[13]

Bisphosphonates are the most commonly used drugs for the treatment of osteoporosis. Since the first such agent was introduced, more than 190 million prescriptions have been written for their use.[14] All patients receiving bisphosphonates should have adequate calcium and vitamin D intake before and during therapy.[15] Some reports have described development of bisphosphonate-induced hypocalcemia in patients with unrecognized hypoparathyroidism, vitamin D deficiency, or impaired renal function.[16]

HYPOCALCEMIA

Hypocalcemia may be defined as a total serum calcium level of less than 8.9 mg/dL and an ionized calcium concentration of less than 4.6 mg/dL. However, it is important to recognize that reporting laboratories often have slightly differing values for normal calcium levels. Hypocalcemia is a common imbalance in critically ill patients. For example, the prevalence of ionized hypocalcemia is reported to range from 60% to 85% in medical, surgical, and trauma patients.[17] Hypocalcemia is a serious imbalance, in that it can potentiate cardiac arrhythmias and seizures.[18] Although mortality is greater in patients with hypocalcemia, this outcome does not appear to be independently associated with the imbalance.[19]

As discussed earlier, hypoalbuminemia can produce a falsely low total serum calcium test result (referred to as pseudohypocalcemia). In this situation, the ionized calcium level remains normal and the patient is asymptomatic and requires no treatment.

Causes

Causes of hypocalcemia vary, but are known to include surgical hypoparathyroidism, acute pancreatitis, magnesium imbalances, hyperphosphatemia, alkalosis, malabsorption syndromes, infusion of citrate in blood products, sepsis, and a variety of drugs (**Table 6-1**). However, hypocalcemia rarely results from decreased intake of calcium alone, as bone reabsorption can maintain normal levels for a prolonged period of time.[20]

Surgical Hypoparathyroidism

Primary hypoparathyroidism causes hypocalcemia, although surgical hypoparathyroidism following thyroidectomy or radical neck dissection is a more common cause. Postsurgical hypoparathyroidism may be either transient or permanent.

The frequency of surgical hypoparathyroidism is partially dependent on the technical skill of the surgeon, who strives to preserve the blood supply to the parathyroid glands. Much lower rates of hypoparathyroidism have been reported in endocrine surgical centers with a high volume of neck surgery than in other settings.[21] Transient hypocalcemia occurs 24 to 48 hours after thyroidectomy but frequently does not require treatment.[22] A recent study of 21 individuals who underwent thyroid surgery revealed that 18 developed hypocalcemia (although only 4 of the 18 were symptomatic).[23] The 4 patients who had symptomatic hypocalcemia had significantly lower intact parathyroid hormone

Table 6-1 Summary of Causes of Hypocalcemia

Cause	Mechanism
Hypoparathyroidism	Calcium shifted from the bloodstream into bone
Hyperphosphatemia	Phosphate binds ionized calcium and removes it from the bloodstream
Alkalosis	Increased binding of ionized calcium to albumin
Pancreatitis	Systemic endotoxins Saponification of fats Faulty PTH feedback loop
Hypomagnesemia	End-organ resistance to PTH Decreased production of PTH
Renal failure	Hyperphosphatemia Decreased active vitamin D
Sepsis	PTH suppression Elevated cytokines Elevated calcitonin
Long-term lack of sunlight	Inadequate vitamin D
Loop diuretics (furosemide)	Increased renal excretion
Phenytoin	Inhibits GI absorption of calcium
Citrate-buffered blood products	Citrate anions bind calcium
Edetate disodium	Chelation of calcium

(iPTH) levels than did the 14 patients without symptoms and the remaining 3 without hypocalcemia. The researchers concluded that a 1-hour postoperative iPTH level of 2.5 pmol/L or less can identify individuals at risk for developing symptomatic hypocalcemia.

The most likely mechanism in terms of causing hypocalcemia after radical neck dissection is ischemia to the parathyroid tissue following dissection and hemostatic maneuvers. It is also possible that trauma to the parathyroid glands precludes PTH from increasing to the level needed to elevate the low serum calcium concentration, thus contributing to the development of hypocalcemia. If permanent parathyroid damage has not occurred, parathyroid insufficiency resolves as edema at the surgical site lessens and revascularization occurs, allowing reestablishment of parathyroid gland integrity. Extensive neck surgery (as in radical neck dissection for cancer) is more likely to be associated with permanent hypoparathyroidism than are less involved surgical maneuvers.

Most patients who develop hypocalcemia after neck surgery are asymptomatic; however, some may develop paresthesias, laryngeal spasm, or tetany. It is common practice to check serum ionized calcium levels at regular intervals in the early postoperative period in patients who have undergone neck surgery.

With the emphasis on cost containment in the current healthcare environment, concerns have been raised that patients who have undergone thyroid or parathyroid gland surgery may be discharged before postoperative hypocalcemia becomes manifest. A retrospective study of 197 patients who had undergone such operations indicated that early postoperative calcium levels give a good indication of whether hypocalcemia is likely to occur.[24] In the study, postoperative calcium levels were plotted as a function of time, and the slope between the first two postoperative calcium levels was examined. The results indicated that an initial upsloping postoperative calcium curve based on these two early postoperative calcium measurements is a strong predictor of a stable postoperative calcium level; conversely, a steeply downsloping initial calcium curve is worrisome for eventual hypocalcemia.

Acute Pancreatitis

Hypocalcemia is not uncommon during acute pancreatitis and is associated with a poor outcome. While it is unclear precisely which mechanisms cause hypocalcemia in this setting, several possibilities have been identified. Inflammation of the pancreas causes release of proteolytic and lipolytic enzymes; it is believed that calcium ions combine with the fatty acids, forming soaps and thereby decreasing the serum calcium concentration.[25] In contrast, other researchers have concluded that systemic endotoxin exposure may play a significant role in the development of hypocalcemia in patients with acute pancreatitis.[26] Other investigators have found that there is an inadequate PTH response to the hypocalcemia caused by acute pancreatitis.[27] In any event, ionized hypocalcemia is a common problem, occurring in as many as 85% of patients with acute severe pancreatitis.[28] See Chapter 20 for a more extensive discussion of this topic.

Magnesium Abnormalities

The serum magnesium level influences both PTH secretion and action and, therefore, the serum calcium level. Severe hypomagnesemia (less than 1 mg/dL) inhibits PTH secretion. One study reported that 22% of the patients with hypocalcemia also had hypomagnesemia.[29] Hypomagnesemic hypocalcemia responds poorly to calcium therapy alone but can be resolved through concurrent calcium and magnesium replacement.

Hyperphosphatemia

Hyperphosphatemia that develops rapidly is associated with hypocalcemia. This condition might be seen in patients who receive excessive hypertonic sodium phosphate enemas. For example, as described in a recent report, a 13-year-old boy with chronic constipation developed severe hyperphosphatemia and hypocalcemia after receiving four hypertonic sodium phosphate pediatric enemas for severe constipation.[30] It is important for clinicians to recognize that these enemas are absorbable and can lead to potentially lethal complications if given improperly. See Chapters 8 and 13 for a more detailed discussion of this topic.

Alkalosis

Blood pH alters Ca^{++} binding to serum proteins. In alkalosis, a greater amount of calcium is bound to plasma proteins, resulting in a smaller percentage of ionized calcium. Thus patients with alkalosis are more susceptible to hypocalcemic tetany.

Inadequate Vitamin D

Inadequate consumption of vitamin D or insufficient exposure to the sun (ultraviolet radiation) can cause reduced calcium absorption, leading to hypocalcemia. Deficiency of vitamin D occurs in malabsorptive states, as described in the next subsection. It is not uncommon for elderly persons to have low vitamin D levels. Breastfed infants born to mothers who are vitamin D deficient are at risk for developing vitamin D deficiency and hypocalcemia; unfortunately, maternal vitamin D deficiency is not uncommon.[31]

Malabsorption Syndromes

Intestinal malabsorptive disorders are likely to lead to hypocalcemia by decreasing the absorption of vitamin D, bile salts, and calcium. In a study involving 82 patients who underwent biliopancreatic bypass from 1988 to 2001, 26% were found to have hypocalcemia and 50% were found to have low vitamin D levels (despite the fact that most took multivitamins).[32]

Infusion of Citrate in Blood Products

Decreases in ionized Ca^{++} during blood transfusion correlate with speed of the transfusion and circulating citrate levels. Hypocalcemia is seen more commonly during the transfusion of plasma and platelets, which have high citrate concentrations.[33] Citrate is added to banked blood to act as an anticoagulant and to preserve the life of the blood. Usually the citrate in blood is rapidly metabolized by the liver as it is transfused and presents no problem for calcium balance. However, when blood is transfused faster than metabolism of the excess citrate can occur, hypocalcemia results. Recall that citrate is a negatively charged ion and that calcium is a positively charged ion; thus the two ions are attracted to each other. Therefore, transient hypocalcemia can occur with massive administration of citrated blood (as in exchange transfusions in neonates), as calcium ions combine with the citrate and are temporarily removed from the circulation (a process referred to as chelation). Citrate metabolism is hindered in patients with liver disease, shock, and hypothermia. Small children and osteoporotic adults are also at increased risk for citrate/calcium imbalances because they tend to have inadequate stores of bone calcium and, therefore, are less able to compensate for declining ionized calcium levels. When citrate intoxication occurs, it may be manifested as circumoral paresthesias, muscle tremors, or tetany.

The infusion of packed red blood cells (instead of whole blood) lowers the amount of citrate infused, thereby decreasing the already low risk for hypocalcemia after transfusions. However, there is sufficient citrate even in packed red blood cells to affect calcium balance. Two cases were reported in which the transfusion of small volumes of packed red blood cells proved sufficient to precipitate symptomatic hypocalcemia.[34] Subsequent investigation revealed that both of the patients had preexisting, untreated, and asymptomatic hypocalcemia (one following partial thyroidectomy years earlier and the other with documented hypocalcemia but without a definitive cause).

As indicated previously, hypocalcemia is more commonly observed during plasmapheresis than during blood transfusions. Ordinarily the citrate anticoagulant used during apheresis procedures is considered a safe medication because it is rapidly metabolized by the donor; however, life-threatening hypocalcemia can occur if the infusion rate of the citrate is too fast. A case was reported in which citrate was inadvertently administered too rapidly to a 54-year-old woman due to malfunction of the anticoagulant line of an apheresis instrument.[35] Seven minutes into the procedure the patient developed muscle spasm, chest pain, and hypotension; her serum ionized calcium level was 0.64 mmol/L (the normal level in the reporting laboratory was in the range of 1.18–1.38 mmol/L).

Drugs

A variety of medications can predispose to hypocalcemia. For example, loop diuretics increase renal excretion of calcium and phenytoin inhibits intestinal absorption of calcium. Phosphate-containing agents bind calcium in the intestinal tract and, therefore, interfere with its absorption. Edetate disodium (EDTA) is a chelating agent used in the treatment of toxic metal poisoning; three deaths were recently reported from hypocalcemia following the administration of this agent.[36]

Alcoholism

Alcoholics are at risk for hypocalcemia for many reasons. Among these are intestinal malabsorption, low levels of 25-hydroxyvitamin D, hypomagnesemia, hypoalbuminemia, respiratory and metabolic alkalosis, and pancreatitis. The most significant of these conditions is probably hypomagnesemia (caused by the toxic effects of alcohol). Magnesium replacement in alcoholics helps to correct hypocalcemia by increasing responsiveness to PTH.

Neonatal Hypocalcemia

Two types of hypocalcemia can occur in newborn infants. The first develops early, during the first 3 days of life. This type is attributed to parathyroid immaturity or maternal hyperparathyroidism (or both), resulting in neonatal parathyroid gland suppression; it most often resolves within the first week of life. Among the predisposing factors for this condition are prematurity, maternal insulin-dependent diabetes mellitus, and asphyxia at birth. A recent study of 381 calcium levels from 111 extremely low birthweight (ELBW) infants during the first 48 hours of life found that the majority (59.9%) had at least one hypocalcemic value.[37] The investigators concluded that serum calcium values are lower in ELBW infants and that the values may be inconsequential; they recommended that hypocalcemia be redefined for ELBW infants.

A second type of neonatal hypocalcemia occurs approximately 1 week after birth and is associated with hyperphosphatemia and hypomagnesemia. Hypocalcemia in infants with this "late-onset" condition can be caused by feeding them milk with a high phosphorus level, leading to hyperphosphatemia and then to hypocalcemia. Low serum calcium levels can persist until the child's parathyroid glands function well enough to respond.

Sepsis

Although hypocalcemia in critically ill, septic patients is common, the underlying basis for this condition is unclear. Researchers have postulated that calcium shifts from the extracellular compartment into the cells and that the hormonal response to the resultant hypocalcemia is inadequate. Possible causes for hypocalcemia in a group of patients with gram-negative sepsis described by Zaloga and Chernow included acquired parathyroid gland insufficiency, dietary vitamin D deficiency, and renal hydroxylase insufficiency.[38] Other sources have reported that hypocalcemia in septic critically ill patients may be related to an inflammatory response.[39]

In experimental settings, calcium administration in sepsis has been shown to increase or have no effect on mortality.[40] It is not known if sepsis-induced hypocalcemia is protective or harmful to the patient; there is no evidence that routine calcium replacement is needed but treatment is generally advocated for symptomatic patients.[41] A review of the literature by Forsythe et al. found no clear evidence that parenteral calcium supplementation affects the outcome of critically ill patients.[42]

Other Factors

Conditions commonly associated with low serum albumin levels (such as cirrhosis of the liver and the nephrotic syndrome) are frequently associated with a low total serum calcium concentration. Often, the ionized calcium concentration is normal and no symptoms of hypocalcemia appear. Medullary thyroid carcinoma may produce hypocalcemia if calcitonin (a calcium-lowering hormone) is secreted by the tumor.

Hypocalcemia was reported in almost 18% of 66 patients with acquired immune deficiency syndrome (AIDS).[43] The researchers postulated that intestinal malabsorption of vitamin D is the most likely cause of hypocalcemia in this patient population.

Clinical Signs

Clinical manifestations of hypocalcemia vary widely among patients and depend on the severity, duration, and rate of development of this condition (**Table 6-2**). The concurrent presence of hypomagnesemia and hypokalemia can potentiate the neurological and cardiac abnormalities associated with hypocalcemia.

Neuromuscular Manifestations

Tetany—the most characteristic manifestation of hypocalcemia—refers to the entire symptom complex induced by increased neural excitability. The increase in nerve mem-

---

Table 6-2 Summary of Clinical Signs of Hypocalcemia

Neuromuscular

- Numbness; tingling of fingers, circumoral region, and toes
- Muscle cramps, which can progress to muscle spasms, tremor, and twitching
- Hyperactive deep-tendon reflexes
- Trousseau's sign
- Chvostek's sign
- Convulsions (usually generalized, but may be focal)
- Spasm of laryngeal muscles

Cardiovascular

- Decreased myocardial contractility with a reduction in cardiac output
- ECG: prolonged QT interval
- Arrhythmias, ranging from bradycardia to ventricular tachycardia and asystole

Mental

- Impaired higher cerebral functioning, such as depression, emotional instability, anxiety, or frank psychoses

Laboratory

- Total serum calcium level less than 8.9 mg/dL
- Ionized calcium level less than 4.6 mg/dL

brane excitability causes fibers to discharge spontaneously, eliciting tetanic contractions. Findings may include sensations of tingling around the mouth (circumoral paresthesia) and in the hands and feet, as well as spasms of the muscles of the extremities and face. Although laryngeal spasms may occur, they rarely result in asphyxia.[44] Ordinarily, tetany occurs when the blood concentration of calcium falls from its normal value to about 6 mg/dL (approximately 35% below the normal calcium concentration).[45]

When hypocalcemic patients fail to show overt signs of tetany, latent tetany can be elicited in two ways. One involves placing a blood pressure cuff on the upper arm and inflating it to above systolic pressure for about 3 minutes and observing for carpal spasm (Trousseau's sign; see Figure 2-3). Trousseau's sign is not specific for hypocalcemia because it is negative in approximately 30% of individuals with latent tetany and positive for a small percentage of healthy individuals. Another test involves tapping over the facial nerve just anterior to the ear and observing for ipsilateral facial muscle contraction (Chvostek's sign). This sign is also not specific for hypocalcemia because it may occur in some healthy adults.

Cardiovascular Manifestations

In some patients, altered cardiovascular hemodynamics may be the most significant effect of hypocalcemia. This outcome is understandable given the important role that calcium ions play in the contraction of cardiac muscle. The cardiovascular effects of hypocalcemia include decreased myocardial contractility leading to reduced cardiac output, hypotension that is refractory to fluid replacement and vasoconstrictive agents, and decreased responsiveness to digitalis.[46] Dysrhythmias associated with hypocalcemia can range from bradycardia to ventricular tachycardia and asystole. Hypocalcemia prolongs the QT interval, predisposing the patient to life-threatening ventricular dysrhythmia. Often cardiac patients are already predisposed to both hypocalcemia and hypomagnesemia because they are taking potent loop diuretics.

Long-standing hypocalcemia can be complicated by reversible cardiomyopathy. In one case, a 46-year-old woman with chronic severe hypocalcemia (associated with untreated hypoparathyroidism) developed severe heart dysfunction.[47] After the hypocalcemia was corrected, near-normal cardiac function returned within a few months. Similar cases have been reported by other authors.[48]

Central Nervous System Manifestations

Convulsions may be the initial symptom of severe hypocalcemia.[49] Hypocalcemia may also cause impaired higher cerebral function, such as anxiety, depression, confusion, and frank psychoses.

Treatment

Treatment of hypocalcemia depends on the underlying cause, the magnitude of the serum calcium deficiency, and the severity of symptoms. Numerous etiological factors are associated with hypocalcemia. Ideally, treatment is directed at alleviating the cause.

Intravenous Calcium Replacement for Acute Hypocalcemia

Acute symptomatic hypocalcemia is a medical emergency, requiring prompt administration of intravenous (IV) calcium. Parenteral calcium salts include calcium gluconate, calcium chloride, and calcium gluceptate. Although calcium chloride produces a significantly higher ionized calcium level than does an equimolar amount of calcium gluconate, it is not used as often because it is more irritating to the vein and can cause tissue sloughing if allowed to infiltrate. Because calcium is very irritating, it should be administered through a central line whenever possible. For symptoms of severe hypocalcemia in an average-sized adult, the physician may prescribe 10 mL of 10% calcium gluconate (90 mg elemental calcium/10 mL), to be administered over a 10-minute period.[50] This dose may be followed by the infusion of additional calcium gluconate diluted in 500 or 1000 mL of 5% aqueous dextrose (D_5W) or 0.9% NaCl. (Calcium should not be mixed with any solution containing bicarbonate because of the possibility of precipitation.) Patients receiving digitalis should be monitored with an electrocardiogram (ECG) during the infusion because calcium administration may produce fatal arrhythmias if the infusion is given too rapidly. The serum calcium level should be monitored every 4 to 6 hours and the infusion rate adjusted to avoid recurrent symptomatic hypocalcemia.

Oral Calcium Replacement for Chronic Hypocalcemia

When oral calcium supplements are tolerated, the oral route of administration is preferred over the IV route because it is safer. Oral calcium can be provided as carbonate, gluconate, lactate, or citrate salts. In some cases, long-term management may require the use of vitamin D preparations. These medications should be used with caution if severe hyperphosphatemia is present because of the danger of calcium phosphate precipitation in the soft tissues. If hyperphosphatemia is present, oral phosphate-binding medications (such as aluminum hydroxide) may be indicated.

Calcium carbonate is the least expensive and most frequently supplied oral calcium salt.[51] However, its rate of absorption is greatly reduced in patients with achlorhydria (unless taken with meals). Patients with achlorhydria, or hypochlorhydria, should be encouraged to take calcium carbonate with meals or to consider taking calcium citrate instead (at any time of the day).[52] Some experts recommend that patients taking proton pump inhibitors take calcium citrate instead of calcium carbonate. Unfortunately, calcium citrate costs approximately 50% more than calcium carbonate.[53]

Clinical Considerations

1. Be aware of patients at risk for hypocalcemia and monitor for its occurrence (see Table 6-2).
2. Be prepared to implement seizure precautions when hypocalcemia is severe.
3. Monitor the patient's airway closely because laryngeal stridor can occur.
4. Take safety precautions if confusion is present.
5. Be aware of factors related to the safe intravenous administration of calcium replacement salts (**Table 6-3**).
6. Educate individuals about recommended calcium dietary intake. Recommended adequate intake for calcium for both men and women aged 19 to 50 years is 1000 mg/day; the recommendation increases to 1200 mg/day for those older than 50 years.[54] The best way for healthy individuals to ensure an adequate calcium intake is to eat a wide variety of foods.
7. Calcium supplements may be necessary for individuals who are unable to consume sufficient calcium in their diets, such as those who do not tolerate milk or dairy products.
8. Individuals with a tendency to form renal stones should be encouraged to increase their fluid intake throughout the day and night. Fluids should be ingested during meals, several hours after meals, before bedtime, and during the night when awakened to void.
9. Inform individuals at risk for osteoporosis about the value of regular physical exercise in decreasing bone

---

Table 6-3 Considerations in the Administration of Intravenous Calcium

1. The dosage of calcium prescribed for a specific hypocalcemic patient depends on the severity of hypocalcemia as well as its cause.
2. The most commonly prescribed calcium preparations for IV use are as follows:
   - *Calcium gluconate*: 10 mL of a 10% solution contains 90 mg (4.5 mEq) of elemental Ca^{++} (suitable for either IV or IM use).
   - *Calcium chloride*: 10 mL of a 10% solution contains 270 mg (13.5 mEq) of elemental Ca^{++} (suitable only for IV use).
3. Calcium preparations may be given undiluted by slow IV push (if indicated) or—preferably—may be diluted with compatible parenteral fluids for slow infusion.
4. Calcium preparations are irritating to veins and may cause venous sclerosis; for this reason, administration through a central vein is recommended.
   - Because calcium gluconate is less irritating to veins than is calcium chloride, it is more frequently prescribed (although it contains only one-third as much elemental calcium as calcium chloride).
   - If a peripheral administration site is necessary, use the largest available vein. Do *not* use small hand veins.
   - Great care should be taken to avoid extravasation of calcium solutions (especially calcium chloride) because they can cause severe soft-tissue damage.
5. Calcium preparations should not be administered with bicarbonate or phosphate because a precipitate will form.
6. Calcium should be administered cautiously (with ECG monitoring) in patients taking digitalis because accidental hypercalcemia induced by too-rapid infusion of calcium could precipitate digitalis toxicity.
7. Frequent monitoring of the patient's response to calcium replacement therapy is indicated.
8. Serum calcium levels should be checked frequently (such as every 1 to 4 hours) and the dosage adjusted accordingly. Adequacy of treatment can also be monitored by observing Chvostek's and Trousseau's signs, the ECG, and hemodynamic parameters.

loss. Walking is well tolerated by all age groups and is an excellent form of exercise, as is bicycling.

10. Discuss the calcium loss associated with the use of alcohol and nicotine. Smoking lowers estrogen levels and interferes with the body's absorption of calcium; as a consequence, women who smoke are at greater risk of developing osteoporosis.

HYPOCALCEMIA CASE STUDIES

Case Study 6-1

A 46-year-old woman with end-stage renal disease was admitted with a secondary diagnosis of seizure activity and multi-infarct dementia. She required dialysis twice a week. On admission, laboratory data from a venous blood sample revealed the following: Na 138 mEq/L, BUN 41 mg/dL, K 5.8 mEq/L, serum creatinine 8.2 mg/dL, total Ca 7.0 mg/dL, albumin 3.0 g/dL, phosphorus 7.1 mg/dL, and HCO_3 13.5 mEq/L.

Commentary. Note the low total calcium level and the presence of hypoalbuminemia. With correction for the low serum albumin level, the serum calcium would be nearer to normal. (Recall that for every gram the serum albumin is below the normal level, 0.8 mg must be added to the reported calcium level.) Using the following equation:

$$\text{Corrected calcium (mg/dL)} = \text{measured serum calcium} + 0.8 \times (4.0 - \text{measured serum albumin g/dL})$$

The corrected total calcium is 7.8 mg/dL. Although the corrected total calcium level is still below normal, the ionized fraction of the calcium was normal; thus symptoms of hypocalcemia were not present. Note that this patient has metabolic acidosis (evidenced by the low serum bicarbonate level); both hypoalbuminemia and acidosis favor increased calcium ionization. Rapid correction, or over-correction, of acidosis in a patient with renal disease predisposes the patient to precipitation of hypocalcemic symptoms. Hyperphosphatemia was present, a major factor in explaining the hypocalcemia in this case.

Case Study 6-2

A hysterical young woman was admitted to the emergency department after an automobile accident in which she fractured her arm. She complained of circumoral paresthesia and then fainted. Arterial blood gas findings included a pH of 7.55 (alkalosis) and an arterial carbon dioxide pressure

($PaCO_2$) of 20 mm Hg (normal, 40 mm Hg), indicating respiratory alkalosis.

Commentary. Hyperventilation secondary to hysteria is a common cause of tetany in the hospital emergency department. In this situation, the tetany resulted from a reduction in the plasma ionized calcium level consequent to respiratory alkalosis. Fainting was due to cerebral ischemia caused by the low $PaCO_2$ (recall that a low $PaCO_2$ causes cerebral vasoconstriction). The total serum calcium level was probably normal, although the ionized fraction decreased. Correction of the hyperventilation (and thus of respiratory alkalosis) will restore the ionized calcium level to normal and alleviate symptoms.

Case Study 6-3

A case was reported in which a 40-year-old female was a first-time apheresis platelet donor.[55] Her history included hypertension, hyperlipidemia, and depression. Medications included bumetanide (a loop diuretic), pravastatin (a cholesterol-lowering drug), and paroxetine (a selective serotonin reuptake inhibitor [SSRI] antidepressant). Thirty minutes after the procedure started, the patient complained of tingling around her mouth, hands, and feet. Shortly thereafter, she developed acute-onset severe facial and extremity tetany. Treatment with intravenous calcium gluconate was started and the muscle contractions subsided over 10 to 15 minutes.

Commentary. These events are consistent with a severe reaction to calcium chelation by the sodium citrate anticoagulant used in the apheresis donation procedure. It is possible that the loop diuretic (bumetanide) contributed to the hypocalcemia. Authors of the reported case study concluded that careful screening is needed to help prevent severe reactions to citrate toxicity; it may be wise to measure pre-procedure calcium levels in selected donors to identify cases requiring extra vigilance. The authors also pointed out the need of maintaining preparedness for managing rare but serious reactions in volunteer apheresis blood donors.[56]

Case Study 6-4

A 32-year-old woman was admitted to an acute care facility with severe hypocalcemia and convulsions. She had undergone a subtotal thyroidectomy two weeks earlier. At the time of admission, her total serum calcium level was 3.2 mg/dL (normal for the reporting laboratory was 8.8 to 10.6 mg/dL).

Commentary. The hypocalcemia associated with thyroidectomy may occur weeks to months after surgery (as evidenced in this case). For this reason, patients should be taught about the symptoms of hypocalcemia and told to report signs early to their healthcare providers.

Case Study 6-5

A case was reported in which a 32-year-old mentally impaired man presented with a year-long history of loss of seizure control (after being seizure-free for 5 years on a regimen of phenytoin and phenobarbital).[57] Physical examination revealed a positive Chvostek's sign and a serum calcium level of 5.9 mg/dL (normal for the reporting laboratory was 8.8 to 10.4 mg/dL). An intravenous infusion of calcium was administered until the patient's serum calcium level reached 8.0 mg/dL. The method of calcium administration was then changed to the oral route. The patient's seizure activity diminished following calcium replacement.

Commentary. Phenytoin can interfere with vitamin D metabolism and impair calcium absorption from the intestinal and mobilization from the bone. The authors of the case report stated that vitamin D and calcium treatment should probably be maintained during the use of antiepileptic drugs.

Case Study 6-6

A case was reported in which a 43-year-old woman with a 20-year history of Crohn's disease presented to the emergency department with fatigue and weight loss.[58] For the past month, she had experienced tetany and muscle cramps as well as peripheral and perioral paresthesia. In addition, she experienced colicky abdominal pain. Upon examination, positive Chvostek's and Trousseau's signs were found. A serum calcium level of 1.3 mmol/L (corrected, 1.7 mmol/L) was found (normal, 2.23–2.57 mmol/L). Also present were hypomagnesemia and hypokalemia. Treatment consisted of electrolyte replacement with intravenous calcium, potassium, and magnesium. Vitamin D was replaced and a semi-elemental tube feeding was started. One month after discharge from the hospital, the patient continued to receive tube feedings and electrolyte replacement therapy. Plasma electrolyte levels normalized and the patient was gaining weight.

Commentary. Short bowel associated with severe Crohn's disease seriously impairs the ability of the bowel to absorb adequate amounts of carbohydrates, proteins, fats, vitamins, minerals, and electrolytes. Note that this patient required replacement of magnesium along with replacement of calcium to allow the serum calcium level to normalize.

HYPERCALCEMIA

Hypercalcemia occurs when calcium enters the extracellular fluid more rapidly than it can be excreted by the kidneys.[59] The incidence of this imbalance depends on the setting in which it occurs.[60] If allowed to become severe, hypercalcemia is associated with significant morbidity and mortality; therefore, it is important to detect this imbalance early.

Causes

Primary hyperparathyroidism and malignancy account for more than 90% of the cases of hypercalcemia in ambulatory and noncritically ill patients.[61] Only a small percentage of hypercalcemia cases are due to immobilization, vitamin A and D intoxication, lithium use, and thiazide diuretics.

Primary Hyperparathyroidism

Primary hyperparathyroidism accounts for more than half of the cases of hypercalcemia in ambulatory patients.[62] This disorder is far more common in women than in men.[63] Due to increased PTH production, hyperparathyroidism causes increased release of calcium from bone, augmented intestinal calcium absorption, and renal reabsorption of calcium. Mild hypercalcemia is found in approximately 10% of patients with thyrotoxicosis.[64]

Malignancies

Approximately 40% of the cases of hypercalcemia in hospitalized patients are associated with cancer.[65] Pathogenesis of the hypercalcemia of malignancy is complex and varies with the type of tumor. The malignancies most often associated with hypercalcemia include breast and lung cancers and hematologic malignancies such as multiple myeloma or lymphoma. Hypercalcemia is usually present only in patients with advanced cancer.[66] In a recent retrospective study, hypercalcemia was found to be a reliable indicator of impending death in cancer patients cared for in a hospice care setting.[67] Chapter 22 provides a more thorough discussion of tumors associated with hypercalcemia.

Immobilization

Bone mineral is lost during immobilization, sometimes causing an elevated total calcium concentration in the bloodstream and resultant calciuria with the possibility of formation of renal stones. Hypercalcemia will result if the rate of bone resorption exceeds the kidneys' ability to excrete the excess calcium. In particular, patients with spinal cord injuries are at risk for immobilization-related hypercalcemia. Notable risk factors in this population include an age less than 21 years, male gender, and extensive cord injury.[68] Immobilization-related hypercalcemia has also been reported in individuals without spinal cord injury, such as those with prolonged illnesses in geriatric and critical care settings.[69, 70] The hypercalcemia of immobilization remits when activity is restored; if treatment is required, bisphosphonates may be the treatment of choice.[71]

Drugs

A variety of drugs can elevate calcium levels (**Table 6-4**). Thiazide-induced hypercalcemia may be partially mediated by volume contraction that increases renal reabsorption of calcium; also, it is thought that thiazides have a direct effect on distal tubular calcium reabsorption. Approximately 5% to 10% of patients treated with lithium develop hypercalcemia.[72] Vitamin D intoxication (with its associated hypercalcemia) is most commonly caused by too-aggressive treatment of hypoparathyroidism, rickets, or osteomalacia. Large doses of vitamin A analogues to treat acne may occasionally be associated with hypercalcemia.

Milk-alkali syndrome can occur in patients with peptic ulcers who are treated for a prolonged period with milk and alkaline antacids, particularly calcium carbonate. This syndrome is characterized by hypercalcemia, hyperphosphatemia, alkalosis, and progressive renal failure.[73] Patients who take large quantities of calcium-containing antacids may present with marked hypercalcemia. The milk-alkali syndrome should also be considered as a cause of hypercalcemia given the current popularity of calcium ingestion as a means to prevent osteoporosis.

Table 6-4 Summary of Hypercalcemia

Causes	Clinical Signs
Hyperparathyroidism	**Neuromuscular**
	• Muscle weakness
Malignant neoplastic disease:	• Decreased deep-tendon reflexes
• Lung tumors, breast tumors, and multiple myeloma account for more than 50% of the cases	**Renal**
	• Polyuria (nephrogenic diabetes insipidus)
Prolonged immobilization	• Hypercalciuria, perhaps leading to renal stones
Drugs:	**Gastrointestinal**
• Thiazide diuretics	• Anorexia
• Lithium	• Nausea
• Calcium supplements	• Vomiting
• Megadoses of vitamin A	• Constipation
• Megadoses of vitamin D	**Cardiovascular**
	• Arrhythmias
	• Heart block
	• ECG: shortened QT interval
	• Increased digitalis sensitivity
	• Hypertension
	Mental
	• Impaired higher cerebral functioning, such as confusion, emotional instability, anxiety, frank psychoses, lethargy, or coma

Clinical Signs

The magnitude of the serum calcium elevation and the time it takes to develop have major effects on clinical findings, as does the underlying cause of hypercalcemia. For example, acute hypercalcemia produces more symptoms than does chronic hypercalcemia. Also, malignancies can present with severe hypercalcemia (serum calcium level ≥ 14 mg/dL) more commonly than with other conditions.[74]

Clinical signs of hypercalcemia are summarized in Table 6-4. In some patients, mild hypercalcemia is found on routine examinations; other patients may present in hypercalcemic crisis. Although there are no firm diagnostic criteria for hypercalcemic crisis, it is generally thought to represent the presence of volume depletion, neurological manifestations, and cardiac arrhythmias in a patient with a serum calcium level greater than 14 mg/dL. As a rule, symptoms of hypercalcemia are proportional to the serum calcium level, although this is not always the case.

Serum calcium levels less than 11.5 mg/dL rarely produce symptoms. By comparison, levels between 11.5 and 13 mg/dL may be associated with lethargy, anorexia, nausea, and polyuria.[75] Further, calcium levels greater than 13 mg/dL constitute severe hypercalcemia and are associated with more severe symptoms (such as muscle weakness, impaired memory, emotional lability, stupor, and coma). A total calcium concentration greater than 14 mg/dL represents hypercalcemic crisis and is a medical emergency.[76]

Neuromuscular Changes

Hypercalcemia reduces neuromuscular excitability because it acts as a sedative at the myoneural junction. Symptoms such as muscular weakness and depressed deep-tendon reflexes may occur.

Gastrointestinal Symptoms

Constipation, anorexia, nausea, vomiting, and adynamic ileus are common symptoms of hypercalcemia. Constipation results from decreased GI motility caused by calcium's action on smooth muscle and nerve conduction, as well as from dehydration.[77] Delayed gastric emptying, nausea, and vomiting are also related to altered motility. Patients with hypercalcemia are predisposed to duodenal ulcer disease because of the increased gastric acid secretion, which is promoted by calcium's action on the parietal cells of the stomach. Pancreatitis is another potential complication of severe hypercalcemia and is probably related to calcium deposits in the pancreatic ducts.

Behavior Changes

Behavior changes associated with hypercalcemia may range from subtle alterations in personality to acute psychosis and may include confusion, impairment of memory, and bizarre behavior. Patients may become inattentive and lose their ability to concentrate; recent memory is affected more dramatically than is distant memory. Other mental status changes sometimes seen in patients with hypercalcemia include lethargy and drowsiness, as well as psychiatric disturbances such as irritability and depression; severe cases are associated with stupor or coma. Although the cause of these symptoms is not known, it has been suggested that increased calcium in the cerebrospinal fluid is involved. The more severe symptoms tend to occur when the serum calcium level approaches or exceeds 15 mg/dL. In a study of eight hypercalcemic inpatients with cancer during a period of 66 patient-days, Mahon found that the most evident changes were those affecting mental status.[78] For example, many subjects could not remember their home telephone numbers or perform simple mathematical computations. Some displayed inappropriate behaviors, such as pulling out a Foley catheter while the balloon was inflated. As serum calcium levels decreased toward normal, the mental symptoms gradually subsided.

Renal Changes

Disturbed renal tubular function produced by hypercalcemia can cause polyuria and polydipsia. More specifically, this disturbed function is a form of nephrogenic diabetes insipidus (NDI) that is usually reversible within 1 to 12 weeks after correction of the imbalance. The concentrating defect may become clinically apparent when the plasma calcium concentration exceeds 11 mg/dL. Renal colic may occur as a result of kidney stones, which may form from the excess calcium presented to the kidneys for excretion. Calcium salts deposited in the kidney can cause renal failure.

Cardiovascular Changes

Calcium is important in cardiac function; it exerts a positive inotropic effect on the heart and reduces heart rate in a way similar to the effect of cardiac glycosides. Calcium administration to patients receiving digitalis must be done with extreme care because it can precipitate severe arrhythmias.

Cardiac effects of hypercalcemia include QT-interval shortening and arrhythmias.[79] Bradycardia; first-, second-, and third-degree heart block; and bundle branch block may occur. Hypercalcemia can also affect the systemic vasculature, perhaps leading to hypertension. The mechanism for the increase in blood pressure may be multifactorial. For example, serum levels of epinephrine and norepinephrine are higher in patients with hypercalcemia than in those with normocalcemia.

Treatment

Treatment should be directed at correcting the underlying cause of hypercalcemia whenever possible. For example, primary hyperparathyroidism is definitively managed by parathyroidectomy; further, when hypercalcemia is caused by malignant disease, treatment is directed at the underlying tumor.[80] When direct treatment of the underlying cause is not feasible, a number of medical treatments are available to treat severe symptomatic hypercalcemia. **Table 6-5** summarizes the treatments for hypercalcemia.

General Conservative Measures

When hypercalcemia is not life-threatening, treatment may be limited to simple actions such as a large fluid intake (unless contraindicated) and eliminating drugs that can contribute to hypercalcemia (such as thiazide diuretics, vitamin D preparations, and calcium-containing antacids). Whenever possible, the patient should be encouraged to be active, because immobility predisposes individuals to hypercalcemia.

0.9% Sodium Chloride and Loop Diuretics

Because most patients with severe hypercalcemia are volume depleted, isotonic saline (0.9% NaCl) is commonly administered to dilute the serum calcium, encourage renal excretion of calcium, and reduce the total serum calcium concentration (such as by 1.5 to 3 0 mg/dL).[81] In the early treatment phase, the rate of 0.9% NaCl and furosemide administration may be adjusted to keep the urine output between 200 and 300 mL/hr.[82] Plasma calcium levels usually will begin to decline within a few hours with the combination of furosemide and normal saline as long as the saline is administered at a sufficient rate.[83] Cardiovascular and renal function should be assessed before rapid saline infusion because fluid overload and congestive heart failure are potential complications. Furosemide should be used as necessary after the plasma volume has been expanded to prevent volume overload and to enhance calcium excretion. (A loop diuretic, such as furosemide, facilitates sodium and calcium excretion; conversely, the thiazide diuretics should not be used because they interfere with calcium excretion and may worsen hypercalcemia.) It may be necessary to monitor the central venous pressure to detect fluid overload, particularly in elderly patients or persons with marginal cardiac reserve; at the very least, breath sounds should be monitored at regular intervals. Hourly intake and output records should be maintained. Losses of potassium and magnesium will result from the large urinary output, which must be corrected as indicated by laboratory data.

Table 6-5 Summary of Treatments for Hypercalcemia

Agent	Mechanism of Action
0.9% sodium chloride solution, IV	Dilutes serum calcium concentration, increases glomerular filtration rate, and increases renal calcium excretion
Furosemide	Increases renal calcium excretion
Calcitonin	Inhibits bone resorption; inhibits renal reabsorption of calcium
Plicamycin	Inhibits bone resorption
Glucocorticoids	Inhibits calcium absorption in the intestine, inhibits bone resorption, inhibits cytokine release, and increases urinary calcium excretion
Phosphate salts	Inhibits bone resorption, interferes with GI absorption of calcium, and inhibits renal synthesis of 1,25-dihydroxyvitamin D
Bisphosphonates	Inhibit bone resorption
Gallium nitrate	Inhibits bone resorption

Bisphosphonates

Bisphosphonates, such as pamidronate and etidronate, inhibit bone resorption and, therefore, can treat hypercalcemia. The bisphosphonate dosage is determined by the severity of the hypercalcemia. Bisphosphonates are the mainstay of treatment for hypercalcemia associated with malignancy. They normalize calcium in more than 70% of patients, although it may take as long as 48 to 72 hours before the full therapeutic effect becomes evident.[84] Serum calcium levels may remain in the normal range for weeks to months after bisphosphonate therapy.

Plicamycin

Plicamycin (an antineoplastic agent) lowers serum calcium by blocking bone resorption. Because of the potential for nephrotoxicity and hepatotoxicity, long-term use of plicamycin is limited; use of this agent should be avoided in patients with underlying renal or liver dysfunction. Since the advent of the bisphosphonates, plicamycin has been used much less often than in the past.[85]

Calcitonin

By inhibiting bone resorption, salmon calcitonin has a slight and short-term effect on plasma calcium levels. The efficacy of calcitonin is largely limited to the first 48 hours after its administration (which limits its use in the control of long-term hypercalcemia).[86] Calcitonin is used largely as adjunctive therapy in controlling hypercalcemia in acute care settings until more powerful (but slower-acting) drugs take effect.[87]

Glucocorticoids

Glucocorticoids can reduce the serum calcium level by inhibiting cytokine release, inhibiting absorption of calcium in the intestine, and increasing urinary calcium excretion.[88] They are effective in reducing serum calcium in hypercalcemia due to sarcoidosis, vitamin D intoxication, multiple myeloma, or other hematologic malignancies. A drawback of glucocorticoids is that clinically significant reductions in serum calcium may not occur until at least 5 to 10 days after therapy is initiated.[89] Possible complications associated with glucocorticoids include hyperglycemia and sodium and water retention.

Gallium Nitrate

Gallium nitrate lowers the serum calcium level by inhibiting bone resorption. It has a delayed action onset of 2 days. This agent carries a significant risk of nephrotoxicity and is contraindicated when the serum creatinine is greater than 2.5 mg/dL.[90]

Phosphate Salts

When ingested orally, phosphate produces a small reduction in the serum calcium level by inhibiting bone resorption, interfering with the GI absorption of calcium, and inhibiting renal synthesis of 1,25-dihydroxy vitamin D. Because of its modest effect on the serum calcium level, oral phosphate use is limited to long-term treatment of mild hypercalcemia. It is important to remember that increasing the serum phosphate concentration alters the extracellular calcium–phosphate equilibrium to promote the formation of calcium-phosphate precipitates, which are then deposited in various body tissues including bone, soft tissues, blood vessels, lung, myocardium, and kidneys. Because of the risk of soft-tissue calcification, phosphate therapy is limited primarily to patients with low serum phosphate levels (less than 3.0 mg/dL) and adequate renal function.

Clinical Considerations

1. Be aware of patients at risk for hypercalcemia and monitor for its presence. (See Table 6-4.)
2. Increase patient mobilization when feasible; recall that immobilization favors hypercalcemia. Hospitalized patients at risk for hypercalcemia should be ambulated as soon as possible; outpatients should be told the importance of frequently moving about.
3. Encourage the oral intake of sufficient fluids to keep the patient well hydrated. Sodium-containing fluids should be given, unless contraindicated by other conditions, because sodium favors calcium excretion. Always consider the patient's preferences when encouraging oral fluids.
4. Encourage adequate bulk in the diet to offset the tendency toward constipation.
5. Take safety precautions if confusion or other mental symptoms of hypercalcemia are present. Explain to the patient and family that the mental changes associated with hypercalcemia are reversible with treatment.
6. Be aware that cardiac arrest can occur in patients with severe hypercalcemia; be prepared to deal with this emergency situation.
7. Be aware that bones may fracture more easily in patients with chronic hypercalcemia because bone resorption has been excessive, weakening the bony structure. Transfer patients cautiously.

8. Educate home-bound oncology patients with a predisposition for hypercalcemia, as well as their families, regarding symptoms that occur with this condition. Instruct them to report symptoms to healthcare providers before they become severe. In a study reported by Mahon, constipation, confusion, anorexia, increasing bone pain, weight loss, and weakness were the symptoms that most frequently caused readmission of patients with cancer. In a study of 22 hospitalized and 18 ambulatory cancer patients,[91] Coward reported that 90% were unaware that hypercalcemia might be a complication of their cancer.[92] Furthermore, only one of the patients knew the symptoms of cancer-induced hypercalcemia. Almost 70% of the patients did not recall being told of measures that might prevent hypercalcemia.

9. Be alert for signs of digitalis toxicity when hypercalcemia occurs in digitalized patients.

10. Be familiar with the treatment modalities for hypercalcemia and associated nursing functions (see the treatment section in this chapter and in Chapter 22).

HYPERCALCEMIA CASE STUDIES

Case Study 6-7

A 47-year-old woman who appeared thin and dehydrated was admitted to the hospital with abdominal pain, weight loss, and a history of vomiting for 3 months. Her body weight of 38 kg was only 84% of her ideal body weight; her mid-arm circumference was 60% of standard. On examination, a nodule was felt near the right lobe of the thyroid gland and was later found to be an adenoma. A serum calcium level was obtained and was found to be high (13.8 mg/dL).

The patient was rehydrated with 0.9% NaCl solution; however, saline diuresis did not represent a long-term solution to this woman's problem of severe hypercalcemia. Thus the right upper parathyroid gland was surgically removed. At the time of discharge from the hospital, the patient's calcium concentration had normalized to 8.7 mg/dL.

Commentary. This patient had hypercalcemia due to a parathyroid adenoma, which is one of the most common causes of hypercalcemia. She received the usual treatment for this disorder—rehydration with isotonic saline and surgical removal of the tumor.

Case Study 6-8

A 49-year-old woman with a history of breast cancer and metastases to the bone and liver was admitted to the hospital with polyuria and polydipsia; her total serum calcium level was 3.08 mmol/L (12.3 mg/dL). A single IV infusion of pamidronate was administered. The serum calcium level returned to normal and did not change until 6 weeks later. Several subsequent recurrences of hypercalcemia were also treated with single infusions of pamidronate given in the outpatient department. The patient was able to continue receiving palliative therapy at home, but died 6 months later from other complications.

Commentary. The polyuria associated with hypercalcemia occurs as a result of a renal concentrating defect; although the precise cause of this abnormality is not certain, a defect in the action of antidiuretic hormone in the collecting ducts and damage to the concentrating segments of the nephrons play a role. Provided the patient is not too nauseated to drink fluids, fluid intake will increase as the patient becomes more thirsty. Treatment of this woman's intermittent bouts of hypercalcemia allowed her to be more comfortable during her remaining months of life.

Case Study 6-9

A 59-year-old woman with carcinoma of the left breast underwent a radical mastectomy and adjuvant chemotherapy. She was later admitted to the hospital for management of hip pain, confusion, and hypercalcemia (corrected serum calcium, 15.2 mg/dL). Isotonic saline was administered IV, and she was given calcitonin subcutaneously every 8 hours. She also received pamidronate IV. The patient remained confused after the serum calcium level normalized. No further treatment was administered when the hypercalcemia recurred, and she died 1 month later from a pulmonary embolus.

Commentary. Because hypercalcemia can impair mental function, it is not unusual to observe confusion in patients with hypercalcemia. However, the behavior changes usually gradually subside once the hypercalcemia is resolved. Therefore, it was concluded that the confusion was due to something other than hypercalcemia.

Case Study 6-10

A 50-year-old man with dysphagia due to an adenocarcinoma in the gastroesophageal junction became acutely confused and reported recent nausea, anorexia, and polyuria. Because of his nausea, he was unable to consume fluids; his skin turgor was poor and his mucous membranes were dry. The ionized serum calcium level was elevated (8.7 mg/dL). Isotonic saline and a single dose of pamidronate were administered IV. The serum calcium level normalized within 3 days and the patient's confusion improved. Later, the confusion returned and he was found to have multiple metastases to the lung, bone, and brain. After consultation with his family, treatment of hypercalcemia was withdrawn, and he was treated palliatively at home until he died 10 days later.

Commentary. Nausea and vomiting are classic symptoms of hypercalcemic states, as is constipation. High serum calcium levels cause slowed GI motility and delayed gastric emptying; these conditions contribute to anorexia, nausea, and vomiting. The polyuria associated with hypercalcemia is related to a renal concentrating defect; inability to replace the large urinary losses with increased oral fluid intake results in fluid volume depletion. Although this patient's confusion was partially alleviated by correction of the serum calcium level, other causes were present that caused it to recur (namely, metastases to the brain).

Case Study 6-11

A case was reported in which a 40-year-old woman was admitted to the emergency department with eclampsia.[93] During her examination, she was found to have profound hypercalcemia and metabolic alkalosis (pH 7.57) secondary to milk-alkai syndrome. The corrected calcium level was 4.71 mmol/L (normal range is 2.23 to 2.57 mmol/L). The patient revealed that she had self-medicated with multiple antacid tablets for dyspepsia. Treatment consisted of aggressive rehydration, bisphosphonates, and discontinuation of antacid tablets. The patient made a full recovery and delivered a normal infant.

Commentary. It is possible to consume enough calcium and alkali with over-the-counter antacids to induce milk-alkali syndrome. Upon questioning, it was learned that the patient had taken approximately 24 antacid tablets per day, in addition to an unknown multivitamin preparation.

Case Study 6-12

A case was reported in which a 32-year-old man had a 3-day history of nausea, vomiting, and constipation.[94] In addition, he complained of muscular weakness and polyuria/polydipsia. Laboratory analysis revealed a serum calcium level of 6.9 mmol/L (equivalent to about 27.6 mg/dL), a hematocrit of 52%, and an extremely high parathyroid hormone concentration (70.2 pmol/L (reference range, 1.6 to 6.8 pmol/L). A parathyroid adenoma was identified and removed.

Commentary. Parathyroid adenoma accounts for 96% of the cases of primary hyperparathyroidism.

Case Study 6-13

A 50-year-old woman with breast cancer and metastases to the bone and lung was admitted with polyuria and polydipsia. Laboratory results showed that her total calcium level was 13.0 mg/dL. Following treatment with a bisphosphonate, her serum calcium level returned to normal for almost 2 months. Several recurrences of hypercalcemia were managed the same way. The patient was able to continue palliative therapy at home before ultimately dying from complications other than hypercalcemia.

Commentary. The polyuria and polydipsia noted in this case were attributable to nephrogenic diabetes insipidus secondary to hypercalcemia. Fortunately, this condition was corrected when the hypercalcemia was treated. The value of bisphosphonates in treating hypercalcemia is immense in that they provide relief from the multiple symptoms of severe hypercalcemia.

Case Study 6-14

A case was reported in which a 69-year-old woman with squamous cancer of the anus was admitted to the hospital in an unresponsive state.[95] She had a 3-day history of lethargy, weakness, obstipation, and emesis of feculent material. A fecal impaction of the transverse and ascending colon was identified. Laboratory results showed a total calcium level of 14.7 mg/dL (corrected for a low albumin level) and a BUN level of 33 mg/dL. The patient was treated with hydration, calcitonin, and a bisphosphonate. The lethargy and bowel dysfunction were ultimately corrected.

Commentary. This case demonstrates the profound effect that hypercalcemia can have on the bowel (slowed bowel function due to smooth muscle depression).

Case Study 6-15

A 70-year-old man presented with progressive weakness over a period of 3 weeks. He had experienced nausea, vomiting, and constipation. The patient had a history of heartburn and self-medicated with 200 antacid (calcium carbonate) tablets per week; in addition, he drank three quarts of milk per day. Laboratory results showed a serum calcium level of 15 mg/dL. Also evident were signs of renal damage (serum creatinine 5.9 mg/dL and BUN 60 mg/dL).

Commentary. This patient presented with evidence of milk-alkali syndrome. A typical calcium carbonate antacid tablet may contain 200 mg of elemental calcium (as calcium carbonate). Multiplying this number by 200 tablets and adding the amount of calcium consumed in three quarts of milk per day shows the extremely high calcium intake consumed by this patient. (One quart of milk contains approximately 1200 mg of calcium.)

Also see Case Studies 14-2, 14-5, and 22-3 for a discussion of other patients with calcium problems.

NOTES

1. Bongard, F. S., Sue, D. Y., & Vintch, J. R. (2008). *Current diagnosis and treatment, critical care* (3rd ed.). New York: McGraw-Hill/Lange, p. 51.
2. Nix, S. (2009). *Williams' basic nutrition and diet therapy* (13th ed.). St. Louis: Mosby Elsevier, p. 126.
3. Holt, P. R. (2008). New insights into calcium, dairy and colon cancer. *World Journal of Gastroenterology, 14*(28), 4429–4433.
4. McPhee, S. J., Papadakis, M. S., & Tierney, L. M. (2008). *2008 current medical diagnosis and treatment.* New York: McGraw-Hill, p. 1394.
5. Bongard et al., note 1, p. 51.
6. McPhee et al., note 4, p. 768.
7. McPherson, R. A., & Pincus, M. R. (2007). *Henry's clinical diagnosis and management by laboratory methods* (21st ed.). Philadelphia: Saunders, p. 172.
8. McPherson & Pincus, note 7, p. 172.
9. Bongard et al., note 1, p. 51.
10. McPhee et al., note 4, p. 994.
11. Orwoll, E. S., Bauer, D. C., Vogt, T. M., & Fox, K. M. (1996). Axial bone mass in older women: Study of osteoporotic fractures research group. *Annals of Internal Medicine, 124*(2), 187–196.
12. McPhee et al., note 4, p. 996.
13. McPhee et al., note 4, p. 996.
14. Recker, R. R., Lewiecki, E. M., Miller, P. D., & Reiffel, J. (2009). Safety of bisphosphonates in the treatment of osteoporosis. *American Journal of Medicine, 122*(2 suppl), S22–S32.
15. Recker et al., note 14.
16. Maalouf, N. M., Heller, H. J., Odvina, C. V., Kim, P. J., & Sakhae, A. (2006). Bisphosphonate-induced hypocalcemia: Report of 3 cases and review of literature. *Endocrine Practice, 12*(1), 48–53.
17. Parrillo, J. E., & Dellinger, R. P. (2008). *Critical care: Principles of diagnosis and management in the adult* (3rd ed.). Philadelphia: Mosby Elsevier, p. 1227.
18. Bongard et al., note 1, p. 52.
19. Parrillo & Dellinger, note 17, p. 1129.
20. Brunicardi, F. C., Andersen, D., Billiar, T. R., Dunn, D. L., Hunter, J. G., Pollock, R. E. et al. (2005). *Schwartz's principles of surgery* (8th ed.). New York: McGraw-Hill, p. 50.
21. Thomusch, O. (2003). The impact of surgical technique on postoperative hypoparathyroidism in bilateral thyroid surgery: A multivariate analysis of 5846 consecutive patients. *Surgery, 133*, 185–188.
22. Klingensmith, M. E., Chen, L. E., Glasgow, S. C., Goers, T. A., & Melby, S. J. (2007). *The Washington manual of surgery* (5th ed.). Philadelphia: Lippincott Williams & Wilkins, p. 347.
23. Lim, J. P., Irvine, R., Bugis, S., Holmes, D., & Wiseman, S. M. (2009). Intact parathyroid hormone measurement 1 hour after thyroid surgery identifies individuals at high risk for development of symptomatic hypocalcemia. *American Journal of Surgery, 197*(5), 648–653.
24. Adams, J., Andersen, P., Everts, E., & Cohen, J. (1998). Early postoperative calcium levels as predictors of hypocalcemia. *Laryngoscope, 108*, 1829–1831.
25. Bongard et al., note 1, p. 53.
26. Ammori, B. J., Barclay, G. R., Larvin, M., & McMahon, M. J. (2003). Hypocalcemia in patients with acute pancreatitis: A putative role for systematic endotoxin exposure. *Pancreas, 26*(3), 213–217.
27. Robertson, G. M., Moore, E. W., Switz, D. M., Sizemore, G. W., & Estep, H. L. (1976). Inadequate parathyroid response to acute pancreatitis. *New England Journal of Medicine, 294*(10), 512–516.
28. Ammori et al., note 26.
29. Whang, R, Oei, T. O., Aikawa, J. K., Vannatta, A., Fryer, J., & Markanich, M. (1984). Predictors of clinical hypomagnesemia. *Archives of Internal Medicine, 144*, 1794–1796.
30. Biebl, A., Grillenberger, A., & Schmitt, K. (2009). Enema-induced severe hyperphosphatemia in children. *European Journal of Pediatrics, 168*(1), 111–112.
31. Camadoo, L., Tibbott, R., & Isaza, F. (2007). Maternal vitamin D deficiency associated with neonatal hypocalcemia and convulsions. *Nutrition Journal, 6*, 23.
32. Newbury, L., Dolan, K., Hatzifortis, M., Low, N., & Fielding, G. (2003). Calcium and vitamin D depletion and elevated parathyroid hormone following biliopancreatic diversion. *Obesity Surgery, 13*(6), 893–895.
33. Perkins, J. G., Cap, A. P., Weiss, B. M., Reid, T. J., & Bolan, C. D. (2008). Massive transfusion and nonsurgical hemostatic agents. *Critical Care Medicine, 36*(suppl), S325–S339.
34. Niven, M., Zohar, M., Shimoni, Z., & Glick, J. (1998). Symptomatic hypocalcemia precipitated by small-volume transfusion. *Annals of Emergency Medicine, 32*(4), 498–501.

35. Uhl, L., Maillet, S., King, S., & Kruskall, M. S. (1997). Unexpected citrate toxicity and severe hypocalcemia during apheresis. *Transfusion, 37,* 1063–1065.

36. Brown, M. J., Wills, T., Omalu, B., & Leiker, R. (2006). Deaths resulting from hypocalcemia after administration of edetate disodium: 2003–2005. *Pediatrics, 118*(2), e534–e536.

37. Altirkawi, K., & Rozycki, H. J. (2008). Hypocalcemia is common in the first 48 hours of life in ELBW infants. *Journal of Perinatal Medicine, 36*(4), 348–353.

38. Zaloga, G., & Chernow, B. Mechanisms for hypocalcemia during gram negative sepsis [abstract]. *Critical Care Medicine, 14,* 405.

39. Lind, L., Carlstedt, F., Rastad, J., Stiernstrom, H., Ljunggren, O., Wide, L., et al. (2000). Hypocalcemia and parathyroid hormone secretion in critically ill patients. *Critical Care Medicine, 28*(1), 93–99.

40. Fink, M. P., Abraham, E., Vincent, J. L., & Kochanek, P. M. (2005). *Textbook of critical care* (5th ed.). Philadelphia: Elsevier Saunders, p. 80.

41. Fink et al., note 40, p. 80.

42. Forsythe, R. M., Wessel, C. B., Billiar, T. R., Angus, D. C., & Rosengart, M. R. (2008). Parenteral calcium for intensive care unit patients. *Cochrane Database of Systematic Reviews, 4,* CD006163.

43. Peter, S. A. (1992). Disorders of serum calcium in acquired immunodeficiency syndrome. *Journal of the National Medical Association, 84,* 626–628.

44. Olinger, M. L (1989). Disorders of calcium and magnesium. *Emergency Medical Clinics of North America, 7,* 795–822

45. Guyton, A. C., & Hall, J. E. (2006). *Textbook of medical physiology* (11th ed.). Philadelphia: W. B. Saunders, p. 979.

46. Yucha, C. B., & Toto, K. H. (1994) Calcium and phosphorus derangements. *Critical Care Nursing Clinics of North America,* 6(4), 747–766.

47. Rallidis, L. S., Gregoropoulos, P., & Papasteriadis, E. (1997). A case of severe hypocalcemia mimicking myocardial infarction. *International Journal of Cardiology, 61,* 89–91.

48. Suzuki, T., Ikeda, U., Fukikawa, H., Saito, K., & Shimada, K. (1997). Hypocalcemic heart failure: A reversible form of heart muscle disease. *Clinical Cardiology, 21,* 227–228.

49. Olinger, note 44.

50. Murray, M. J. Coursin, D. B, Pearl, R. G., & Prough, D.S. (2002). *Critical care medicine: Perioperative management* (2nd ed.). Philadelphia: Lippincott Williams & Wilkins, p. 218.

51. Steichen, O. (2008). Use of oral calcium to treat hypocalcemia. *British Medical Journal, 336*(7658), 1298–1392.

52. Steichen, note 51.

53. Steichen, note 51.

54. Nix, note 2, p. 126.

55. Bell, A. M., Nolen, J. D., Knudson, C. M., & Raife, T. J. (2007). Severe citrate toxicity complication volunteer donor apheresis platelet donation. *Journal of Clinical Apheresis, 22*(1), 15–16.

56. Bell et al., note 55.

57. Ali F. E, Al-Bustan, M. A, Al-Busairi, W. A, & Al-Mulla, F. A. (2004). Loss of seizure control due to anticonvulsant-induced hypocalcemia. *Annals of Pharmacotherapy, 38,* 1002–1005.

58. Kelly, A. P., Robb, B. J., & Gearry, R. B. (2008). Hypocalcaemia and hypomagnesaemia: A complication of Crohn's disease. *New Zealand Medical Journal, 121,* 77–79.

59. Murray et al., note 55, p. 219.

60. Parrillo & Dellinger, note 17, p. 1229.

61. Parrillo & Dellinger, note 17, p. 1229.

62. Parrillo & Dellinger, note 17, p. 1230.

63. Gardner, D. G., & Shoback, D. (2007). *Greenspan's basic and clinical endocrinology* (8th ed.). New York: McGraw-Hill, p. 300.

64. Gardner & Shoback, note 63, p. 308.

65. Parrillo & Dellinger, note 17, p. 1230.

66. Parrillo & Dellinger, note 17, p. 1230.

67. Alsirafy, S. A., Sroor, M. Y., & Al-Shahri, M. Z. (2009). Predictive impact of electrolyte abnormalities on the admission outcome and survival of palliative care cancer referrals. *Journal of Palliative Medicine, 12*(2), 177–180.

68. Maynard, F. M. (1986). Immobilization hypercalcemia following spinal cord injury. *Archives of Physician Medicine & Rehabilitation, 67*(1), 41–44.

69. Wick, J. Y. (2007). Immobilization hypercalcemia in the elderly. *Consultant Pharmacist, 22*(11), 892–905.

70. Alborzi, F., & Leibowitz, A. B. (2002) Immobilization hypercalcemia in critical illness following bariatric surgery. *Obesity Research. 12*(6), 871–873.

71. Gardner & Shoback, note 63, p. 309.

72. Parrillo & Dellinger, note 17, p. 1230.

73. Fink et al., note 40, p. 1124.

74. Edelson, G. W., & Kleerekoper, M. (1995). Hypercalcemic crisis. *Medical Clinics of North America, 79,* 79–92.

75. Murray et al., note 55, p. 219.

76. Edelson & Kleerekoper, note 74.

77. Edelson & Kleerekoper, note 74.

78. Mahon, S. M. (1987). Symptoms as clues to calcium levels. *American Journal of Nursing, 87,* 354.

79. Klingensmith et al., note 22, p. 80.

80. Kaye, T. B. (1995). Hypercalcemia: How to pinpoint the cause and customize treatment. *Postgraduate Medicine, 97,* 153.

81. Murray et al., note 55, p. 219.

82. Klingensmith et al., note 22, p. 80.

83. Bongard et al., note 1, p. 56.

84. McPhee & Papadakis, note 4, p. 771.

85. Bongard et al., note 1, p. 56.

86. Govindan, R. (2008). *The Washington manual of oncology* (2nd ed.). Philadelphia: Lippincott Williams & Wilkins, p. 405.

87. Gardner & Shoback, note 63, p. 883.

88. Cooper, D. H., Krainik, A. J., Lubner, S. J., & Reno, H. E. (2007). *The Washington manual of medical therapeutics* (32nd ed.). Philadelphia: Lippincott Williams & Wilkins, p. 81.

89. Cooper et al., note 88, p. 81.

90. Cooper et al., note 88, p. 81.

91. Mahon, note 78.

92. Coward, D. D. (1988). Hypercalcemia knowledge assessment in patients at risk for developing cancer-induced hypercalcemia. *Oncology Nursing Forum, 15,* 471–476.

93. Bailey, C. S., Weiner, J. J., Gibby, O. M., & Penney, M. D. (2008). Excessive calcium ingestion leading to milk-alkai syndrome. *Annals of Clinical Biochemistry, 45,* 527–529.

94. Marienhagen, K., Due, J., Hanssen, T., & Svartberg, J. (2005). Surviving extreme hypercalcemia: A case report and review of the literature. *Journal of Internal Medicine, 258*(1), 86–89.

95. Bush, E., & Friedman, I. (2004). Case report: An unusual case of constipation. *American Journal of Hospital & Palliative Medicine, 21,* 455–456.

Chapter 7

Magnesium Imbalances

MAGNESIUM BALANCE

Approximately 99% of the body's magnesium is found in the bone matrix or inside the cells.[1] Of the skeletal magnesium, approximately one-third is exchangeable and serves as a reservoir for maintaining a normal serum magnesium concentration.[2] Only 1% of the body's magnesium is located in the extracellular fluid (and less than 0.3% is in the serum). Of the magnesium found in the serum, approximately 55% is available in the ionized form (the portion that influences myoneural function); the remainder is bound to albumin and other anions. The normal serum magnesium level can be expressed in milliequivalents per liter, millimoles per liter, or milligrams per deciliter (**Table 7-1**).

Functions

Magnesium is an important constituent of intracellular fluid, where it affects multiple cellular functions. It participates in more than 300 enzymatic reactions, especially those processes involving the production and utilization of adenosine triphosphate (ATP). Extracellular magnesium is implicated in neuronal control, neuromuscular transmission, and cardiovascular tone. Its high concentration in bone means that magnesium levels are closely related to calcium and phosphorus levels. However, because it is a major intracellular ion, magnesium levels are also closely related to potassium levels. Disorders of magnesium may lead to impaired energy production and substrate utilization.[3]

Homeostasis

Magnesium balance depends on gastrointestinal absorption and renal excretion. The recommended daily magnesium allowance in adults is approximately 200 mg.[4] Because magnesium is a major constituent of chlorophyll, it is plentiful in green vegetables. Other good sources of magnesium include grains, cereals, meat, and seafood. Approximately one-third of the magnesium ingested in the diet is absorbed in the jejunum and ileum. Little is known about factors that control the intestinal absorption of magnesium.

The kidneys are the primary route of magnesium excretion. Daily renal excretion of magnesium is in the range of 120–140 mg in an individual on a normal diet.[5] Fortunately, the kidneys are capable of conserving magnesium efficiently in times of need, and excreting it when it is not needed. Sustained hypermagnesemia is difficult to maintain when normal renal function exists because renal magnesium excretion increases in proportion to the load presented to the kidney.

Laboratory Assessment

Like calcium, magnesium exists in serum in two forms: ionized and bound to anions (mainly albumin). Laboratory tests may measure either the total magnesium concentration or just the ionized form. Similar to calcium, ionized magnesium measurement is affected by pH. When pH is

Table 7-1 Normal Serum Magnesium Levels

Expression of Measurement	Normal Range
Milliequivalents per liter (mEq/L)	1.3 to 2.1
Millimoles per liter (mmol/L)	0.65 to 1.1
Milligrams per 100 mL (mg/dL)	1.6 to 2.5

increased, magnesium ionized is decreased. Conversely, when pH is decreased, magnesium ionization is increased.

A less than normal serum magnesium level is most often indicative of total body magnesium deficiency; however, a normal serum magnesium concentration may exist in some individuals with a total body magnesium deficiency. A high index of suspicion is required for patients whose clinical condition suggests magnesium depletion but whose serum magnesium is normal or only slightly reduced according to laboratory tests. The serum magnesium level may not fall until several hours after the onset of an acute illness (such as myocardial infarction [MI]).

Magnesium levels can be measured within the red blood cells and in skeletal muscle. Erythrocyte magnesium concentration is approximately three times higher than that found in the serum.[6] Several groups of investigators have found low cellular levels of magnesium in patients who had normal serum magnesium levels.[7,8] This finding demonstrates that cells can be deficient in magnesium even when there is no evidence of a magnesium deficit on blood tests.

Another type of test of magnesium balance involves measuring 24-hour urinary magnesium excretion. This test is helpful because patients with magnesium deficiency can be expected to conserve magnesium, so that they excrete less magnesium in the urine per day than individuals with a normal magnesium balance. Under normal circumstances, given average magnesium intake and total body stores, 24-hour urinary magnesium excretion ranges from 120 to 140 mg.[9] In the absence of agents or conditions that promote magnesium excretion, a 24-hour urinary magnesium excretion of less than 25 mg suggests magnesium deficiency.[10] A more elaborate test is the magnesium load test, which involves obtaining a 24-hour baseline urine magnesium determination, followed by the intravenous administration of a magnesium load; urine is collected for 24 hours from the beginning of the infusion. Patients with normal total magnesium stores are expected to excrete 60% to 80% of the administered magnesium, whereas patients with magnesium deficiency will excrete less than 50%.

A curious relationship exists between magnesium and calcium. Although low serum levels of these electrolytes produce similar effects (i.e., increased neuromuscular irritability), their actions sometimes antagonize each other. For example, magnesium narcosis can be antagonized by parenteral calcium administration.

HYPOMAGNESEMIA

Hypomagnesemia is a common clinical problem, both in ambulatory and hospitalized patients. For example, it has been estimated that approximately 10% of hospitalized patients have hypomagnesemia; the incidence may be as high as 40% in patients who have other electrolyte imbalances.[11]

Causes

Gastrointestinal Losses

An important route for magnesium loss is the gastrointestinal (GI) tract. Losses may take the form of drainage from nasogastric suction, diarrhea, or fistulas. Because fluid from the lower GI tract is richer in magnesium (10–14 mEq/L) than is fluid from the upper tract (1–2 mEq/L), losses from diarrhea and intestinal fistulas are more likely to induce magnesium deficits than are losses from gastric suction.[12] Nevertheless, hypomagnesemia may occur in patients with prolonged nasogastric suction, especially if parenteral fluids are magnesium free.

Because the distal small bowel is the major site of magnesium absorption, any disruption in small bowel function (such as occurs in intestinal resection or inflammatory bowel disease) can lead to hypomagnesemia. One study reported that 15 of 42 patients with malabsorption syndromes had subnormal serum magnesium levels; the degree of hypomagnesemia showed a rough correlation with the degree of steatorrhea.[13] In the presence of steatorrhea, it is believed that magnesium ions are excreted in the stool in the form of magnesium soaps. In a study reported in 1981, 50% of 191 patients developed hypomagnesemia in the first postoperative year after bowel resection for the treatment of morbid obesity.[14]

Alcoholism

Chronic alcoholism is the most common cause of hypomagnesemia in the United States. One study found that 30% of all alcoholics and 86% of patients with delirium tremens had hypomagnesemia during the first 1 to 2 days of hospitalization.[15] Although there are no convincing data to indicate that hypomagnesemia causes delirium tremens, it is likely that magnesium deficiency aggravates alcohol withdrawal. For this reason, it is recommended that the serum magnesium level be measured every 2 or 3 days in hospitalized alcoholic patients who are undergoing withdrawal. Although the serum magnesium level may be normal on these patients' admission, it can fall as a result of metabolic changes associated with therapy (such as the intracellular shift of magnesium associated with intravenous glucose administration).

Decreased dietary intake of magnesium is a major factor in the development of hypomagnesemia in alcoholics. Other factors include increased GI losses (due to episodic emesis and diarrhea) and intestinal malabsorption. In addition, alcohol ingestion increases renal loss of magnesium (by interfering with tubular reabsorption of magnesium).[16]

A recent randomized trial of alcoholics found that those who received 500 mg of magnesium as opposed to a placebo had less severe liver damage (as evidenced by lower aspartate aminotransferase levels).[17] The researchers concluded that magnesium treatment may decrease the risk of death from alcoholic liver disease.

Refeeding After Starvation

In the catabolic state, the protein structure of cells is metabolized as energy sources; as a result, intracellular ions are lost and total body concentrations of these ions (magnesium, potassium, and phosphate) are decreased. Conversely, during nutritional repletion, these electrolytes are taken from the serum and deposited into newly synthesized cells. Thus, if the enteral or parenteral feeding formula is deficient in magnesium content, serious hypomagnesemia will occur. Serum levels of these primarily intracellular ions should be measured at regular intervals during the administration of IV total parenteral nutrition (TPN) and even during enteral feedings, especially in patients who have experienced a period of starvation. See Chapters 11 and 12 for further discussions of this topic.

Drugs Disrupting Magnesium Homeostasis

The loop diuretics (furosemide, bumetanide, and ethacrynic acid) increase urinary magnesium excretion. Although these agents are the most potent magnesuric diuretics, long-term use of thiazide diuretics may also lead to mild hypomagnesemia.

Although the exact mechanism is not clear, it has been demonstrated that aminoglycosides (such as gentamycin, tobramycin, and kanamycin) are associated with urinary magnesium wasting.[18] Amphotericin B (an antifungal agent) can also cause hypomagnesemia.

Cisplatinum (cisplatin) administration is associated with hypomagnesemia secondary to increased urinary excretion of magnesium. This potentially nephrotoxic chemothera-

peutic agent appears to cause hypomagnesemia in a dose-related manner. Cyclosporine usage in renal transplant patients may produce a significant drop in the serum magnesium concentration, presumably by increasing renal magnesium wasting.

Citrate is a preservative that is added to collected blood to prolong its longevity. Rapid administration of citrated blood can temporarily decrease the ionized magnesium level because citrate chelates circulating magnesium ions (and calcium ions). This outcome is most likely to occur when citrate clearance is diminished by renal or hepatic disease or by hypothermia.

Other Factors

Magnesium deficiency is often seen in patients with diabetic ketoacidosis. It is primarily the result of increased renal excretion of magnesium during osmotic diuresis (caused by the high glucose load) and of the shifting of magnesium into cells that occurs with insulin therapy. (See Chapter 18.)

Some causes of renal disease, such as glomerulonephritis, pyelonephritis, and renal tubular acidosis, may produce hypomagnesemia by impairing renal magnesium reabsorption. In the setting of advanced renal disease (glomerular filtration rate [GFR] less than 10–25 mL/hr), however, hypermagnesemia usually results from impaired renal magnesium excretion.

Pancreatitis may cause hypomagnesemia in much the same way that it causes hypocalcemia. (See Chapter 20.) In addition, any condition associated with hypercalcemia (such as excessive doses of vitamin D or calcium supplements) may result in renal magnesium loss. Magnesium and calcium share a common route of absorption in the intestinal tract and appear to have a mutually suppressive effect; thus, if calcium intake is unusually high, calcium will be absorbed in preference to magnesium, and vice versa.

Magnesium deficiency has also been described in burn patients, where its occurrence may be related to loss of magnesium during debridement and bathing of denuded skin. Other conditions believed to predispose to hypomagnesemia include sepsis and hypothermia. Postoperative patients may have increased magnesium loss in the urine due to increased aldosterone release associated with stress from the operative procedure.

Administration of magnesium-free, sodium-rich IV fluids to induce extracellular fluid expansion can cause hypomagnesemia. In fact, any condition predisposing patients to excessive calcium or sodium in the urine can augment renal excretion of magnesium because magnesium is normally reabsorbed in the kidney with calcium and sodium.

Clinical Signs

Some of the effects of hypomagnesemia are directly caused by the low serum magnesium level, whereas others are due to secondary changes in potassium and calcium metabolism. Manifestations of magnesium deficiency do not usually occur until the serum magnesium level is less than 1 mEq/L. However, because the serum magnesium concentration may underestimate intracellular magnesium depletion, a high index of suspicion for magnesium deficiency is warranted.[19]

Neuromuscular Changes

Neuromuscular hyperexcitability with tremors and athetoid movements may be seen in conjunction with hypomagnesemia. Other manifestations may include tetany, generalized tonic–clonic or focal seizures, laryngeal stridor, and positive Chvostek's and Trousseau's signs. The neuromuscular symptoms of hypomagnesemia are similar to those occurring in hypocalcemia and result mainly from increased neuronal excitability. Because severe hypomagnesemia may ultimately lead to hypocalcemia and hypokalemia, it is possible that the symptoms may be partly due to these disturbances. Vague but nonspecific GI symptoms have been described; for example, dysphagia may develop.

Cardiovascular Effects

Magnesium is important for normal cardiac function; therefore, it is understandable that hypomagnesemia is associated with a high frequency of cardiac arrhythmias and sudden death. Because standard antiarrhythmic drugs and defibrillation may be ineffective in controlling ventricular arrhythmias associated with magnesium deficiency, refractory arrhythmias should be treated with IV magnesium salts. Intracellular magnesium depletion in the myocardium is even more likely to predispose to arrhythmias if hypokalemia is also present. Eelctrocardiographic (ECG) changes observed in severe hypomagnesemia include PR- and QT-interval prolongation, widened QRS complex, ST-segment depression, and diminution of the T-wave.

Digitalis Toxicity. Increased susceptibility to digitalis toxicity is associated with low serum magnesium levels. An experiment with animals found that the uptake of digoxin by myocardial cells was enhanced by magnesium depletion.[20] One report indicated that hypomagnesemia was present twice as often in digitalis-toxic patients (21%) as in nontoxic patients (10%).[21] This is important because patients receiving digoxin are also likely to be on diuretic therapy, which predisposes patients to renal loss of magnesium.

Hypertension. An inverse relationship between serum magnesium levels and blood pressure has been implicated in experimental and epidemiological studies.[22] It appears that magnesium affects blood pressure by modulating vascular tone and reactivity. Although most epidemiological and experimental studies suggest that low magnesium levels play a role in the pathophysiology of hypertension, data from clinical studies have been less convincing.[23]

Central Nervous System Changes

Because decreased serum magnesium increases irritability of nerve tissue, convulsions may occur. Disorientation is common. Other changes may include ataxia, vertigo, depression, and psychosis.

Associated Imbalances

Hypomagnesemia may occur with and contribute to other imbalances, such as hypokalemia, hypocalcemia, and hypophosphatemia. Hypokalemia is a relatively common finding in hypomagnesemic patients because the kidneys are not able to conserve potassium when magnesium deficiency exists. Hypokalemia accompanying hypomagnesemia is often refractory to potassium replacement alone, instead requiring the replacement of both potassium and magnesium before correction of the imbalance can occur. The plasma magnesium concentration should always be measured in patients with otherwise unexplained hypokalemia. It is likely that hypocalcemia and hypophosphatemia occur in conjunction with hypomagnesemia because severe magnesium depletion interferes with the secretion of parathyroid hormone (PTH), which is needed to return calcium and phosphorus levels to their normal ranges. A study of 35 adult patients who exhibited profound hypomagnesemia, hypokalemia, and hypocalcemia on admission found that alcoholism and cisplatin administration were the most common causes of this combination of electrolyte imbalances.[24]

Glucose and Insulin Homeostasis

Hypomagnesium influences glucose and insulin homeostasis and is associated with insulin resistance.[25] A high prevalence of hypomagnesemia has been found in epidemiological studies of diabetic subjects, especially in those with poor glycemic control.[26] Low magnesium intake and increased magnesium losses have been found to be associated with magnesium deficits in diabetic subjects.[27] It is possible that hyperglycemia has a role in the increased urinary magnesium excretion contributing to magnesium depletion in diabetics.[28]

Treatment

Magnesium replacement may be indicated even when the serum magnesium concentration is normal, given that total body magnesium stores may be decreased despite normomagnesemia. Magnesium deficiency is treated by correcting the cause of the imbalance (when possible) and supplying magnesium to correct the deficit. Serum magnesium levels may normalize rather quickly, but sustained magnesium replacement for several days is usually needed to replace cellular magnesium deficits. Provided the patient is able to eat, dietary sources of magnesium should be encouraged; especially magnesium-rich foods include green vegetables, seafood, nuts, and grains. When symptoms of hypomagnesemia are absent, it is best to administer magnesium orally to avoid causing abrupt increases in the plasma magnesium level. Magnesium salts in tablet form (such as magnesium oxide) can be given orally to replace continuous excessive losses. Unfortunately, diarrhea is a side effect that can interfere with the usefulness of oral magnesium preparations.

Magnesium may be given intravenously or by deep intramuscular injection (although this route of administration is painful) when indicated. Parenteral magnesium is especially helpful in patients with symptomatic hypomagnesemia or malabsorption. Before magnesium administration, renal function should be assessed because the kidneys are primarily responsible for the elimination of magnesium. When renal function is impaired in those receiving magnesium, blood levels should be closely monitored. During parenteral magnesium replacement, serum magnesium levels should be monitored, as should deep-tendon reflexes. Marked depression of deep-tendon reflexes signals too high a serum magnesium level and is an indication that no further magnesium should be administered. Reports of serum levels at which loss of the patellar reflex occurs vary, but most agree that it is decreased at 4 to 6 mEq/L and is lost at a range of 6 to 10 mEq/L. Because deep-tendon reflexes disappear before respiratory paralysis and heart block occur, frequent assessment of deep-tendon reflexes is reasonable to help detect hypermagnesemia before it reaches a critical level.

Controversial Conditions for Magnesium Replacement

Myocardial Infarction. Magnesium has properties that could benefit patients with acute myocardial infarction; among these are possible prevention of arrhythmias, antiplatelet effect, vasodilation, and possible reduction of infarct size. Adverse events associated with magnesium supplementation include bradycardia and generalized vasodilatation that can cause hypotension and increase risk of shock and extension of myocardial necrosis.[29] Currently available data do not support the routine use of magnesium in patients with myocardial infarction.[30] However, this does not preclude magnesium administration to rectify serum magnesium deficits in patients with myocardial infarction.[31] Patients with myocardial infarction may have hypomagnesemia for reasons that are not explainable by renal or other increased excretion of magnesium.[32] Treatment with magnesium has beneficial effects in such patients by reducing the frequency and consequences of ventricular arrhythmias.[33]

Hypertension. The therapeutic value of magnesium in the management of hypertension is unclear.[34] More data from clinical trials are needed to consider magnesium as a nonpharmacologic tool for treating hypertension.

Menstrual Migraine Headaches. Deficiencies in magnesium may play an important role in the pathogenesis of menstrual migraine headaches.[35] Magnesium supplementation has been investigated as an option for the treatment of menstrual migraine headaches and shown to be effective for short-term prevention of menstrual migraines.[36,37] In one small study, patients who received magnesium (versus those who received a placebo) had a significant reduction in pain scores and number of days with headache.[38]

Diabetes Mellitus. The effects of magnesium supplements on the metabolic profile of patients with type 2 diabetes mellitus are unclear; some studies have shown a benefit from this therapy, whereas others have not.[39,40] At present, there does not appear to be sufficient clinically based evidence to support the routine use of magnesium supplementation in type 2 diabetes and its use for this purpose remains controversial.[41] It has been suggested that because the most frequent origin of micronutrient deficiencies is an inadequate diet, healthcare providers should emphasize nutrition counseling rather than focusing on micronutrient supplements.[42] Certainly there is need for long-term trials to determine the role of magnesium supplementation in type 2 diabetes treatment.

Clinical Considerations

1. Be aware of patients at risk for hypomagnesemia and monitor for its presence. **Table 7-2** summarizes the causes and clinical signs of hypomagnesemia.

2. Assess patients who are receiving digitalis and who are at risk for hypomagnesemia especially closely for symptoms of digitalis toxicity, because a deficit of magnesium predisposes them to such toxicity.

Table 7-2 Summary of Hypomagnesemia

Causes	Clinical Signs
Inadequate Intake	*Neuromuscular*
• Prolonged administration of magnesium-free fluids	• Muscle weakness
• Starvation	• Muscle twitching, cramps
• Total parenteral nutrition without adequate magnesium supplementation	• Paresthesias
• Chronic alcoholism	• Chvostek's sign
	• Trousseau's sign
Increased Gastrointestinal Losses	*Cardiovascular*
• Diarrhea	• Increased sensitivity to digitalis
• Laxative abuse	• Hypertension
• Fistulas	• Arrhythmias
• Prolonged nasogastric suction	• Coronary artery spasm
• Vomiting	
• Malabsorbtion syndromes	ECG changes:
	• Prolonged QT and PR intervals
Increased Renal Losses from Drugs	• Widened QRS complex
• Loop and thiazide diuretics	• Depressed ST segment
• Mannitol	
• Cisplatin	*Metabolic*
• Cyclosporine	• Hypocalcemia
• Aminoglycosides	• Hypokalemia
• Carbenicillin	• Hypophosphatemia
• Amphotericin B	• Insulin resistance
Increased Renal Losses from Diseases	*Central Nervous System*
• Uncontrolled diabetes mellitus	• Depression
• Hyperaldosteronism	• Agitation
	• Confusion
Changes in Magnesium Distribution	• Psychosis
• Pancreatitis	
• Thermal injury	
Drugs Causing Magnesium Shift into Cells	
• Insulin	
• Glucose	
• Catecholamines	
Citrate Chelation	
• Citrated blood products	
• Plasmapheresis	

3. Be prepared to take seizure precautions when hypomagnesemia is severe.

4. Monitor the condition of the patient's airway because laryngeal stridor can occur.

5. Take safety precautions if confusion is present.

6. Be familiar with magnesium replacement salts and factors related to their safe administration. **Table 7-3** provides information regarding the intravenous administration of magnesium.

7. Be aware that magnesium-depleted patients may experience difficulty in swallowing. (Dysphagia is probably related to the athetoid or choreiform movements associated with magnesium deficit.) If difficulty in swallowing is suspected, test the ability to swallow with water before offering oral medications.

8. When magnesium deficit is due to abuse of diuretics or laxatives, educating the patient may help alleviate the problem. Part of the nursing assessment should be directed toward identifying problems amenable to prevention through education.

9. Be aware that most commonly used IV fluids (such as 0.9% sodium chloride, 0.45% sodium chloride, and lactated Ringer's solution) contain no magnesium. Prolonged use of magnesium-free parenteral fluids with no oral intake of magnesium and abnormal losses of magnesium by the GI or renal route will eventually lead to hypomagnesemia. When indicated, discuss the need for magnesium replacement with the physician.

10. For patients experiencing abnormal magnesium losses who are able to consume a general diet, encourage the intake of magnesium-rich foods, such as green vegetables, meat, seafood, dairy products, and cereal.

Table 7-3 Nursing Considerations in Administering IV Magnesium

1. Recall that magnesium sulfate ($MgSO_4$) is available in concentrations of 10%, 20%, and 50%, where 1 g of $MgSO_4$ is contained in 10 mL of a 10% solution, 5 mL of a 20% solution, and 2 mL of a 50% solution. Serious errors can occur if the wrong concentration is used.

2. Never accept order for "amps" or "vials" without further specifications.

3. Carefully check the order for IV magnesium. Be sure that it stipulates one of the following:
   - Concentration of the solution to be administered (as well as the number of milliliters), the IV fluid in which it is to be diluted, and the time frame over which it is to be given. For example: "Give 2 mL of 50% $MgSO_4$, diluted in 100 mL of 0.9% sodium chloride, over 1 hr."
   - Number of grams of $MgSO_4$ to be administered, along with the required dilution and the time frame over which it is to be administered. For example: "Give 1 g of $MgSO_4$, diluted in 100 mL of 0.9% sodium chloride, over 1 hr."

4. Use IV magnesium with great caution in patients with impaired renal function (as evidenced by an elevated serum creatinine level)

5. Monitor urine output at regular intervals throughout the magnesium infusion. Therapy is generally not continued if urinary output is less than 100 mL every 4 hours. An output less than this amount raises the question of adequate urinary elimination of magnesium.

6. Check deep-tendon reflexes (such as patellar "knee jerk") before each dose of magnesium, or periodically during continuous infusion of the drug. If reflexes are absent, do not give additional magnesium and notify the physician. (Because deep-tendon reflexes are decreased before adverse respiratory and cardiac effects occur, the presence of knee jerks can usually be relied on to indicate that life-threatening hypermagnesemia is not present.)

7. Therapeutic doses of magnesium can produce flushing and sweating because magnesium acts peripherally to produce vasodilation. Inform the patient that these side effects might occur to minimize concern.

8. Check blood pressure, pulse, and respirations every 15 minutes and monitor the serum magnesium level at regular intervals. Look for a sharp fall in blood pressure and respiratory distress; both are signs of hypermagnesemia. (These outcomes can be induced rather easily with improper doses of magnesium.) Patients receiving very aggressive magnesium therapy should receive close cardiac monitoring.

9. If the patient displays signs of severe hypermagnesemia, stop IV administration of magnesium and run in the IV solution from the primary line (as appropriate) to keep the vein open. Notify the physician and be prepared to administer artificial ventilation and IV calcium (if prescribed).

10. Because magnesium is primarily an intracellular ion, it may take several days to completely correct cellular deficits. Therefore, normal serum magnesium values do not necessarily imply that the magnesium depletion has been corrected.

HYPOMAGNESEMIA CASE STUDIES

Case Study 7-1

A 65-year-old emaciated woman with carcinoma of the stomach was started on a TPN protocol because she was unable to eat or tolerate enteral tube feedings. On the seventh day, when electrolytes were checked for the first time, the serum magnesium was 0.8 mEq/L (normal range is 1.3 to 2.1 mEq/L). The patient was lethargic and had coarse tremors, most notably in the arms. TPN was stopped and 12 mL of 50% magnesium sulfate was added to 1 L of 10% glucose in water and infused over 3 hours. Additional magnesium was administered over the next 2 days. TPN was slowly restarted with adequate magnesium supplementation.

Commentary. Serum electrolytes should be measured regularly during TPN to detect abnormalities before they become severe. Requirements for the intracellular ions (potassium, magnesium, and phosphate) vary with calorie and nitrogen intake and the nutritional state of the patient. As the anabolic state is achieved with TPN, these ions are incorporated into the newly synthesized cells. In this way, extracellular deficits will develop if inadequate amounts are provided in the nutrient solution.

Case Study 7-2

A 50-year-old man with a history of chronic alcoholism was admitted for treatment. He had been on a diet of only alcoholic beverages for a week and then stopped drinking for a few days. Because of nausea, he ate very little. On examination, he was noted to have hyperactive knee jerks. Laboratory findings included a serum magnesium level of 0.7 mEq/L (normal range is 1.3 to 2.1 mEq/L).

Commentary. Hypomagnesemia is a frequent occurrence in alcoholic patients. One reason for its tendency to occur in this population is their often poor dietary intake. Another reason is the increased renal loss of magnesium associated with excessive alcohol intake.

Case Study 7-3

A 40-year-old man developed a high-output intestinal fistula after treatment for an intestinal obstruction. For 2 weeks he received only isotonic saline (0.9% NaCl) and 5% dextrose in water with added KCl. The patient developed choreiform movements of the arms and muscle twitching.

In addition, he was noted to be confused. Laboratory findings included serum Na 140 mEq/L, K 3.3 mEq/L, and Mg 0.7 mEq/L

Commentary. Although the serum sodium level is normal, the magnesium is far below normal and a mild degree of hypokalemia is present, despite addition of KCl to the IV fluids. Recall that intestinal fluid contains 10 to 12 mEq/L of magnesium; these losses were not replaced because the IV fluids were magnesium-free. With a negative magnesium balance, hypokalemia is often present (even when potassium intake is adequate).

Case Study 7-4

A 50 year-old woman with carcinoma of the cervix was treated with radiotherapy and six courses of cisplatin.[43] Twelve weeks after receiving the last dose of cisplatin, she was admitted to the hospital with sudden blindness associated with an occipital headache. Myoclonic jerking was noted in both arms. An extremely low serum magnesium level was reported (0.1 mmol/L; normal for reporting laboratory, 0.7–1.2 mmol/L). A diagnosis of functional blindness was considered. The patient was treated with 40 g of magnesium sulfate over the next 36 hours; within 72 hours of treatment, her cognitive ability improved, myoclonic jerking decreased, and her vision returned to almost normal.

Commentary. Cisplatin therapy may be associated with ophthalmologic toxicity. The neurotoxicity associated with cisplatin therapy may include peripheral neuropathy, auditory impairment, and visual disturbances.[44] The authors reporting this case study state that the relationship between the correction of hypomagnesemia and resolution of blindness in their patient supports the supposition that cisplatin-induced hypomagnesemia caused this patient's blindness.

HYPERMAGNESEMIA

Although hypermagnesemia is much less common than hypomagnesemia, it may occur more frequently than previously thought. In one study, as many as 86% of patients with laboratory-diagnosed hypermagnesemia were not clinically identified.[45] Serum magnesium concentrations tend to be good predictors of total body magnesium excess. Most causes of hypermagnesemia are treatment related.

Causes

Renal Failure

Hypermagnesemia is most likely to occur in patients with renal insufficiency (especially if creatinine clearance is less than 30 mL/min).[46] This relationship is understandable because magnesium is primarily excreted by the kidneys. The predisposition of patients with renal failure to hypermagnesemia is aggravated if they are given magnesium to control convulsions or if they take one of the many commercial magnesium-containing antacids or laxatives. Elderly persons are at greater risk for hypermagnesemia because they often have age-related reduced renal function and tend to consume more magnesium-containing preparations (such as antacids or mineral supplements) than younger individuals. Also, elderly patients may have GI disorders (e.g., gastritis and colitis) that alter the GI mucosal barrier, thereby increasing absorption of magnesium.[47] Renal dialysis patients may develop hypermagnesemia if an excessive amount of magnesium is used in the dialysate (either because of inadvertent use of hard water or an error in manufacturing of the concentrate).

Excessive Magnesium Intake

Although hypermagnesemia most often occurs in patients with renal insufficiency, it may also arise when magnesium administration exceeds the renal tolerance of patients with normal renal function. For example, a case was reported in which a massive dose of a seemingly harmless magnesium-containing cathartic resulted in profound hypermagnesemia (21.7 mg/dL) and cardiopulmonary arrest in a patient with

normal kidney function.[48] Examples of over-the-counter laxatives containing magnesium include citrate of magnesia and milk of magnesia. In addition, many antacids contain magnesium, and patients should be instructed to read the labels of these products if they need magnesium restriction.

Magnesium sulfate is commonly used in obstetrical cases and can result in serious overdoses if used improperly. See Chapter 23 for a discussion of the use of magnesium sulfate in pregnancy.

Clinical Signs

Because magnesium is not measured as routinely as most other electrolytes, healthcare providers must maintain a high index of suspicion for hypermagnesemia in at-risk patients. The clinical manifestations of hypermagnesemia largely reflect the magnesium ion's action on the nervous and cardiovascular systems. Because hypermagnesemia diminishes neuromuscular transmission, it can depress skeletal muscle function and cause neuromuscular blockade. Cardiovascular effects of hypermagnesemia are related to its "calcium-channel blocker" effect on cardiac conduction and smooth muscle of blood vessels. Arrhythmias occurring with hypermagnesemia may include bradycardia, atrioventricular block, and asystole. Changes seen on ECG tracings may include prolongation of the PR interval and widening of the QRS complex; when severe, the QT interval may be prolonged. Hypotension tends to occur early in hypermagnesemia and is related to vasodilation.

Table 7-4 lists some approximate relationships between serum magnesium levels and expected symptoms. Note that

Table 7-4 Summary of Hypermagnesemia

Causes	Clinical Signs
Acute and chronic renal failure (particularly when magnesium-containing medications are used)	*Serum Magnesium Levels (mEq/L)**
	3–5: Peripheral vasodilation with facial flushing, sense of warmth, and tendency for hypotension; nausea and vomiting
Excessive magnesium administration during treatment of eclampsia or to delay labor (affects both mother and fetus)	4–7: Drowsiness; decreased deep-tendon reflexes; muscle weakness
Excessive doses of magnesium during treatment of hypomagnesemia	5–10: More severe hypotension and bradycardia
Excessive use of magnesium-containing antacids or laxatives by elderly persons (who have age-related decreased renal function)	7–10: Loss of patellar reflex
Adrenal insufficiency	10: Respiratory depression
	10–15: Respiratory paralysis; coma
Hemodialysis with excessively hard water or with a dialysate high in magnesium content	15–20: Cardiac arrest

*These are only general ranges; precise levels at which signs and symptoms are expected to develop are not uniformly defined. Reports in the literature vary widely in regard to symptoms and the level at which they appear.

authorities do not agree on precise serum magnesium levels at which specific symptoms will occur, with the disagreement arising largely because patients respond differently to elevated serum magnesium levels. There is good agreement that deep-tendon reflexes will diminish and disappear well before respiratory paralysis or cardiac arrest occurs. For this reason, deep-tendon reflexes are monitored closely during magnesium infusions to prevent potentially life-threatening outcomes.

Rizzo et al. reported a case in which a 27-year-old woman with diabetes was inadvertently given a massive overdose of magnesium sulfate over a 6-hour period for treatment of hypomagnesemia.[49] Profound hypermagnesemia (9.85 mmol/L) resulted and caused total neuromuscular blockade and a pseudocoma state that mimicked a midbrain syndrome. Fortunately, the patient eventually recovered.

Treatment

The best treatment for hypermagnesemia is prevention. This goal can be accomplished by avoiding administration of magnesium to patients with renal insufficiency and by administering magnesium salts very carefully to seriously ill patients. In the presence of hypermagnesemia, any parenteral or oral magnesium salt should be discontinued; this step may be all that is needed if the deep-tendon reflexes are still present. Neuromuscular and cardiac toxicity of hypermagnesemia can be antagonized transiently by the IV administration of 10 to 20 mL of 10% calcium gluconate over 10 minutes. (Recall that calcium acts as a direct antagonist to magnesium.) Mechanical ventilation may be needed for patients with impaired respiratory function from hypermagnesemia. A temporary pacemaker may be needed if bradyarrhythmias have emerged. Dialysis (either peritoneal or hemodialysis) may be needed for treating hypermagnesemic patients with renal failure.

Safety Issues with Administration of Magnesium Sulfate

There is serious risk for harm when errors are made during the administration of magnesium sulfate. For this reason, magnesium sulfate is on the "List of High-Alert Medications" developed by the Institute of Safe Medication Practices (ISMP).[50] Consequences related to medication errors with magnesium sulfate are potentially deadly. See Chapter 23 for a discussion of the use of magnesium during pregnancy.

Magnesium sulfate is available in 10%, 20%, and 50% solutions, where1 g of magnesium sulfate is equivalent to 2 mL of a 50% solution, 5 mL of a 20% solution, and 10 mL of a 10% solution. Reports of severe hypermagnesemia resulting from improperly written or executed orders for IV magnesium sulfate emphasize the need for extreme caution in administering magnesium.[51] Three cases of severe hypermagnesemia were attributed to the inadvertent use of 50-mL vials of 50% magnesium sulfate. In two cases, the orders called for "one amp" of 50% magnesium sulfate by slow IV infusion. Although the prescriber intended that a 2-mL ampule be given, a 50-mL ampule was substituted. In the third case, the order was for a 50-mL vial of 50% dextrose; instead, a 50-mL vial of magnesium sulfate was mistakenly used. The author emphasizes the need to recognize the potency of currently available electrolyte solutions and the importance of physicians writing precise orders pertaining to their use. Certainly, orders containing terms such as "amp" or "vial" without further specification should not be written by physicians or accepted by nurses. The third case emphasizes the need to read product labels carefully before use. Never rely solely on the size, shape, or label design of the container for product identification.

An audit carried out over 3 weeks in an adult neuroscience critical care unit in the United Kingdom sought to establish whether a relationship exists between the quality of syringe labeling and drug preparation and variability in concentrations of drug infusions.[52] Magnesium was one of the drugs studied. These investigators found a number of the magnesium syringes contained as much as four to five times too much magnesium, presumably because of confusion about converting millimoles to grams.

Clinical Considerations

1. Be aware of patients who are at high risk for hypermagnesemia and assess for its presence. Table 7-4 summarizes the causes and clinical signs of hypermagnesemia.
2. When hypermagnesemia is suspected, assess the following parameters:
   - Vital signs: Look for low blood pressure and shallow respirations with periods of apnea.
   - Patellar reflexes: If these reflexes are absent, notify the physician because this usually implies a serum magnesium level greater than 6 mEq/L. If this imbalance is allowed to progress, cardiac or respiratory arrest could occur.

- Level of consciousness: Look for drowsiness, lethargy, and coma.
3. Do not give magnesium-containing medications to patients with renal failure or renal insufficiency. Be particularly careful in following "standing orders" for bowel preparation for radiography because some of these solutions contain magnesium citrate.
4. Caution patients with renal disease to check with their healthcare providers before taking over-the-counter medications.
5. Be aware of factors related to safe parenteral administration of magnesium salts. Table 7-3 provides guidelines for the intravenous administration of magnesium.

HYPERMAGNESEMIA CASE STUDIES

Case Study 7-5

A 43-year-old woman was awaiting a kidney transplant when an order was written for a barium enema. Routine orders for bowel preparation in the institution included the administration of magnesium citrate as a laxative. Without considering the need to modify directives for a renal patient, healthcare providers administered the preparation to her. Shortly after administration of the magnesium citrate, the patient became very lethargic and developed muscular weakness.

Commentary. Magnesium salts should never be given to patients with advanced acute or chronic renal disease because diseased kidneys are incapable of eliminating magnesium. Blindly following standing orders caused serious problems for this patient. Hemodialysis was performed on an emergency basis.

Case Study 7-6

A 62-year-old woman with chronic glomerulonephritis took Maalox (a magnesium-containing antacid) to alleviate gastric discomfort. She developed lethargy and difficulty in breathing. On admission to an acute care facility, her serum magnesium level was 7.8 mEq/L (normal, 1.3–2.1mEq/L). Calcium gluconate was administered to alleviate respiratory depression. Hemodialysis was initiated.

Commentary. Magnesium-containing medications are contraindicated in patients with acute or chronic renal disease. Patient education should emphasize checking with care providers before using any over-the-counter drugs.

Case Study 7-7

A 42-year-old schizophrenic woman was admitted to the emergency department with confusion, abdominal pain, vomiting, and constipation. Before admission, she had been treated with milk of magnesia (30 mL) each night and Maalox (30 mL) three times daily. Her abdomen was distended and diffusely tender, and she would respond only briefly to voice or painful stimuli. Laboratory results revealed severe hypermagnesemia (9.1 mEq/L; normal range, 1.3–2.1 mEq/L). The patient's BUN was 16 mg/dL and her serum creatinine was 0.9 mg/dL. A laparotomy was performed and an adhesive band from a previous surgery was found to be compressing the sigmoid colon. Despite successful treatment of the hypermagnesemia with calcium, IV fluids, and furosemide, the patient died from cardiac problems on the second postoperative day.

Commentary. This patient had normal renal function (as indicated by the serum creatinine and BUN values); however, she still developed serious hypermagnesemia following the excessive use of magnesium-containing medications.

Also see Case Studies 22-4, 23-3, and 23-4 for a discussion of other patients with magnesium problems.

NOTES

1. McPherson, R. A., & Pincus, M. R. (2007). *Henry's clinical diagnosis and management by laboratory methods* (21st ed.). Philadelphia: Saunders, p. 173.
2. McPherson & Pincus, note 1, p. 173.
3. Bongard, F. S., Sue, D. Y., & Vintch, J. R. (2008). *Current diagnosis and treatment, critical care* (3rd ed.). New York: McGraw-Hill/Lange, p. 47.
4. Alpers, D. H., Stenson, W. F., Taylor, B. E., & Bier, D. M. (2008). *Manual of nutritional therapeutics* (5th ed.). Philadelphia: Wolters Kluwer/Lippincott Williams & Wilkins, p. 244.
5. McPherson & Pincus, note 1, p. 173.
6. McPherson & Pincus, note 1, p. 173.
7. Fiaccadori, E., Del Canale S, Coffrini, E., Melej, R., Vitali, P., Guariglia, A., et al. (1988). Muscle and serum magnesium in pulmonary intensive care unit patients. *Critical Care Medicine, 16,* 751–760.
8. Ryzen, E., Elkayam, U., & Rude, R. K. (1986). Low blood mononuclear cell magnesium in intensive cardiac care unit patients. *American Heart Journal, 111,* 475–480.
9. White, J. R., & Campbell, R. K. (1993). Magnesium and diabetes: A review. *Annals of Pharmacotherapy, 27,* 775–780.
10. Matz, R. (1993). Magnesium deficiencies and therapeutic uses. *Hospital Practice, 28:* 79.

11. Murray, M. J., Coursin, D. B, Pearl, R. G, & Prough, D. S. (2002). *Critical care medicine: Perioperative management* (2nd ed.). Philadelphia: Lippincott Williams & Wilkins, p. 220.

12. Chernow, B, Smith, J., Rainey, T. J., & Finton, C. (1982). Hypomagnesemia: Implications for the critical care specialist. *Critical Care Medicine, 10,* 193–196

13. Booth, C. C, Babouris, N., Hanna, S. & MacIntyre, I. (1963). Incidence of hypomagnesemia in intestinal malabsorption. *British Medical Journal, 2,* 141–144.

14. Hallberg, D. (1981). Magnesium problems in gastroenterology. *Acta Medica Scandinavica, 661,* 19–20.

15. Sullivan, J. F, Langford, H. G, Swartz, M. J, & Farrell, C. (1963). Magnesium metabolism in alcoholism. *American Journal Clinical Nutrition, 63,* 297.

16. Bongard et al., note 3, p. 48.

17. Poikolainen, K., & Alho, H. (2008). Magnesium treatment in alcoholics: A randomized clinical trial. *Substance Abuse Treatment, Prevention, & Policy, 3,* 1.

18. Zaloga, G. P., & Chernow, B. (1983). Magnesium metabolism in critical illness. *Critical Care Nursing Quarterly, 6,* 22–27.

19. Olerich, M. A., & Rude, R. K (1994). Should we supplement magnesium in critically ill patients? *New Horizons, 2,* 186–192.

20. Goldman, R. H., Kleiger, R. E., Schweizer, E., & Harrison, D. C. (1971). The effect of myocardial 3H-digoxin of magnesium deficiency. *Proceedings of the Society for Experimental Biology & Medicine, 136*(3), 747–749.

21. Beller, G. A, Hood, W. B, Smith, T. W., Abelmann, W. H., & Wacker, W. E. C. (1974). Correlation of serum magnesium levels and cardiac digitalis intoxication. *American Journal of Cardiology, 33,* 225–229.

22. Sontia, B., & Touyz, R. M. (2007). Role of magnesium in hypertension. *Archives of Biochemistry & Biophysics, 458*(1), 33–39.

23. Sontia & Touyz, note 22.

24. Elisaf, M., Miliniois, H., & Siamopoulos, K. C. (1997). Hypomagnesemic hypokalemia and hypocalcemia: Clinical and laboratory characteristics. *Mineral Electrolyte Metabolism, 23,* 105–112.

25. Sontia & Touyz, note 22.

26. Sjogren, A., Floren, C. H., & Nilsson, A. (1988). Magnesium, potassium and zinc deficiency in subjects with type II diabetes mellitus. *Acta Medica Scandinavica, 224,* 461–466.

27. Barbagallo, M., Dominques, L. J., & Resnick, L. M. (2007). Magnesium metabolism in hypertension and type 2 diabetes mellitus. *American Journal of Therapeutics, 14*(4), 375–385.

28. Barbagallo et al., note 27.

29. Seelig, M. S., & Elin, R. J. (1995). Reexamination of magnesium infusions in myocardial infarction. *American Journal of Cardiology, 76*(3), 172–173.

30. Li, J., Zhang, Q., Zhang M, & Egger, M. (2007). Intravenous magnesium for acute myocardiac infarction. *Cochrane Database of Systematic Review, 2,* CD002755.

31. Gowda, R. M., & Khan, I. A. (2004). Magnesium in treatment of acute myocardial infarction. *International Journal of Cardiology, 96*(3), 467–469.

32. Bongard et al., note 3, p. 49.

33. Bongard et al., note 3, p. 49.

34. Barbagallo et al., note 27.

35. Sun-Edelstein, C., & Mauskop, A. (2009). Role of magnesium in the pathogenesis and treatment of migraine. *Expert Review of Neurotherapeutics, 9*(3), 369–379.

36. Martin, V. (2007). Targeted treatment strategies for menstrual migraine. *Journal of Family Practice,* 56: 13–22.

37. Silberstein, S. D., & Goldgerg, J. (2007). Menstrually related migraine: Breaking the cycle in your clinical practice. *Journal of Reproductive Medicine, 52*(10), 888–895.

38. Facchinetti, F., Sances, G., Borella, P., Genazzani, A. R., & Nappi, G. (1991). Magnesium prophylaxis of menstrual migraine: Effects on intracellular magnesium. *Headache, 31,* 298–301.

39. Rodriguez-Moran, M., & Guerrero-Romero, F. (2003). Oral magnesium supplementation improves insulin sensitivity and metabolic control in type 2 diabetic subjects: A randomized double-blind controlled trial. *Diabetes Care, 26,* 1147–1152.

40. deValk, H. W., Verkaaik, R., van Rijn, H. J., Geerdink, R. A., & Struyvenberg, A. (1998). Oral magnesium supplementation in insulin-requiring type 2 diabetic patients. *Diabetes Medicine, 15,* 503–507.

41. Guerrero-Romero, F. & Rodriquez-Moran, M. (2005). Complementary therapies for diabetes: The case for chromium, magnesium, and antioxidants. *Archives of Medical Research, 36*(3), 250–257.

42. Guerrero-Romero & Rodriquez-Moran, note 41.

43. Al-Tweigeri, T., Magliocco, A. M., & DeCoteau, J. F. (1999). Cortical blindness as a manifestation of hypomagnesemia secondary to cisplatin therapy: Case report and review of literature. *Gynecologic Oncology, 72,* 120–122.

44. Al-Tweigeri et al., note 43.

45. Rude, R. K. (1993). Magnesium metabolism and deficiency. *Endocrinology Metabolism Clinics of North America, 22,* 377–395.

46. Toto, K. H., & Yucha, C. B. (1994). Endocrine and metabolic disturbances in the critically ill. *Critical Care Clinics of North America, 6,* 767–783.

47. Clark, B., & Brown, R. (1992). Unsuspected morbid hypermagnesemia in elderly patients. *American Journal of Nephrology, 12,* 336.

48. Qureshi, T., & Melonakos, T. K. (1996). Acute hypermagnesemia after laxative abuse. *Annals of Emergency Medicine, 28,* 552–555.

49. Rizzo, M. A, Fisher, M., & Lock, J. P. (1993). Hypermagnesemic pseudocoma. *Archives of Internal Medicine, 153,* 1130–1132

50. Institute for Safe Medication Practices. (2005). Preventing magnesium toxicity in obstetrics. *ISMP Medication Safety Alert, 10*(21), 1–2.

51. Hoffman, R. S., Smilkstein, M. J., & Rubenstein, F. (1989). An amp by any other name: The hazards of intravenous magnesium dosing [letter]. *Journal of the American Medical Association, 261,* 557.

52. Wheeler, D. W., Degnan, B. A., Sehmi, J. S., Burnstein, R. M., Menon, D. K., Gupta, A. K., et al. (2008). Variability in the concentrations of intravenous drug infusions prepared in a critical care unit. *Intensive Care Medicine, 34*(8), 1441–1447.

Chapter 8

Phosphorus Imbalances

PHOSPHORUS BALANCE

Functions and Distribution

Phosphorus plays a major role in cellular metabolism. For example, it forms part of the adenosine triphosphate (ATP) molecule that serves as a reservoir of energy in cells to fuel muscle contractility, neuronal transmission, electrolyte transport, and conversion of dietary nutrients into energy. Phosphorus also forms part of the 2,3-diphosphoglycerate (2,3-DPG) enzyme in red blood cells, a substance that facilitates release of oxygen from hemoglobin to tissues.

Approximately 85% of the body's phosphorus is located in bone, where it is necessary for skeletal integrity. About 14% of the body's phosphorus is located intracellularly; only 1% is located extracellularly. Because phosphorus plays an essential role in many facets of normal physiology, it is understandable how phosphorus imbalances (either too low or too high levels) would cause diverse signs and symptoms.[1]

Terminology and Normal Laboratory Values

The terms "phosphorus" and "phosphate" are often used interchangeably, although the term "phosphate" actually refers to the inorganic, freely available form.[2] Laboratories generally report the inorganic component as "phosphorus."[3] The normal serum phosphorus level in adults ranges from 2.5 to 4.5 mg/dL (0.81–1.45 mmol/L). Levels are greater in children, because of the higher rate of skeletal growth in this population.[4] Phosphorus circulates in the bloodstream in three major forms: protein bound (12%), complexed (33%), and ionized (55%). The ionized form is physiologically active, but most laboratories measure total phosphorus.

Serum levels may fluctuate throughout the day. For example, glucose intake, insulin administration, and hyper-ventilation may all lower the serum phosphorus concentration by causing phosphorus to shift into the cells. Because phosphorus is primarily an intracellular ion, serum levels do not always reflect the total body stores. As a consequence, hypophosphatemia does not necessarily imply a total body phosphate depletion. Conversely, a normal serum phosphate level does not necessarily mean the total body phosphate stores are normal. Nonetheless, in clinical settings, measurement of the serum phosphate level is the most widely used measure of body phosphate stores. It is best to measure serum phosphorus in a fasting patient in the morning.[5] Because phosphorus has a high cellular concentration, hemolyzed blood samples are unacceptable for testing purposes because they produce falsely elevated serum phosphorus results.[6]

Dietary Intake

The usual dietary intake of phosphate ranges between 1000 and 1200 mg/day.[7] Adequate dietary intake is ensured by a normal diet because phosphorus is plentiful in many foods, including red meat, fish, poultry, eggs, milk products, whole grains, nuts, and legumes. Cola beverages and prepackaged fast foods contain extra phosphorus as a preservative.[8] In fact, phosphorus-based additives in commercially prepared foods and beverages are a rapidly growing source of dietary phosphorus and may provide as much as one-third of overall phosphorus intake in the general population.[9] Because phosphorus is so widely used as a food additive/preservative, it is very difficult to accurately predict dietary intake of phosphorus.[10] Some authors caution that a high phosphorus intake may be harmful to the general public.[11] For example, the dietary phosphorus intake of individuals in the United States has been increasing while calcium intake has been decreasing;[12] these intake patterns interfere with calcium balance and may, in turn, adversely affect bone mass.[13]

Most dietary phosphorus is absorbed in the duodenum and jejunum. Absorption can be impaired by certain medications (such as phosphate-binding antacids) or by malabsorptive disorders.

Routes of Excretion

Maintenance of normal phosphate balance requires an efficient renal conservation mechanism because the kidneys are responsible for roughly two-thirds of the total amount of phosphorus excreted daily; the remaining one-third is excreted in the stool.[14] During times of low phosphate intake, the kidneys retain more phosphorus.

Regulation by Hormones

Parathyroid hormone lowers the serum phosphate level by increasing renal excretion of phosphorus; thus hyperparathyroidism can cause hypophosphatemia. In contrast, thyroid hormone and growth hormone increase serum levels by reducing renal excretion of phosphorus. Vitamin D increases the serum phosphorus level by increasing intestinal absorption and renal retention of phosphorus.[15]

HYPOPHOSPHATEMIA

Hypophosphatemia in an adult refers to a serum phosphorus concentration below the lower limit of normal (less than 2.5 mg/dL); it is considered to be severe at a concentration of less than 1.0 mg/dL. This imbalance may occur in the presence of a total body phosphorus deficit or merely reflect a temporary shift of phosphorus into the cells. Severe hypophosphatemia is associated with a high mortality rate.[16] A recent report indicated that even mild to moderate hypophosphatemia was associated with an increased mortality rate in a group of 125 older hospitalized women.[17] Hypophosphatemia occurs more often than hyperphosphatemia in hospitalized and critically ill patients.[18]

Approximately 2% to 3% of hospitalized patients and as many as 30% of patients in intensive care units develop hypophosphatemia.[19] In a study of 208 consecutive patients admitted to a surgical intensive care unit, 60 (28.8%) had hypophosphatemia.[20] A number of reasons explain why hypophosphatemia is so prevalent in this population. For example, patients in intensive care settings may be chronically malnourished as a result of their pre-admission illness, and they often receive drugs that increase phosphate loss (such as loop diuretics). Stress may add to the problem by increasing catecholamine release, which in turn may produce a shift of phosphate into the cells.

When doubt exists about the presence of phosphorus depletion, it is helpful to measure phosphorus in a 24-hour urine collection. When hypophosphatemia is present, the kidneys should retain phosphorus. A urinary phosphorus excretion less than 100 mg over a 24-hour period, indicates that gastrointestinal phosphorus losses or shifting of phosphorus from the extracellular space into the cells are occurring.[21]

Causes

A wide variety of clinical disorders and therapeutic interventions can cause hypophosphatemia. Patients at especially high risk are those with malnutrition, uncontrolled diabetes mellitus, sepsis, and chronic alcoholism.[22] **Table 8-1** summarizes the causes and clinical signs of hypophosphatemia.

Table 8-1 Summary of Causes and Clinical Signs of Hypophosphatemia

Causes	Clinical Signs
Alcoholism	Paresthesias
Refeeding syndrome	Muscle weakness (perhaps manifested as decreased strength of hand grasp and difficulty speaking)
Malabsorption and chronic diarrhea	
Respiratory alkalosis	Muscle pain and tenderness (due to breakdown of muscle tissue)
Vitamin D deficiency	Mental changes, such as apprehension, confusion, delirium, and coma
Phosphate-binding antacids	Decreased cardiac contractility
Recovery phase after severe burns	Acute respiratory failure (related to chest muscle weakness)
Starvation or anorexia	Seizures
Glucose/insulin administration	Decreased tissue oxygenation
Diabetic ketoacidosis	Serum phosphate < 2.5 mg/dL

Essentially, causes of hypophosphatemia fall into one of three categories: (1) shift of phosphate from the extracellular fluid (ECF) into the cells; (2) decreased absorption of phosphate from the gastrointestinal tract; and (3) increased renal phosphate losses. Usually at least two, and often all three, of these mechanisms are present in a given situation. Many of the precipitating causes are related to treatment. For example, one group of investigators reported that medications contributed to hypophosphatemia in 82% of the patients in their study; among the implicated medications were intravenous (IV) glucose, antacids, anabolic steroids, and diuretics.[23]

Refeeding Syndrome

Refeeding syndrome (also referred to as *nutritional recovery syndrome*) occurs when malnourished patients are started on an overly aggressive refeeding program (either orally, by feeding tube, or by the parenteral route). Even the consumption of calories in normally required amounts by patients with severe protein-calorie malnutrition can result in serious electrolyte imbalances, one of the most serious of which is hypophosphatemia. This condition more frequently occurs with total parenteral nutrition (TPN) and tube feedings than with oral feedings. Individuals who are especially at risk of developing hypophosphatemia include patients with chronic alcoholism, anorexia nervosa, and other causes of chronic malnutrition.[24]

A chronically malnourished patient is usually in a catabolic state, which itself causes muscle breakdown and depletion of intracellular phosphate stores. Despite these changes in the body, the extracellular (serum) phosphate level tends to remain relatively normal until a large glucose load is administered, as in TPN or tube feeding. Glucose administration causes the pancreas to release more insulin, which in turn promotes the transport of both glucose and phosphorus into the cells (primarily of the skeletal muscle and liver) as the patient becomes anabolic. Delivery of exogenous insulin in an attempt to control hyperglycemia intensifies the shift of phosphorus from the bloodstream into the cells by promoting glycolysis. In a study reported by Van Landingham et al., hypophosphatemia was found in 30% of tube-fed patients.[25] This imbalance primarily occurred in patients who were treated with insulin for hyperglycemia (causing intracellular transport of phosphate).

The development of severe hypophosphatemia in malnourished patients receiving TPN without adequate phosphorus replacement has been well documented and may occur within the first 24 hours, although it often becomes evident only after 2 to 3 days of treatment (see Case Study 8-1).

As indicated earlier, refeeding syndrome can occur in a wide variety of adult patients (such as those with anorexia nervosa or alcoholism and elderly debilitated patients). It has also been observed in children. For example, a 3-year-old boy was admitted after having been starved by an abusive parent; he was started on a regular diet by mouth and consumed an average 140 kcal/kg/day and rapidly gained weight.[26] On admission, his serum phosphorus concentration was normal for his age (7.0 mg/dL); however, on the twentieth day, it was low for his age (2.8 mg/dL). Fortunately, this patient's imbalance was relatively minor and was easily correctable with phosphate replacement.

Alcoholism

Alcoholism is one of the most common causes of severe hypophosphatemia. In one study, hypophosphatemia was found in 30.4% of alcoholic patients admitted to medical services (as compared to only 1.8% of matched non-alcoholic patients).[27] Factors contributing to phosphate depletion in alcoholics include poor food intake, vomiting, use of antacids, marked phosphaturia, and diarrhea. (Because phosphate is absorbed in the small bowel, chronic diarrhea predisposes individuals to development of hypophosphatemia.)

Excessive Pharmacological Phosphate Binding

Absorption of phosphate from the small bowel can be blocked by phosphate-binding antacids commonly available over-the-counter (such as aluminum-, calcium-, and magnesium-containing antacids). Further, their chronic use can result in hypophosphatemia, particularly when there is poor dietary intake of phosphorus. Phosphate binders are more likely to produce hypophosphatemia when other conditions associated with this imbalance are present, such as diuretic therapy, renal tubular defects, or hyperparathyroidism.

Hyperventilation and Respiratory Alkalosis

A decrease in serum phosphate associated with alkalosis occurs secondary to increased cellular uptake of phosphate. Prolonged, intense hyperventilation can depress serum phosphorus to values in the vicinity of 0.5 mg/dL, presumably by inducing respiratory alkalosis. Hyperventilation may be caused by sepsis, withdrawal from chronic alcoholism, fever, pain, anxiety and many other causes. Even normal persons with severe hyperventilation ($PaCO_2 < 20$ mm Hg) may exhibit serum phosphate concentrations less than 1.0 mg/dL.[28]

Diabetic Ketoacidosis

Patients with poorly controlled diabetes who have glycosuria, ketonuria, and polyuria lose phosphate excessively in the urine. Although patients with untreated ketoacidosis may have normal or slightly elevated serum phosphorus levels, administration of insulin and parenteral fluids quickly causes serum phosphorus levels to drop below normal (see Chapter 18). As indicated previously, insulin administration favors shifting of phosphate from the bloodstream into the cells.

Other Factors

Primary and Secondary Hyperparathyroidism. Because parathyroid hormone causes the kidneys to excrete phosphorus, hypophosphatemia is a common finding in patients with primary or secondary hyperparathyroidism. All diuretic drugs (but especially acetazolamide) increase the excretion of phosphate in the urine.[29]

Panic Disorders. Patients with panic disorders may have a significant incidence of hypophosphatemia, at least partly due to respiratory alkalosis.[30, 31] See Case Study 8-3.

Organ Transplantation. For reasons that are unclear, hypophosphatemia frequently develops after live-donor right hepatectomy.[32] This electrolyte imbalance is also common after kidney transplant and may represent persistent hyperparathyroidism, renal phosphate wasting, or even malnutrition.[33] Although hypophosphatemia usually resolves during the first few months following renal transplant surgery, in some cases it may persist indefinitely. The worst consequence of post-renal-transplant hypophosphatemia is a significant decrease in bone mineral density, with the loss occurring most rapidly in the first 6 to 12 months post-surgery.[34] Women lose bone mainly from the lumbar spine, while men lose bone primarily from the femoral neck.

Chronic Obstructive Pulmonary Disease. Patients with chronic obstructive pulmonary disease and asthma often have hypophosphatemia, perhaps because of malnutrition and the use of xanthine derivatives (such as theophylline), which cause extracellular phosphorus to shift into the cells.[35] Another factor contributing to the development of this imbalance is the use of diuretics. The muscle weakness associated with hypophosphatemia intensifies the respiratory difficulties that are already so prevalent in these patients.

Thermal Burns. Hypophosphatemia is common in patients with extensive burns and usually appears within several days after injury. The mechanism by which it develops is

not clear. Because burn patients often hyperventilate, it is possible that respiratory alkalosis occurs and results in acceleration of glycolysis, thereby causing hypophosphatemia. It has also been postulated that urinary loss of phosphate may occur during the diuresis of salt and water or that phosphorus may be taken up by the cells as the burned patient becomes anabolic.

Clinical Signs

Most signs and symptoms of phosphorus deficiency result from a deficiency of ATP (adenosine triphosphate) or 2,3-DPG (2,3-diphosphoglycerate) or both. Cellular energy resources in virtually all organ systems are impaired by ATP deficiency, and oxygen delivery to tissues is impaired by 2,3-DPG deficiency.

Muscle Weakness

Profound muscular weakness has been described in severely hypophosphatemic patients, as has muscular pain. Actual muscle damage may develop as the ATP level in the muscles declines. This change is manifested clinically by muscle weakness, release of creatinine phosphokinase (CPK), and, at times, acute rhabdomyolysis (disintegration of striated muscle). Elevations in CPK levels have been reported in patients whose serum phosphate concentrations remain at less than 1 mg/dL for 1 to 2 days. While muscle weakness primarily occurs in large muscles, it may also manifest as dysphagia (difficulty swallowing), diplopia, low cardiac output, and depression of respiratory muscles.

Ventilatory Changes

Weakness of chest muscles has long been recognized as a consequence of hypophosphatemia.[36] In patients with this type of electrolyte imbalance, ventilatory muscle fatigue may arise from cellular depletion of ATP, impaired cellular oxygenation, and central respiratory depression. Respiratory failure is most likely to occur in patients with underlying lung disease. The possibility of hypophosphatemia should be considered in all patients who develop acute ventilatory failure or have difficulty weaning from mechanical ventilation.[37] In some cases, patients can be removed from the ventilator soon after phosphate repletion has been achieved.

A case of hypoxic respiratory failure was recently reported in a young bulimic woman with severe hypophosphatemia.[38] The patient presented with severe hyperventilation, acute onset of dyspnea, paresthesias, SpO_2 of 74%, and a serum phosphate level of less than 1.0 mg/dL. Fortunately, this patient's condition rapidly improved with parenteral administration of phosphorus.

Central Nervous System Changes

Patients with hypophosphatemia may have a wide range of neurological symptoms, including irritability, apprehension, weakness, numbness, paresthesias, ataxia, lack of coordination, confusion, unequal pupils, nystagmus, convulsive seizures, and coma. The basic cause of these disturbances is not clear, but is likely related to a decreased availability of phosphate, which in turn causes reduced ATP synthesis in the brain.

Hematological Changes

Hypophosphatemia affects all the blood cells, but changes in the red blood cells are most pronounced. A decline in 2,3-DPG levels in erythrocytes occurs in hypophosphatemia. Recall that 2,3-DPG is an enzyme in red blood cells that normally interacts with hemoglobin to promote the release of oxygen. Thus low levels of 2,3-DPG reduce the delivery of oxygen to peripheral tissues, resulting in tissue hypoxia. Hemolytic anemia may also occur because the red cells are more fragile and easily destroyed as a result of low ATP levels. This circumstance is particularly significant in critically ill patients who cannot tolerate even modest decreases in oxygen delivery.

Hypophosphatemia may depress the chemotactic and phagocytic activity of granulocytes, thereby increasing the patient's risk of infection. These abnormalities are apparently reversible with correction of the hypophosphatemia. It is thought that hypophosphatemia impairs granulocytic function by interfering with ATP synthesis. Platelet dysfunction may also be present in hypophosphatemic patients and contribute to bleeding.[39]

Cardiac Changes

Patients with severe hypophosphatemia may develop cardiomyopathy that can be corrected with phosphorus replacement.[40] In addition, hypophosphatemic patients may have an increased incidence of arrhythmias as well as a decreased sensitivity to inotropic and vasoconstrictive medications.[41, 42]

Treatment

Mild to Moderate Hypophosphatemia

Treatment of hypophosphatemia varies with the cause and severity of the imbalance. If mild and asymptomatic, it may be managed adequately by treatment of the primary disor-

der. Because phosphorus is plentiful in the average diet, improved nutrition may suffice. Oral replacement of phosphorus is preferable to intravenous replacement because the latter can lead to extraskeletal calcification.[43] Milk products are good sources of phosphorus; for example, one quart of skim milk provides approximately 1000 mg of phosphorus. For patients who are unable to tolerate dairy products, a number of preparations of oral sodium phosphate and potassium phosphate are commercially available.[44] Nausea and diarrhea are side effects that may limit dosage of these agents.

Severe Hypophosphatemia

Severe hypophosphatemia (phosphorus level less than 1 mg/dL) is dangerous and requires IV replacement. Use of a weight-based and serum phosphate-based algorithm for intravenous phosphate repletion has resulted in better achievement of normal serum phosphorus levels compared to reliance on a nonstandardized approach.[45,46] Two IV preparations are available, relying on sodium phosphate and potassium phosphate. If a patient is oliguric, sodium salts rather than potassium salts should be administered. Dosage is guided by serial determinations of serum phosphorus levels (such as every 6 hours) and clinical response. Possible dangers of IV phosphorus administration include hyperphosphatemia and hypocalcemia. Another consideration is that calcium and phosphate should not be administered in the same IV infusion because of the risk of precipitation. Phosphorus replacement in patients receiving TPN is discussed in Chapter 11; replacement in patients with diabetic ketoacidosis is discussed in Chapter 18.

Clinical Considerations

1. Identify patients at risk for hypophosphatemia and monitor for signs of this imbalance. (See Table 8-1.)
2. Be aware that severely hypophosphatemic patients are thought to be at greater risk for infection because of changes in white blood cells. Take precautions to prevent infections (as in meticulous care of central lines for TPN patients).
3. Administer IV phosphate products cautiously and monitor clinical response as well as serum phosphate levels. Because it is possible to give too much phosphorus, monitor for signs of hyperphosphatemia and of the salt in which it is administered. For example, excessive administration of potassium phosphate could cause paresthesias of the extremities, flaccid paralysis, listlessness, confusion, weakness,

arrhythmias, heart block, and electrocardiographic abnormalities.

4. Be aware that a sudden increase in the serum phosphorus level during treatment can cause hypocalcemia. For this reason, serum calcium levels should be monitored. Watch for twitching around the mouth, laryngospasm, positive Chvostek's sign, and paresthesias.

5. Be aware of the need to introduce TPN and tube feedings gradually in patients who are malnourished.

HYPOPHOSPHATEMIA CASE STUDIES

Case Study 8-1

A 40-year-old woman with a prolonged history of severe diarrhea, nausea, and anorexia was admitted. Two months earlier, she had undergone a bilateral salpingo-oophorectomy for ovarian cancer and radium implant. A 30-lb weight loss was sustained over the previous 4 months. The patient's weight on admission was 88 lb. A retroperitoneal small bowel fistula was found, and surgical repair of the fistula and a colostomy were performed. After the patient suffered a multitude of postoperative complications, TPN was begun; at this time, her serum electrolytes were all within normal range.

Eight days later, the patient's condition markedly deteriorated. Glucose intolerance (blood glucose of 270 mg/dL) was treated with regular insulin, 20 units, every 6 hours. Inflammation was noted at the central line insertion site. At this time, her serum phosphorus level was 0.4 mg/dL (normal range, 2.5–4.5 mg/dL). Assessment revealed slurred speech and drooping of the mouth and tongue. The patient appeared restless and anxious and complained of numbness all over. The next day, muscle twitching and gross abnormal movements were noted. She was unable to grasp objects with her hands and was too weak to raise her arms. She complained of pain whenever anything touched her skin. At this time, her serum phosphorus level was 0.2 mg/dL. A nutritional consultation was made and IV phosphorus administration was started.

Two days later the patient's speech remained slurred, spastic movements continued, and intense sensitivity to touch remained. However, her glucose intolerance had improved. Slowly, over a period of days, her hand grasps became perceptibly stronger and the muscle pain diminished. Numbness eventually disappeared. Three weeks later, the patient was discharged with a serum phosphorus level of 4.5 mg/dL.

Commentary. The patient's initial laboratory work was normal, even though she was greatly malnourished; such findings are not uncommon in starving patients. As is typical in such patients, overzealous refeeding can cause refeeding syndrome, especially when inadequate cellular electrolytes (such as phosphate) are added to the TPN solution. Note that this patient's serum phosphorus concentration reached extremely low levels before it was noticed and treated. Typical signs of hypophosphatemia were present. Even after the serum phosphorus concentration was raised to a normal level, it took several days for the clinical manifestations to begin to resolve (indicating sustained cellular deficits) and weeks for the patient to fully recover. In this case, this patient was allowed to become critically ill before the cause of her problem was diagnosed and treated.

Case Study 8-2

A 50-year-old woman with a series of complications after gallbladder surgery received phosphate-binding antacids for epigastric burning.[47] Oral intake was poor and enteral feedings were not tolerated; thus the patient was treated with dextrose solutions for 5 days and later with TPN for 10 days. For the first 2 days; no phosphorus was added to the TPN solution; after that, only 10 mmol/L was added. On transfer to another facility, the patient had slurred speech and difficulty swallowing. She complained of weakness, perioral paresthesia, and numbness and tingling of both hands. Although she was very weak, she could move all extremities against gravity with better strength distally. Laboratory tests revealed serum phosphorus levels ranging from 0.4 to 0.6 mg/dL (normal range in the reporting laboratory was 2.4–4.4 mg/dL). After appropriate phosphate replacement, the patient showed marked improvement in 3 weeks.

Commentary. In addition to receiving TPN with insufficient phosphate, this patient received phosphate-binding antacids. (See Chapter 11 for a discussion of the relationship between phosphate and TPN.) Fortunately, her symptoms responded to phosphorus replacement over a period of weeks—it took that long to replace the large cellular deficits of phosphorus. The profound hypophosphatemic neuropathy observed in this patient was caused by decreased nerve oxygen and energy supply. (Recall that hypophosphatemia causes a decrease in ATP and in 2,3-DPG in the red blood cells, which in turn increases red blood cell affinity for oxygen while diminishing tissue oxygen supply.)

Case Study 8-3

A case was reported in which a 31-year-old man with a history of panic disorder experienced a recurrence of panic symptoms.[48] Among his symptoms were paresthesias and continuous hiccups. During the period in which panic attacks were present, his serum phosphorus levels ranged between 1.3 and 1.9 mg/dL (reference range, 2.5 to 4.5 mg/dL). The patient was treated with a combination of pharmacologic and behavioral therapies and eventually was free of panic attacks. Following the elimination of panic attacks, his serum phosphorus levels returned to near normal (2.3 mg/dL) and then normal (2.8 to 3.0 mg/dL).

Commentary. Paresthesias in this patient were likely due to hypophosphatemia (secondary to the sustained hyperventilation of anxiety). The authors concluded that serum phosphate levels appear to mirror the clinical course of panic disorder.[49] Recall that hyperventilation causes respiratory alkalosis, which can in turn temporarily force phosphorus into cells.

HYPERPHOSPHATEMIA

By definition, hyperphosphatemia in an adult refers to a higher than normal serum phosphorus level (defined as greater than 4.5 mg/dL in most laboratories). Moderate hyperphosphatemia in an adult exists when the serum phosphate level is in the range of 4.6 to 6.0 mg/dL; severe hyperphosphatemia exists when the serum phosphate level is greater than 6.0 mg/dL. Normal values for phosphorus in children vary with the child's age (as discussed earlier in this chapter).

Causes

Three basic mechanisms can lead to hyperphosphatemia: (1) reduced renal phosphate excretion; (2) shifting of phosphorus from the intracellular space into the ECF; and (3) increased phosphate intake or absorption. **Table 8-2** summarizes the causes and clinical signs of hyperphosphatemia.

Renal Failure: Decreased Renal Excretion of Phosphorus

Because phosphorus is primarily eliminated via the kidneys; an increase in the serum phosphorus concentration is observed when the glomerular filtration rate (GFR) is 25 mL/min or less. Hyperphosphatemia that is present for more than 12 hours is seen almost exclusively in the setting of acute kidney disease.[50] In general, this imbalance is highly prevalent in patients with both acute and chronic kidney disease.

A serum phosphorus level greater than 5.5 mg/dL is independently associated with a 20% to 40% increase in mortality risk for patients with end-stage renal disease (ESRD).[51] Some evidence indicates that a high serum phosphorus level is a predictor of mortality in patients with a renal transplant.[52] An elevated serum phosphate level has been identified as an important contributor to the vascular calcification seen in patients with chronic kidney disease.[53]

High Phosphate Intake

While hyperphosphatemia is more likely to occur in patients with impaired renal function, it can also occur in patients with normal renal function. See Case Studies 8-5, 8-6, and 8-7.

Table 8-2 Summary of Causes and Clinical Signs of Hyperphosphatemia

Causes	Clinical Signs
Renal failure	Short-term consequences: symptoms of tetany, such as tingling of fingertips and around mouth, numbness, and muscle spasms
Chemotherapy, particularly for acute lymphoblastic leukemia and lymphoma (tumor lysis syndrome)	
Overzealous administration of phosphorus supplements, orally or IV	Long-term consequences: precipitation of calcium phosphate in non-osseous sites, such as the kidney, heart, arteries, skin, or cornea
Excessive use of Fleet's phosphosoda as enema solution or laxative, particularly in children and individuals with slow bowel elimination	
High vitamin D intake (increases phosphorus absorption)	Serum phosphate > 4.5 mg/dL
Use of cow's milk in infants	

Phosphate-Containing Laxatives and Nephrotoxicity. Use of phosphate-containing laxatives may be associated with hyperphosphatemia and even phosphate nephropathy in some patients.[54,55] Risk factors for acute phosphate nephropathy include advanced age, kidney disease, decreased intravascular volume, and use of medications that affect renal perfusion or function (e.g., diuretics, angiotensin-converting enzyme [ACE] inhibitors, angiotensin-receptor blockers, and possibly nonsteroidal anti-inflammatory drugs [NSAIDs]). See Case Study 8-7 for an example of the inappropriate use of oral sodium phosphate in an infant.

Phosphate-Containing Enemas. Hyperphosphatemia can also result from the improper use of phosphate-containing enemas (especially in patients with slowed colonic motility or megacolon). For example, a case of hyperphosphatemia was reported in a 13-year-old, developmentally delayed boy following multiple phosphate-containing pediatric ene-mas.[56] On the day prior to his admission to the hospital, this patient was given four phosphate-containing enemas to treat chronic constipation. Within 24 hours, the child developed severe hyperphosphatemia (17.75 mmol/L; reference range, 0.81–1.45 mmol/L), hypertonic dehydration (Na = 171 mEq/L; reference range, 135–145 mEq/L), and severe hypocalcemia (Ca = 0.56 mmol/L; reference range, 2.23–3.57 mmol/ L). With intervention, the child survived without sequelae. **Table 8-3** provides guidelines for the safe administration of hypertonic sodium–phosphate enemas. Also see Case Studies 8-4, 8-5, and 8-6.

Phosphate-containing enemas are not appropriate for patients with ESRD who require dialysis. For example, severe hyperphosphatemia was reported in a 39-year-old man with ESRD who erroneously received a hypertonic phosphate enema in preparation for a colonoscopy.[57] The patient recovered after daily dialysis and administration of intravenous calcium. Other conditions that may contraindicate the use of phosphate-containing enemas include dehydration, an elec-

Table 8-3 Considerations for the Safe Use of Fleet Sodium Phosphate Enemas

Manufacturer's Recommendations for Dosage, According to Age

Enema Type	Age Recommendations	Dosing Recommendations
Fleet Pedia-Lax Enema and Fleet Enema for Children (contains 2.25 fl oz per bottle)	Intended for children ages 2 to 11 years Do *not* use in children younger than 2 years of age	For ages 2 to 4 years, half of the bottle or as directed by doctor. For ages 5 to 11 years, full bottle or as directed by a doctor.
Fleet Enema Adult Size (contains 4.5 fl oz per bottle) Intended for adults and children 12 years and older	Do *not* use in children younger than 12 years of age	One bottle.
Fleet Enema Extra (contains 7.8 fl oz per bottle) Intended for adults and children 12 years and older	Do *not* use in children younger than 12 years of age	One bottle.

Examples of Information for Patients and Warnings Provided by the Manufacturer

- Follow guidelines for the type of enema to use according to age (see above).
- Fleet Pedia-Lax Enema and Fleet Enema for Children should be used with caution in children of any age; careful consideration of the use of enemas in children in general is recommended.
- More than one enema in a 24-hour period may lead to severe electrolyte disturbances.
- If, after the enema solution is administered, the retention time exceeds 10 minutes or there is no return of liquid, contact a physician immediately, as electrolyte disturbances and consequent serious side effects could occur.
- Enema solutions are not intended for oral intake

Source: Reprinted with permission of PDR Network, LLC from the *Physician's Desk Reference,* 64th edition. (2010). Montvale, NJ; p. 1143.

trolyte imbalance, congestive heart failure, and ascites. Patients with megacolon or ileus are more likely to absorb the enema solution than are those without these conditions.

High Milk Intake. Hyperphosphatemia may develop in infants who are fed cow's milk, which contains more phosphate than human milk. Patients who consume large quantities of milk as a means of peptic ulcer management may also develop increased serum phosphorus levels. Large intake of vitamin D, either therapeutic or self-administered, causes increased phosphorus absorption that, together with impaired renal function, can result in hyperphosphatemia.

Shift of Intracellular Phosphate to Extracellular Fluid

Tumor Lysis Syndrome. Large quantities of phosphates may be released into the circulation when chemotherapy is administered for neoplastic conditions (particularly acute lymphoblastic leukemia and lymphoma). These releases are the result of cell destruction and liberation of intracellular phosphates ("tumor lysis").

Other Causes. A shift of phosphorus from the cellular space to the ECF can also occur when sepsis, severe hypothermia, and rhabdomyolysis are present. Recall that muscle tissue contains the bulk of soft-tissue phosphate. Therefore, necrosis of muscle is a potent cause of hyperphosphatemia. Situations associated with rhabdomyolysis include direct trauma, viral infections, and heat stroke.

Clinical Signs

Table 8-2 summarizes the clinical signs of hyperphosphatemia. These are primarily the same symptoms associated with hypocalcemia, because both conditions are induced as the elevated serum phosphate combines with ionized calcium. Insoluble calcium phosphate is formed when the calcium–phosphate product becomes too high (such as 60–70 mg/dL).[58] The calcium-phosphate product is obtained by multiplying the serum calcium value times the serum phosphate value. For example, if a patient has a serum calcium value of 8 mg/dL and a serum phosphate value of 6 mg/dL, the calcium-phosphate product would be 48 mg/dL. Multiple reports have described patients who developed kidney disease related to renal calcium–phosphate precipitates several months following the administration of laxatives containing sodium phosphate in preparation for colonoscopy.

Hypocalcemia and Tetany

Because of the reciprocal relationship between phosphorus and calcium levels in the body, a high serum phosphorus level tends to cause a low calcium concentration in the serum. Tetany can result and present as sensations of tingling in the tips of the fingers and around the mouth. These sensations may increase in severity, spread proximally along the limbs and to the face, and be followed by numbness. Muscle spasms and pain may occur as well. Because patients with renal disease often have some degree of acidosis, they are less prone to develop symptoms of hypocalcemia because acidosis favors increased calcium ionization.

Soft-Tissue Calcification

High levels of serum inorganic phosphate are harmful because they promote precipitation of calcium phosphate in non-osseous sites. One such site is the kidney, where precipitation of calcium phosphate can result in progressive renal impairment. Other sites vulnerable to this problem include the heart, lungs, skin, and cornea. Hyperphosphatemia has been linked to vascular calcification, which is one cause of cardiovascular problems contributing to the high mortality associated with chronic kidney disease.[59]

Calcification of soft tissue is seen primarily in patients with chronic renal failure and long-term serum phosphate elevations. In such cases, an attempt is made to control the hyperphosphatemia and thus keep the concentration of the calcium–phosphate product at a level less than 60 to 70 mg/dL. Recall that normal serum levels of calcium (8.9–10.3 mg/dL) and phosphate (2.5–4.5 mg/dL) have a product concentration in the range of 30 to 40 mg/dL.

Other Effects

One effect of hyperphosphatemia is an increase in 2,3-DPG levels in the red blood cells. In patients with chronic renal failure, hyperphosphatemia helps protect against the adverse effects of anemia on tissue oxygenation. Recall that 2,3-DPG favors the release of oxygen from hemoglobin to the tissues.

Treatment

Treatment for hyperphosphatemia focuses on reducing phosphate intake and enhancing removal of excess phosphate.

Dietary Restriction

When possible, treatment is directed at the underlying disorder. If the hyperphosphatemia is due to excessive phosphate administration in drugs or in milk, the disorder is rather easily remedied by eliminating these products from the diet or medication regimen. Less easily managed is the "hidden" presence of phosphorus-containing additives in many prepared foods. Education of patients with ESRD needs to include information about how to avoid these additives.

Oral Phosphate Binders

Phosphate-binding agents are frequently used to decrease serum phosphate levels in patients with renal disorders. In the past, aluminum-containing agents were widely used for this purpose; however, they are largely avoided now because of their proven toxicity. More commonly used phosphate-binding agents include the calcium-based salts; however, there is growing concern about their association with hypercalcemia and vascular calcification.[60] Although associated with fewer adverse events than are calcium salts, sevelamer hydrochloride is associated with a large pill burden and high cost.[61] Sevelamer carbonate is also available as a phosphate-binding agent and may be more appropriate than sevelamer hydrochloride for patients at risk for metabolic acidosis who require phosphate binders that do not contain calcium or aluminum.[62] A newer agent, lanthanum carbonate, appears to be well tolerated and effective in reducing phosphorus levels in dialysis patients; however, it is relatively expensive.[63]

Other Treatments

In acute hyperphosphatemia, IV infusions of saline may promote renal phosphate excretion, provided the patient has functional kidneys. Diuretics that work on the proximal tubules, such as acetazolamide, enhance phosphate excretion.[64] It may be necessary to administer hypertonic dextrose in conjunction with regular insulin to temporarily drive phosphorus into the cells. Either hemodialysis or peritoneal dialysis may be needed for patients with compromised renal function.

Clinical Considerations

1. Identify patients who are at high risk for hyperphosphatemia and monitor them for signs of this imbalance. (See Table 8-2.)
2. Administer prescribed enteral and IV phosphate supplements cautiously, and monitor serum phosphate levels periodically during their use.
3. Instruct patients that improper use of phosphate-containing laxatives may result in acute phosphate poisoning.

4. Instruct patients that improper use of phosphate-containing enemas may result in acute phosphate poisoning. Ensure that patients are familiar with the various sizes of phosphate-containing enemas (pediatric and adult). Also ensure that patients and their families are familiar with the instructions provided by the manufacturer for safe use of phosphate-containing enemas. (See Table 8-3.)

HYPERPHOSPHATEMIA CASE STUDIES

Case Study 8-4

An elderly woman was admitted to the hospital with abdominal pain and constipation that had been present for 5 days.[65] Abdominal radiography revealed multiple fecal impactions. Over a period of 12 hours, six phosphosoda enemas were administered to attempt to correct the constipation; however, no relief was obtained. The patient's condition deteriorated and she had positive Chvostek's and Trousseau's signs. Blood test revealed a serum phosphorus level of 22 mg/dL (normal, 2.5–4.5 mg/dL) and a total serum calcium level of 5.4 mg/dL (normal, 8.9–10.3 mg/dL). IV fluids were maintained using central venous monitoring and calcium gluconate was administered by continuous infusion. In the first 24 hours, 6.7 L of fluids was administered. Within 24 hours, serum electrolyte levels returned to near normal values (phosphorus, 4.7 mg/dL; calcium, 9.3 mg/dL). The paralytic ileus resolved slowly, after the fecal impactions were manually removed, with the assistance of isotonic saline enemas. The patient was discharged to an extended care facility in 2 weeks.

Commentary. Most cases of hyperphosphatemia due to phosphate enemas have occurred in young children. However, severe electrolyte abnormalities can also occur in adults, particularly when conditions are present that cause prolonged retention of the enema solution. In this case, paralytic ileus and fecal impaction promoted retention of the phosphate solution and precipitated the extreme hyperphosphatemia and hypocalcemia described. Both of these imbalances were directly caused by the retained hypertonic phosphate solution. The high phosphorus content of the enema, which was absorbed through the colon, caused a rise in the serum phosphorus level; the elevated serum phosphorus level caused a reciprocal drop in the serum calcium level. Elderly patients with atonic colons and poor renal function are particularly at risk for hyperphosphatemia. In these patients, use of enemas should be carefully supervised, and whenever possible, isotonic saline enemas should be used.

Case Study 8-5

A case was reported in which a 64-year-old man was to undergo a colostomy revision to correct an area of stenosis.[66] The evening before surgery, a standard oral bowel preparation with 4 L of polyethylene glycol solution was ordered, along with maintenance IV fluids to prevent dehydration. The next morning, it was discovered that the patient did not drink all of the lavage solution; therefore, an order was given for "Fleet's enemas" through the end colostomy "until clear." It was later discovered that a total of 11 sodium phosphate–based enema preparations (approximately 1100 mL) were administered over a period of 2 hours. While being readied for transport to the operating room, the patient was confused, ashen, and very weak. His heart rate was 60 beats/min and he was tachypneic. He was immediately moved to the surgical intensive care unit, where IV resuscitation and oxygen therapy were initiated. A series of tests (including serum electrolytes) were performed. Laboratory results revealed the following findings: Na 157 mEq/L; K 6.5 mEq/L; phosphorus 10.4 mg/dL; Ca 4.4 mg/dL; arterial blood gases: pH 6.94, HCO_3 6.9 mEq/L, and $PaCO_2$ 37 mm Hg. Despite vigorous attempts to correct the patient's severe metabolic disturbances, he died of shock and multisystem organ failure approximately 8 hours after the enemas were given.

Commentary. This tragic case was due to an improperly written order and failure of the staff to consider the danger of administering large doses of sodium phosphate enemas to a patient unable to evacuate the solution normally. Under normal circumstances, the enema solution would be evacuated in 2 to 15 minutes, resulting in minimal absorption from the bowel; in this case, the authors concluded, the stenotic colostomy prevented this from occurring. The 11 adult-sized enemas given to this patient resulted in a dose of approximately 209 g sodium biphosphate, 77 g sodium phosphate, and a total of 48.4 g sodium over 2 hours. Absorption of phosphate from the enema caused binding of serum calcium and ultimately resulted in hyperphosphatemia and hypocalcemia. This, in turn, led to severe cardiovascular collapse with hypoperfusion, metabolic acidosis, and finally multisystem organ failure.

When the house staff and nursing personnel were interviewed, it was found that the term "Fleet's enema" was used variably to describe true sodium phosphate–based enema preparations, simple isotonic saline enemas, or as a generic term encompassing all types of enemas. (This practice is not unlike calling all facial tissues "Kleenex" or all feeding tubes "Dobbhoff's.") Of course, referring to all enemas as "Fleet's enemas" should be avoided because there are vast differences between the various types of enema solutions. The authors of the article in which this case was reported emphasized the need for all healthcare personnel to be fully aware of the potential for clinically significant hyperphosphatemia and hypocalcemia with the use of sodium phosphate–based enema preparations. Indeed, the manufacturer of Fleet's enemas carefully explains the precautions needed to use its products safely. (See Table 8-3.)

Case Study 8-6

A case was recently reported in which a 66-year-old woman received oral sodium phosphate solution prior to a colonoscopy to determine the source of bloody loose stools.[67] The patient had a history of hypertension and was managed with lisinopril (an ACE inhibitor) and hydrochlorothiazide (a diuretic). Baseline renal function was deemed to be normal, based on a serum creatinine level of 0.8 mg/dL. Following colonoscopy, colitis was identified and resolved without treatment. One week after the colonoscopy, the patient presented with acute renal failure (serum creatinine of 10.2 mg/dL). Her serum phosphate level was 25.4 mg/dL and her urinary specific gravity was 1.010. Untrasonography demonstrated large kidneys. Widespread intratubular calcific concretions were identified on renal biopsy. A diagnosis of phosphate nephropathy with mild acute tubular necrosis was made. Following treatment with phosphate binders, the patient's serum phosphorus level improved and her creatinine level eventually stabilized at 2.6 mg/dL.

Commentary. While phosphate nephropathy is especially problematic in patients with preexisting renal disease, it may also occur in patients with normal renal function (as indicated in the case reported here).[68] The authors pointed out that their patient's recent diarrheal illness and documented colitis may have been a contraindication to the administration of sodium phosphate. Volume depletion is a recognized risk factor for precipitation of calcium phosphate in the renal tubules. Use of ACE inhibitors predisposes patients to phosphate nephropathy by impairing renal perfusion in the presence of volume depletion and by enhancing urinary alkalinization (thereby increasing precipitation of calcium and phosphorus).[69]

Case Study 8-7

A case was recently reported in which a 3-month-old boy was admitted to the emergency department with respiratory distress and fever (40.2°C).[70] The infant had intermittent muscular spasms and stiffness of all four extremities (interpreted as possible seizure activity). Among the laboratory results were the following findings: Na 155 mEq/L, Cr 0.9 mg/dL (reference range, 0.2 to 0.4 mg/dL), Ca 5.1 mg/dL (reference range, 8.5 to 11.0 mg/dL), phosphorus 38.3 mg/dL (reference range, 3.2 to 6.3 mg/dL), and an elevated anion gap (29 mEq/L; reference range varies but is generally considered to be 12 ± 2 mEq/L). Calcium gluconate was administered intravenously and the infant was transferred to a pediatric intensive care unit. At this time, the ionized calcium level was found to be 2.3 mg/dL (reference range, 4.6 to 5.3 mg/dL). A central venous catheter was placed and additional calcium was administered along with aggressive fluid hydration. All cultures were negative. The phosphorus level returned to normal within 20 hours of initial presentation. A complete recovery ensued and the infant was discharged from the PICU on hospital day 3.

Commentary. Upon questioning, the infant's parents admitted to giving him a phosphate-containing laxative because they thought he was constipated. During the 7 days prior to admission, the child was given 2 mL of Purgasol (DLC Marketing Company, Paramount, CA) every 4 hours with each feeding. The parents had also administered peppermint herb tea (8 oz/day), simethicone drops, and slivers of Ivory soap rectally.[71] This case illustrates the need for caregivers to educate parents not to administer laxatives or enemas to infants without medical consultation. Healthcare providers in this case provided fluid therapy to promote urinary excretion of phosphate; for example, during the first day of hospitalization, the infant's urine output was maintained at level of more than 2 mL/kg/hr. The seizure activity was apparently due to hypocalcemia (recall that a high phosphate level causes the serum calcium level to decrease because the negatively charged phosphate ions combine with the positively charged calcium ions). Calcium was administered through a central line. The elevated anion gap was indicative of a high-anion-gap metabolic acidosis, secondary to the high serum phosphate level. (Recall that phosphate is an anion normally present in fairly low amounts.) The anion gap declined as the serum phosphate level was corrected.

Also see Case Studies 13-4 and 13-6, which concern patients with phosphate imbalances.

NOTES

1. Parillo, J. E., & Dellinger, R. P. (2008). *Critical care medicine: Principles of diagnosis and management in the adult* (3rd ed.). Philadelphia: Mosby, p. 1234.

2. Moe, S. M. (2008). Disorders involving calcium, phosphorus, and magnesium. *Primary Care Clinics in Office Practice, 35*(2), 215–237.

3. Moe, note 2.

4. Worley, G., Claerhout, S. J., & Combs, S. P. (1998). Hyphosphatemia in malnourished children during refeeding. *Clinical Pediatrics, 37*, 347–352.

5. McPherson, R. A., & Pincus, M. R. (2007). *Henry's clinical diagnosis and management by laboratory methods* (21st ed.). Philadelphia: Saunders, p. 173.

6. McPherson & Pincus, note 5, p. 173.

7. Hruska, K. A., Mathew, S., Lund, R., Qiu, P., & Pratt, R. (2008). Hyperphosphatemia of chronic kidney disease. *Kidney International, 74*(2), 148–157.

8. Moe, note 2.

9. Sullivan, C., Sayre, S. S, Leon, J. B., Machekano, R., Love, T. E., Porter, D., et al. (2009). Effect of food additives on hyperphosphatemia among patients with end-stage renal disease: A randomized controlled trial. *Journal of the American Medical Association, 301*(6), 629–635.

10. Moe, note 2.

11. Sullivan et al., note 9.

12. Calvo, M. S., & Park, Y. K. (1996). Changing phosphorus content of the US diet: Potential for adverse effects on bone. *Journal of Nutrition, 126*(4 suppl), 1168S–1180S.

13. Sullivan et al., note 9.

14. Moe, note 2.

15. McPherson & Pincus, note 5, p. 173.

16. Hoffmann, M., Zemlin, A. E., Meyer, W. P., & Erasmus, R. T. (2008). Hypophosphatemia at a large academic hospital in South Africa. *Journal of Clinical Pathology, 61*, 1104–1107.

17. Sumukadas, D., Jenkinson, F., & Witham, M. D. (2009). Associations and consequences of hypophosphatemia in older hospitalized women. *Age and Aging, 38*, 112–115.

18. Parillo & Dellinger, note 1, p. 1234.

19. Crook, M. A. (2009). Management of severe hypophosphatemia. *Nutrition, 25*, 368–369,

20. Zazzo, J., Troche, G., Ruel, P., & Maintenant, J. (1995). High incidence of hypophosphatemia in surgical intensive care patients: Efficacy of phosphorus therapy on myocardial function. *Intensive Care Medicine, 21*, 826–831.

21. Moe, note 2.

22. Zazzo et al., note 20.

23. Halevy, J., & Bulvik, S. (1988). Severe hypophosphatemia in hospitalized patients. *Archives of Internal Medicine, 148,* 153–155.

24. Parillo & Dellinger, note 1, p. 1235.

25. Vanlandingham, S., Simpson, S., Daniel P., & Newmark, S. R. (1981). Metabolic abnormalities in patients supported with enteral tube feeding. *Journal of Parenteral & Enteral Nutrition, 5,* 322–324.

26. Worley et al., note 4.

27. Ryback, R. S., Eckardt, M., & Pautler, C. P. (1980). Clinical relationship between serum phosphorus and other blood chemistry values in alcoholics. *Archives of Internal Medicine, 140,* 673–677.

28. Moe, note 2.

29. Parillo & Dellinger, note 1, p. 1236.

30. Balon, R., Yeragani, V. K., & Pohl, R. (1988). Relative hypophosphatemia in patients with panic disorders. *Archives of General Psychiatry, 45,* 294–295.

31. Roestel, C., Hoeping, W., & Deckert, J. (2004). Hypophosphatemia in panic disorder [letter]. *American Journal of Psychiatry, 161,* 8.

32. Lee, H. W., Suh, K. S., Kim, J., Shin, W. Y., Cho, E. H., Yi, N. J., et al. (2008). Hypophosphatemia after live donor right hepatectomy. *Surgery, 144*(3), 445–453.

33. Feehally, J., Floege, J., & Johnson, R. J. (2007). *Comprehensive clinical nephrology* (3rd ed.). Philadelphia: Mosby Elsevier, p. 1095.

34. Levi, M. (2001). Post-transplant hypophosphatemia. *Kidney International, 59,* 2377–2387.

35. McPhee, S. J., Papadakis, M. A., & Tierney, M. L. (2008). *Current medical diagnosis and treatment.* New York: McGraw-Hill/Lange, p. 772.

36. Newman, J. H., Neff, T. A., & Ziporin, P. (1977). Acute respiratory failure associated with hypophosphatemia. *New England Journal of Medicine, 297,* 1101–1103.

37. Varsano, S., Shapiro, M., Taragan, R., & Bruderman, I. (1983). Hypophosphatemia as a reversible cause of refractory ventilator failure. *Critical Care Medicine, 11,* 908–909.

38. Oud, L. (2009). Transient hypoxic respiratory failure in a patient with severe hypophosphatemia. *Medical Science Monitor, 15*(3), C49–C53.

39. Bongard, R. S., Sue, D. Y., & Vintch, J. R. (2008). *Current diagnosis and treatment: Critical care* (3rd ed.). New York: McGraw-Hill/Lange, p. 44.

40. O'Connor, L. R., Wheeler, W. S., & Bethune, J. E. (1977). Effect of hypophosphatemia on myocardial performance in man. *New England Journal of Medicine, 297,* 901–903.

41. DeFronzo, R. A., & Lang, R. (1980). Hypophosphatemia and glucose intolerance: Evidence for tissue insensitivity to insulin. *New England Journal of Medicine, 303,* 1259–1263.

42. Venditti, F. J., Marrota, C., Panezai, F. R., Oldewurtel, H. A., & Regan, T. J. (1987). Hypophosphatemia and cardiac arrhythmias. *Mineral Electrolyte Metabolism, 13,* 19–25.

43. Moe, note 2.

44. Brunelli, S. M., & Goldfarb, S. (2007). Hypophosphatemia: Clinical consequence and management. *Journal of the American Society of Nephrology, 18,* 1999–2003.

45. Brunelli & Goldfarb, note 44.

46. Taylor, B. E., Huey, W. Y., Buchman, T. G., Boyle, W. A., & Coopersmith, C. M. (2004). Treatment of hypophosphatemia using a protocol based on patient weight and serum phosphorus level in a surgical intensive care unit. *Journal of the American College of Surgeons, 198,* 198–204.

47. Siddiqui, M. F, & Bertorini, T. E. (1998). Hypophosphatemic-induced neuropathy: Clinical and electrophysiologic findings. *Muscle & Nerve, 21,* 650–652.

48. Roestel et al., note 31.

49. Roestel et al., note 31.

50. Moe, note 2.

51. Sullivan et al., note 9.

52. Connolly, G. M., Cunningham, R., McNamee, P. T., Young, I. S., & Maxwell, A. P. (2009). Elevated serum phosphate predicts mortality in renal transplant recipients. *Transplantation, 87*(7), 1040–1044.

53. Block, G. A., Hulbert-Shearon, T. E., Levin, N. W., & Port, F. K. (1998). Association of serum phosphorus and calcium × phosphate product with mortality risk in chronic hemodialysis patients: A national study. *American Journal of Kidney Diseases, 31*(4), 607–617.

54. FDA Alerts. (2006, May 5). Fleet Phospho-Soda and Fleet Accu-Prep.

55. FDA Alerts. (2008, December 11). Oral sodium phosphate (OSP) products for bowel cleansing (marketed as Viscol and Osmo-Prep, and oral sodium phosphate products available without a prescription).

56. Biebl, A., Grillenberger, A., & Schmitt, K. (2009). Enema-induced severe hyperphosphatemia in children. *European Journal of Pediatrics, 168*(1), 111–112.

57. Azad, B. B., & Cordtz, J. (2009). Acute hyperphosphatemia in a dialysis patient after administration of sodium phosphate. *Ugeskrift for Laeger, 171*(17), 1414.

58. McPhee et al., note 35, p. 797.

59. Hruska et al., note 7.

60. Hutchinson, A. J. (2009). Oral phosphate binders. *Kidney International, 75,* 906–914.

61. Hutchinson, note 60.

62. Pai, A. B., & Shepler, B. M. (2009). Comparison of sevelamer hydrochloride and sevelamer carbonate: Risk of metabolic acidosis and clinical implications. *Pharmacotherapy, 29*(5), 554–561.

63. Hutchinson, note 60.

64. Feehally et al., note 33, p. 73.

65. Korzets, A., Dicker, D., Chaimoff, C., & Zevin, D. (1992). Life-threatening hyperphosphatemia and hypocalcemic tetany following the use of fleet enemas. *Journal of the American Geriatrics Society, 40*(6), 620–621.

66. Pitcher, D. E., Ford, R. S., Nelson, M. T., & Dicenson, W. E. (1997). Fatal hypocalcemic, hyperphosphatemic, metabolic acidosis following sequential sodium phosphate-based enema administration. *Gastrointestinal Endoscopy, 46,* 266–268.

67. Beyea, A., Block, C., & Schned, A. (2007). Acute phosphate nephropathy following oral sodium phosphate solution to cleanse the bowel for colonoscopy. *American Journal of Kidney Diseases, 50*(1), 151–154.

68. Beyea et al., note 67.

69. Beyea et al., note 67.

70. Domico, M. B., Huyndh, V., Anand, S. K., & Mink, R. (2006). Severe hyperphosphatemia and hypocalcemic tetany after oral laxative administration in a 3-month-old infant. *Pediatrics, 118*(5), e1580–e1583.

71. Domico et al., note 70.

Chapter 9

Acid–Base Imbalances

This chapter describes the four simple acid–base imbalances as well as a variety of mixed imbalances. Acid–base problems, with answers, are provided at the end of the chapter to allow the reader to practice evaluating arterial blood gases in relation to clinical situations. Before the discussion of acid–base imbalances, however, it is helpful to review some basic facts about acid–base balance.

REGULATION OF ACID–BASE BALANCE

By definition, pH is the concentration of hydrogen ions: The more hydrogen ions, the more acidic the solution (**Table 9-1**). As shown in **Figure 9-1**, the pH of body fluids varies widely (with the pH of blood being slightly over 7). The body has the remarkable ability to maintain arterial pH within the narrow normal range of 7.35 to 7.45. It does so by means of chemical buffering mechanisms and homeostatic regulation by the kidneys and lungs. The plasma pH range that is considered to be compatible with life (6.8–7.8) represents a 10-fold difference in hydrogen ion concentration in plasma.

Chemical Buffering Mechanisms

Chemical buffers are substances that prevent major changes in the pH of body fluids by removing or releasing hydrogen ions; they can act within a fraction of a second to prevent excessive changes in hydrogen ion concentration.

Table 9-1 Relationship Between pH and Hydrogen Ion Concentration

pH	Hydrogen ion concentration (moles/liter)
1	0.1
2	
3	
4	
5	
6	
7	
8	
9	
10	
11	
12	
13	
14	0.00000000000001

(Note that H^+ concentration *decreases* as pH increases)

Bicarbonate–Carbonic Acid Buffer System

The major buffer system in the extracellular fluid (ECF) is the bicarbonate–carbonic acid (HCO_3–H_2CO_3) buffer:

$$H^+ + HCO_3 \leftrightarrow H_2CO_3 \leftrightarrow CO_2 + H_2O$$

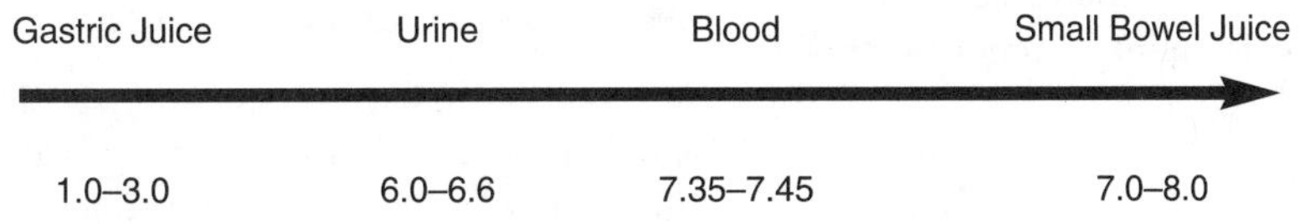

Gastric Juice	Urine	Blood	Small Bowel Juice
1.0–3.0	6.0–6.6	7.35–7.45	7.0–8.0

Figure 9-1 Differences in pH in various body fluids.

An example of this buffer system is when a strong acid (present in a patient with metabolic acidosis) is buffered by bicarbonate, resulting in the formation of carbon dioxide (which is then excreted by the lungs) and water (which is eventually excreted by the kidneys).[1] During respiratory imbalances, the bicarbonate buffer system has no role in buffering; in these situations, only the non-bicarbonate buffers act to stabilize pH.[2]

Other Buffer Systems

Other buffer systems in the ECF include the plasma proteins (primarily albumin) and inorganic phosphates. Hemoglobin, although technically an intracellular buffer, also has a relatively important impact on the pH of extracellular fluid. Phosphate is the least important of the major non-bicarbonate buffers in the extracellular fluid.[3] Buffers are also found inside the cells and act to keep the internal pH of cells stable. The two major intracellular buffers are protein molecules and phosphate groups.[4]

Homeostatic Organs

Lungs

Disruptions in ventilation affect acid–base balance. For example, hypoventilation causes the lungs to retain excessive amounts of carbon dioxide (resulting in respiratory acidosis), whereas hyperventilation causes excessive elimination of carbon dioxide (resulting in respiratory alkalosis).

The lungs have primary importance in maintaining normal pH by regulating the concentration of carbon dioxide (CO_2) in the extracellular fluid. For example, in the presence of metabolic acidosis (low bicarbonate level), hyperventilation occurs to lower the CO_2 concentration in blood. Conversely, in the presence of metabolic alkalosis (high bicarbonate level), hypoventilation occurs, causing retention of CO_2. Of course, the lungs are unable to compensate for metabolic pH disturbances when severe pulmonary dysfunction is present. It has been estimated that body metabolism normally produces 13,000 mEq of hydrogen ions per day; all but 1% of this amount is excreted by the lungs. This relationship emphasizes the importance of the lungs in eliminating hydrogen ions and controlling acid–base balance. Cessation of breathing for minutes produces critical acid–base changes.

Kidneys

The kidneys regulate the concentration of bicarbonate (HCO_3) in the extracellular fluid. They do so by reabsorbing bicarbonate from the renal tubular cells and regenerating bicarbonate, as needed. In the presence of respiratory acidosis, the kidneys excrete hydrogen ions and conserve bicarbonate ions to help restore balance. In the presence of respiratory alkalosis, these organs retain hydrogen ions and excrete bicarbonate ions to help restore balance. Renal compensation for imbalances is slow (a matter of hours or days).

CLASSIFICATION OF ACID–BASE IMBALANCES

Simple Versus Mixed Imbalances

Acid–base imbalances range from simple to complex. By definition, a simple acid–base imbalance is defined as a single primary imbalance with its appropriate compensatory change. In contrast, a mixed imbalance is one in which there is more than one primary (simple) imbalance.

Four Simple Acid–Base Imbalances

The four simple acid–base imbalances and their primary causes are listed here and summarized in **Table 9-2**:

1. Metabolic acidosis (deficit of bicarbonate)
2. Metabolic alkalosis (excess of bicarbonate)
3. Respiratory acidosis (excess of carbon dioxide)
4. Respiratory alkalosis (deficit of carbon dioxide)

Two of these imbalances are due to "metabolic" problems and the other two are due to "respiratory" problems. To avoid confusion, it is important to recognize that "respiratory" imbalances refer to a primary change in carbon dioxide, while "metabolic" imbalances refer to a primary change in bicarbonate. For example, a pathologic increase in CO_2 is called "respiratory acidosis," while a pathologic decrease in CO_2 is called "respiratory alkalosis." Conversely, a pathologic increase in HCO_3 is called "metabolic alkalosis," while a pathologic decrease in HCO_3 is called "metabolic acidosis." It is sometimes helpful to visualize the lungs when thinking of respiratory imbalances, and to visualize the kidneys when thinking of metabolic imbalances (**Figure 9-2**).

Mixed Acid–Base Imbalances

It is possible to have coexistent double imbalances (such as respiratory acidosis and metabolic acidosis) or even triple imbalances (such as respiratory acidosis, metabolic acidosis, and metabolic alkalosis). However, it is not possible to have quadruple imbalances because the two respiratory imbal-

Table 9-2 Four Simple Acid–Base Imbalances: Primary Causes and Compensatory Changes

Imbalance	Pathologic (Primary Change)	Compensatory Change	Mechanism of Compensation
Metabolic acidosis	↓ Low HCO_3	↓ Low $PaCO_2$	Hyperventilation (blow off CO_2)
Metabolic alkalosis	↑ High HCO_3	↑ High $PaCO_2$	Hypoventilation (retain CO_2)
Respiratory acidosis	↑ High $PaCO_2$	↑ High HCO_3	Renal retention of HCO_3
Respiratory alkalosis	↓ Low $PaCO_2$	↓ Low HCO_3	Renal excretion of HCO_3

The compensatory change for an imbalance goes in the same direction as the primary change. For example, the primary problem in metabolic acidosis is a low bicarbonate level; to compensate for this disturbance, the lungs blow off more carbon dioxide, thereby lowering the carbon dioxide concentration in the bloodstream.

ances cannot exist at the same time: Obviously, the lungs cannot hypoventilate and hyperventilate at the same time.[5]

Acute Versus Chronic Imbalances

Respiratory imbalances are classified as "acute" or "chronic." Acute respiratory acidosis occurs when ventilation is abruptly depressed (as in an overdose of a respiratory depressant). Respiratory acidosis becomes "chronic" when it is present for an extended period of time (as in chronic pulmonary obstructive disease). Similarly, respiratory alkalosis can be classified as "acute" or "chronic." In acute respiratory alkalosis, there is an abrupt cause of hyperventilation (such as a sudden stressful situation). Respiratory alkalosis becomes chronic if it is present for an extended period of time (as in chronic hyperventilation due to a central nervous system disorder).

Compensation for Acid–Base Imbalances

The relationship between $PaCO_2$ and HCO_3 is important in determining pH, not the absolute value of either one alone. For example, a patient with a $PaCO_2$ of 40 mm Hg and an arterial HCO_3 of 24 mEq/L will have an arterial pH of 7.4. The same would be true if both values were doubled (such as a $PaCO_2$ of 80 mm Hg and an arterial HCO_3 of 48

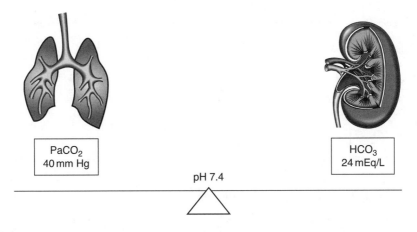

PaCO$_2$
40 mm Hg

HCO$_3$
24 mEq/L

pH 7.4

Figure 9-2 Normal acid-base balance.

mEq/L), or if both values were halved (such as a $PaCO_2$ of 20 mm Hg and a HCO_3 of 12 mEq/L). These relationships are used by the body in a strategy called "compensation." That is, if a pathologic change causes the HCO_3 or $PaCO_2$ level to change, the body institutes measures to bring about a change in the same direction of the other variable. For example:

- If the HCO_3 drops (metabolic acidosis), the lungs will hyperventilate and lower the $PaCO_2$ concentration.
- If the HCO_3 increases (metabolic alkalosis), the lungs will hypoventilate and retain more $PaCO_2$ (thereby elevating its concentration).
- If the $PaCO_2$ increases (respiratory acidosis), the kidneys will retain more HCO_3.
- If the $PaCO_2$ decreases (respiratory alkalosis), the kidneys will excrete more HCO_3.

Note that the compensatory change is always in the *same direction* as the pathologic (primary) change. (See Table 9-2.) However, it is important to recognize that compensatory changes do not always match the degree of the primary change. For example, a 50% primary change might be matched by a 40% secondary change. As such, even compensated acid–base disturbances are accompanied by some alteration in pH (albeit not as severe as what would be observed if no compensation occurred). The following terms are sometimes used when referring to compensation for an imbalance:

- Uncompensated imbalance: pH remains in the abnormal range.
- Partly compensated imbalance: pH remains in the abnormal range but compensation has been initiated.

- Fully compensated imbalance: pH has reached the limits of normal—that is, between 7.35 and 7.45.

As indicated earlier, respiratory compensation for metabolic imbalances starts almost immediately. In contrast, renal compensation for respiratory imbalances occurs more slowly.

The lungs are less able to compensate for metabolic imbalances than the kidneys are for respiratory imbalances. For example, assume a patient has metabolic alkalosis (a high HCO_3 concentration): The compensation for this condition would be hypoventilation to elevate the $PaCO_2$. Yet, while they are retaining CO_2, the lungs are not taking in oxygen. Thus, to avoid a dangerous drop in oxygenation, the lungs will usually not allow the $PaCO_2$ to exceed 55 mm Hg in compensation for metabolic alkalosis. In other words, oxygen need takes precedence over compensation at some point.

MEASUREMENT OF ACID–BASE BALANCE

The best way to evaluate acid–base balance is to measure arterial blood gases (ABGs). The analysis of ABGs (**Table 9-3**) allows the sampling of blood that has come from various parts of the body—not just one extremity, as is the case with venous blood. Also, arterial blood gives information as to how well the lungs are oxygenating the blood.

Note in Table 9-2 that only two of the listed measures are actually gases ($PaCO_2$ and PaO_2). However, reporting the non-respiratory component (bicarbonate) is essential to understanding the respiratory measures. To review the key points, the $PaCO_2$ is controlled by the lungs and refers to the pressure exerted by dissolved CO_2 gas in arterial blood.

Table 9-3 Normal Blood Gas Values

Term	Normal Range	Midpoint	Definition/Implications
pH	7.35–7.45	7.4	Reflects H^+ concentration • pH < 7.35 (acidosis) • pH > 7.45 (alkalosis)
$PaCO_2$	35–45 mm Hg	40 mm Hg	Partial pressure of CO_2 in arterial blood
PaO_2	80–100 mm Hg	90 mm Hg	Partial pressure of O_2 in arterial blood
Standard HCO_3	22–26 mEq/L	24 mEq/L	HCO_3 concentration in plasma of blood that has been equilibrated at a $PaCO_2$ of 40 mm Hg, and with O_2 to fully saturate the hemoglobin

Carbon dioxide should be considered as an acid substance because, when dissolved in water, it forms carbonic acid (H_2CO_3). The PaO_2 refers to the pressure exerted by dissolved oxygen in the blood.

Venous Blood "CO_2 Content"

The venous blood CO_2 content value is usually included with routine plasma electrolyte determinations in *venous* blood. Although listed on the laboratory report as "CO_2 content," it is actually a measure of the sum of bicarbonate (24 mEq/L) and dissolved CO_2 gas (1.2 mEq/L). Thus, in normal situations, the "CO_2 content" in venous blood should be 25.2 mEq/L. Because "CO_2 content" primarily reflects the concentration of bicarbonate, it is largely a measure of the non-respiratory (or metabolic) component of acid–base balance. Instead of merely using "CO_2" as a term, it is important to clarify whether it refers to the gas ($PaCO_2$) in arterial blood or the "CO_2 content" in venous blood.

METABOLIC ACIDOSIS

Metabolic acidosis is a clinical disturbance characterized by a low pH (increased hydrogen concentration) and a low plasma bicarbonate concentration. It can be produced by a gain of hydrogen ions or a loss of bicarbonate. In patients with intact ventilatory responses, metabolic acidosis causes compensatory hyperventilation to decrease the $PaCO_2$ concentration (movement in the same direction as the primary bicarbonate disturbance).

Causes

To understand the causes of metabolic acidosis, it is necessary to first define "anion gap" because the causes of metabolic acidosis are classified as either "high anion gap" or "normal anion gap."

Anion Gap

The anion gap (AG) represents the difference between the number of readily measured cations and anions. It can be calculated by the following formula:

$$\text{Anion gap (AG)} = Na^+ - (Cl^- + HCO_3^-) = 12 \pm 2 \text{ mEq/L}$$

As this equation demonstrates, sodium represents the major cation in body fluids, and chloride and bicarbonate represent the two major anions. Of course, other cations (including calcium, magnesium, and potassium) and other anions (including albumin, phosphate, sulfate, and other organic

acids) are present. Normally, the sum of these unmeasured anions should be no greater than 12 ± 2 mEq/L. However, in some situations, the amounts of these anions are markedly increased and the AG is greater than expected. These situations are referred to as "high AG metabolic acidosis." In contrast, if the primary problem is direct loss of bicarbonate, gain of chloride, or decreased renal ammonia production, the AG will be within normal limits (12 ± 2 mEq/L). One form of a normal AG acidosis is hyperchloremic acidosis (due to a rise in chloride).[6] **Table 9-4** lists causes of metabolic acidosis classified as either high or normal AG.

Normal values for AG may vary according to the laboratory performing the assays; therefore, clinical laboratories need to establish the AG reference interval for the analyzer used in their laboratory. A number of factors can affect the accuracy of AG measurement. For example, in hypoalbuminemia, a 2 mEq/L drop in anion gap will occur for each 1 g/dL decrease in serum albumin.[7] Other causes for AG error include hyponatremia or hypernatremia.[8] Most often, a decreased AG is due to either severe dilution or hypoalbuminemia. Hypoalbuminemia is not a surprising cause because albumin accounts for most of the non-chloride or non-bicarbonate anions in the blood. Other causes of a decreased AG include an increase in unmeasured cations (as in hyperkalemia, hypercalcemia, hypermagnesemia, or lithium intoxication).

High Anion Gap Acidosis

The three most common disorders associated with high AG acidosis are lactic acidosis, ketoacidosis, and renal failure. The next most frequent cause is the ingestion of toxins (especially methanol, ethylene glycol, or salicylates).

Table 9-4 Causes of Metabolic Acidosis Classified as High Anion Gap or Normal Anion Gap

High Anion Gap (Gain of Unmeasured Anions)	Normal Anion Gap
Diabetic ketoacidosis	Diarrhea
Starvational ketoacidosis	Biliary or pancreatic fistulas
Alcoholic ketoacidosis	Excessive administration of isotonic saline or ammonium chloride
Lactic acidosis	
Renal failure	Ureteroenterostomies
Poisonings:	Renal tubular acidosis
• Methanol	
• Ethylene glycol	Acetazolamide (Diamox)
• Salicylates	

Although there are varied ranges in the AG with these causes, the largest gaps are caused by ketoacidosis, lactic acidosis, and methanol or ethylene glycol ingestion.

Lactic Acidosis. Because lactic acid is formed as a product of anaerobic metabolism, its production is increased when oxygen delivery is impaired.[9] This condition is most commonly seen in patients with significant cardiopulmonary problems, sepsis, and shock. Correlation of elevated lactate levels with mortality in critically ill patients is well established. For example, a high mortality rate is associated with an arterial lactate level greater than 10 mmol/L. (The normal arterial lactate level is less than 2.5 mmol/L.) Lactate is a credible clinical indicator of tissue hypoxia because it reflects anaerobic metabolism.

Example: The high AG in a patient with lactic acidosis:

Na = 131 mEq/L
HCO_3 = 9 mEq/L
Cl = 86 mEq/L
AG = Na^+ − (HCO_3^- + Cl^-) or 131 − (9 + 86) = 36 mEq/L (elevated above normal)

Ketoacidosis. Simply stated, ketoacidosis refers to metabolic acidosis caused by the overproduction of ketoacids (beta-hydroxybutyrate and acetoacetate). These ketones are derived from oxidation of fatty acids in the liver. Patients who commonly exhibit this problem include uncontrolled insulin-dependent diabetes, alcoholics, and (to a lesser extent) starving patients.[10] Accumulation of ketonic anions causes a reciprocal decrease in bicarbonate and an increase in the AG. A common scenario for alcoholics who develop ketoacidosis is a recent drinking binge and little food intake. Alcoholic ketoacidosis is reported to occur in two vastly different populations: chronic alcoholics and young children. In children, alcoholic ketoacidosis typically occurs when a small child who has fasted overnight awakens and samples an alcoholic drink left out by the parents the previous evening.

Renal Failure. Metabolic acidosis is a frequent complication of both acute and chronic renal failure. As the failing kidneys are unable to excrete phosphate, sulfate, and various other organic acids, the levels of these anions become elevated in the bloodstream and cause a reciprocal drop in the serum bicarbonate level. Usually the AG does not rise appreciably until the glomerular filtration rate (GFR) has fallen to 20% of normal.

Example: The high AG associated with chronic renal failure:

Na = 139 mEq/L
HCO_3 = 14 mEq/L
Cl = 105 mEq/L
AG = Na − (HCO_3 + Cl)
AG = 139 − (14 + 105) = 20 mEq/L (elevated above normal)

Exogenous Intake of Toxic Substances. Ingestion of toxic substances such as methanol (wood alcohol), ethylene glycol (an ingredient in most radiator antifreeze solutions), and salicylates (usually in the form of plain aspirin) produces metabolites that cause metabolic acidosis with a high AG. Metabolism of methanol and ethylene glycol produces acids that dissociate in body fluids and consume bicarbonate.[11] Salicylate intoxication results in metabolic acidosis and respiratory alkalosis; the latter imbalance develops first in most patients. The respiratory alkalosis is often mild in children younger than 10 years of age. Individuals older than age 10 are more likely to have both imbalances co-equally.

Normal Anion Gap Acidosis

The most frequent causes of normal AG acidosis are diarrhea and renal tubular acidosis. Although renal failure typically causes a high AG acidosis, it may also present with a normal AG when renal function is still adequate to allow the excretion of unmeasured anions.

Diarrhea. Diarrhea causes direct loss of bicarbonate in the stool, ECF volume depletion, and concentration of the remaining serum chloride, resulting in hyperchloremic acidosis. Because no change is apparent in the "unmeasured" anions, the AG remains within normal limits. The same mechanism is seen in pancreatic and biliary fistulas, where bicarbonate-rich fluid is lost through external drainage.

Excessive Chloride. Excessive infusion of chloride-containing fluids, such as isotonic sodium chloride (0.9% NaCl) or ammonium chloride, can cause hyperchloremic acidosis. Other causes include renal tubular acidosis and carbonic anhydrase inhibitors. Renal tubular acidosis exists in various forms and can be characterized by either bicarbonate loss in the urine or inability to generate new bicarbonate. As the plasma bicarbonate level decreases, the chloride level increases. Carbonic anhydrase inhibitors (such as acetazolamide) cause renal bicarbonate wasting. Hyperchloremic acidosis often develops in patients with urinary diversion into the sigmoid colon. This condition appears to be associated with bicarbonate secretion into the colon in exchange for the reabsorption of urinary chloride. The same changes may occur with urinary diversion to an ileal segment.

Example: The normal AG in a patient with ureterosigmoidostomy:

Na = 134 mEq/L
HCO_3 = 10 mEq/L
Cl = 115 mEq/L
AG = Na − (HCO_3 + Cl)
134 − (10 + 115) = 9 mEq/L (normal AG; fall in HCO_3 is due to a reciprocal rise in Cl)

Clinical Signs

Causes and clinical signs of metabolic acidosis are outlined in **Table 9-5**. An example of blood gases in patients with metabolic acidosis is presented here.

Example: Patient with diabetic ketoacidosis:

pH = 7.05
HCO_3 = 5 mEq/L (primary disturbance is decreased bicarbonate level)
$PaCO_2$ = 12 mm Hg (represents compensatory hyperventilation to decrease CO_2)
Acidemia depresses myocardial contractility, lowers the fibrillation threshold, and blunts the pressor response to catecholamines. At the same time, it enhances tissue oxygenation by shifting the oxyhemoglobin dissociation curve to the right.

Treatment

Because many conditions may lead to the development of metabolic acidosis, it is reasonable that treatment must vary, at least somewhat, according to the cause of the imbalance. For example, insulin administration and fluid replacement are frequently sufficient to correct even very low pH values in patients with ketoacidosis. Also, dialysis may be needed for the patient with extremely acidotic renal failure. In general, the administration of sodium bicarbonate to patients with metabolic acidosis is controversial; the possible risks associated with this therapy must be weighed against the benefits. Among the possible risks are hypernatremia, hyperosmolality, and conversion of the administered HCO_3 to CO_2, which may diffuse into the cells and lower intracellular pH.[12] Bicarbonate therapy is indicated in patients with diarrhea or high-output intestinal fistulas who have lost substantial amounts of HCO_3 and subsequently have pH values less than 7.2.[13] In contrast, there is no evidence to support the use of bicarbonate to treat patients with lactic acidosis.[14] Bicarbonate administration may be needed in patients with methanol and ethylene glycol poisoning.[15]

METABOLIC ALKALOSIS

Metabolic alkalosis is a clinical disturbance characterized by a high pH (decreased hydrogen concentration) and a high

---

Table 9-5 Summary of Metabolic Acidosis (Base Bicarbonate Deficit)

Causes	*Clinical Signs*
Normal anion gap: • Diarrhea • Intestinal fistulas • Ureteroenterostomy • Acidifying drugs (such as ammonium chloride) • Renal tubular acidosis	Headache
	Confusion
	Drowsiness
	Increased respiratory rate and depth (may not become clinically evident until HCO_3 is quite low)
High anion gap: • Diabetic ketoacidosis • Starvational ketoacidosis • Alcoholic ketoacidosis • Lactic acidosis • Renal failure • Ingestion of toxins (such as salicylates, ethylene glycol, and methanol)	Nausea and vomiting
	Peripheral vasodilatation (may be present, causing warm, flushed skin)
	Decreased cardiac output when pH falls below 7.1
	Arterial blood gases: • Fall in pH (< 7.35) • HCO_3 low (primary) • $PaCO_2$ low (compensation by lungs)

plasma bicarbonate concentration. It can be produced by a gain of bicarbonate or a loss of hydrogen ion. In compensation, the lungs hypoventilate to increase the $PaCO_2$ concentration, thereby producing movement in the same direction as the primary bicarbonate disturbance. Metabolic alkalosis can be acute or chronic.

Causes

Table 9-6 outlines the causes and clinical signs of metabolic alkalosis. Probably the most common cause of metabolic alkalosis is vomiting or gastric suction, both of which result in loss of hydrogen and chloride anions. Metabolic alkalosis occurs frequently in pyloric stenosis because only gastric fluid is lost in this disorder. Recall that gastric fluid usually has an acid pH (usually less than 4); loss of acidic fluid, of course, increases alkalinity of body fluids. Vomiting related to other conditions sometimes involves loss of both gastric and alkaline upper small intestinal fluid; when this occurs, the severity of the pH change is tempered.

Other factors predisposing individuals to metabolic alkalosis include the loss of potassium, such as that caused by certain diuretics (e.g., thiazides, furosemide, and ethacrynic acid) and the presence of excessive adrenal corticoid hormones (as in hyperaldosteronism and Cushing's syndrome). Hypokalemia produces alkalosis in two ways:

- In the presence of hypokalemia, the kidneys conserve potassium and thus increase hydrogen ion excretion. Recall that these ions compete for renal excretion.

- Cellular potassium shifts out into the extracellular fluid in an attempt to maintain near-normal serum levels: As potassium leaves the cell, hydrogen must enter to maintain electroneutrality.

Excessive alkali ingestion, as in the use of bicarbonate-containing antacids (e.g., Alka-Seltzer) can also cause metabolic alkalosis. Metabolic alkalosis due to high-dose sodium bicarbonate administration during cardiopulmonary resuscitation was a common finding a decade ago. Abrupt relief of a chronically high CO_2 level in the plasma (e.g., assisted ventilation) results in a "lag period" before the chronically high serum bicarbonate level can be corrected by the kidneys.

Clinical Signs

Alkalosis is manifested primarily by symptoms related to decreased calcium ionization, such as tingling of the fingers and toes, dizziness, and hypertonic muscles. Respirations are depressed as a compensatory action by the lungs.

Arterial blood gases show an increased pH (greater than 7.45) and an elevated bicarbonate level (greater than 26 mEq/L), the primary disorder. To help temper the severity of the imbalance, compensatory hypoventilation occurs (elevating the $PaCO_2$); it is more pronounced in semiconscious, unconscious, or debilitated patients than in alert patients. Debilitated patients may develop marked hypoxemia as a result of hypoventilation.

Table 9-6 Summary of Metabolic Alkalosis (Base Bicarbonate Excess)

Causes	Clinical Signs
Vomiting or gastric suction	Signs related to decreased calcium ionization:
Hypokalemia	• Dizziness
Hyperaldosteronism	• Tingling of fingers and toes
Cushing's syndrome	• Circumoral paresthesia
Potassium-losing diuretics (e.g., thiazides, furosemide, ethacrynic acid)	• Carpopedal spasm
	• Hypertonic muscles
Alkali ingestion (bicarbonate-containing antacids)	Depressed respiration (compensatory action by lungs)
Parenteral NaHCO$_3$ administration for cardiopulmonary resuscitation	Arterial blood gases:
Abrupt relief of chronic respiratory acidosis, which allows bicarbonate to remain elevated until the kidneys can excrete the excess level	• pH > 7.45
	• Bicarbonate elevated (primary)
	• PaCO$_2$ elevated (compensatory)
	Serum Cl relatively lower than Na

Example: Patient with vomiting:

pH = 7.62
HCO$_3$ = 45 mEq/L (primary disturbance is high bicarbonate level)
PaCO$_2$ = 48 mm Hg (compensatory elevation in CO$_2$)

Other laboratory values are also disrupted in metabolic alkalosis. The serum potassium concentration is often—although not always—below 3.5 mEq/L. This finding is especially likely if the cause of the alkalosis is also associated with potassium loss (as in use of potassium-losing diuretics or vomiting). The serum chloride is relatively lower than the serum sodium, as an elevation in the serum bicarbonate level causes the chloride level to drop. (Recall that as the concentration of one anion increases, the concentration of another ion tends to decrease to maintain electroneutrality.)

The ionized fraction of serum calcium decreases in the presence of alkalosis as more calcium combines with serum proteins. Because it is the ionized fraction of calcium that influences neuromuscular activity, it is understandable why symptoms of hypocalcemia are often the predominant ones of alkalosis.

Urinary chloride concentration is sometimes measured to determine the cause of metabolic alkalosis; usually, it is less than 15 mEq/L when metabolic alkalosis is due to vomiting, gastric suction, or prolonged diuretic use. Conversely, it is usually greater than 20 mEq/L when metabolic alkalosis is due to hyperaldosteronism, Cushing's syndrome, or profound potassium depletion (serum potassium < 2.0 mEq/L).

Treatment

Treatment in cases of metabolic alkalosis is aimed at reversal of the underlying disorder. It is important to replenish any fluid deficit with 0.9% sodium chloride (normal saline) and to supplement potassium to achieve a high normal level of this electrolyte.[16] It is also important to recognize that metabolic alkalosis is generally associated with hypokalemia.

RESPIRATORY ACIDOSIS

An elevated PaCO$_2$ that leads to acidosis is referred to as respiratory acidosis; this condition can be either acute or chronic. Hypoventilation is the primary cause of this imbalance, and the compensatory change (retention of HCO$_3$) is initiated slowly by the kidneys. Plasma bicarbonate remains in the normal range during the early phase of acute respiratory acidosis; as a consequence, the high PaCO$_2$ can quickly produce a sharp decrease in plasma pH. When respiratory acidosis is chronic, as in chronic obstructive pulmonary disease (COPD), the kidneys have plenty of time to elevate the plasma HCO$_3$ level and attenuate the level of acidity. Although COPD patients with chronic respiratory acidosis are not seriously acidemic, they are in a precarious position. That is, any acute medical stress that elevates the PaCO$_2$ (on top of the chronically elevated PaCO$_2$) can cause acute-on-chronic ventilatory failure.[17]

Causes

Table 9-7 outlines the causes and clinical signs of respiratory acidosis. As indicated earlier, respiratory acidosis is always due to hypoventilation (inadequate excretion of CO$_2$), resulting in increased plasma CO$_2$ levels and, therefore, increased carbonic acid levels. Pulmonary disease may be at fault, although the most common cause of respiratory acidosis is decreased central drive due to overdose of drugs that suppress ventilation and lead to hypercapnea (CO$_2$ excess). In addition to an elevated PaCO$_2$ level, hypoventilation usually causes a decrease in PaO$_2$.

Acute respiratory acidosis is associated with certain emergency situations (such as acute pulmonary edema, aspiration of a foreign object, atelectasis, pneumothorax, overdosage of sedatives, and severe pneumonia). Chronic respiratory acidosis is associated with chronic situations such as emphysema, bronchiectasis, and bronchial asthma. Other causes of respiratory acidosis are listed in Table 9-7.

Clinical Signs

Clinical signs vary for acute and chronic respiratory acidosis; they are summarized in Table 9-7.

Acute Respiratory Acidosis

A sudden rise in the PaCO$_2$ concentration can cause increased pulse and respiratory rate, increased blood pressure, mental cloudiness, and a feeling of fullness in the head. The latter effect occurs because the increased PaCO$_2$ causes cerebrovascular vasodilation and increased cerebral blood flow, particularly when more than 60 mm Hg.

Table 9-7 Summary of Respiratory Acidosis (Carbonic Acid Excess)

Causes	Clinical Signs

Acute respiratory acidosis:
• Acute pulmonary edema
• Aspiration of a foreign body
• Atelectasis
• Pneumothorax, hemothorax
• Overdosage of sedatives or anesthetic
• Position on operating table that interferes with respiration
• Cardiac arrest
• Severe pneumonia
• Laryngospasm
• Improperly regulated mechanical ventilation
 	
Chronic respiratory acidosis:
• Emphysema
• Cystic fibrosis
• Advanced multiple sclerosis
• Bronchiectasis
• Bronchial asthma
 	
Factors favoring hypoventilation:
• Obesity
• Tight abdominal binders or dressings
• Postoperative pain (as in high abdominal or chest incisions)
• Abdominal distention from cirrhosis or bowel obstruction
	Acute respiratory acidosis:
	• Feeling of fullness in the head ($PaCO_2$ causes cerebrovascular vasodilatation and increased cerebral blood flow, particularly when higher than 60 mm Hg)
	• Mental cloudiness
	• Dizziness
	• Palpitations
	• Muscular twitching
	• Convulsions
	• Warm, flushed skin
	• Unconsciousness
	• Ventricular fibrillation may be the first sign in an anesthetized patient (related to hyperkalemia)
	• Arterial blood gases:
	  pH < 7.35
	  $PaCO_2$ elevated (primary)
	  HCO_3 (normal or only slightly elevated)
	Chronic respiratory acidosis:
	• Weakness
	• Dull headache
	• Symptoms of underlying disease process
	• Arterial blood gases:
	  pH < 7.35 or lower limits of normal
	  $PaCO_2$ elevated (primary)
	  HCO_3 elevated (compensatory)

Ventricular fibrillation may be the first sign of respiratory acidosis in the anesthetized patient. Respiratory acidosis may occur as soon as 15 minutes after the initiation of anesthesia and is most likely to occur in patients with chronic pulmonary disease. Changes in the ABGs occur immediately when ventilation is abruptly altered. The pH may reach a level of 7 or less in a few minutes. In such a case, the $PaCO_2$ is greater than 45 mm Hg and may reach 120 mm Hg or higher. The bicarbonate is normal or only slightly elevated because there has been little time for renal compensation (an exception would be the patient with COPD who has a chronically elevated bicarbonate level; in that situation, it would not be high enough to compensate for the sudden increase in $PaCO_2$). The PaO_2 (oxygenation) is below normal when the patient is breathing room air and is the result of hypoventilation.

Example: Patient with acute respiratory acidosis:

pH = 7.26
$PaCO_2$ = 56 mm Hg (primary problem is high CO_2)
HCO_3 = 24 mEq/L (kidneys have not yet started to compensate by retaining bicarbonate)

Chronic Respiratory Acidosis

Before discussing chronic respiratory acidosis, it is helpful to review the relationship between ventilation and levels of carbon dioxide and oxygen. In normal individuals, a rise in the arterial carbon dioxide concentration is a much more powerful stimulant to respiration than is a decreased arterial oxygen concentration. The stimulatory effect of increased CO_2 reaches its peak within a few minutes; however, it gradually declines for the next 1 or 2 days to as little as 20% of the initial effect. Therefore, after several days, elevation of blood CO_2 has only a weak effect as a respiratory stimulant. This relationship is of significance in patients with COPD; in these patients, the primary drive to ventilation is a depressed PaO_2. A decreased PaO_2 will not stimulate alveolar ventilation significantly until it falls to very low levels.

The patient with chronic respiratory acidosis may complain of weakness, dull headache, and the symptoms of the underlying disease process. The ABGs reveal a pH less than 7.35 or within the lower limit of normal (if complete compensation has occurred). The $PaCO_2$ is higher than normal:

It is often 60 mm Hg or higher. Patients with COPD who gradually accumulate CO_2 over a prolonged period (days to months) may not develop symptoms of carbon dioxide excess (hypercapnia) because compensatory changes have had time to occur. For example, an emphysematous patient kept alive with oxygen therapy for more than 1 year may be mentally alert even though his $PaCO_2$ is 140 mm Hg. In the healthy person, a rapid rise in the $PaCO_2$ to 140 mm Hg would surely produce unconsciousness. The patient with chronic respiratory acidosis has had time for partial or complete renal compensation; therefore, the bicarbonate level is higher than normal.

Example: Patient with chronic respiratory acidosis:

pH = 7.38
$PaCO_2$ = 76 mm Hg (primary disturbance is high CO_2)
HCO_3 = 42 mEq/L (kidneys have compensated by retaining bicarbonate)

When the $PaCO_2$ is chronically elevated above normal, the respiratory center becomes relatively insensitive to CO_2 as a respiratory stimulant, leaving hypoxemia as the major drive for respiration. Therefore, excessive oxygen administration removes the stimulus of hypoxemia and the patient develops acute ventilatory failure unless the situation is quickly reversed.

Treatment

Treatment of respiratory acidosis is directed at improving ventilation; exact measures vary with the cause of inadequate ventilation. Pharmacological agents are used as indicated. For example, bronchodilators help reduce bronchial spasm; antibiotics are administered to treat respiratory infections. Pulmonary hygiene measures are used, when necessary, to rid the respiratory tract of mucus and purulent drainage. Adequate hydration (2–3 L/day) is indicated to keep the mucous membranes moist, thereby facilitating removal of secretions. Supplemental oxygen is used as necessary.

A mechanical ventilator, used cautiously, may improve pulmonary ventilation. Overzealous use of a mechanical ventilator, however, may cause such rapid excretion of CO_2 that the kidneys will be unable to eliminate excess bicarbonate with sufficient rapidity to prevent alkalosis and convulsions.

RESPIRATORY ALKALOSIS

Causes

Respiratory alkalosis is characterized by a low $PaCO_2$ (hypocarbia) and an elevated pH. This imbalance is always due to hyperventilation, which causes excessive "blowing off" of CO_2 and, therefore, an elevation in pH. A low $PaCO_2$ can be "normal" in pregnancy, owing to stimulation of the respiratory center by progesterone. This condition emerges early in pregnancy and continues until birth, when plasma progesterone falls to pre-pregnancy levels.[18] Also, respiratory alkalosis sometimes occurs in individuals who are exposed to high altitudes to which they are unaccustomed; the relatively low atmospheric oxygen causes hyperventilation.

Rather common causes of respiratory alkalosis are anxiety and pain. In these situations, a variety of cortical and possibly subcortical influences can produce hyperventilation. Another cause is hypoxemia (a low PaO_2). Arterial hypoxemia is sensed by chemoreceptors in the aorta and carotid artery; these receptors stimulate the respiratory center in the brain and increase ventilatory drive. While this reaction results in increased PaO_2, it unfortunately causes a reduced $PaCO_2$ as well. The presence of edema fluid in the lung is a major stimulus to ventilation, as is a pulmonary embolus. Hyperventilation with respiratory alkalosis is also common in patients with sepsis (perhaps secondary to stimulation of respiratory chemoreceptors by cytokines).[19] Serious, chronic liver disease may be associated with a fall in $PaCO_2$ (a decrease between 5 and 10 mm Hg is typical).[20] **Table 9-8** summarizes causes of respiratory alkalosis.

Clinical Signs

Acute respiratory alkalosis causes vasoconstriction of cerebral vessels. This relative degree of ischemia can cause lightheadedness and fainting; it can also impair higher mental functioning.

Abnormal sensations are also common in patients with respiratory alkalosis; for example, peri-oral numbness may be present, as may a tingling sensation in the fingers and toes. Occasionally, seizures may occur, possibly as a result of alkalemia and cerebral ischemia. Patients with preexisting coronary disease and acute respiratory alkalosis may be more likely to experience atrial and ventricular arrhythmias.

Respiratory alkalosis can be either acute or chronic. (See Table 9-8.) Examples of arterial blood gases in a patient with acute respiratory alkalosis and one with chronic respiratory alkalosis are presented below. Patients with acute respiratory alkalosis tend to have high pH values because the renal compensatory response is quite slow.

Table 9-8 Summary of Respiratory Alkalosis (Carbonic Acid Deficit)

Causes	Clinical Signs
Extreme anxiety (most common cause)	Lightheadedness (a low $PaCO_2$ causes cerebral vasoconstriction and, therefore, decreased cerebral blood flow)
High fever	Inability to concentrate
Hypoxemia	Signs of decreased calcium ionization: numbness and tingling of extremities and circumoral paresthesia (more likely to occur if respiratory alkalosis develops rapidly)
Early salicylate intoxication (stimulates the respiratory center)	Hyperventilation syndrome:
Gram-negative bacteremia	• Tinnitus
	• Palpitations
Central nervous system lesions involving respiratory center	• Sweating
	• Dry mouth
	• Tremulousness
Pulmonary emboli	• Precordial pain (tightness)
Thyrotoxicosis	• Nausea and vomiting
	• Epigastric pain
Excessive ventilation by mechanical ventilators	• Blurred vision
	• Convulsions and loss of consciousness (may be partly due to cerebral ischemia, caused by cerebral vasoconstriction)
Pregnancy (high progesterone level sensitizes the respiratory center to CO_2; physiological)	Arterial blood gases:
	• pH > 7.45
	• $PaCO_2$ low (primary)
	• HCO_3 low (compensatory)

Example: Patient with acute respiratory alkalosis:

pH = 7.52
$PaCO_2$ = 30 mm Hg (primary problem is low CO_2)
HCO_3 = 24 mEq/L (kidneys have not started compensatory change as yet)

In contrast, in the chronic form of respiratory alkalosis, the kidneys have had time to lower the bicarbonate level.

Example: Patient with chronic respiratory alkalosis:

pH = 7.40
$PaCO_2$ = 30 mm Hg (primary problem is low CO_2)
HCO_3 = 18 mEq/L (compensatory decrease in bicarbonate)

Treatment

In general, treatment of respiratory alkalosis is directed at diagnosing and correcting the underlying disorder. For example, in a mechanically ventilated patient, this issue may be simply handled by adjusting the ventilator settings to decrease ventilation. If the cause of respiratory alkalosis is anxiety, the patient should be made aware that the abnormal breathing practice is responsible for the symptoms accompanying this condition. Instructing the patient to breathe more slowly (to cause accumulation of CO_2) may be helpful.

Breathing into a paper bag increases the $PaCO_2$ and is sometimes recommended to correct the hypocapnea.[21] However, this practice is not recommended by some emergency room physicians because it may result in hypoxia.[22]

GUIDELINES FOR ASSESSING ACID–BASE BALANCE

Table 9-9 provides suggestions of ways to systematically assess arterial blood gases. It is important to master the interpretation of simple imbalances before moving on to the assessment for mixed acid–base imbalances.

Mixed Acid–Base Imbalances

The preceding discussions have described single acid–base imbalances. These single imbalances do occur often in clinical settings, but it is also not unusual for patients to have two or more primary acid–base disturbances simultaneously (**Table 9-10**). It isn't always easy to detect the presence of mixed imbalances. One useful method is to use the "rule of thumb" numeric calculations presented in **Table 9-11** to determine if expected compensatory changes have occurred (or if they have gone too far, or not far enough).

Table 9-9 Suggestions for Systematic Assessment of Arterial Blood Gases

The following steps are recommended to evaluate arterial blood gas values. They are based on the assumption that the average values are as follows:

pH = 7.4 (midpoint of 7.35 to 7.45)
$PaCO_2$ = 40 mm Hg (midpoint of 35 to 45 mm Hg)
HCO_3 = 24 mEq/L (midpoint of 22 to 26 mEq/L)

1. Look at the pH. It can be high, low, or normal:
pH > 7.45 (alkalosis)
pH < 7.35 (acidosis)
pH = 7.35–7.45 (normal range)

A normal pH may indicate perfectly normal blood gases, or it may be an indication of a compensated imbalance. A compensated imbalance is one in which the body has been able to correct the pH by either respiratory or metabolic changes (depending on the primary problem).

2. Determine the primary cause of the disturbance by evaluating the $PaCO_2$ and HCO_3 in relation to the pH.

For example, if pH > 7.45 (alkalosis):
- If $PaCO_2$ < 40 mm Hg, the primary disturbance is respiratory alkalosis.
- If HCO_3 > 24 mEq/L, the primary disturbance is metabolic alkalosis

For example, if pH < 7.35 (acidosis):
- If $PaCO_2$ > 40 mm Hg, the primary disturbance is respiratory acidosis.
- If HCO_3 < 24 mEq/L, the primary disturbance is metabolic acidosis.

3. Determine if compensation has begun by looking at the value other than the primary disorder.

If it is moving in the same direction as the primary value, compensation is under way.

Table 9-10 Examples of Combinations of Imbalances (Mixed Imbalances)

Combination of Imbalances	Two Primary Changes	Explanation
Cardiopulmonary arrest • Metabolic acidosis • Respiratory acidosis	HCO_3 low; $PaCO_2$ high	Hypoxemia produces lactic acidosis with decrease in HCO_3. Respiratory arrest causes CO_2 retention.
Vomiting during pregnancy • Metabolic alkalosis • Respiratory alkalosis	HCO_3 high; $PaCO_2$ low	Vomiting causes the loss of H^+ and Cl^- ions and, therefore, an increase in HCO_3. A progesterone increase during pregnancy stimulates respirations and causes a decrease in CO_2.
Vomiting with COPD • Metabolic alkalosis • Respiratory acidosis	HCO_3 high; $PaCO_2$ high	Vomiting causes a loss of H^+ and Cl^- ions and, therefore, an increase in HCO_3. COPD is associated with sustained elevation of CO_2.
Salicylate intoxication • Metabolic acidosis • Respiratory alkalosis	HCO_3 low; $PaCO_2$ low	Salicylates alter peripheral metabolism and cause overproduction of organic acids, with a resultant decrease in HCO_3. Salicylates stimulate the respiratory center and cause hyperventilation.

COPD = chronic obstructive pulmonary disease.

Table 9-11 "Rules of Thumb" for Determining if the Level of Compensation Is Appropriate

Imbalance	Primary Change	Compensatory Change
Metabolic acidosis	HCO₃ decreased	Expected $PaCO_2$ = 1.5 (HCO_3) + 8 ± 2
Metabolic alkalosis	HCO₃ increased	0.5 mm Hg increase in $PaCO_2$ for every 1 mEq/L rise in HCO_3
Respiratory acidosis		
• Acute	PaCO₂ increased	0.1 mEq/L increase in HCO_3 for every 1 mm Hg rise in $PaCO_2$
• Chronic	PaCO₂ increased	0.4 mEq/L rise in HCO_3 for every 1 mm rise in $PaCO_2$
Respiratory alkalosis		
• Acute	PaCO₂ decreased	0.2 mEq/L decrease in HCO_3 for every 1 mm fall in $PaCO_2$
• Chronic	PaCO₂ decreased	0.5 mEq/L decrease in HCO_3 for every 1 mm Hg fall in $PaCO_2$

For example, assume a patient has a metabolic acidosis with a HCO_3 level of 12 mEq/L. Using the equation Expected $PaCO_2$ = 1.5 (HCO_3) + 8 ± 2, it is found that the expected $PaCO_2$ in this situation ranges between 24 and 28 mm Hg. If the actual $PaCO_2$ is 40 mm Hg, the patient has respiratory acidosis (in addition to metabolic acidosis). If the actual $PaCO_2$ is 20 mm Hg, patient also has respiratory alkalosis (in addition to metabolic acidosis).

RELATIONSHIP BETWEEN pH AND POTASSIUM BALANCE

Acid–base imbalances can produce changes in potassium distribution between the cells and the extracellular fluid. In general, the following relationships hold:

- Acidemia causes potassium to shift *from* the cells to the extracellular fluid, thus elevating the plasma concentration of potassium.
- Alkalemia causes potassium to shift *into* the cells, thus lowering the plasma concentration of potassium.

Potassium and Alkalemia

When alkalosis is present, hydrogen ions (H^+) are released from the cellular buffers and move into the extracellular fluid to help correct the elevated pH. In turn, to preserve electroneutrality, extracellular potassium enters the cells. Although the effect of alkalemia on potassium itself is relatively small, hypokalemia is commonly present in patients with metabolic alkalosis. This effect partly occurs because common causes of hypokalemia (such as use of potassium-losing diuretics and vomiting) also cause loss of hydrogen ions, thereby inducing alkalosis. Apparently there is little change in plasma potassium concentration with respiratory alkalosis.

Potassium and Acidemia

When acidosis is present, hydrogen ions leave the extracellular fluid and shift into the cells to help correct the acidic pH in the extracellular fluid. In turn, to preserve electroneutrality, cellular potassium moves from the cells into the extracellular fluid. Respiratory acidosis is a weaker stimulus for potassium shifting than is metabolic acidosis.

Other Factors Affecting pH and Potassium Balance

The cause of metabolic acidosis affects the extent to which the plasma potassium concentration will become elevated:

- Hyperkalemia typically occurs in untreated diabetic ketoacidosis, but it is due more to a lack of insulin and the presence of hyperosmolality than it is to acidemia.
- Lactic acidosis typically does not cause hyperkalemia.
- Plasma potassium concentration is usually low when metabolic acidosis is caused by diarrhea, because the actual loss of potassium in the liquid stools predominates over the amount of potassium shifted from the cells into the extracellular fluid. The shift of cellular potassium to the bloodstream in a patient with diarrhea becomes clinically important because it may result in normokalemia (masking the true state of potassium deficit, and perhaps leading to inadequate potassium replacement therapy).

PRACTICE ACID–BASE PROBLEMS

Table 9-12 provides a series of acid–base problems. Answers and explanations are provided for all of the problems.

Table 9-12 Acid–base practice problems.

Review the following situations and determine the primary acid–base problem as well as the compensatory change. Also, determine whether the imbalance is compensated or uncompensated. Answers are provided below the exercises. All values are arterial. For purposes of working the problems, use a pH range of 7.35 to 7.45 (midpoint 7.4), a $PaCO_2$ midpoint of 40 mm Hg, and a HCO_3 midpoint of 24 mEq/L.

	1	2	3	4	5	6
pH	7.54	7.20	7.55	7.35	7.36	7.15
$PaCO_2$	29	34	58	95	25	80
HCO_3	24	15	49	49	15	28

1. The pH is above normal (greater than 7.45); therefore, this is alkalosis. Two conditions can produce a high pH: low $PaCO_2$ and high HCO_3. The $PaCO_2$ is below the lower limit of normal and is the primary change. The HCO_3 is unchanged (remember—the kidneys are slow to respond in compensation for respiratory problems). In time, the HCO_3 will decrease, following the direction of the primary problem. Because the pH is not within the normal range, this imbalance is *uncompensated respiratory alkalosis*. One might see a set of blood gases like this in an anxious patient who is hyperventilating.

2. The pH is below normal (less than 7.35); therefore, this is acidosis. Two conditions can produce a low pH: high $PaCO_2$ and low HCO_3. The HCO_3 is below normal and is the primary change. The $PaCO_2$ has started to decrease below normal and is a compensatory change, following the direction of the primary change. Because the pH is not within the normal range, this imbalance is *uncompensated metabolic acidosis*. One might see a set of blood gases like this in a patient with diabetic ketoacidosis.

3. The pH is above normal (greater than 7.45); therefore, this is alkalosis. Two conditions can produce a high pH: low $PaCO_2$ and high HCO_3. The HCO_3 is far above normal and is the primary change. The $PaCO_2$ has increased above normal and is a compensatory change, following the direction of the primary change. Because the pH is not within the normal range, this imbalance is *uncompensated metabolic alkalosis*. One might see a set of blood gases like this in a patient who has been vomiting.

4. The pH is within the normal range, but just barely. Because the pH is on the low side of the 7.4 midpoint, one would look for changes that might produce acidosis. Two conditions can produce a low pH: high $PaCO_2$ and low HCO_3. The $PaCO_2$ is far above normal and is the primary change. The HCO_3 has increased dramatically to compensate for the very high $PaCO_2$, following the direction of the primary change. Because the pH is within the normal range, this imbalance is *compensated respiratory acidosis*. This set of blood gas values is often seen in patients with chronic obstructive pulmonary disease (COPD).

5. The pH is within the normal range, but just barely. Because the pH is on the low side of the 7.4 midpoint, one would look for changes that might produce acidosis. Two conditions can produce a low pH: high $PaCO_2$ and low HCO_3. The HCO_3 is far below normal and is the primary change. The $PaCO_2$ has decreased to compensate for the low HCO_3, following the direction of the primary change. Because the pH is within normal range, this imbalance is *compensated metabolic acidosis*. One might see a set of blood gases like this following diarrhea or in a patient with diabetic ketoacidosis or lactic acidosis.

6. The pH is below the normal range (less than 7.35); therefore, this is acidosis. Two conditions can produce a low pH: high $PaCO_2$ and low HCO_3). The $PaCO_2$ is far above normal and is the primary change. The HCO_3 has increased slightly to help compensate for the high $PaCO_2$, following the direction of the primary change. In time, the kidneys will retain even more HCO_3 to further compensate for the primary excessive retention of $PaCO_2$. Because the pH is below the normal range, this imbalance is *uncompensated respiratory acidosis*. One might see a set of blood gases like this in a patient who is hypoventilating because of a respiratory depressant drug overdose.

Additional Problems

7. The following set of blood gases occurred in a patient with emphysema who recently developed an acute respiratory infection:
   pH = 7.20
   $PaCO_2$ = 55 mm Hg
   HCO_3 = 20.5 mEq/L
   PaO_2 = 55 mm Hg

   Note that the patient has a high $PaCO_2$ and a low HCO_3—both conditions produce acidosis. Thus, there are two concurrent imbalances: respiratory acidosis and metabolic acidosis. If the only problem were respiratory acidosis, the HCO_3 would have elevated as a compensatory action. If the only problem were metabolic acidosis, the $PaCO_2$ would have decreased as a compensatory action. The patient in this example had emphysema, which caused respiratory acidosis. The associated metabolic acidosis was likely due to the low PaO_2 (lactic acidosis associated with hypoxemia).

continues

Table 9-12 Acid–base practice problems—Continued.

8. The following set of blood gases was found in a diabetic young man admitted to the emergency department with Kussmaul breathing and an irregular pulse:
   pH = 7.05
   $PaCO_2$ = 15 mm Hg
   HCO_3 = 6 mEq/L

   This patient has *uncompensated metabolic acidosis* (note the extremely low HCO_3 level). The below-normal $PaCO_2$ is due to compensatory hyperventilation. The expected $PaCO_2$ in this patient should be between 15 to 19 mm Hg, as calculated by the following formula:

   $$\text{Expected } PaCO_2 = 1.5 \, (HCO_3) = 8 \pm 2$$

   Thus this is a single imbalance. The pH is dangerously low; the HCO_3 is also dangerously low, most likely due to an accumulation of ketone acids associated with a lack of insulin.

9. The following set of blood gases was found in a young woman who entered the emergency department with a broken ankle and multiple contusions:
   pH = 7.55
   $PaCO_2$ = 25 mm Hg
   HCO_3 = 22 mEq/L

   Note that the combination of a high pH and a low $PaCO_2$ indicates uncompensated respiratory alkalosis. In acute respiratory alkalosis (as in this case), the expected decrease in HCO_3 is 0.2 mEq/L for every 1 mm Hg decrease in the $PaCO_2$. The $PaCO_2$ is 15 mm Hg below the normal level (40 mm Hg): 40 − 25 = 15; 15 × 0.2 = 3. Thus the expected compensatory decrease in HCO_3 would be 3.0 mEq/L. The actual HCO_3 is 2 mEq/L below normal (close enough).

10. The following set of blood gases was found in a man who had been vomiting for several days:
    pH = 7.56
    $PaCO_2$ = 49 mm Hg
    HCO_3 = 40 mEq/L

    Note that combination of a high pH and a high HCO_3 indicates uncompensated metabolic alkalosis. The expected compensatory change for metabolic alkalosis would be an increase in $PaCO_2$ by about 0.5 mm Hg for every 1 mEq/L rise in the HCO_3. The HCO_3 is 16 mEq/L higher than it should be (40 − 24 = 16); 0.5 × 16 = 8. Thus the expected change in $PaCO_2$ has occurred (40 + 8). Note that the expected compensatory change did not produce a normal pH. As indicated earlier in the chapter, compensatory changes do not consistently match the primary changes.

11. A patient was admitted to the emergency department with no history and the following set of ABGs:
    pH = 7.11
    $PaCO_2$ = 40 mm Hg
    HCO_3 = 12 mEq/L

    Note that the pH is very low (uncompensated acidosis). The HCO_3 is half of the normal level; this case involves metabolic acidosis. Respiratory acidosis is also present. Recall that the lungs begin compensation for metabolic imbalances very quickly. The fact that the $PaCO_2$ has not decreased is evidence of respiratory acidosis. Thus this scenario is a mixed imbalance: metabolic and respiratory acidosis.

12. An insulin-dependent patient with uncontrolled diabetes mellitus and severe vomiting is admitted to the emergency department with the following set of blood gases:
    pH = 7.54
    $PaCO_2$ = 49 mm Hg
    HCO_3 = 40 mEq/L
    Na = 139 mEq/L
    Cl = 50 mEq/L

    The combination of a high pH and a high HCO_3 indicates uncompensated metabolic alkalosis. The expected compensatory change in the $PaCO_2$ would be 0. 5 mm Hg for every 1 mEq elevation of HCO_3. The bicarbonate is 16 mEq/L above the normal level (40 − 24 = 16); 16 × 0.5 = 8. Note that the actual $PaCO_2$ is close to the expected level. However, there is more information in this case that needs to be explored. An insulin-dependent patient with uncontrolled diabetes mellitus would be expected to have ketosis. If one calculates the anion gap [AG = Na − (Cl + HCO_3)], it is evident that the AG is elevated: 139 − (40 + 50) = 49. This patient actually has two metabolic imbalances: metabolic alkalosis from vomiting (loss of chloride) and metabolic acidosis from uncontrolled diabetes mellitus (gain of ketones).

Table 9-12 Acid–base practice problems—Continued.

13. A patient with primary hyperaldosteronism is admitted with the following set of ABGs:
    pH = 7.54
    $PaCO_2$ = 45 mm Hg
    HCO_3 = 36 mEq/L

    The pH clearly indicates alkalosis. The elevated HCO_3 indicates metabolic alkalosis. The expected compensatory change for metabolic alkalosis is an increase in $PaCO_2$ by 0.5 mm Hg for every 1 mEq/L the HCO_3 is elevated. The HCO_3 is 12 mEq/L above the normal level (36 − 24); 12 × 0.5 = 6. Thus one would expect the $PaCO_2$ to be approximately 46 mm Hg (which is close to the actual value). Recall that hyperaldosteronism is associated with hypokalemia; hypokalemia, in turn, can lead to metabolic alkalosis. That is likely what occurred in this case.

14. Assume a patient with chronic encephalitis has the following set of ABGs:
    pH = 7.5
    $PaCO_2$ = 18 mm Hg
    HCO_3 = 14 mEq/L

    The combination of a high pH and a low $PaCO_2$ clearly indicates uncompensated respiratory alkalosis. The expected compensatory change in chronic respiratory alkalosis is a decrease in the HCO_3 of 0.5 mEq/L for every 1 mm Hg the $PaCO_2$ is below normal. The $PaCO_2$ is 22 mm Hg below the normal level (40 − 18 = 22); 22 × 0.5 = 11. Thus the HCO_3 is expected to drop by 11 (24 − 11 = 13). Note that the actual HCO_3 is close to this value. Note that although the expected compensatory change has occurred, the pH remains abnormal. As indicated earlier, the level of expected compensation does not necessarily match the level of the primary change.

15. An 18-year-old boy was admitted to the emergency department with an acute onset of severe epigastric pain. The following set of ABGs was available:
    pH = 7.57
    $PaCO_2$ = 24 mm Hg
    HCO_3 = 24 mEq/L

    The combination of a high pH and a low $PaCO_2$ clearly indicates that uncompensated respiratory alkalosis is present. Severe pain is a frequent cause of hyperventilation. The expected compensatory change in the HCO_3 is a 0.2 mEq/L decrease for every 1 mm Hg decrease in the $PaCO_2$. Because the $PaCO_2$ is 16 mm Hg below the normal level (40 = 24 = 16), one would expect to see a decrease in the HCO_3 of 3.2 mEq/L (24 − 3.2 = 20.8). However, the HCO_3 has not changed (likely because the kidneys are very slow in initiating compensation).

NOTES

1. Abelow, B. (1998). *Understanding acid–base.* Baltimore: Williams & Wilkins, p. 129.

2. Abelow, note 1, p. 130.

3. Abelow, note 1, p. 42.

4. McPhee, S. J., Papadakis, M. S., & Tierney, M. L. (2008). *2008 current medical diagnosis and treatment.* New York: McGraw-Hill, p. 776.

5. McPhee et al., note 4, p. 776.

6. Bongard, R. S., Sue, D. Y., & Vintch, J. R. (2008). *Current diagnosis and treatment: Critical care* (3rd ed.). New York: McGraw-Hill/Lange, p. 60.

7. McPhee et al., note 4, p. 777.

8. McPhee et al., note 4, p. 777.

9. Abelow, note 1, p. 142.

10. Abelow, note 1, p. 145.

11. McPhee et al., note 4, p. 780.

12. McPhee et al., note 4, p. 780.

13. Marik, P. E. (2001). *Handbook of evidence-based critical care.* New York: Springer, p. 247.

14. Marik, note 13, p. 247.

15. Marik, note 12, p. 247.

16. Marik, note 12, p. 249.

17. Abelow, note 1, p. 187.

18. Abelow, note 1, p. 196.

19. Abelow, note 1, p. 195.

20. Abelow, note 1, p. 195.

21. Rose, B. D., & Post, T. W. (2001). *Clinical physiology of acid–base and electrolyte disorders* (5th ed.). New York: McGraw-Hill, p. 680.

22. Ma, O. J., Cline, D. M, Tintinalli, J. E., Kelen, G. D., & Stapczynski, M.D. (2004). *Emergency medicine manual* (6th ed.). New York: McGraw-Hill, p. 45.

Parenteral and Enteral Nutrition

Chapter 10

Parenteral Fluids

Described in this chapter are a variety of fluids administered by the intravenous route (including water and electrolyte solutions, colloids, and blood). Intraosseous fluid administration is discussed in Chapters 15 and 24. Information regarding the administration of subcutaneous fluids (hypodermoclysis) is provided in Chapters 24 and 25.

PURPOSES OF INTRAVENOUS FLUID THERAPY

Intravenous fluid therapy is administered for three major purposes:

- Provide usual maintenance fluid needs
- Replace abnormal fluid losses
- Correct existing electrolyte disturbances

Provision of Usual Maintenance Needs

The average healthy adult requires approximately 2600 mL of fluid daily to replace fluid lost in urine, stool, exhalation, and radiation from the skin. For an adult with normal renal function who requires IV fluids for a week or less, a typical intravenous fluid prescription for maintenance purposes is as follows:

- 2000 to 3000 mL of fluid per day
- 50 to 150 mEq of sodium per day
- 40 to 60 mEq of potassium per day

An example of a 24-hour fluid prescription to meet these needs in the typical adult is 2 L of 0.45% NaCl with 20 mEq of KCl added to each liter. Because 1 L of 0.45% NaCl contains 77 mEq of sodium, 2 L would provide 154 mEq (easily meeting the daily sodium requirement of most adults). Addition of 20 mEq of KCl to each liter of fluid would provide the typically needed 40 mEq of potassium per day.

Although 2000 to 3000 mL of water per day for the average healthy adult is a useful figure to keep in mind, it is important to realize that this amount may need to be adjusted downward for smaller adults. Usually 50 g of dextrose (providing 170 calories) is added to each liter of 0.45% NaCl, yielding D_5/0.45% NaCl. Thus the hypothetical infusion of 2 L of D_5/0.45NaCl would also provide 340 calories per day. Although this represents a small fraction of the daily caloric need, it is far better than none in terms of warding off the ketosis of starvation. As indicated in Chapter 11, sophisticated solutions are available to meet the nutritional needs of patients requiring prolonged parenteral therapy and of patients needing a large caloric intake due to hypermetabolism (such as occurs in trauma or burns).

Maintenance needs for sodium and potassium were briefly discussed above. Remember that calcium, magnesium, and phosphorus will need to be added to infusions if parenteral therapy is prolonged for more than one or two weeks. For patients who are unable to consume oral nutrients over a prolonged period, long-term provisions for nutrient intake are warranted. In such situations, the introduction of total parenteral nutrition via a central line (see Chapter 11) or the introduction of a feeding tube into the gastrointestinal tract (see Chapter 12) is indicated.

Replacement of Abnormal Fluid Losses

More than maintenance fluids are needed in the patient who is losing fluid by an abnormal route, such as gastric suction, vomiting, diarrhea, excessive sweating, or hyperventilation. The amount of fluid that must be replaced is partially determined by fluid intake and output measurements.

Water needs are also greater in patients with decreased renal concentrating ability because relatively more water is required to eliminate wastes. Finally, fluid requirements are greatly increased in patients with shock, multiple trauma, and sepsis (either because of direct fluid loss or because of pooling of fluid in the capillaries or interstitial space). The electrolyte content of the replacement fluids must reflect that of the electrolyte content of the lost fluids. For example, gastric fluid loss is usually replaced with 0.9% NaCl because of its high chloride content. In contrast, lactated Ringer's (LR) solution may be favored to replace diarrheal fluid losses because LR contains lactate (a substance readily converted to bicarbonate by the liver).

Correction of Existing Electrolyte Disturbances

Providing maintenance fluid and electrolytes is more complicated if the patient has electrolyte disturbances that need correction. The task becomes one of safely providing maintenance fluids while also adjusting their volume and electrolyte content to correct existing electrolyte disturbances. Most important in determining what and how much to give

are laboratory results and clinical observations. The therapy for specific fluid and electrolyte imbalances is discussed in Chapters 3 through 9.

DESCRIPTION OF WATER AND ELECTROLYTE SOLUTIONS

Table 10-1 lists some several commercially available water and electrolyte solutions; note that each of these solutions has the same number of cations as anions. For example, 1 L of 0.9% NaCl contains 154 mEq of sodium (a cation) and 154 mEq of chloride (an anion). This balance is required by the law of electroneutrality: The number of cations must equal the number of anions. These and other fluids are discussed in this section.

Dextrose and Water Solutions

Dextrose and water solutions are available in 2.5%, 5%, 10%, 20%, and 50% concentrations. A 5% dextrose in water solution may be used cautiously to treat hypernatremia.

Table 10-1 Contents of Selected Water and Electrolyte Solutions with Comments About Their Use

Solution (liters)	Na (mEq)	K (mEq)	Ca (mEq)	Mg (mEq)	Cl (mEq)	Lactate (mEq)	Glucose (grams)	Calories	Osmolality (mOsm/L)	General Comments
5% dextrose in water							50	170	252	Supplies calories and free water. Should not be used to expand plasma volume; should not be used in patients with high antidiuretic hormone levels (predisposes patients to hyponatremia).
0.9% sodium chloride	154				154				308	Commonly used to expand plasma volume in hypovolemic patients. Because of the high chloride content, it is sometimes used to treat mild metabolic alkalosis. Because of the high chloride content, excessive use can lead to hyperchloremia (metabolic acidosis).
0.45% sodium chloride	77				77				154	Provides NaCl and free water; commonly used maintenance fluid.
0,33% sodium chloride	56				56					More hypotonic than half-strength saline; provides NaCl and free water. Often used to gradually lower sodium level in hypernatremic patients.

Table 10-1 Contents of Selected Water and Electrolyte Solutions with Comments About Their Use—Continued

Solution (liters)	Na (mEq)	K (mEq)	Ca (mEq)	Mg (mEq)	Cl (mEq)	Lactate (mEq)	Glucose (grams)	Calories	Osmolality (mOsm/L)	General Comments
Lactated Ringer's (LR) solution	130	4	3		109	28			274	A roughly isotonic fluid commonly used to expand the plasma volume in hypovolemic patients. Provides approximately 110 mL free water; calcium interferes with using LR with blood transfusions.
3% sodium chloride	513				513				1026	Grossly hypertonic solution used to treat severe hyponatremia; used only in ICU settings.
5% sodium chloride	855				855				1710	Grossly hypertonic solution used to treat severe hyponatremia; used only in ICU settings.

More concentrated dextrose solutions may be used to correct hypoglycemia. Dextrose concentrations in the range of 25% to 35% are commonly used in total parenteral nutrition formulations to provide calories.

Distilled water without additives cannot be infused intravenously because it will cause hemolysis of red blood cells; indeed, deaths have occurred from inadvertent IV administration of this fluid. Five percent dextrose in water is a roughly isotonic (252 mOsm/L) fluid given to provide free water. The dextrose in D_5W is metabolized to carbon dioxide and water, leaving a solution that is physiologically equivalent to distilled water but that does not cause hemolysis.

For each liter of D_5W given IV, no more than 100 mL remains in the intravascular space after 1 hour. Thus D_5W is never used to expand the extracellular fluid (ECF) volume. Too much D_5W can seriously dilute serum sodium, especially in a patient who has high antidiuretic hormone (ADH) activity (as in the immediate postoperative period).

Dextrose is often added to electrolyte solutions to help meet caloric needs. Theoretically, because each gram of carbohydrate supplies 4 calories, the 50 g in 1 L of D_5W should supply 200 calories. However, because dextrose in parenteral solution provides only 3.4 calories per gram, 1 L of D_5W provides 170 calories and 1 L of $D_{10}W$ provides 340 calories. As indicated earlier, this small amount of dextrose is often enough to stave off the ketosis of starvation, which is why dextrose is frequently added to electrolyte solutions. Electrolyte solutions without added nutrients have essentially no calories. Examples of dextrose and electrolyte solu-

tions include 5% dextrose in 0.9% NaCl, 5% dextrose in 0.45% NaCl, and 5% dextrose in lactated Ringer's solution. As discussed in Chapter 11, a typical total parenteral nutrition (TPN) solution for central vein administration has a 25% to 35% glucose concentration. **Table 10-2** summarizes the caloric content and osmolality of selected dextrose solutions. The extent to which dextrose solutions are used in intensive care settings is affected by the current emphasis on maintaining tight control of blood glucose levels to help reduce mortality and morbidity.

Table 10-2 Caloric Content and Osmolality of Selected Dextrose Solutions

| Concentration | Dextrose | | |
	Grams per Liter	Kilocalories per Liter	Approximate Osmolality
5%	50	170	252
10%	100	340	505
15%	150	510	758
20%	200	680	1010
25%	250	850	1263
30%	300	1020	1510
50%	500	1710	2525

Each gram of dextrose provides 3.4 kcal.

Sodium Chloride Solutions

Isotonic Saline

A liter of a solution of 0.9% sodium chloride contains 154 mEq sodium and 154 mEq chloride; 0.9% NaCl is commonly referred to as either isotonic saline or normal saline (NS). NS is an isotonic solution because the sum of total cations (Na^+) and anions (Cl^-) is 308 mEq/L; this level of tonicity is very similar to that of body fluids. Addition of 50 g of dextrose to 1 L of isotonic saline results in a solution with an approximately osmolality of 560 mOsm/L; however, the dextrose is quickly metabolized to water and carbon dioxide as the fluid is being infused.

When infused IV, isotonic saline is distributed in the ECF compartment; none enters the intracellular fluid (ICF). One liter of isotonic saline adds 1 L to the ECF, theoretically expanding the plasma volume in the average adult by 0.25 L and the interstitial volume by 0.75 L by 1 hour after administration.

The ECF normally contains 140 mEq sodium and 100 mEq chloride per liter—amounts that are smaller and in different proportions from those in 0.9% NaCl. The greater amount of chloride than normally present in plasma imposes an excess chloride load on the kidneys and can result in hyperchloremic metabolic acidosis if large volumes of NS are infused. For example, researchers have reported that hyperchloremic acidosis was observed more often in a group of surgical patients who received 0.9% sodium chloride than in those who receive lactated Ringer's solution.[1] A potential problem associated with acidosis is a shift of potassium from the cells into the plasma, elevating the plasma potassium concentration.[2]

In contrast, the excess of chloride in 0.9% sodium chloride makes it an ideal fluid for patients with fluid volume deficit that coexists with hyponatremia, hypochloremia, and metabolic alkalosis (such as in patients with excessive vomiting or gastric suction loss). Because of its high sodium content, however, isotonic saline is used cautiously in patients whose renal or other regulatory mechanisms are compromised.

Half-Strength Saline (0.45% NaCl)

As its name implies, 1 L of half-strength saline provides half the electrolytes found in 1 L of isotonic saline—that is, 77 mEq each of sodium and chloride. It is frequently used as a basic fluid for maintenance needs. It is also used to treat hypovolemic patients who have hypernatremia—that is, those individuals who have a greater water deficit than sodium deficit.

Other, more hypotonic sodium chloride solutions are available commercially. For example, a liter of 0.11% sodium chloride solution provides 19 mEq of sodium and of chloride, while a solution of 0.33% provides 56 mEq/L of each electrolyte. Excessive use of these hypotonic solutions can cause dilutional hyponatremia, especially in people who tend to retain water.

Hypertonic Saline

A 3% or 5% sodium chloride solution is used to treat severe symptomatic hyponatremia. Small volumes are infused slowly and with great caution to avoid causing severe volume overload with pulmonary edema. Hypertonic saline should be used only in settings where the patient can be closely monitored because it requires frequent assessment for pulmonary edema, worsening neurological signs, and serum sodium levels. As indicated in Table 10-1, a liter of a 3% solution contains 513 mEq each of sodium and chloride; a liter of a 5% solution contains 855 mEq each of sodium and chloride. General considerations in the administration of hypertonic saline are provided in Table 4-4.

Hypertonic saline may also be used in resuscitation of patients with hemorrhagic shock, burns, or sepsis.[3] Far less volume is required to provide resuscitation when hypertonic saline is used (when compared to the volume required with isotonic sodium solutions). Fluid is drawn into the plasma from other body compartments, thus increasing the overall plasma volume by up to fourfold that of the volume infused.[4] The effects are short-lived unless a colloid is also administered with the hypertonic saline; for that reason, hypertonic saline is admixed with a colloid to help maintain the expanded plasma volume. Hypertonic saline may have favorable immunomodulatory effects. For example, in an animal study, reduced bacterial counts were noted in animals resuscitated with hypertonic saline, as opposed to those resuscitated with lactated Ringer's solution.[5]

Lactated Ringer's Solution

Considered a near-physiological solution, the electrolyte content of lactated Ringer's solution is similar to that of plasma. (See Table 10-1.) Because of its relatively high sodium concentration (130 mEq/L), LR is often used to expand the plasma volume in hypotensive conditions and to correct isotonic fluid volume deficit (as in hypovolemia due to third-space fluid shift after major trauma or surgery). Although LR is generally considered an isotonic fluid, each liter provides approximately 110 ml of free water (a consideration in patients at risk for cerebral edema). The lactate provided in LR is quickly metabolized into bicarbonate by the normal liver; thus this solution can be used to treat many forms of metabolic acidosis. The lactate content in lactated Ringer's solution apparently does not potentiate the lactic acidosis associated with hemorrhagic shock.

Although isotonic saline (0.9% NaCl) and lactated Ringer's solution are apparently equivalent in the treatment of moderate hemorrhage, LR may be favored because it does not impose an excessive chloride load (as is observed with administration of 0.9% sodium chloride because of its high chloride content). As indicated earlier, isotonic saline can predispose patients to hyperchloremic acidosis because it has a relatively high chloride content (154 mEq/L), in relation to the normal plasma concentration of chloride (100 mEq/L).

Current standards stipulate that no solution, other than normal saline, should be added to blood components during administration, unless approved by the FDA or unless there is evidence that the blood component is not adversely affected.[6] Lactated Ringer's solution is not recommended for administration with citrated blood because its calcium content could cause clotting when mixed with citrate. Even if the IV line does not become occluded, there is the possibility of transfusing small clots or microaggregates. As stated by authors of a recent literature review on this topic, there is insufficient evidence to suggest that lactated Ringer's solution is safe to administer with red blood cells.[7]

Numerous other balanced electrolyte solutions are available commercially in a wide array of electrolyte combinations. Some solutions are designed for maintenance needs, whereas others are formulated to replace specific body fluids. Each manufacturer usually affixes its own trade name to these solutions, making it necessary to refer to the label to review the specific content. It is common to refer to these fluids by the number of cations in the solution. For example, a liter of electrolyte #48 contains 25 mEq sodium, 20 mEq potassium, and 3 mEq calcium.

Premixed Potassium Solutions

Premixed potassium-replacement solutions are available in a variety of strengths, furnishing amounts ranging from 10 to 40 mEq of potassium chloride per liter. Concentrated potassium solutions are also available in ampules for addition to parenteral fluids (such as D_5W, 0.9% NaCl, and 0.45% NaCl). Potassium solutions should be prepared in the pharmacy (not on the nursing units). Concentrated potassium chloride solutions from ampules are *not* meant for direct IV

injection because they would cause fatal cardiac arrhythmias. Factors to consider when administered potassium solutions intravenously are described in Table 5-4.

COLLOIDS

Colloids contain substances of high molecular weight that do not readily migrate across capillary walls. By increasing the osmotic pressure within the bloodstream, colloids draw fluid in from other compartments, thereby increasing the vascular volume. On a milliliter per milliliter basis, colloids cause greater plasma volume expansion than do isotonic crystalloid solutions (such as isotonic saline and lactated Ringer's solution). Further, colloids tend to remain in the intravascular space longer than crystalloid solutions. Albumin is a natural colloid; examples of artificial colloids include hydroxyethyl starches (HES), dextran, and gelatins. Although smaller volumes of colloids are needed (relative to crystalloids) to provide volume expansion, they are more expensive. In addition, the potential for poor outcomes may be greater with colloids than with crystalloids. Notably, colloids have the potential to leak into the interstitial space if the capillary wall permeability is increased.[8]

Albumin

Albumin provides approximately 80% of the plasma colloid osmotic pressure in healthy adults. Albumin for therapeutic uses is prepared from donor plasma and is available as either 5% or 25% solutions. The 5% albumin solution is osmotically and oncotically equivalent to plasma; the 25% albumin solution is hyperoncotic. The sodium content of the various albumin preparations is approximately 145 mEq/L.

The major clinical use of albumin is as a plasma volume expander in the treatment of shock caused by blood or plasma loss. Both 25% albumin (100 mL) and 5% albumin (500 mL) preparations cause the intravascular volume to expand by an equivalent amount (approximately 400–500 mL). The use of 25% albumin is particularly helpful in patients who show clinical evidence of both edema and hypovolemia. Albumin may be useful in treating burns and third-space fluid shifts caused by acute peritonitis, intestinal obstruction, or radical surgical procedures. It is also prescribed for acute volume depletion associated with paracentesis, dialysis, or over-aggressive diuresis in patients with chronic diseases such as cirrhosis and nephrotic syndrome. Less than 10% of a 5% albumin infusion leaves the vascular space within 2 hours of its administration.[9]

Albumin will not correct chronic hypoalbuminemia caused by malnutrition and should not be used for this purpose. Using albumin as a source of nutritional protein is not only inefficient, but also expensive; nutritional repletion is best accomplished with parenteral fluids designed for this purpose (see Chapter 11). Compared to artificial colloids, albumin may offer several advantages—for instance, lower risk for impaired hemostasis, reduced incidence of anaphylactic reactions, less risk for pruritus, and less restrictive dose limitations.[10]

Albumin costs much more than crystalloid solutions; therefore, unless specifically needed, albumin is less likely to be used than the latter option. Reported side effects of albumin include urticaria, flushing, chills, fever, headache, and circulatory overload with pulmonary edema (with rapid infusion).

Hydroxyethyl Starches

Hydroxyethyl starch (HES) is used as a blood volume expander. For example, HES was recently found to be effective in preventing hypotension in women undergoing spinal anesthesia for cesarean delivery.[11] The first HES product (Hespan) became available in the United States in the 1970s.[12] Voluven (hydroxyethyl starch [130/0.4]), is a newly developed third-generation HES product with low molecular weight.[13]

Problems sometimes associated with the administration of HES solutions include increased risk for bleeding, increased risk for renal damage, and severe pruritus. The mechanisms whereby HES can impair coagulation include an efflux of coagulation factors from the bloodstream to the interstitial space, and interference with clot formation.[14–17] A bleeding or blood clotting disorder is a contraindication to the use of HES solutions. All HES solutions, even at low dosages, seem to be inherently nephrotoxic.[18] As a consequence, HES solutions are contraindicated in patients with renal failure and oliguria not related to hypovolemia; moreover, these solutions should be used cautiously in patients with renal transplantation and sepsis because of a risk for acute kidney injury in these groups.[19–21] Severe pruritus can occur days after the administration of HES products (perhaps due to the deposition of HES in the Schwann cells of cutaneous nerves).[22]

Compared to first- and second-generation HES solutions, it seems that the third-generation product (Voluven) impairs the coagulation system to a lesser extent.[23] Also, it has been suggested that the lower molecular weight of the modern tetrastarches is associated with a reduced incidence of pruritus and perhaps even decreased risk of renal dysfunction.[24]

Dextran

Dextrans are polysaccharides that have a similar colloidal activity to that of albumin when given IV; they are available as low-molecular-weight dextran (dextran 40) and high-molecular-weight dextran (dextran 70).[25] Both solutions may be used for volume expansion; however, dextran 70 is generally preferred for this purpose because it remains in the intravascular space for a longer period of time.

Possible complications associated with dextran include renal failure and bleeding.[26] Anaphylactoid reactions have been reported to occur in approximately 1% to 5% of patients receiving dextran.[27] Administration of dextran in volumes exceeding 20% of blood volume can interfere with blood typing and cross-matching.[28] If it is necessary to draw blood for typing and cross-matching, that task should be completed before dextran is started.

In addition to dextran's indication for treating hypovolemia, it may be used for thromboembolism prophylaxis and promotion of peripheral perfusion.[29] For example, dextran can improve microvascular circulation by decreasing blood viscosity and minimizing platelet and red blood cell aggregation.[30]

Gelatins

Gelatin solutions have an oncotic power close to that of plasma and are widely used in Europe.[31] Unlike with other colloids, the daily dose of gelatin solutions is not limited.[32] Like HES solutions, gelatin solutions can negatively influence hemostatic competence, apparently by binding of von Willebrand factor to gelatin, and impairment with platelet aggregation.[33] Anaphylactoid reactions (0.15%) are the most common complication of gelatin products.[34] Gelatins do not appear to be associated with renal failure.[35]

ASSESSMENT OF PATIENTS RECEIVING PARENTERAL FLUID THERAPY

A major nursing responsibility is the provision of precise intake and output records and daily weight charts. The accuracy of this information is crucial to the correct formulation of fluid replacement regimens, especially in critically ill patients. In addition, nurses must share the responsibility for detecting undesirable trends in these data. Keeping in mind the contents of the fluids being administered, it is important to consider the following parameters when evaluating the patient's response to fluid therapy:

- Comparison of intake and output measurements (positive or negative fluid balance)
- Body weight (rapid gain or loss)
- Vital signs (signs of hypovolemia or hypervolemia)
- Hemodynamic measurements (such as central venous pressure, pulmonary arterial pressure, pulmonary capillary wedge pressure, and cardiac output in critically ill patients)
- Urinary specific gravity (high or low)
- Laboratory values (especially BUN, creatinine, and electrolyte concentrations)

Refer to Chapter 2 for a review of these indices and to Chapters 13 through 25 for specific clinical conditions. Chapters 3 through 9 also present specific information regarding assessment of patients receiving parenteral fluids.

Adequacy of Fluid Volume

Giving the right amount of fluid depends on calculating measurable fluid losses, estimating insensible and third-space losses, factoring in the functional ability of key homeostatic organs, and revising fluid prescriptions according to current indicators of the patient's fluid and electrolyte status. Standing fluid orders are never acceptable. For typical patients, fluid orders are readjusted every 24 hours. However, this practice is not sufficient for many critically ill patients whose fluid status is subject to rapid change. For these patients, it may be necessary to readjust fluid directives every 8 hours (or even more frequently). Fluid orders are best written as the desired number of milliliters per hour over a specific period (such as 100 mL per hour over the next 24 hours). Failure to adhere to this simple rule can have disastrous results.

Nurses are responsible for assuring that the desired hourly flow rate is maintained. Unfortunately, evidence suggests that accuracy in flow rates is a problem in some clinical areas. For example, a recent prospective study in the United Kingdom examined flow rates over a 4-week period in patients requiring continuous IV fluids.[36] A total of 207 IV bags were monitored; only 26% were administered at the prescribed flow rate (percentage error +10% to −10%). Most of the bags (67%) were administered too slowly, although 16% were administered too quickly. The investi-

gators concluded that marked inaccuracies in IV infusion rates are relatively common and not viewed as important by staff. In this study, infusion rate errors were reduced when infusion pumps were used.

Too Little Fluid

Signs of too little fluid include hypotension, tachycardia, poor skin turgor, and acute weight loss. Providing too little fluid can result in oliguria associated with pre-renal azotemia. If oliguria is allowed to persist, the patient may develop acute tubular necrosis (ATN). To differentiate between these conditions, a fluid load is infused over a short period and the patient is observed closely. If urine output improves, the problem was simple fluid volume deficit; if urine flow is not reestablished, the problem is likely to be renal insufficiency. A fluid challenge test to distinguish simple fluid volume deficit from a deficit complicated by ATN is described in Chapter 3. These two conditions must be differentiated because prompt treatment of pre-renal azotemia can prevent ATN. Treatment of a patient with adequate renal function is simplified greatly if sufficient water and electrolytes are provided because healthy kidneys can select the needed substances and maintain normal fluid and electrolyte balance.

Too Much Fluid

It is also possible to administer too much fluid. An early indication of such an imbalance is an acute weight gain. Both peripheral edema and pulmonary edema may occur as well (especially if the fluid has a high sodium content). Perioperative weight gain has been shown to be related to patient mortality; although it is unclear whether the fluid gain is a cause of mortality or if it is merely the effect of some other condition associated with increased mortality.[37] Nonetheless, it is important to infuse only enough fluid to maintain normal physiologic functioning. In regard to the volume of blood transfusions needed in a specific situation, the following recommendation is plausible: "Until more data become available, it appears rational to transfuse as much as necessary, and as little as possible."[38]

Adequacy of Potassium Intake

For patients unable to obtain potassium by the gastrointestinal route, potassium must be administered intravenously. For the typical adult, 40 to 60 mEq per day suffices (if there are no abnormal losses). An attempt is made to replace sufficient potassium to keep the serum potassium level within the normal range (such as 3.5 to 5.0 mEq/L). If the patient has cardiac disease, the physician may prefer that the serum potassium level be kept at or above 4.0 mEq/L (of course, without exceeding the upper limit of normal). Table 5-4 summarizes nursing considerations in administering intravenous potassium.

Adequacy of Magnesium Intake

Recall that routine intravenous fluids are lacking in magnesium. While this lack may be tolerated for a week or two, it cannot be tolerated on a long-term basis. Either parenteral or enteral nutrition must be implemented if the patient remains unable to take adequate nutrients by mouth for more than 1 to 2 weeks. The need for magnesium replacement is increased when diarrhea or a high-output intestinal fistula is present; conversely, a reduced magnesium intake is indicated for patients with renal disease. A variety of magnesium salts are commercially available in concentrated forms for addition to IV fluids; most commonly used is magnesium sulfate. To monitor the adequacy of magnesium replacement, serum magnesium levels are monitored (normal range in an adult is approximately 1.6 to 2.5 mg/dL). Nursing considerations in the administration of intravenous magnesium are described in Table 7-3. A discussion of the use of magnesium infusions in pregnancy is provided in Chapter 23.

Adequacy of Calcium Intake

Like magnesium, calcium is not provided in most routine IV solutions. Even though calcium is present in LR, its concentration in this solution is far too low (3 mEq/L) to meet long-term calcium needs. Thus, if routine IV fluids are needed for more than 1 to 2 weeks, it will likely be necessary to provide calcium (as well as magnesium and phosphorus) in tube feeding formulas or specially formulated parenteral nutrition formulas. Calcium is primarily available in two forms for parenteral use: calcium gluconate and calcium chloride. Table 6-3 identifies nursing considerations in the administration of intravenous calcium.

IMBALANCES ASSOCIATED WITH BLOOD TRANSFUSIONS

Blood transfusions are primarily used to increase the oxygen-carrying capacity of the recipient's blood, replace hemostatic components, and expand the circulating intravascular volume. Although blood transfusion can be life-saving therapy when indicated, it should not be undertaken lightly because the transfusion process has a number of inherent risks, including electrolyte problems associated with storage of the transfused blood.

Hyperkalemia

Continual destruction of red blood cells occurs when blood is stored; as a result, potassium is released from the destroyed red blood cells and is also transferred from intact red blood cells into the surrounding plasma. This leakage of potassium is related to loss of cell membrane integrity resulting from hypoxia. For example, the extracellular potassium concentration may average 12 mEq/L at 7 days of storage and reach as high as 32 mEq/L after 21 days of storage.[39] When the stored blood is infused into the recipient, the blood cells are re-oxygenated and take up the leaked potassium; however, before this uptake occurs, transient hyperkalemia can develop if massive blood transfusion is required. Risk factors for hyperkalemia identified in 131 trauma victims included an initial plasma potassium level of 4.0 mEq/L or greater and transfusion of 20 or more units of cell- or plasma-based transfusion products.[40]

It has been recommended that blood be transfused from lines as distal as possible from the right atrium to allow greater mixture of the transfused blood with the recipient's blood before it reaches the right atrium.[41] The use of fresh blood helps to prevent hyperkalemia (because the leakage of potassium from the cells is not as advanced as occurs in blood that has been stored for a period of time). Once hyperkalemia develops, its management is essentially the same as for other conditions. (See Chapter 5.)

Hypocalcemia

Citrate (a negatively charged ion) is used as an anticoagulant in blood products. In some situations, such as in massive transfusions, the citrate anions may combine with the positively charged calcium ions circulating in the patient's bloodstream. In most cases, the citrate in stored blood causes no problem because the patient's liver rapidly converts it to bicarbonate as it is being transfused. Further, calcium is mobilized from the bone to help correct the deficit of ionized calcium in the bloodstream. Citrate-induced hypocalcemia is usually transient and cause no hemodynamic effect.

Although the overall incidence of transfusion-related hypocalcemia is thought to be quite small, certain patients are at increased risk. For example, metabolism of citrate to bicarbonate by the liver may be dramatically impaired during hypothermia, poor perfusion, or liver damage. Patients with impaired metabolism of citrate will manifest symptoms of hypocalcemia (such as tetany, hypotension, prolonged QT interval, and decreased myocardial contractility).

During later stages of pregnancy, serum ionized calcium and magnesium are normally decreased.[42] If rapid infusion of blood products is required during this period, tetany and muscle rigidity (as well as other symptoms of hypocalcemia and hypomagnesemia) may be precipitated. For this reason, ionized calcium and magnesium are closely monitored in women who require large blood transfusions during the later stages of pregnancy.

Most liver transplant patients are anhepatic for part of the surgical procedure and, therefore, cannot metabolize the citrate they receive in blood transfusions during this time. In such patients, calcium supplementation may be needed to prevent decreased ventricular function and hypotension. A study reported in 2003 indicated that hypocalcemia is a problem in liver transplant patients even when citrated blood products are not administered; as such, the researchers recommended that calcium ionization be monitored during liver transplants (regardless of whether the patient is receiving citrated blood products or noncitrated products, such as 5% albumin during the operative procedure).[43]

Calcium replacement (in the form of calcium chloride or calcium gluconate) is usually limited to patients in whom symptomatic hypocalcemia develops. Patients with underlying cardiac problems are at increased risk for complications such as hypotension or heart failure; as such, this group of patients is more likely to require calcium replacement therapy than are patients without these conditions.

Acid–Base Changes

The pH of 3-week-old stored red blood cells decreases to about 6.8 as a result of cellular metabolism. If shock is present, the patient is less able to metabolize the accumulated acids in the transfused blood; in turn, any existing acidosis (as from hypoxia and poor tissue perfusion) is made worse. It is important to remember that the acidosis seen in massively transfused patients is more likely due to hypoxemia and poor tissue perfusion, rather than the blood itself. Thus the key is to provide adequate volume restoration and perfusion (which will help correct the acidosis). Acidosis predisposes to dysrhythmias, decreased cardiac contractility, and hypotension. Also, clotting factors may be adversely affected by the decreased plasma pH.

A retrospective study of 23 patients who required transfusions of more than 50 units of plasma-poor red cells or whole blood was conducted to determine factors that affected survival.[44] Among the six patients who survived, the lowest arterial pH values ranged from 6.87 to 7.28; among those who did not survive, the range was 6.77 to 7.27. The authors concluded that the severity of acidosis was not a predictor of outcome.

Although an initial metabolic acidosis may occur during rapid transfusion, metabolic alkalosis may eventually result, because the citrate in stored blood is eventually converted to bicarbonate by the liver. Patients with normal renal function can readily excrete the excess bicarbonate load; however, those with decreased renal function (secondary to hypovolemia) may have difficulty excreting the excess alkali load.

Fluid Volume Overload

Fluid volume overload is a possible complication of blood transfusions. Most commonly red blood cells (RBCs) are administered as packed RBCs (which are obtained by centrifuging whole blood and drawing off 200 to 225 mL of plasma). Although packed RBCs have a reduced plasma volume, it is necessary to use a slow infusion rate for patients with impaired cardiopulmonary function (especially given that isotonic saline is administered with the RBCs). When too much fluid is given or the transfusion is too fast, acute left ventricular failure may occur, accompanied by dyspnea, tachypnea, cough, basal lung crackles, hypotension, and tachycardia. The onset of circulatory overload is usually gradual, with symptoms becoming more severe as the transfusion continues.

Summary of Key Points

- The most commonly used IV fluid for maintenance needs is 0.45% sodium chloride; this fluid provides 77 mEq of sodium per liter as well as free water to help eliminate wastes via the kidneys. It is often referred to as "half-strength" saline.

- The fluids most commonly used to replace sodium and expand the plasma volume are 0.9% sodium chloride solution (also called isotonic saline and normal saline) and lactated Ringer's (LR) solution.

- Lactated Ringer's solution contains slightly less sodium than normal saline (130 mEq/L as compared to 154 mEq/L). As such, each liter of LR provides a small amount (approximately 110 mL) of free water.

- 0.9% sodium chloride (normal saline) can be administered in the same line as blood and is recommended for this purpose. Lactated Ringer's solution contains a small amount of calcium; therefore, it should not be used in the same IV line as blood (because it could cause the line to clog)

- Both 3.0% and 5.0% sodium chloride solutions are extremely hypertonic as compared to the tonicity of body fluids. These solutions are used sparingly and only when necessary to treat hyponatremia associated with neurologic changes. They are also used in some settings to expand the plasma volume in patients with shock. They should be administered only in settings where the patient can be closely monitored.

- The 5% dextrose in water solution, which is often referred to as D$_5$W, contains no electrolytes. This fluid can cause serious hyponatremia in patients with high antidiuretic hormone levels, such as postoperative patients. Use of this fluid in practice settings is usually limited to mixing with medications to be administered IV.

- Dextrose is often added to electrolyte solutions to provide calories. For example, a 5% solution of dextrose provides 170 calories per liter.

- A number of products (other than isotonic sodium solutions and blood) are available to expand the plasma volume. Among these are albumin, hydroxyethyl starch, dextran, and gelatins.

- Blood transfusions may be life-saving; however, they can also be associated with electrolyte disturbances, such as hyperkalemia when a large volume of stored blood is administered rapidly.

NOTES

1. Waters, J. H., Gootlieb, A., Schoenwald, P., Popovich, M. J., Sprung, J., & Nelson, D. R. (2001). Normal saline versus lactated Ringer's solution for intraoperative fluid management in patients undergoing abdominal aortic aneurysm repair: An outcome study. *Anesthesia & Analgesia, 93*, 817–822.

2. O'Malley, C. M., Frumento, R. J., Hardy, M. A., Benvenisty, A. I., Brentjens, T. E., Mercer, J. S., et al. (2005). A randomized, double-blind comparison of lactated Ringer's solution and 0.9% NaCl during renal transplantation. *Anesthesia & Analgesia, 100*, 1518–1524.

3. Singh, A., Carlin, B. W., Shade, D., & Kaplan, P. D. (2009). The use of hypertonic saline for fluid resuscitation in sepsis: A review. *Critical Care Nursing Quarterly, 32*(1), 10–13.

4. Singh et al., note 3.

5. Shields, C. J., O'Sullivan, A. W., Wang, J. H., Winter, D. C., Kirwan, W. O., & Redmond, H. P. (2003). Hypertonic saline enhances host response to bacterial challenge by augmenting receptor-independent neutrophil intracellular superoxide formation. *Annals of Surgery, 238*, 249–257.

6. Price, T.H. (ed.). (2008). *Standards for blood banks and transfusion services* (25th ed.). American Association of Blood Banks. Bethesda, MD.

7. Saidenberg, E., & Tinmouth, A. (2009). Ringer's lactate and red blood cells: Is there sufficient evidence to recommend for routine use? *Canadian Journal of Anaesthesia, 56*(5), 343–347.

8. Reilly, R. F., & Perazella, M. A. (2007). *Acid–base, fluids and electrolytes.* New York: McGraw-Hill, p. 8.

9. Marik, P. E. (2001). *Handbook of evidence-based critical care.* New York: Springer, p. 117.

10. Groeneveld, A. B. (2000). Albumin and artificial colloids in fluid management: Where does the clinical evidence of their utility stand? *Critical Care, 4*(suppl 2), S16–S20.

11. Carvalho, B., Mercier, F. J., Riley, E. T., Brummel, C., & Cohen, S. E. (2009). Hetastarch co-loading is as effective as pre-loading for the prevention of hypotension following spinal anesthesia for cesarean delivery. *International Journal of Obstetric Anesthesia, 18*(2), 150–155.

12. Westphal, M., James, M. F., Kozek-Langenecker, S., Stocker, R., Guidet, B., & Van Aken, H. (2009). Hydroxyethyl starches: different products – different effects. *Anesthesiology, 111*(1), 187–202.

13. Jin, S. L., & Yu, B.W. (2009). Effects of artificial colloids on haemostasis. *British Journal of Hospital Medicine, 70*(2), 101–103.

14. Jin & Yu, note 13.

15. Lucas, C. E., Denis, R., Ledgerwood, A. M., & Grabow, D. (1988). The effects of Hespan on serum and lymphatic albumin, globulin, and coagulant protein. *Annals of Surgery, 207*, 416–420.

16. Nielsen, V. G. (2005). Colloids decrease clot propagation and strength: Role of factor XIII-fibrin polymer and thrombin-fibrinogen interactions. *Acta Anaesthesiologica Scandinavica, 49*, 1163–1171.

17. Nielsen, V. G. (2006). Hemodilution modulates the time of onset and rate of fibrinolysis in human and rabbit plasma. *Journal of Heart and Lung Transplantation, 25*, 1344–1352.

18. Davidson, I. J. (2009). Acute kidney injury by hydroxyethyl starch: Can the risks be mitigated? *Critical Care Medicine, 37*(4), 1499–1501.

19. Schortgen, F., Lacherade, J. C., Bruneel, F., Cattaneo, I., Hemery, F., Lemaire, F., et al. (2001). Effects of hydroxyethylstarch and gelatin on renal function in severe sepsis: A multicentre randomized study. *Lancet, 357*, 911–916.

20. Brunkhorst, F. M., Engel, C., Bloos, F., Meier-Hellmann, A., Ragaller, M., Weiler, N., et al. (2008). Intensive insulin therapy and pentastarch resuscitation in severe sepsis. *New England Journal of Medicine, 358*, 125–139.

21. Davidson, note 18.

22. Dettori, N., & Spahn, D. R. (2003). Hydroxyethyl starches and pruritus: A real problem? *Transfusion Alternatives in Transfusion Medicine, 5*(4), 401–404.

23. Kellum, J. A., Cerda, J., Kaplan, L.J., Nadim, M. K., & Palevsky, P. M. (2008). Fluids for prevention and management of acute kidney injury. *International Journal of Artificial Organs, 31*(2), 96–110.

24. Langeron, O., Doelberg, M., Ang, E. T., Bonnet, F., Capdevila, X., & Coriat, P. (2001). Voluven, a lower substituted novel hydroxyethyl starch (HES 130/0.4) causes fewer effects on coagulation in major orthopedic surgery than HES 200/0.5. *Anesthesia and Analgesia, 92*, 855–862.

25. James, M. F. (2008). The role of tetrastarches for volume replacement in the perioperative setting. *Current Opinion in Anaesthesiology, 21*(5), 674–678.

26. Bongard, F. S., Sue, D. Y., & Vintch, J. R. (2008). *Current diagnosis & treatment critical care* (3rd ed.). New York: McGraw-Hill, p. 229.

27. Hahn, R. G., Prough, D. S., & Svensen, C. H. (2007). *Perioperative fluid therapy*. London: Informa Healthcare, p. 273.

28. Hahn et al., note 27, p. 254.

29. Klingensmith, M. E., Glasgow, S. C., Goers, T. A., & Melby, S. J. (2008). *The Washington manual of surgery* (5th ed.). Philadelphia: Lippincott Williams & Wilkins, p. 85.

30. Hahn et al., note 27, p. 273.

31. Bongard et al., note 26, p. 229.

32. Jin & Yu, note 13.

33. Jin & Yu, note 13.

34. Bongard et al., note 26, p. 229.

35. Bongard et al., note 26, p. 229.

36. Rooker, J. C., & Gorard, D. A. (2007). Errors in intravenous fluid infusion rates in medical patients. *Clinical Medicine, 7*(5), 482–485.

37. Schuller, D., Mitchell, J. P., Calandrino, F. S., & Schuster, D. P. (1991). Fluid balance during pulmonary edema: Is fluid gain a marker or a cause of poor outcome? *Chest, 100*(4), 890–892.

38. Frenzel, T., Van Aken, H., & Westphal, M. (2008). Our own blood is still the best thing to have in our veins. *Current Opinion in Anaesthesiology, 21,* 657–663.

39. Perkins, J. G., Cap, A. P., Weiss, B. M., Reid, T. J., & Bolan, C. D. (2008). Massive transfusion and nonsurgical hemostatic agents. *Critical Care Medicine, 36*(7 suppl), S325–339.

40. Perkins et al., note 39.

41. Perkins et al., note 39.

42. Powner, D. J., & Bessinger, V. J. (2002). Tetany following resuscitation after abruption placentae. *Obstetrics & Gynecology, 99*(5, Pt 2, suppl), 885–886.

43. Jawan, B., de Villa, V., Luk, H. N., Cheng, Y. F., Huang, T. L., Eng, H. L., et al. (2003). Ionized calcium changes during living-donor liver transplantation in patients with and without administration of blood-bank products. *Transplant International, 16*(7), 510–514.

44. Hakala, P., Hippala, S., Syriala, M., & Randell, T. (1999). Massive blood transfusion exceeding 50 units of plasma poor red cells or whole blood: The survival rate and the occurrence of leucopenia and acidosis. *Injury, 30*(9), 619–622.

Chapter 11

Parenteral Nutrition

Specialized nutrition support is indicated for a patient who has been without nourishment for at least a week and who is unlikely to be able to eat soon. If tube feeding can be tolerated, it is the preferred route. If not, nutrients can be delivered intravenously by either a peripheral vein (peripheral parenteral nutrition [PPN]) or a central vein (central parenteral nutrition). Central parenteral nutrition is also referred to as total parenteral nutrition (TPN). While potentially lifesaving, a number of serious metabolic problems (including fluid and electrolyte imbalances) can occur with TPN.

INDICATIONS FOR PARENTERAL NUTRITION

Parenteral nutrition is used less frequently than tube feedings because the latter are thought to be more physiologic and associated with fewer metabolic problems. However, despite the preference for enteral feedings, certain patients require parenteral nutrition because they are unable to meet their nutritional needs by the gastrointestinal (GI) route. Indications for parenteral nutrition include the following:

- Inadequate small-bowel surface area to absorb nutrients (as in massive small-bowel resection or severe radiation enteritis). For example, nutritional supplements are likely to be needed when less than 200 cm of small bowel remains.[1]
- Need for temporary "bowel rest" during recovery from a primary gastrointestinal disease condition.
- Any condition in which the patient is unable to consume adequate calories via the GI route.

PERIPHERAL PARENTERAL NUTRITION

Occasionally patients need intravenous nutrients for only a relatively short period of time (such as less than 7 days),

making it impractical to access a central vein. In this situation, nutrients may be administered via a peripheral vein. A typical solution administered for this purpose might consist of 5% to 10% glucose, 2% to 5% amino acids, and variable quantities of electrolytes (according to individual need). Fat emulsions may be "piggybacked" simultaneously into the primary line.

Peripheral veins have a relatively low rate of blood flow (such as less than 100 mL/min). See **Figure 11-1**. For this reason, a solution with a high osmolality causes venous irritation. A peripheral vein can likely tolerate a formula with an osmolality of 600 mOsm/L without venous damage; the maximal osmolality tolerated in a peripheral vein is 900 mOsm/L.[2] Even when the osmolality of the solution is limited to this level, phlebitis will eventually occur at the

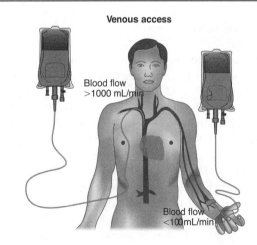

Venous access

Blood flow >1000 mL/min

Blood flow <100 mL/min

Figure 11-1 Comparison of rates of blood flow through peripheral and central veins.
Source: Adapted from American Gastroenterology Association.

infusion site. The onset of this complication may be slowed by decreasing the nutrient density of the formula or by decreasing its flow rate. Unfortunately, these maneuvers also decrease the caloric intake.

It is usually necessary to move the infusion site daily as a measure to avoid phlebitis. Over time, venous access becomes increasingly difficult.

In summary, peripheral parenteral nutrition is contraindicated in patients who have large nutrient or electrolyte needs, significant malnutrition, severe metabolic stress, and need for prolonged parenteral nutrition (greater than 2 weeks).[3]

CENTRAL ADMINISTRATION OF TOTAL PARENTERAL NUTRITION

When prolonged intravenous nutrient support is needed, a central vein is the necessary delivery site. Delivery of the solution into the superior vena cava can be accomplished by introducing a catheter through a subclavian or jugular vein, or via a peripherally inserted central venous catheter. Because the rate of blood flow through a central vein is high (usually more than 1000 mL/min), a high-osmolality, high-caloric solution can be tolerated when administered in this way.

Continuous Versus Cyclic Method

Some patients receive their TPN formula continuously over the 24-hour day, whereas others may receive it only for a period of 12 hours or so per day. The type of infusion method is selected according to individual patient characteristics.

Continuous infusion is the most common method for delivering the total parenteral solution, especially to hospitalized patients. When TPN is initiated, the rate is gradually increased until the caloric goal is achieved; the rate is then maintained evenly over 24 hours. If metabolic problems arise, the flow rate and composition of the formula may need to be adjusted.

After a patient receiving TPN is deemed to be metabolically stable, cyclic infusion of the solution may be considered. This method is especially desirable for patients receiving TPN at home. For these individuals, the solution is infused for 12 hours (usually at night) and then is turned off for the remainder of the 24-hour period. The cyclic method frees the patient from the infusion for the major part of the day and allows for normal activities. In a report

of 36 patients receiving home cyclic TPN through Broviac or Hickman catheters, researchers noted that 80% were able to return to work, school, or housekeeping activities, or at least to care for themselves unaided.[4]

Compared to continuous TPN, cyclic TPN may be associated with less liver complications. Cyclic TPN may not be suitable for patients with diabetes (because of the risk for hypoglycemia) and those with heart failure (who may not be able to tolerate the higher rate of fluid administration).[5]

Composition and Appearance of TPN Solutions

In most facilities in the United States, TPN formulations are prepared in the pharmacy, according to specifications provided by the physicians for individual patients. A typical formulation has an osmolality of 1800 mOsm/L or greater. Fortunately, because the vena cava has a high rate of blood flow, the solution is rapidly diluted and is not harmful to the vessel. The American Society for Parenteral and Enteral Nutrition (ASPEN) recommends that a standardized order form be used for adult and pediatric parenteral nutrition formulations; in this way, prescribers will be better able to meet each patient's estimated daily nutrition requirements and improve order clarity.[6]

Fluid requirements vary widely, based on the individual patient's clinical status. An adult patient with normal fluid volume typically requires approximately 30 mL of fluid per kilogram of body weight per day. Factors that increase fluid demands include fever, frequent vomiting or diarrhea, or high output from fistulas or drains. While central parenteral nutrition is in progress, peripheral infusions may occasionally be necessary to correct newly developed electrolyte imbalances. Of course, fluid administered via all routes is included in the fluid intake/output calculations. Nutrients available for TPN infusion include amino acids (protein), dextrose (carbohydrate), and fat emulsions.

A formulation that consists of dextrose and amino acids (with added electrolytes, vitamins, and trace elements) is clear and easily identifiable as an intravenous solution; it is sometimes referred to as a "2-in-1" formulation. A fat emulsion may be administered in a separate container via piggyback into the IV line in which the "2-in-1" solution is infusing. When the fat emulsion is added to the dextrose and amino acid solution in a single bag, it is referred to as a total nutrient admixture (or as a "3-in-1" TPN formulation). An advantage of the "3-in-1" formulation is reduced risk for infection because of less manipulation of the central line.

A "3-in-1" formulation has an appearance similar to that of some tube feeding formulas. Unfortunately, this can cause caregivers to confuse the two solutions. For example, a case was reported in which a nurse confused a bag of ready-to-hang tube feeding formula with a bag of TPN solution.[7] The enteral formula was then inadvertently administered into the central IV line of a young pregnant woman; both she and her fetus died as a result of this action. Other potential disadvantages of a "3-in-1" solution include a greater risk for infection because lipid emulsions are a good medium for bacterial and fungal growth, the incompatibility with some medications with the formula, difficulty in visualizing precipitated salts, and potential breakdown of the emulsion.[8] A "3-in-1" solution should be inspected for deterioration before hanging, and it should not hang at room temperature for longer than 24 hours.[9]

Premixed parenteral nutrition products are commercially available; some include two compartments (one with amino acids and the other with dextrose). An advantage of these products is time saved by pharmacists; a disadvantage is that they are not prepared for the specific needs of individual patients.[10]

Dextrose

Carbohydrate is usually the primary source of calories in humans.[11] Dextrose (glucose) is the primary carbohydrate used in parenteral nutrition solutions, furnishing 3.4 kcal of energy per gram delivered. Glucose is required (or preferentially used) by the brain, blood cells, and renal medulla.[12] Among the complications associated with excessive glucose administration are increased risk for infections, hyperosmolar complications, and excess carbon dioxide production.[13] Thus, while it is important to provide therapeutic levels of dextrose, it is imperative to guard against giving too much of this nutrient. Critically ill patients are less tolerant of glucose than are stable hospitalized patients.[14]

Recall that CO_2 is an end product of carbohydrate metabolism. When CO_2 retention is a problem, excessive carbohydrate administration can lead to respiratory acidosis. For example, investigators observed a rise in $PaCO_2$ within 12 hours after TPN was initiated in a patient maintained on a fixed mechanical ventilator setting; the $PaCO_2$ rose from 43 to 93 mm Hg and the serum pH fell from 7.4 to 7.25 within 24 hours after the carbohydrate intake increased from 1500 to 2500 kcal/day.[15] To minimize excessive CO_2 production, healthcare providers should make an effort to avoid administering excessive calories (particularly in the form of glucose) to patients at risk for hypercapnia (excessive $PaCO_2$).

Another adverse effect from giving too much dextrose is hepatic steatosis.[16] Fatty infiltration of the liver (steatosis) may develop after 7 to 21 days of parenteral nutrition and is usually asymptomatic. In severe cases, however, it may be associated with hepatomegaly and upper right quadrant pain.[17]

Amino Acids

A variety of amino acids are available as a protein source for TPN solutions; they vary in concentration from 3.5% to 10%. Under most conditions, conventional amino acid formulations are the optimal form of intravenous amino acid therapy. Disease-specific amino acids are available for patients with liver and renal failure. In general, these formulations are not recommended for use longer than 2 weeks because they do not provide a complete amino acid profile.[18]

Fat Emulsions

Intravenous fat emulsions are available in concentrations of 10%, 20%, and 30% (prepared from soybean or safflower oil in combination with glycerol and emulsifiers).[19] A 10% emulsion supplies 1.1 kcal/mL, while a 20% emulsion provides 2.0 kcal/mL. Fat emulsions are contraindicated in patients with a triglyceride concentration exceeding 400 mg/dL; also, patients who are allergic to eggs should not receive fat emulsions because egg phospholipids are used as an emulsifier.[20] Currently available fat emulsions contain one-half to two-thirds of their fatty acids as linoleic acid and 5% to 10% as linolenic acid.[21] This content has important implications, in that these essential fatty acids are required for all patients receiving parenteral nutrition. Most intravenous fat emulsions contain vitamin K (a factor of interest when patients are receiving anticoagulant therapy with warfarin.)[22]

Because fat emulsions are isotonic, they help reduce the osmolality of the infused parenteral nutrition (either by direct mixture with the base solution or by infusion in a piggybacked peripheral line). Patients with diabetes may require a higher percentage of fat calories to prevent hyperglycemia; patients with respiratory failure may require more fat (and less glucose) calories to minimize CO_2 production. The latter consideration is particularly important when attempting to wean patients off ventilators.

Electrolytes

Electrolyte requirements vary during a course of TPN therapy, depending on the patient's clinical status. Particul attention should be paid to the major intracellular electrolytes (potassium, phosphate, and magnesium) because these electrolytes are required for the anabolic process (i.e., the formation of new cells). Clinical conditions that may warrant cautious use of parenteral nutrition include the presence of hypokalemia (such as potassium < 3 mEq/L), hypophosphatemia (such as phosphorus < 2 mg/dL), and hypernatremia (such as sodium > 150 mEq/L).[23] See the discussion of electrolyte abnormalities in the next section for more details.

Trace Minerals.

Trace minerals, such as zinc, chromium, copper, manganese, zinc, and selenium, are available commercially for addition to parenteral nutrient solutions. While patients do not require daily supplementation with these substances, deficits can occur if the trace minerals are omitted during long-term parenteral nutrition. Trace element deficiency is relatively uncommon in patients receiving parenteral nutrition, but can occur when intake is insufficient over a prolonged period of time The patient's clinical status influences the need for specific trace minerals. For example, the need for zinc supplementation is greater when large zinc losses are occurring (as from diarrhea or ileostomy output).

Vitamins

Vitamins are usually given daily or every other day from the initiation of parenteral nutrition. Among the vitamins administered are thiamine, riboflavin, pyridoxine, niacin, folic acid, pantothenic acid, biotin, ascorbic acid, and vitamins A, D, E, and K. Thiamine is especially important, in that it is a coenzyme for carbohydrate metabolism. Daily replacement of this vitamin is important during parenteral dextrose administration because thiamine is not stored by the body. Failure to administer adequate thiamine as part of parenteral nutrition can precipitate Wernicke's encephalopathy. Replacement of thiamine is especially important in alcoholic patients.

METABOLIC DERANGEMENTS ASSOCIATED WITH TPN

Virtually any metabolic disturbance may occur during TPN, and they are largely reflective of the patient's underlying disease state, which may sometimes interfere with the ability to metabolize or excrete the infused nutrients. Metabolic derangements are also influenced by the contents of the parenteral nutrient solution (i.e., too much or too little of a specific component).

Electrolyte Abnormalities

Essentially, expected abnormalities fall into two categories. First, the addition of too little of an essential electrolyte or nutrient can result in a deficiency state. Second, an excess of the electrolytes or nutrients in the parenteral solution may lead to toxicity when they exceed the body's normal metabolic and excretory capacity. To guard against either type of imbalance, baseline electrolyte values should be obtained before the initiation of central TPN and serious abnormalities corrected before TPN is initiated.

Electrolyte abnormalities in patients receiving TPN are primarily detected by evaluating daily laboratory results. When detected early, the imbalances can usually be rectified by altering the electrolyte composition of the formula. For this reason, it is customary to monitor serum electrolytes frequently. For example, electrolytes may be monitored daily in critically ill patients receiving TPN, and one or two times per week in stable patients. An imbalance should be quickly called to the attention of the physician.

Hypophosphatemia

Hypophosphatemia is probably the most common imbalance in patients receiving TPN. Although the incidence of this condition is only 0.5% to 3% in the general hospital population, it is as high as 31% in patients receiving specialized nutritional support.[24] Hypophosphatemia occurs as a result of new tissue synthesis and a shift of phosphate from the extracellular to the intracellular compartment. (See the discussion of refeeding syndrome later in this chapter.) Hypophosphatemia can even occur in patients who chronically have elevated phosphate levels (such as patients with renal failure) during the aggressive administration of TPN.[25]

To avoid precipitation of calcium phosphate, the amounts of calcium and phosphate that are added to a TPN mixture must be controlled. Therefore, significant hypophosphatemia (less than 1 mg/dL) should be corrected with supplemental phosphate in a separate IV. Preparations containing either sodium phosphate or potassium phosphate are available, with selection of the most appropriate salt being based on the patient's serum potassium concentration and the state of renal function. Clinical signs of hypophosphatemia are described in Chapter 8.

Hyperphosphatemia

Although rare, hyperphosphatemia in patients receiving TPN is possible. This imbalance is most likely to occur in patients whose kidneys are unable to adequately excrete phosphate. Hyperphosphatemia can also occur when too much phosphate is added to the formulation. For example, this imbalance was reported in a septic female patient whose TPN formulation unintentionally contained triple the amount of required phosphate.[26] Her serum phosphate concentration increased as a result to 3.02 mmol/L (normal, 0.76–1.46 mmol/L). Hyperphosphatemia contributed to calcification of her arteries and resulted in widespread infarcts of the skin. See Chapter 8 for a more detailed discussion of the consequences and clinical signs of hyperphosphatemia.

Hypokalemia

Hypokalemia in patients receiving TPN can occur as cells take up additional potassium to synthesize new tissue. (See the discussion of refeeding syndrome later in this chapter.) Also, cellular uptake of potassium is increased by elevated catecholamine levels in stressed patients. If insufficient potassium is contained in the solution, a significant fall in the serum concentration of potassium may occur as early as 6 to 12 hours after beginning TPN. Serum potassium levels must be monitored closely during the initiation of TPN and the amount of potassium added to the TPN formula adjusted as necessary. Patients who receive insulin for hyperglycemia need to be monitored especially closely for hypokalemia because insulin facilitates transport of potassium into cells and further depresses the serum potassium concentration. (Refer to Chapter 5 for a review of the clinical signs of hypokalemia as well as its treatment.)

Hyperkalemia

Addition of too much potassium to the TPN solution, or large intake from other sources without cutting back the amount added to the solution, can lead to hyperkalemia (particularly in patients with impaired renal ability to excrete potassium). Tissue necrosis and systemic sepsis also predispose to hyperkalemia. Further, metabolic acidosis favors a shift of potassium from the cells to the bloodstream. Medications associated with increased risk of hyperkalemia include potassium-sparing diuretics and angiotensin-converting enzyme (ACE) inhibitors. See Chapter 5 for a more detailed discussion of potassium imbalances.

Hypomagnesemia

Hypomagnesemia is seen in patients who are chronic alcoholics, severely malnourished, receiving drugs associated with renal magnesium wasting (such as diuretics, amphotericin B, cisplatin, or cyclosporine), or experiencing large losses of intestinal fluid. As indicated in the discussion of refeeding syndrome (later in this chapter), hypomagnesemia is part of the triad of imbalances associated with this syndrome. Clinical signs of hypomagnesemia are described in Chapter 7.

Hypermagnesemia

Hypermagnesemia can occur if excessive magnesium is supplied in the parenteral formula, especially in patients with renal insufficiency. Symptoms of hypermagnesemia are described in Chapter 7. This imbalance is treated by decreasing the magnesium load in the parenteral nutrient solution. If the derangement is severe, dialysis may be necessary to rectify it.

Hyponatremia

Hyponatremia in a patient receiving TPN is most often due to the excessive administration of hypotonic fluid. For example, a young adult trauma patient receiving TPN became hyponatremic because of the daily administration of almost 3 L of D_5W in a peripheral vein as a diluent for antimicrobial agents administered for sepsis.[27] Other possible causes of hyponatremia in patients receiving TPN include syndrome of inappropriate antidiuretic hormone secretion, congestive heart failure, cirrhosis, and adrenal insufficiency. Dilutional hyponatremia is usually managed by decreasing the fluid intake; if sodium intake is inadequate, additional sodium may be given.

Hypernatremia

Hypernatremia occurs infrequently during TPN infusions. When this imbalance does occur, it is usually due to excessive water loss (as in fever or hyperventilation) or inadequate water intake. To help correct hypernatremia, free water intake should be increased (either in the TPN solution or through another route).

Hypocalcemia

Because most patients receiving TPN are malnourished and, therefore, have low serum albumin levels, their total serum calcium levels are also likely to be below normal. However, because ionization of calcium usually remains normal in hypoalbuminemic patients, this "hypocalcemia" is not physiologically significant and will not result in paresthesias or other signs of tetany. Other causes of hypocalcemia include inadequate vitamin D intake and hypomagnesemia. (Recall that hypomagnesemia causes decreased mobilization of calcium from the bone by inhibiting the release of parathyroid hormone.)

Hypercalcemia

Hypercalcemia can occur in patients receiving TPN for extended periods. Possible causes are metabolic bone disease associated with long-term TPN and excessive infusion of calcium or vitamin A and D supplements. When hypercalcemia occurs, it is necessary to consider other causes as well, such as neoplasm or primary or secondary hyperparathyroidism.

Fluid Volume Imbalances

It is important to monitor for fluid volume problems in patients who are receiving TPN. These imbalances can best be detected by maintaining accurate fluid intake and output records as well as body weight records. Some patients have difficulty tolerating the relatively large fluid load required as part of TPN; when this problem occurs, it may be necessary to switch to a more concentrated solution to decrease the fluid volume. Other patients may need additional fluids to meet their needs. Recall that a sudden increase in urine output could be a sign of osmotic diuresis associated with hyperglycemia. An excessive amount of protein in the parenteral nutrition solution results in increased metabolic demand on the body for excreting by-products of protein metabolism. An increased blood urea nitrogen (BUN) level can result, especially if the patient's fluid status is low.

Refeeding Syndrome

Refeeding syndrome (RFS) consists of a constellation of metabolic derangements that can occur when any type of nutritional intervention is implemented in a patient who has been malnourished for days to weeks.[28] Among the potential metabolic derangements are hypophosphatemia, hypomagnesemia, hypokalemia, fluid and sodium retention, hyperglycemia, thiamine deficiency, and neurologic and hematolic complications, occurring within the first few days of feeding a starving patient.[29] While the pathophysiology of RFS is complex, it is primarily the result of an acute intracellular shift of electrolytes, increased demand for phosphate during tissue anabolism, and formation of high-energy intracellular bonds.[30] Potentially life-threatening complications of RFS include cardiac arrhythmias, heart failure, respiratory failure, and hematologic derangements (see Case Study 11-3.) Refeeding syndrome is also discussed in Chapter 12.

Hyperglycemia

Hyperglycemia is one of the most common metabolic derangements caused by TPN. Some have speculated that this condition is a key factor in the increased rate of complications associated with parenteral nutrition as opposed to enteral nutrition.[31]

Common causes of hyperglycemia include too rapid or uneven administration of the high-dextrose solution and increased levels of glucose-elevating stress hormones (associated with a number of illnesses and injury states). The development or worsening of glucose intolerance may be a harbinger of sepsis or another complicating condition (such as myocardial infarction). Indeed, hyperglycemia may precede other signs of infection by 18 to 24 hours. When hyperglycemia occurs despite careful management, its cause should be carefully investigated.

Hyperglycemia causes an osmotic diuresis and predisposes patients to both fluid volume deficit and increased renal loss of electrolytes (such as potassium and magnesium). The increased serum tonicity associated with hyperglycemia can lead to intracellular dehydration in the brain and, eventually, to coma.[32] A retrospective study of 457 patients receiving TPN found that hyperglycemia was significantly correlated with increased morbidities and mortality.[33] Another retrospective study of 357 adults admitted for initial autologous or allogenic transplantation compared outcomes in those who received TPN versus those who did not; researchers found that the broad use of TPN was associated with profound hyperglycemia and higher morbidity.[34] Still another group of investigators reported longer need for artificial ventilation in septic premature infants who developed hyperglycemia while receiving TPN.[35]

Other adverse effects of hyperglycemia include exacerbation of inflammation, impaired neutrophil chemotaxis and phagocytosis, and impaired wound healing.[36] Hyperglycemia is more likely to occur in patients receiving more than the required number of calories. Not surprisingly, patients with diabetes mellitus are also at higher risk.

Uncontrolled hyperglycemia can lead to hyperosmotic hyperglycemic syndrome (HHS). Fortunately, due to frequent blood glucose monitoring for hyperglycemia, this complication is seen less frequently today than in the past. When it occurs, the source is often underlying diabetes mellitus and preexistent negative water balance. For example, in a study of 200 patients receiving TPN, 6 individuals developed HHS; all had familial histories of diabetes mellitus and had negative water balance with hyperglycemia for several days preceding the development of the syndrome.[37] See Chapter 18 for a detailed discussion of HHS and it management.

Detection of Hyperglycemia

During TPN administration, the patient should be closely monitored for glucose intolerance, especially during the early days of this intervention. In acute care settings, glucose tolerance is usually measured by checking capillary blood sugars at regular intervals. There is no universal agreement about the most desirable upper level of serum glucose in a patient receiving TPN; however, a reasonable level appears to be no greater than 140 mg/dL.

Insulin Therapy for Hyperglycemia

All patients who receive parenteral nutrition should have their blood glucose measured frequently (such as every 4 hours) by a glucometer during the infusion. In the presence of hyperglycemia, it is usually necessary to administer insulin. Regimens for insulin administration vary, one method is to administer insulin subcutaneously on a sliding scale. Another option is to add insulin to the TPN solution to achieve more even blood sugar control; in this way, an increase or decrease in the TPN flow is accompanied by a similar change in insulin administration. Other providers prefer to infuse insulin via a separate line so that blood glucose can be controlled without disturbing the rate of the parenteral nutrient solution (based on frequent glucometer readings). Diabetics may have basal insulin requirements added to their TPN solution while breakthrough elevations in blood glucose are covered with subcutaneous injections. Oral hypoglycemics should be discontinued when TPN is started.[38]

Prevention of Hyperglycemia

Deciding how much dextrose to add to the parenteral nutrient solution falls under the purview of the physician and dietitian. The nurse can contribute to the prevention of hyperglycemia by recognizing the need for introducing the nutrient solution slowly and gradually advancing its rate as tolerated. By monitoring blood glucose levels on a frequent basis, the nurse can provide valuable information about how the patient is tolerating the infusion.

If, for some reason, the infusion falls behind, its flow should not be abruptly increased to compensate for the deficiency. A common cause of transient hyperglycemia in patients on TPN is inadvertent rapid administration of the TPN solution due to equipment malfunction or operator error. For patients receiving cyclic TPN, it is customary to begin with a reduced flow rate for 2 hours before initiating the full infusion rate and then to taper the rate of flow for 2 hours before discontinuance. As indicated earlier, this method is usually reserved for patients who are metabolically stable.

When patients receiving TPN are scheduled to have surgery for a major procedure, medical orders should be clear about what to do with the infusion rate. Although physician preferences vary greatly, the rate of glucose infusion is usually decreased because patients often become less glucose tolerant when subjected to the major stress of surgery.

Discontinuing Parenteral Nutrition

At present, there is no consistent protocol for discontinuing parenteral nutrition. It is possible for hypoglycemia to occur if the parenteral nutrient solution is discontinued abruptly (especially after the infusion rate has recently been increased, resulting in increased endogenous insulin production). However, studies have provided conflicting findings regarding the effect of abrupt discontinuation of a parenteral nutrient solution. For example, a small randomized trial compared the effects of tapered TPN discontinuation over 90 minutes in 10 patients to the effects seen in 11 patients in which TPN was discontinued abruptly; symptoms of hypoglycemia were not evident in either group.[39] However, in a study of 11 children who had TPN abruptly discontinued, 6 developed hypoglycemia (glucose concentration less than 40 mg/dL).[40] Hypoglycemia can be likely be prevented by tapering the flow rate over 1 to 2 hours prior to discontinuation. In most instances, an effort is made to ensure that adequate nutrients (i.e., 75% of maintenance calories) are consumed by the enteral route before TPN is stopped.

Clinically, there is a rarely a reason to discontinue the nutrient solution abruptly. Even when quick discontinuation is needed, there is usually time to taper the solution's flow rate over an hour or more. If this is not possible, coverage with a 10% dextrose solution at the previous TPN flow rate in a peripheral vein generally presents no risk and could be beneficial. Obtaining a capillary glucose reading 30 minutes to 1 hour after TPN is discontinued is helpful in identifying rebound hypoglycemia.[41]

CASE STUDIES

Case Study 11-1

A case was reported in which a 45-year-old man was admitted for elective resection of a large temporal arteriovenous malformation.[42] Because of severe hemorrhage during the procedure, he required massive blood transfusions. The patient was mechanically ventilated but self-extubated himself on the first postoperative day; during this time, he suffered aspiration and required reintubation. He soon developed acute respiratory distress syndrome (ARDS) and required high positive end-expiratory pressure and fraction of inspired oxygen to maintain adequate oxygenation. He also required chemical paralysis and sedation to minimize oxygen consumption and to control airway pressures.

On the second postoperative day, TPN was started. The caloric intake was increased gradually and a low volume of enteral formula was started via a nasojejunal feeding tube. The total caloric intake from both routes was 3370 kcal/day. The patient's ARDS became progressively more difficult to manage. Hypercapnea ($PaCO_2$ ranged between 65 and 70 mm Hg) was present and was assumed to be due, at least in part, to overfeeding. TPN was discontinued and the enteral feeding was adjusted to deliver 1440 kcal/day. Within 36 hours of these changes, the $PaCO_2$ dropped to 43 mm Hg and other ventilatory parameters improved. Weekly indirect calorimetry was performed to guide adjustments in nutrient delivery. The patient's ARDS gradually resolved and no further ventilatory support was required by the 59th postoperative day. The patient was discharged 5 weeks later.

Commentary. This patient's high total caloric intake generated excess CO_2. The high production of CO_2, coupled with his lung pathology, resulted in ineffective clearing of CO_2 and eventually led to hypercapnea. Fortunately, the healthcare providers' recognition of overfeeding allowed this patient to ultimately recover.

Case Study 11–2

A recent case report described a previously healthy 15-year-old boy with an intentional weight loss of 110 pounds over approximately one year.[43] When his pediatrician suggested that he maintain a 3000-calorie diet, the patient attempted to adhere to this recommendation one week before a follow-up visit with the pediatrician. Because of abnormal vital signs observed during the visit, the boy was admitted to an emergency department. He had a low body temperature (93.0°F), a heart rate of 46 beats per minute, and a blood pressure of 83/53 mm Hg. His eyes were sunken and his lower extremities were cool. At this time, his serum phosphate was 3.7 mg/dL and his serum magnesium was 2.5 mg/dL (both within normal limits). Eight hours later, the serum phosphate was 2.7 mg/dL and the serum magnesium was 2.2 mg/dL. The authors concluded that the boy was

experiencing early refeeding syndrome and admitted him for further care.

Commentary. The patient in this case study was fortunate to have been diagnosed with early refeeding syndrome so that potentially life-threatening complications associated with this syndrome could be prevented. He was transferred 8 days later to an outpatient hospitalization program for individuals with an eating disorder.

Case Study 11–3

A recent case report described a 56-year-old bedridden woman receiving continuous ambulatory peritoneal dialysis (CAPD) who developed electrolyte problems after starting TPN.[44] Her past history consisted of rheumatic heart disease and cerebrovascular disease. Because of a cloudy dialysate and abdominal fullness, she was admitted to the hospital with a diagnosis of peritonitis associated with CAPD. Prior to admission, her serum phosphate level was 5.27 mmol/L (equivalent to approximately 16.3 mg/dL); phosphate lowering medications had not been ordered. Upon admission, the patient's serum sodium level was low (130 mEq/L), as was her serum potassium level (2.5 mEq/L). She was treated with antibiotics and an attempt was made to deliver tube feedings because of her poor oral intake. Enteral feedings failed because of an ileus, and parenteral nutrition was started on the 11th hospital day.

The parenteral nutrient solution contained a low quantity of phosphate because the patient was uremic and had experienced previous hyperphosphatemic episodes. On the third day of parenteral nutrition, the following serum values were recorded: Na, 131 mEq/L; K, 2.9 mEq/L; albumin, 1.5 g/dL; phosphate, 0.3 mg/dL (normal range, 2.5–4.5 mg/dL). Recall that a phosphate concentration less than 1.0 mEq/L is potentially life-threatening. Although potassium phosphate was administered immediately to treat the severe hypophosphatemia, the patient was found unconscious and suffered a cardiac arrest on the morning of the fourth hospital day. Despite intensive cardiopulmonary resuscitation, she did not survive.

Commentary. Because patients with renal failure characteristically have high serum phosphate levels, it is understandable why the amount of phosphate added to this patient's TPN solution was limited. This case illustrates that even a patient with a history of high serum phosphate levels can develop hypophosphatemia related to cellular uptake of phosphate and other electrolytes during refeeding syndrome. The authors of this case report pointed out that malnutrition affects as many as 50% of patients on chronic dialysis therapy. (Recall that malnutrition is a risk factor for refeeding syndrome.) Complications associated with a serum phosphate level less than 1.0 mg/dL can include cardiac arrhythmias, heart failure, and sudden death.

Case Study 11–4

A case was reported in which a 23-year-old man with a leg amputation was given TPN because of an intestinal ileus.[45] He later developed sepsis and required antimicrobial medications, which were administered in a solution of 5% dextrose in water (resulting in an addition of 3 L of free water each day to his fluid intake). When the patient developed hyponatremia, more sodium was added to his TPN solution. After 14 days, the antimicrobial agents were discontinued; however, the high sodium content in the TPN solution was not adjusted. Subsequently, the patient developed hypernatremia.

Commentary. The authors of this case report pointed out that the most appropriate management of this patient would have involved changing the fluids in which the antimicrobial agents were diluted to a saline solution (and not modifying the sodium content of the TPN solution). This action would have prevented hyponatremia and the resultant treatment that led to the development of hypernatremia. The lesson to be learned from this case is that sodium and fluid can be adjusted by means other than the TPN solution, including medication admixtures and maintenance intravenous fluids.

Also see Case Studies 5-2, 7-1, 8-1, and 8-2 for a discussion of patients receiving TPN who experienced fluid and electrolyte problems.

Summary of Key Points

- Total parenteral nutrition (TPN) is reserved for use in patients who cannot tolerate oral or tube feedings. Nutrients that can be delivered by the intravenous route include carbohydrates, amino acids, fat emulsions, vitamins, and electrolytes.
- The low rate of blood flow in peripheral veins (less than 100 mL/min) limits the administration of nutrient formulations to those having an osmolality less than 900 mOsm/L. This factor, in turn, limits the amount of calories that can be administered by the peripheral route (largely because phlebitis is a frequent problem).
- A typical TPN solution may have an osmolality that exceeds 1800 mOsm/L. (Recall that the osmolality of body fluids is approximately 290 mOsm/L.) A central vein can tolerate a high-osmolality fluid because of its high rate of blood flow (more than 1000 mL/min).
- Refeeding syndrome can occur when aggressive TPN is given to a malnourished patient. The major electrolyte imbalances associated with this condition are hypophosphatemia, hypokalemia, and hypomagnesemia.
- TPN solutions should be administered via a volumetric pump. The solutions should be introduced gradually and flow rates increased incrementally until the desired rate is achieved. If the flow rate falls behind, it should be adjusted to the prescribed rate; no attempt should be made to "catch up" by exceeding the prescribed flow rate.
- Close monitoring of serum electrolyte levels is indicated during the administration of TPN.
- Hyperglycemia is a potential complication of TPN infusions. Insulin therapy may be needed. Often, the insulin is administered via a separate IV line—a helpful maneuver when frequent adjustments of insulin doses must be made to keep the serum glucose level within the desired range.
- A TPN solution is usually discontinued gradually as the patient becomes able to tolerate enteral feedings. If TPN must be discontinued abruptly, it is usually reasonable to provide a 10% dextrose solution in a peripheral vein for an hour or two (using the same flow rate as the TPN that was discontinued).
- Because "3-in-1" TPN solutions may have a similar appearance to some tube feeding formulas, it is imperative to assure that a tube feeding formula is not inadvertently connected into a central venous line.
- When attempts are made to wean a patient from mechanical ventilation, the number of calories attributable to carbohydrates may be decreased to reduce the work of breathing; carbohydrate metabolism generates carbon dioxide (CO_2).

NOTES

1. Nightingale, J., & Woodward, J. M. (2006). Small Bowel and Nutrition Committee of the British Society of Gastroenterology: Guidelines for management of patients with a short bowel. *Gut*, 55(suppl iv), 1–12.

2. Merritt, R. (2005). *The A.S.P.E.N. nutrition support manual* (2nd ed.). Silver Spring, MD: American Society for Parenteral and Enteral Nutrition.

3. Mirtallo, J. M. (2007). Overview of parenteral nutrition. In: M. M. Gottschlich (Ed.), *The A.S.P.E.N. nutrition support core curriculum*. Silver Spring, MD: American Society for Parenteral and Enteral Nutrition, p. 267.

4. Freund, H. R, Rimon, B., Sullam, M. M., & Gimmon, Z. (1991). A decade of experience with home total parenteral nutrition. *Harefuah, 121(9)*, 294–297.

5. Alpers, D. H., Stenson, W. F., Taylor, B. E., & Mier, D. M. (2008). *Manual of nutritional therapeutics* (5th ed.). Philadelphia: Lippincott Williams & Wilkins, p. 398.

6. Kochevar, M., Guenter, P., Holcombe, B., Malone, A., Mirtallo, J., & ASPEN Board of Directors and Task Force on Parenteral Nutri-

tion Standardization. (2007). ASPEN statement on parenteral nutrition standardization. *Journal of Parenteral and Enteral Nutrition, 31*(5), 441–448.

7. Guenter, P., Hicks, R. W., Simmons, D., Crowley, J., Joseph, S., Croteau, R., et al. (2008). Enteral feeding misconnections: A consortium position statement. *The Joint Commission Journal on Quality and Patient Safety, 34*(5), 285–292.

8. Alpers et al., note 5, p. 391.

9. Alpers et al., note 5, p. 391.

10. Miller, S. J. (2009). Commercial premixed parenteral nutrition: Is it right for your institution? Nutrition in Clinical Practice, 24(4), 459–469.

11. Parrillo, J. E., & Dellinger, R. P. (2008). *Critical care: Principles of diagnosis and management in the adult* (3rd ed.). Philadelphia: Mosby Elsevier, p. 1712.

12. Alpers et al., note 5, p. 389.

13. Parrillo & Dellinger, note 11, p. 1712

14. Alpers et al., note 5, p. 389.

15. Covelli, H. D., Black, J. W., Olsen, M. S., & Beekman, J. F. (1981). Respiratory failure precipitated by high carbohydrate loads. *Annals of Internal Medicine, 95,* 579–581.

16. Parrillo & Dellinger, note 11, p. 1712.

17. Parrillo & Dellinger, note 11, p. 1722.

18. Alpers et al., note 5, p. 384.

19. Alpers et al., note 5, p. 389.

20. Alpers et al., note 5, p. 389.

21. Alpers et al., note 5, p. 382.

22. Alpers et al., note 5, p. 389.

23. Mirtallo, note 3, p. 268.

24. Clark, C. L, Sacks, G., Dickerson, R., Kudsk, K. A., & Brown, R. O. (1995). Treatment of hypophosphatemia in patients receiving specialized nutrient support using a graduated dosing scheme: Results from a prospective clinical trial. *Critical Care Medicine, 23,* 1504–1511.

25. Duerksen, D. R., & Papineau, N. (1998). Electrolyte abnormalities in patients with chronic renal failure receiving parenteral nutrition. *Journal of Parenteral and Enteral Nutrition, 22,* 102–104.

26. Janigan, D. T., Perey, B., Marrie, T. J., Chiasson, P. M., & Hirsch, D. (1997). Skin necrosis: An unusual complication of hyperphosphatemia during total parenteral nutrition therapy. *Journal of Parenteral and Enteral Nutrition, 21,* 50–52.

27. Sunyecz, L., & Mirtallo, J. M. (1993). Sodium imbalance in a patient receiving total parenteral nutrition. *Clinical Pharmacy, 12*(2), 138–149.

28. Marinella, M. A. (2009). Refeeding syndrome: An important aspect of supportive oncology. *Journal of Supportive Oncology, 7*(1), 11–16.

29. Miller, S. J. (2008). Death resulting from overzealous total parenteral nutrition: The refeeding syndrome revisited. *Nutrition in Clinical Practice, 23*(2), 166–171.

30. Marinella, note 28.

31. Fink, M. P., Abraham, E., Vincent, J. L., & Kochanek, P. M. (2005). *Textbook of critical care* (5th ed.). Philadelphia: Elsevier Saunders, p. 948.

32. Mizock, B. A. (2003). Blood glucose management during critical illness. *Reviews in Endocrine & Metabolic Disorders, 4*(2), 187–194.

33. Lin, L. Y., Lin, H. C., Lee, P. C., Ma, W. Y., & Lin, H. D. (2007). Hyperglycemia correlates with outcomes in patients receiving total parenteral nutrition. *American Journal of the Medical Sciences, 333*(5), 261–265.

34. Sheean, P. M., Freels, S. A., Helton, W. S., & Braunschweig, C. A. (2006). Adverse clinical consequences of hyperglycemia from total parenteral nutrition exposure during hematopoietic stem cell transplantation. *Biology of Blood & Marrow Transplantation, 12*(6), 656–664.

35. Alaedeen, D. I., Walsh, M. C., & Chwals, W. J. (2006). Total parenteral nutrition-associated hyperglycemia correlates with prolonged mechanical ventilation and hospital stay in septic infants. *Journal of Pediatric Surgery, 41*(1), 239–244.

36. Fink et al., note 31, p. 948.

37. Kaminski, M.V. (1979). A review of hyperosmolar hyperglycemic nonketotic dehydration: Etiology, pathophysiology and prevention during intravenous hyperalimentation. *Journal of Parenteral and Enteral Nutrition, 2,* 690–698.

38. Alpers et al., note 5, p. 394.

39. Nirula, R., Yamada, K., & Waxman, K. (2000). The effect of abrupt cessation of total parenteral nutrition on serum glucose: A randomized trial. *American Surgeon, 66*(9), 866–869.

40. Bendorf, K., Friesen, C. A, & Roberts, C. C. (1996). Glucose response to discontinuation of parenteral nutrition in patients less than 3 years of age. *Journal of Parenteral and Enteral Nutrition, 20,* 120–122.

41. Gottschlich, M. M. (2007). *The A.S.P.E.N. nutrition support core curriculum.* Silver Spring, MD: American Society for Parenteral and Enteral Nutrition, p. 325.

42. Sullivan, D. J, Marty, T. L., & Barton, R. G. (1995). A case of overfeeding complicating the management of adult respiratory distress syndrome. *Nutrition, 11,* 375–378.

43. Tresley, J., & Sheean, P. M. (2008). Refeeding syndrome: Recognition is the key to prevention and management. *Journal of the American Dietetic Association, 108*(12), 2105–2108.

44. Lin, K. K., Lee, J. J., & Chen, H. C. (2006). Severe refeeding hypophosphatemia in a CAPD patient: A case report. *Renal Failure, 28*(6), 515–517.

45. Sunyecz & Mirtallo, note 27.

Chapter 12

Fluid and Electrolyte Disturbances Associated with Tube Feedings

Clinicians generally agree with the philosophy that "When the gut works, use it." That is, if gastrointestinal function is present, enteral feedings should be favored over parenteral nutrition. Aside from being less expensive, enteral feedings are associated with better preservation of both immune function and intestinal function. Nevertheless, tube feedings are not without problems. Primarily, these problems arise because many tube-fed patients have preexisting fluid and electrolyte imbalances associated with their underlying illnesses. A multitude of enteral products are available; some are "disease specific" and others are "standard" (suitable for most patients). It is important to review some of the characteristics of enteral formulas to understand their potential impact on fluid and electrolyte balance.

FORMULA OSMOLALITY

Osmolality is an important characteristic of an enteral formula; it is primarily a function of the number and size of molecular and ionic particles in a given volume. **Table 12-1** shows the wide variance in osmolalities of some commercially available tube feeding formulas. Whereas some formulas approximate the osmolality of plasma (300 mOsm/kg) and, therefore, are deemed isotonic, others have considerably higher osmolalities and are referred to as "hypertonic." Isotonic formulas are generally well tolerated; in contrast, hypertonic formulas can slow gastric emptying and cause nausea, vomiting, and distention. When hypertonic formulas are administered in the small bowel,

Table 12-1 Characteristics of Selected Enteral Formulas

Formula	Cal/mL	Osmolality	Content (mg) per 8 Ounces of Formula				
			Na	K	Ca	P	Mg
Glucerna 1.0	1.0	355	220	370	170	170	67
Glucerna 1.5	1.5	875	330	600	240	240	95
Jevity 1.0	1.0	300	220	375	215	180	72
Osmolite 1.0	1.0	300	220	370	180	180	72
Osmolite 1.5	1.5	525	330	425	240	240	95
Pulmocare	1.5	475	310	465	250	250	100
Two-Cal HN	2.0	725	345	580	250	250	100
Vital HN	2.0	500	170	420	200	200	80

Notes: All of the formulas are made by Abbott Laboratories, Abbott Park, Illinois. Formulations may have changed since this table was prepared; refer to the manufacturer's literature.

they create an osmotic gradient that pulls water into the intestine. If the fluid is not adequately absorbed, cramping and diarrhea may result. For this reason, hypertonic formulas are introduced slowly until the body has time to adapt to them.

A formula's osmolality affects the renal solute load and thus the water requirements. Renal solute load can be defined as the sum of substances that must be excreted by the kidneys (such as urea, potassium, sodium, and chloride). A high renal solute load (created by nutrient use) requires a large water volume for excretion. If enough water is not provided, the patient will become dehydrated. Therefore, the renal solute load imposed by a formula should be considered in patients with impaired renal function and in those with increased losses of body fluids (such as from fever or diarrhea).

A number of liquid medications administered via feeding tubes are hyperosmolar and can cause osmotic diarrhea if given undiluted, especially into the small intestine. Among these products are acetaminophen, potassium chloride, and phosphosoda. For example, the osmolality of an acetaminophen solution can range between 3000 and 6000 mOsm/kg. The delivery of hyperosmolar preparations should be limited to the stomach; even then, the medications should be diluted before administration and water flushes given through the tube before and after delivery. This action not only dilutes the medication, but also enhances its absorption. Of course, it is important to keep any fluid restrictions in mind. At times, the parenteral route may be necessary for electrolyte supplements when they are not tolerated by the GI tract.

TYPES OF FORMULAS

Commercial sources supply standardized as well as specialized products targeted to patients with specific problems, such as renal, hepatic, and respiratory failure. Because numerous enteral formula products are available, it is important to read the literature supplied by manufacturers. Enteral formulas are classified as standard, elemental, or specialized, with multiple formulas available in each category.[1]

Standard Formulas

A standard formula contains intact protein and is similar to an average diet for healthy individuals; it can be administered to patients with normal digestion. These formulas are available with and without added fiber. Unless there is evidence to the contrary, a standard formula is the product of choice for the majority of tube-fed patients.[2]

Calorie-Dense Formulas

A calorie-dense formula usually contains 2.0 kilocalories per milliliter of fluid and is used in patients who require fluid restriction—for example, patients with congestive heart failure, syndrome of inappropriate antidiuretic hormone (SIADH), or renal failure. For instance, for a patient requiring 1800 kcal/day, the amount of water delivered in the formula could be reduced by 900 mL merely by converting from a 1.0 calorie per milliliter formula to a 2.0 calories per milliliter formula.[3]

Fiber-Containing Formulas

Fiber-containing formulas may be helpful in patients with diarrhea or constipation. The fiber added to the formula increases stool bulk and helps to regulate bowel transit time.[4] Recall that the colon is the final site of water and electrolyte absorption and ultimately determines fecal composition. In patients who can tolerate high-residue formulas, use of a high-fiber formula is thought to increase the sodium and water absorptive ability of the colon, thereby minimizing fecal fluid loss. For example, in a study of a group of 20 critically ill patients randomized to either a soluble fiber formula or a fiber-free formula, the number of liquid stools was significantly lower in the fiber group.[5] It has been recommended that this type of formula be considered in patients for whom tube feedings will be the sole source of nutrition for a long period of time, especially if intestinal disease is present.[6]

Elemental Formulas

An elemental formula contains hydrolyzed protein and simple sugars; further, it has a low fat content.[7] This type of formula is administered to patients with severe malabsorption, such as may be seen with intestinal atrophy or loss of absorptive surface associated with profound malnutrition, critical illness, and acquired immune deficiency syndrome (AIDS).

Research reports focusing on the efficacy of elemental diets provide mixed findings. For example, several studies have indicated that peptide-based formulas are helpful in avoiding diarrhea in hypoalbuminemic, critically ill patients.[8,9] In contrast, a larger prospective study did not demonstrate any advantage in a peptide-based formula over a standard, polymeric formula.[10] Further, a meta-analysis of 10 trials involving a total of 334 patients found no significant difference in the efficacy of elemental versus non-elemental formulas.[11] One group of investigators recommended that the use of elemental formulas be limited to specific conditions in which absorption has been definitely shown to be impaired.[12] Another group of investigators indicated that enteral feeding with elemental diets can lessen diarrhea in patients infected with human immunodeficiency virus (HIV).[13] Elemental formulas are more expensive than standard formulas and have an unpleasant taste and odor.

Specialized Formulas

Formulas for Renal Disease

Compared to standard enteral formulas, formulas designed specifically for renal patients are calorically dense, are lower in protein, and have lower concentrations of potassium, magnesium, and phosphorus. Such a formulation is used because patients with renal failure have difficulty excreting urea (the end product of protein metabolism), electrolytes (especially potassium, phosphorus, and magnesium), and fluid. Thus an enteral formula for a renal failure patient not receiving dialysis should be calorically dense and restricted in protein and minerals. The renal enteral formula contains a high percentage of essential amino acids (allowing for protein synthesis with minimal production of urea). Patients with renal failure who are being tube fed require frequent monitoring of electrolyte values and fluid status. Standard enteral formulas are usually acceptable for patients with mild renal impairment or those who are on dialysis.[14]

Formulas for Chronic Obstructive Pulmonary Disease

Compared to standard formulas, enteral formulas for patients with chronic obstructive pulmonary disease (COPD) are lower in carbohydrate and higher in fat—a formulation intended to lower carbon dioxide production and, therefore, improve pulmonary status. Recall that metabolism of carbohydrate yields more carbon dioxide than does metabolism of fat. Lessening the formation of carbon dioxide reduces the workload on the lungs, which are responsible for eliminating carbon dioxide.

It has been pointed out that the amount of carbon dioxide generated is more a function of the number of calories delivered than of the formula's fat-to-carbohydrate ratio.[15] For this reason, it is important to not overfeed pulmonary patients. Moreover, it is more difficult to wean a patient from a mechanical ventilator when excessive calories are delivered.

Formulas for Hepatic Disease

For patients with hepatic insufficiency who cannot tolerate the protein contained in standard enteral formulas, specialized products are available that are calorically dense and low in protein (to minimize ammonia production). Hepatic formulas contain increased amounts of branched chain amino acids and reduced amounts of aromatic amino acids.[16] Theoretically, hepatic enteral formulas should reduce the neurological symptoms that occur with hepatic encephalopathy.[17] These products are expensive, however, and their use is generally limited to patients with hepatic failure associated with encephalopathy.

Formulas for Diabetes

The carbohydrate content in standard enteral formulas may not be tolerated by patients with diabetes or stress-induced glucose intolerance. Thus use of a formula with complex carbohydrates (such as fructose) and fiber improves blood sugar control by delaying gastric emptying and reducing intestinal transit time.[18] Trends toward better glycemic control with the use of specialized diabetic formulas have been reported in several small studies.[19–21] However, it is unclear if the difference in glycemic control between specialized diabetic formulas and standard formulas is clinically significant. Given the current emphasis on tight blood glucose control via insulin drips in critically ill patients, special diabetic formulas may be used less often.

FLUID AND ELECTROLYTE DISTURBANCES ASSOCIATED WITH TUBE FEEDINGS

Tube-fed patients tend to have the fluid and electrolyte disturbances associated with their underlying disease and treatment conditions. Theoretically, then, it should be possible to observe all types of electrolyte disturbances in tube-fed patients. In addition, factors related to the enteral formula itself can produce disturbances if these products are used incorrectly. A combination of electrolyte imbalances is associated with refeeding syndrome, a potentially deadly complication.

Refeeding Syndrome

Definition

Refeeding syndrome (RFS) comprises a constellation of metabolic derangements that can occur when either parenteral or enteral nutrients are administered to a patient who has been malnourished for a period ranging from days to weeks.[22] Although parenteral nutrition has received more attention as a precipitator of RFS, enteral feedings are not without risk. For example, the sudden deaths of four malnourished children within 6 to 9 days of starting high-caloric enteral feedings have been reported.[23]

The major electrolyte imbalances in RFS are hypophosphatemia, hypokalemia, and hypomagnesemia (discussed separately later in this chapter). These imbalances are associated with many of the symptoms of RFS (**Table 12-2**). Other problems associated with this syndrome include fluid and sodium retention, hyperglycemia, thiamine deficiency, and neurologic and hematolic complications, occurring within the first few days of feeding a starving patient.[24] While the pathophysiology of RFS is complex, it is primarily the result of an acute intracellular shift of electrolytes (phosphate, potassium, and magnesium), increased demand for phosphate during tissue anabolism, and formation of high-energy intracellular bonds.[25]

Potentially life-threatening complications of RFS include cardiac arrhythmias, heart failure, respiratory failure, and hematologic derangements. (See Case Study 11-3.) **Table 12-3** summarizes selected risk factors associated with this syndrome.

Major Electrolyte Problems

Hypophosphatemia. As indicated previously, refeeding causes phosphates to shift into the cells during tissue synthesis; when this happens, the plasma phosphate level may drop precipitously. Hypophosphatemia tends to occur less often in enterally fed patients than in those who receive total parenteral nutrition (TPN), because enteral nutrition solutions usually contain adequate phosphate for patients with normal phosphate stores. However, this imbalance remains a serious problem during aggressive enteral feeding of starving patients. Despite the phosphate content in enteral formulas, patients with protein-energy malnutrition can develop severe hypophosphatemia during enteral feedings; additive risk factors include chronic alcoholism and intestinal malabsorptive conditions.[26] For this reason, it is important to monitor serum phosphate levels daily for at least 1 week after commencement of feedings in malnourished patients.

Hypokalemia. Hypokalemia is a component of the refeeding syndrome. Adding to the problem are other causes of hypokalemia, including the use of potassium-losing diuretics and diarrhea. As shown in Table 12-1, the potassium content of tube feeding formulas varies. Hypokalemia can result if the potassium intake is chronically less than body requirements.

Hypomagnesemia. Hypomagnesemia is another component of RFS. As with the other primary cellular electrolytes (potassium and phosphorus), extracellular magnesium deficiency may result if inadequate amounts are present in the formula or added as supplements (either enterally or parenterally).

Sodium and Water Retention. For an unknown reason, the body retains fluid during RFS, causing the extracellular space to expand. This fluid retention increases cardiac workload, to the point that it may precipitate heart failure in patients with cardiovascular disease. The increased fluid retention, coupled with the adverse cardiac effects of hypophosphatemia, hypokalemia, and hypomagnesemia, places all patients with this syndrome at risk for adverse cardiac events.

Table 12-2 Selected Clinical Features of Refeeding Syndrome and Associated Imbalances

Clinical Feature	Probable Associated Imbalances
Paresthesias and muscle weakness	Hypokalemia, hypophosphatemia
Cardiac dysrhythmias	Hypokalemia, hypomagnesemia
Decreased cardiac muscle strength	Hypophosphatemia
Respiratory failure	Hypophosphatemia, hypokalemia
Congestive heart failure	Hypophosphatemia, salt and water retention
Rhabdomyolysis, muscle pain	Hypophosphatemia
Dysfunction of erythrocytes, leukocytes, and platelets	Hypophosphatemia
Slowed gastrointestinal motility	Hypokalemia

Table 12-3 Selected Risk Factors for Refeeding Syndrome

Patient Characteristics
- Poor food intake for a period of more than 10 days
- Weight less than 70% of ideal body weight

Disease Conditions
- Anorexia nervosa
- Alcoholism
- Malignancy
- Intestinal malabsorption
- Recent major surgery

Thiamine Deficiency. Malnourished patients may also become deficient in thiamine (vitamin B_1), an important cofactor for carbohydrate metabolism. Wernicke's encephalopathy and lactic acidosis may develop if patients who are deficient in thiamine are refed carbohydrates without prior adequate thiamine replacement.

Clinical Signs

Clinical signs of RFS may be nonspecific and difficult to recognize (see Table 12-2). Most prominent are the symptoms of hypophosphatemia, the primary electrolyte problem in RFS patients. Other signs may reflect those associated with deficits of potassium and magnesium (also prominent in RFS). Rhabdomyolysis may result from severe hypophosphatemia and hypokalemia, resulting in muscle pain and weakness. Weakness of the diaphragm associated with hypophosphatemia in conjunction with RFS may make it difficult to wean these patients from mechanical ventilation.[27] Cardiomyopathy is another possible complication, as are seizures, a disturbed mental state, and renal tubular impairment. Hematological effects associated with severe hypophosphatemia include thrombocytopenia, abnormal clotting process, and impaired leukocyte function.[28] Sodium and water retention may become manifest as edema associated with the rapid administration of carbohydrate to a starving patient. The most feared sequela is the potential for cardiac and respiratory arrest associated with RFS.

Prevention

Failure to detect and treat RFS can result in serious and even fatal consequences. Thus early recognition and interventions to prevent the syndrome is critical to protect patients from harm:

1. Recognize "at-risk" patients, such as those with chronic cachexia due to prolonged starvation or any patient who has been chronically deprived of adequate nutrition (see Table 12-3). For example, a patient whose weight is less than 70% of ideal is at greater risk than is a patient whose weight is near normal.[29] It is important to be aware that malnutrition is a major problem in hospitalized patients.
2. Advocate the testing of plasma electrolytes before initiating nutritional support in at-risk patients, either orally, enterally, or intravenously. Advocate replacing electrolyte deficits *before* starting feedings.
3. Begin nutritional repletion *slowly* and keep increases in calories modest during the first week.
4. Advocate daily assessments of serum sodium, potassium, magnesium, and phosphorus levels until the patient is stable.

Other Electrolyte Imbalances

Hyponatremia

Hyponatremia is probably the most common imbalance seen in tube-fed patients. Contributing factors include water-retaining states (e.g., SIADH) and abnormal routes of sodium loss (primarily diarrhea or diuretic use). In the presence of excessive antidiuretic hormone (ADH) activity, large water supplements (by any route) can cause dilution of the serum sodium level, particularly when hypotonic or isotonic feedings are used. Although water boluses via the tube are usually charted, it is often difficult to determine the volume of flush solutions used to maintain tube patency and the volume of fluid in which medications are administered. The latter factor can be a significant source of fluid intake; thus the diluent fluid volume should be measured and recorded on the intake and output (I & O) record. Intravenous fluids also should be considered as a source of free water (such as in the use of D_5W as a diluent for intravenous medications).

Hypernatremia

Hypernatremia is less common today than it was in the past when high-protein, high-osmolality formulas (approximately 1000 mOsm/kg) were often used. Ingestion of large solute loads with too little water can result in dehydration (hypernatremia) and azotemia (uremia). Although formulas in use today typically have lower osmolalities, hypernatremia can still develop in patients who are given inadequate water supplements. Hypernatremia is most prevalent in patients who are unable to make their thirst known (such as those who are unconscious, very young, aphasic, elderly, or debilitated). Elderly patients are notably more prone to developing hypernatremia because of their decreased renal concentrating ability, which makes it difficult for them to conserve needed water. The very young may also have difficulty in concentrating urine because of immature renal function. With decreased ability to concentrate urine, patients need more fluid to eliminate body wastes. If this fluid is not provided through the feeding tube or the IV route, it is taken from internal fluid reserves.

Hyperkalemia

If potassium supplements are given in addition to the enteral formula, hyperkalemia could result, particularly in high-risk patients (such as those with renal failure). Even standard formulas may contain more potassium than some patients can tolerate.

Hyperphosphatemia

Although hypophosphatemia is far more common, hyperphosphatemia has also been observed in tube-fed patients who have renal disease. This incidence reflects the parallel between electrolyte abnormalities and underlying disease states in tube-fed patients.

Hypermagnesemia

Patients with renal failure are at risk for hypermagnesemia if the amount of magnesium contained in the formula exceeds the ability of the kidneys to excrete magnesium. Use of magnesium-containing medications adds to the risk.

Fluid Volume Overload

It is possible to cause fluid volume overload when attempting to provide sufficient calories to a patient with renal, cardiac, or hepatic disease. For such patients, a formula supplying 2 kcal/mL is often selected (as opposed to one supplying only 1 kcal/mL). In addition, special low-sodium formulas are available for such patients. As noted in Table 12-1, some formulas contain considerably more sodium than others.

Edema can also occur when a high-carbohydrate formula is fed to a previously fasting patient.[30] This is because refeeding with carbohydrate causes an abrupt decrease in urinary sodium excretion in patients who have fasted for as little as 3 days. Fluid retention is most pronounced during the first few days of refeeding. Contributing to edema in tube-fed patients may be the presence of hypoalbuminemia, which favors shifting of fluid from the vascular to the interstitial space.

Fluid Volume Deficit Associated with Hyperglycemia

Tube-fed patients are at risk for hyperglycemia because of the high carbohydrate content of some formulas and because of the relative insulin resistance commonly present in acute illness. Patients with mild to moderate hyperglycemia need extra fluid to replace increased urinary fluid losses until their disorder can be controlled by hypoglycemic agents. (When insulin is administered, it is important to remember its contributory effect on the shifting of potassium, phosphorus, and magnesium from the extracellular fluid into the cells.) Occasionally, tube feedings will cause severe hyperglycemia that may progress to a hyperosmolar reaction.

Zinc Deficiency

Although several trace element deficiencies may occur in patients receiving long-term enteral feedings as their only nutritional source, zinc deficiency has probably received the most attention. Zinc deficiency has been described in two patients who received tube feedings for 4 and 7 months, respectively.[31] Both patients developed skin rashes around the groin and under the breasts and axilla; after supplementation with zinc sulfate, these rashes disappeared and the patients' serum zinc levels returned to normal.

Monitoring Metabolic Status

Routine Laboratory and Clinical Monitoring

Although clinical assessment is important, electrolyte disturbances are usually detected by laboratory analysis. Recommendations vary regarding the frequency of metabolic monitoring in tube-fed patients; however, it seems reasonable to measure serum sodium, potassium, glucose, blood urea nitrogen (BUN), and creatinine daily for the first week and once a week thereafter, and serum phosphorus, magnesium, and calcium at least twice weekly during the first week and once a week subsequently. As evidence of stabilization is gathered, the testing frequency can be gradually decreased. In many situations, the severity of illness dictates how frequently laboratory values are obtained. For example, it may be necessary to check all electrolytes daily in critically ill patients.

Fluid I & O should be monitored and recorded every 8 hours (or hourly in acute situations, such as when the patient experiences a hyperosmolar reaction). Body weight should be measured and recorded daily. In acute care settings, capillary blood glucose should be checked regularly until the patient is stable. If exogenous insulin is administered, capillary blood glucose should be measured every 4 hours. If blood glucose levels are markedly elevated, urine acetone levels should also be tested.

Hydration Status

Because tube-fed patients may develop either fluid volume deficit or fluid volume excess, with or without sodium imbalances, it is necessary to monitor the hydration status closely (**Table 12-4**). A perplexing problem for the nurse is determining how much free water is needed for each tube-fed patient. The previous discussion identified several variables affecting this decision. Some key questions to consider include the following:

- Is there a need for fluid restriction due to SIADH or renal or cardiac disease?
- Is extra fluid required due to delivery of high-osmolality, high-protein feedings, or increased loss from other routes, such as diarrhea, fistula or wound drainage, hyperventilation, or fever?
- Is the patient receiving significant amounts of fluid through the IV route?
- How does the I & O record look?
- What is the serum sodium concentration?

All of these factors must be considered individually.

Table 12-4 Summary of Assessment of Hydration Status of Tube-Fed Patients

Assessment	Description
Fluid intake and output	Record volume and type of all fluids given by mouth, tube, and IV; include water used to flush tube to maintain patency and to administer medications.
	Record all fluid losses, including those from the following sources: • Urine • Liquid feces • Vomitus • Drainage from fistulas, wounds
	Consider fluid losses associated with fever, perspiration, hyperventilation, and dry environmental conditions.
Urine concentration	• In addition to volume of urine, record its color (ranging from dark amber to pale or colorless).
	• If necessary, measure urinary specific gravity with a urinometer or refractometer.
Body weight	• Measure body weight daily (using the same scales and the same clothing).
	• A slight increase in weight is anticipated in the anabolic patient; for example, a weight gain of 1 to 1.5 lb per week may be the result of increased nutrients.
	• Daily increases in weight may indicate fluid gain.
Edema	• Look for dependent edema in the feet and ankles of ambulatory patients and in the backs of bedfast patients.
	• Assess breath sounds for pulmonary edema.
Sensorium	• Assess for changes in sensorium (from baseline) after feedings are initiated. Sodium derangements (high or low) can affect responsiveness and level of consciousness.
Blood chemistries	• Examine serum sodium level: If high, it indicates a need for free water; if low, it indicates a need for water restriction.
	• Examine BUN/Cr ratio: If > 20:1, fluid volume deficit likely exists.
	• Look for elevated blood sugar level: If present, the patient is at increased risk for osmotic diuresis and fluid volume deficit.

Water Replacement Guidelines

Given these qualifiers, a rough guideline for the free water requirements of normal afebrile adults receiving tube feedings is 30 to 35 ml of water per kilogram of body weight per day. Another consideration in determining the amount of extra water to provide is the amount of water included in the formula itself. For example, most formulas that provide 1 calorie/mL contain 800 to 850 mL of water per liter of formula; more calorically dense formulas may contain only 600 mL per liter of formula. After determining how much water is provided by the enteral formula, it is necessary to calculate how much IV fluid is infused as well as how much water is given through the feeding tube with medications or as flushes to maintain tube patency. Subtracting what is given from what is needed provides the amount of extra water that should be provided.

Diarrhea

Diarrhea is a frequent complication in tube-fed patients.[32] Although in some cases the cause of diarrhea is unknown, it can often be traced back to the enteral delivery of medications, such as antibiotics, potassium and phosphate supplements, and sorbitol-based drugs. Intestinal infections (e.g., *Clostridium difficile*) are also frequent causes of diarrhea. For example, a recent study of 20 patients started on nasogastric tube feedings found that 10 patients (50%) developed diarrhea and that these individuals had significantly higher concentrations of clostridia.[33] Yet another cause of diarrhea is the rapid delivery of a formula with a high osmolality.

If not corrected, diarrhea may necessitate the cessation of enteral nutritional support.[34] One way to minimize diarrhea is to prevent microbial contamination of the enteral formula and the delivery system. For example, a study of a large cohort of tube-fed patients found that the rate of diarrhea was significantly lower in those individuals for whom strict adherence to delivery-set washing-and-changing procedures was observed.[35] If diarrhea is due to enteral-delivered medications, it may be necessary to change the medications to the intravenous forms. Also, it may be necessary to select a different enteral formula, such as one without osmotically active, poorly absorbed short-chain carbohydrates.[36] Switching from a hyperosmolar formula to an isotonic formula may be sufficient to reduce diarrhea. Use of a fiber-containing formula is sometimes recommended to minimize diarrhea.[37]

CASE STUDIES

Case Study 12-1

The condition of a 75-year-old woman admitted to the ICU with shortness of breath progressively worsened over a period of 1 week.[38] The patient's medical history included hypertension, interstitial lung disease, and alcohol abuse. She showed no clinical evidence of liver disease or of drinking in the week preceding her admission to the ICU. On physical examination, the patient was alert and fully oriented, but moderately malnourished. A chest x-ray showed pulmonary congestion. Rales were present. A diagnosis of congestive heart failure was made. The patient responded to diuretics, and serum electrolytes were found to be within normal range. After she was stabilized, enteral feedings were started and progressively advanced to 42 kcal/kg/day. On the third day of feedings, the patient's serum phosphorus level began to drop and she became drowsy. On the fourth day of feeding, she developed coma and respiratory failure and required intubation and mechanical ventilation. Her serum phosphorus level on day 5 was 0.5 mg/dL (normal range is 2.5 to 4.5 mg/dL). Despite subsequent correction of the hypophosphatemia, the patient did not regain consciousness and died on the eleventh hospital day. It was surmised that hypophosphatemia initiated the chain of events that ultimately led to her death.

Commentary. Central to the pathophysiology of refeeding syndrome is a block in the synthesis of adenosine triphosphate and 2,3-diphosphoglycerate, which ultimately leads to neurological and muscular dysfunction. Metabolic encephalopathy associated with hypophosphatemia can cause lethargy and coma; further, respiratory failure can be a consequence of severe hypophosphatemia. Like most malnourished patients, this patient had a normal serum phosphorus concentration on admission, even though her total body phosphorus content was likely diminished by chronic malnutrition. This deficit was unmasked by the initiation of enteral feedings when her body was called on to metabolize the nutrients (especially carbohydrates).

Case Study 12-2

A 22-year-old woman with a history of anorexia nervosa was admitted to the hospital for enteral feedings because she had sustained a large weight loss over the previous few months.[39] She was easily tired on exertion and complained of generalized weakness. Her admission body weight was 59 lb and she was 5 ft 1 in. tall. Lying flat, her blood pressure was 90/50 mm Hg; it dropped to 70/50 mm Hg when she sat upright. Her pulse rate was 50 beats/min. Because her serum phosphorus level was low (0.47 mmol/L; approximately 1.46 mg/dL), the patient was given oral phosphate 500 mg, twice daily. Tube feedings were started and advanced over several days to full strength at a rate of 100 mL/hr. Although she felt stronger, the patient became tachycardic on the fourth day. At that time, her serum phosphorus concentration was 0.18 mmol/L (roughly equivalent to 0.6 mg/dL). To counteract this imbalance, she was started on potassium phosphate supplements intravenously. On the sixth day, her serum phosphorus level had dropped to 0.16 mmol/L (0.5 mg/dL) and she developed symptoms of heart failure. Oxygen was started and the patient was given furosemide IV; her tube feedings were discontinued. In addition, her phosphate supplement was increased orally and IV. By the seventh day, her electrocardiogram was essentially normal and she no longer required oxygen. As she improved, the patient was restarted on enteral feedings and continued on oral phosphate supplements only. No further complications were noted.

Commentary. The cardiac decompensation noted in this patient during refeeding was likely caused by hypophosphatemia, and then enhanced by the cardiac changes associated with severe malnutrition. Fortunately, the changes were reversible. The authors of this case study emphasize the need to monitor serum electrolyte levels closely in anorectic patients during refeeding, especially during the first week. Further, they indicate a need to start feedings gradually, implementing graded increases in the caloric content of the feeds.

Case Study 12-3

A case was recently reported in which an obese 60-year-old man with carcinoma of the esophagus and dysphagia was admitted to the hospital for placement of a jejunostomy feeding tube via a mini-laparotomy.[40] Upon admission, his serum electrolyte levels were within normal range, although he had undergone an unintentional weight loss of approximately 40 lb within months prior to his admission. Initially, a solution of 10% dextrose was administered at a rate of 10 mL/hr via the feeding tube. At this time, the patient's serum K level decreased to 3.0 mEq/L (normal range, 3.5 to 5.0 mEq/L); further, his serum Mg level decreased to 1.6 mg/dL (normal range in the reporting laboratory, 1.8–2.7 mg/dL).

These deficiencies were treated with supplemental potassium and magnesium. A polymeric tube feeding formula was then started at a rate of 10 mL/hr. Over a period of 48 hours, the rate of the enteral formula was increased to 65 mL/hr. At this point, the patient complained of severe dyspnea and abdominal pain. Laboratory results showed a K level of 2.7 mEq/L, a Mg level of 1.5 mg/dL, and a serum phosphate level of 0.7 mg/dL (normal range, 2.5–4.5 mg/dL); recall that a concentration less than 1.0 mg/dL can be life-threatening. The patient was transferred to an ICU where he could be intubated and mechanically ventilated. Intravenous replacement of phosphorus and other electrolytes successfully normalized his serum electrolyte levels over the following 4 days. Jejunostomy feedings were started slowly again after 36 hours in the ICU and gradually advanced to a rate of 50 mL/hr. The patient was gradually weaned from the ventilator but later required a tracheostomy. He was transferred out of the ICU after 35 days; at that time, he was free of ventilatory support and was tolerating jejunostomy feedings.

Commentary. While refeeding syndrome is usually thought to occur in starving patients with a low body weight, this case demonstrates that it can occur even in obese patients who have lost a large percentage of their body weight over a short period of time. As noted in the case description, this patient had sustained a significant recent weight loss.

Case Study 12-4

A case was reported in which a 70-year-old woman was admitted to the hospital with shortness of breath and difficulty swallowing.[41] Although she had lost weight recently, she did not know how much. The patient was tachycardic (pulse rate, 120/min) and had a respiratory rate of 26 breaths/min. On room air, her O_2 saturation was 75%. She complained of dry eyes and mouth. All of her blood work was normal except for a white blood cell count of 13,500. This patient was diagnosed with connective tissue disease leading to myositis and dysphagia.

Upon transfer to an intensive care unit, the patient was mechanically ventilated because of worsening respirations. A nasogastric tube was inserted and feedings were started, using a high-energy enteral formula. Twelve hours after the start of feedings, the patient suffered a cardiac arrest from which she was successfully resuscitated. In the following days, she remained drowsy and had severe muscle weakness; attempts to wean her from mechanical ventilation failed.

Upon consultation with a clinical nutrition team, the patient was diagnosed as having severe malnutrition complicated by refeeding syndrome. On day 1 of the ICU admission, the patient's serum phosphate level was below normal (1.3 mg/dL; normal range, 2.4–4.5mg/dL). Also, her serum magnesium, potassium, and calcium levels were slightly below normal. Following 3 days of repletion of these electrolytes, along with a change to an enteral formula with a reduced carbohydrate content, she was able to be weaned from ventilator. She was later allowed to return home on a normal diet with oral nutritional supplements.

Commentary. This patient fits the picture of a patient at increased risk for refeeding syndrome; that is, she had suffered a recent significant weight loss and was unable to eat due to dysphagia. Upon initiation of a high-energy formula, her serum phosphate, potassium, and magnesium levels dropped below normal. The respiratory weakness that prevented weaning from the ventilator did not subside until these imbalances were corrected and the enteral formula was changed to a low-carbohydrate formula. Recall that a high carbohydrate intake contributes to intracellular shifting of phosphate, potassium, and magnesium from the bloodstream.

Summary of Key Points

- Enteral feedings are commonly used to nourish patients in acute and chronic care facilities.

- A wide variety of formulas are available; their contents are listed on their labels.

- Many formulas provide 1 kcal/mL, while others provide 2 kcal/mL. The latter options are useful in patients who need fluid restriction.

- Hyponatremia is the most common electrolyte imbalance in tube-fed patients, especially those with high antidiuretic (ADH) levels. Contributing factors include excessive water administration during tube flushes and mixing with medications given via the tube.

- Hypophosphatemia, hypokalemia, and hypomagnesemia are imbalances associated with refeeding syndrome. This syndrome is a potential problem when malnourished patients receive aggressive enteral feedings.

- Feedings should be initiated slowly and advanced according to tolerance in malnourished patients to prevent refeeding syndrome.

- Plasma electrolytes should be closely monitored, especially when tube feedings are first initiated.

- Careful monitoring of intake and output is necessary to detect fluid volume imbalances associated with tube feedings.

- Frequent weighing of patients will help healthcare providers detect developing fluid volume imbalances.

- Hyperglycemia is possible with tube feedings, especially in patients with insulin resistance. Therefore, glucose monitoring is indicated during the early phase of feeding in acutely ill patients.

- Hyperosmolar medications should be diluted prior to administration via a feeding tube. The probability of diarrhea is decreased when the medication is administered into the stomach instead of the small bowel.

NOTES

1. Malone, A. M. (2005, June). Enteral formula selection: A review of selected product categories. *Nutrition Issues in Gastroenterology, Series #28. Practical Gastroenterology*, p. 44.

2. Malone, note 1.

3. Malone, note 1.

4. Alpers, D. H., Stenson, W. F., Taylor, B. E., & Bier, D. M. (2008). *Manual of nutritional therapeutics* (5th ed.). Philadelphia: Lippincott Williams & Wilkins, p. 341.

5. Rushdi, T. A., Pichard, C., & Khater, Y. H. (2004). Control of diarrhea by fiber-enriched diet in ICU patients on enteral nutrition: A prospective randomized controlled trial. *Clinical Nutrition, 23*, 1344–1352.

6. Alpers et al., note 4, p. 342.

7. Alpers et al., note 4, p. 342.

8. Brinson, R. R., Curtis, W. D., & Singh, M. (1987). Diarrhea in the intensive care unit: The role of hypoalbuminemia and the response to a chemically defined diet. *Journal of the American College of Nutrition, 6*, 517–523.

9. Brinson, R. R, & Kolts, B. E. (1988). Diarrhea associated with severe hypoalbuminemia: A comparison of a peptide-based chemically defined diet and standard enteral alimentation. *Critical Care Medicine, 16*, 130–132.

10. Mowatt-Larssen, C. A, Brown, R. O., Wojtsiak S. L., & Kudsk, K. A. (1992). Comparison of tolerance and nutritional outcome between a peptide and a standard enteral formula in critically ill, hypoalbuminemic patients. *Journal of Parenteral and Enteral Nutrition, 16*, 20–24.

11. Zachos, M., Tondeur, M., & Griffiths, A. M. (2007). Enteral nutrition therapy for induction of remission in Crohn's disease: Update of *Cochrane Database Systematic Review* (3)CD000542. *Cochrane Database of Systematic Reviews, 1*, CD000542.

12. Dietscher, J. E., Foulks, C. J., & Smith, R. W. (1998). Nutritional response of patients in intensive care unit to an elemental formula vs a standard enteral formula. *Journal of the American Dietetic Association, 98*, 335–336.

13. Salomon, S. B., Jung, J., Voss, T., Suguitan, A., Rowe, W. B., & Madsen, D. C. (1998). An elemental diet containing medium-chain triglycerides and enzymatically hydrolyzed protein can improve gastrointestinal tolerance in people infection with HIV. *Journal of the American Dietetic Association, 98*, 460–462.

14. Alpers et al., note 4, p. 343.

15. Alpers et al., note 4, p. 342.

16. Malone, note 1.

17. Malone, note 1.

18. Alpers et al., note 4, p. 343.

19. Craig, L. D., Nicholson, S., Silverstone, F. A., & Kennedy, R. D. (1998). Use of a reduced-carbohydrate, modified-fat enteral formula for improving metabolic control and clinical outcomes in long-term care residents with type 2 diabetes: Results of a pilot trial. *Nutrition, 14,* 529–534.

20. Leon-Sanz, M., Garcia-Luna, P. P., Sanz-Paris, A., Gomez-Candela, C., Casimiro, C., Chamorro, J., et al. (2005). Glycemic and lipid control in hospitalized type 2 diabetic patients: Evaluation of 2 enteral nutrition formulas (low carbohydrate-high monounsaturated fat vs high carbohydrate). *Journal of Parenteral and Enteral Nutrition, 29,* 21–29.

21. McCargar, L. J., Innis, S. M., Bowron, E., Leichter, J., Dawson, K., Toth, E., et al. (1998). Effect of enteral nutritional products differing in carbohydrate and fat on indices of carbohydrate and lipid metabolism in patients with NIDDM. *Molecular and Cellular Biology, 188,* 81–89.

22. Marinella, M. A. (2009). Refeeding syndrome: An important aspect of supportive oncology. *Journal of Supportive Oncology, 7*(1), 11–16.

23. Patrick, J. (1977). Death during recovery from severe malnutrition and its possible relationship to sodium pump activity in the leukocyte. *British Medical Journal, 1,* 1051–1054.

24. Stanga, Z., Brunner, A., Leuenberger, M., Grimble, R. F., Shenkin, A., Allison, S. P., et al. (2008). Nutrition in clinical practice—the refeeding syndrome: Illustrative cases and guidelines for prevention and treatment. *European Journal of Clinical Nutrition, 62,* 687–694.

25. Marinella, note 22.

26. Maier-Dobersberger, T., & Lochs, H. (1994). Enteral supplementation of phosphate does not prevent hypophosphatemia during refeeding of cachectic patients. *Journal of Parenteral and Enteral Nutrition, 18,* 182–184.

27. Patel, U., & Sriram, K. (2009). Acute respiratory failure due to refeeding syndrome and hypophosphatemia induced by hypocaloric enteral nutrition. *Nutrition, 25*(3), 364–367.

28. Patel & Sriram, note 27.

29. Alpers et al., note 4, p. 114.

30. Havala, T., & Shronts, E. (1990). Managing the complications associated with refeeding. *Nutrition in Clinical Practice, 5,* 23–29.

31. Jhangiani, S., Prince, L., Holmes, R., & Agardwal, N. (1986). Clinical zinc deficiency during long-term total enteral nutrition. *Journal of the American Geriatric Society, 34,* 385–388.

32. Thorson, M. A., Bliss, D. Z., & Savik, K. (2008). Re-examination of risk factors for non-*Clostridium difficile*–associated diarrhoea in hospitalized patients. *Journal of Advanced Nursing, 62*(3), 354–364.

33. Whelan, K., Judd, P. A., Tuohy, K. M., Gibson, G. R., Preedy, V. R., & Taylor, M. A. (2009). Fecal microbiota in patients receiving enteral feeding are highly variable and may be altered in those who develop diarrhea. *American Journal of Clinical Nutrition, 89*(1), 240–247.

34. Trabal, J., Leyes, P., Hervas, S., Herrera, M., & de Tallo Forga, M. (2008). Factors associated with nosocomial diarrhea in patients with enteral tube feeding. *Nutricion Hospitalaria, 23*(5), 500–504.

35. Luft, V. C., Beghetto, M. G., de Mello, E. D., & Polanczyk, C. A. (2008). Role of enteral nutrition in the incidence of diarrhea among hospitalized adult patients. *Nutrition, 24*(6), 528–535.

36. Barrett, J. S., Shepherd, S. J., & Gibson, P. R. (2009). Strategies to manage gastrointestinal symptoms complicating enteral feeding. *Journal of Parenteral and Enteral Nutrition, 33*(1), 21–26.

37. Alpers et al., note 4, p. 360.

38. Vaszar L. T., Culpepper-Morgan, J. A., & Winter, S. M. (1998). Refeeding syndrome induced by cautious enteral alimentation of a moderately malnourished patient. Gastroenterologist. 6, 79–81

39. Vaszar et al., note 38.

40. Patel & Sriram, note 27.

41. Gariballa, S. (2008). Refeeding syndrome: A potentially fatal condition but remains underdiagnosed and undertreated. *Nutrition, 24*(6), 604–606.

UNIT IV

Clinical Situations Associated with Fluid and Electrolyte Problems

Chapter 13

Gastrointestinal Problems

Gastrointestinal (GI) fluid loss is a common cause of fluid and electrolyte disturbances. This is because of the large volume of fluid within the GI tract and the many ways in which it can be lost, such as vomiting, diarrhea, suction drainage, fistulas, and third-spacing into an obstructed bowel. Along with the possibility of fluid volume deficit (FVD), there is the potential for various electrolytes and acid–base imbalances.

CHARACTER OF GASTROINTESTINAL FLUIDS

In healthy individuals, approximately 3 to 5 L of gastric, pancreatic, biliary, and intestinal secretions is secreted into the GI lumen each day. Counting normal fluid intake and endoge-nous GI secretions in adults, approximately about 9 L of fluid enters the upper intestinal tract each day. Most of these fluids are then reabsorbed in the ileum and proximal colon, resulting in daily loss of only 100 to 200 mL water in feces.

With the exception of saliva, the GI secretions are iso-tonic with the extracellular fluid (ECF). In addition, material entering the GI tract tends to become isotonic during the course of its absorption. Because many liters of ECF pass into the GI tract and back again as part of the normal digestive process, this movement is sometimes referred to as the "gastrointestinal circulation." The electrolyte content of GI secretions is summarized in **Table 13-1**. The usual pH of GI secretions is listed in **Table 13-2**.

Table 13-1 Volume and Composition of Gastrointestinal Secretions

Secretion	Volume (mL/24 hr)	Na+ (mEq/L)	K+ (mEq/L)	Cl− (mEq/L)	HCO3− (mEq/L)
Saliva	1500 (500–2000)	10 (2–10)	26 (20–30)	10 (8–18)	30
Gastric	1500 (100–4000)	60 (9–116)	10 (0–32)	130 (8–154)	0
Duodenal	(100–2000)	140	5	80	0
Ileal	3000 (100–9000)	140 (80–150)	5 (2–8)	104 (43–137)	30
Colonic		60	30	40	0
Pancreatic	Variable (100–800)	140 (113–185)	5 (3–7)	75 (54–95)	115
Bile	Variable (50–800)	145 (131–164)	5 (3–12)	100 (89–180)	35

Values in parentheses represent ranges.

Source: Reprinted with permission from Faber, M. D., Schmidt, R. J., Bear, R. A., et al. Management of fluid, electrolyte, and acid–base disorders in surgical patients. In: Narins, R. F. (Ed.), *Clinical disorders of fluid and electrolyte metabolism*. New York: McGraw-Hill,1994:1424.

Table 13-2 Gastrointestinal Secretions and Their Usual pH

Secretion	pH
Saliva	6.0–7.0
Gastric juice	1.0–3.5*
Pancreatic juice	8.0–8.3
Bile	7.8
Small intestine	7.5–8.0
Large intestine	7.5–8.0

*Gastric pH will probably be higher than 3.5 in patients receiving gastric acid-inhibiting agents.

VOMITING AND GASTRIC SUCTION

Fluid and Electrolyte Disturbances

Major electrolytes in gastric juice are hydrogen (H^+), chloride (Cl^-), potassium (K^+), and sodium (Na^+). Gastric juice is the most acidic of the GI secretions, with a pH of 1.0 to 3.5 in the fasting state. The following imbalances are most often associated with the loss of gastric juice:

- Fluid volume deficit
- Metabolic alkalosis
- Hypokalemia

Others may include sodium imbalances and hypomagnesemia.

Fluid Volume Deficit

If vomiting or gastric suction is prolonged and fluid replacement therapy is inadequate, severe FVD may result. Among the clinical signs of this condition are decreased urinary output, postural hypotension, tachycardia, elevated hematocrit, and elevated blood urea nitrogen (BUN)/creatinine ratio.

Metabolic Alkalosis

Excessive loss of gastric juice by vomiting or suction causes metabolic alkalosis (base bicarbonate excess). This occurs because secretions from the stomach contain high concentrations of H^+ and Cl^- ions. With loss of Cl^-, there is a compensatory increase in bicarbonate ions.[1] (Each milliequivalent of hydrochloric acid lost from the stomach represents 1 mEq of bicarbonate added to the ECF.) Consequently, symptoms generally reflect decreased calcium ionization related to the alkaline plasma—recall that calcium ionization is decreased in alkalosis. Because it is the ionized fraction of calcium that controls neuromuscular excitability, symptoms of tetany can occur.

Hypokalemia

As noted in Table 13-1, gastric fluid contains approximately 10 mEq of potassium per liter. While the direct loss of potassium from vomiting or gastric suction is a contributor to hypokalemia, the major cause of this imbalance is metabolic alkalosis (described previously). As the kidneys strive to correct the metabolic alkalosis by retaining hydrogen ions, they excrete more potassium ions (an exchange of one cation for another).

Sodium Imbalances

Gastric fluid is usually isotonic or mildly hypotonic; therefore, the plasma sodium level will remain essentially normal unless other factors are present that alter it. For example, in the hospital setting, if excessive amounts of free water (such as 5% dextrose in water) are given, the plasma sodium concentration may drop below normal. This scenario is particularly likely to occur in the patient who is vomiting because nausea is a potent stimulus for the release of antidiuretic hormone (ADH), thus causing water retention. Hyponatremia is less likely to occur in the homebound patient because vomiting usually precludes oral fluid intake until the problem is resolved. Of course, in the presence of other factors that increase free water loss (e.g., fever and hyperventilation), the plasma sodium level could become elevated.

Hypomagnesemia

Prolonged vomiting or gastric suction can contribute to magnesium depletion—an imbalance that is less likely to occur than those mentioned previously because the magnesium concentration in gastric juice is relatively low (1–2 mEq/L). Nevertheless, this deficiency can be a problem if losses are prolonged (lasting several weeks) and no magnesium is supplied in the IV fluids. Unfortunately, most routine electrolyte replacement solutions do not contain magnesium (e.g., lactated Ringer's solution and isotonic saline have none).

Management of Vomiting

When vomiting is present, it may be helpful to instruct patients to drink small quantities of clear liquids frequently; among recommended liquids are clear soup broth, juice, and lemon-lime soda. It is important to avoid drinking large quantities of water in the scenario of persistent vomiting, because water can dilute plasma sodium and predispose the patient to other electrolyte problems. It is important to instruct patients to seek treatment when vomiting precludes oral fluid intake. At times, oral medications for nausea can be retained; if not, rectal suppositories may be helpful. If vomiting is not controlled by either method, intravenous fluid replacement may be necessary.

Treatment of gastric fluid loss requires replacement of fluid, sodium chloride, and potassium to correctFVD, hypochloremic metabolic alkalosis and hypokalemia. One author recommends replacing gastric fluid losses with 5% dextrose in 0.45% NaCl with 20 mEq KCl per liter, given milliliter for milliliter of gastric fluid lost in the previous 24 hours.[2] Isotonic saline (0.9% NaCl) may be used to replace gastric fluid loss, especially if the patient is hypotensive.

Irrigation of Gastric Suction Tubes

Sometimes when vomiting is severe, it may be necessary to temporarily rest the stomach and apply intermittent gastric suction. When hyponatremia is present, it may be helpful to irrigate gastric suction tubes with isotonic saline (0.9% sodium chloride) instead of water. Recall that it is difficult to remove all of the fluid instilled as an irrigating solution; thus at least some of this fluid may be absorbed by the stomach. Also, ice chips should be used sparingly because this water is also absorbed by the stomach and can worsen hyponatremia.

DIARRHEA

Fluid and Electrolyte Disturbances

Diarrhea is characterized by increased frequency of stools with excessive water content. It can have many causes, such as infectious agents (viral, bacterial, and parasitic), toxins, and certain drugs. Viral enteritis and bacterial infections with organisms such as *Escherichia coli, Shigella, Salmonella, Campylobacter,* and *Yersinia* are the most common causes of diarrhea.[3] Frequent causes of diarrhea in hospitalized patients are antibiotics and fecal impactions. Examples of medications associated with diarrhea include antimicrobial agents, antacids, and cardiac medications (such as digitalis and quinidine).[4]

Diarrhea is classified into several categories, including osmotic, secretory, structural, and primary motility disorders. Examples of causes of osmotic diarrhea are ingestion of poorly absorbable solutes (e.g., lactulose, sorbitol, man-nitol, magnesium sulfate, magnesium hydroxide, and sodium phosphate), generalized malabsorption or maldigestion, and certain infections. Secretory diarrhea is caused by abnormal secretion of water and electrolytes into the bowel lumen and may be the result of enterotoxigenic bacteria (e.g., *E. coli* and *Vibrio cholerae*) and partial or recently relieved intestinal obstruction.[5] Diarrhea secondary to structural changes occur in inflammatory bowel disease, collagen vascular disease, and sprue.

The following imbalances are likely to be associated with diarrhea:

- Fluid volume deficit
- Hypokalemia
- Hypomagnesemia
- Sodium imbalances

Fluid Volume Deficit

Volume depletion occurs secondary to sodium and water loss in the diarrheal fluid. Severe diarrhea can lead to a daily loss of 2 to 10 L of fluid, together with large quantities of electrolytes. Obviously, prolonged diarrhea poses a serious threat to water and electrolyte balance.

Metabolic Acidosis

Intestinal fluids have a high bicarbonate content; thus, diarrhea causes a loss of bicarbonate and a reciprocal elevation in serum chloride concentration (a form of metabolic acidosis referred to as hyperchloremic acidosis). Metabolic acidosis is by far the most common disorder associated with diarrhea and is especially likely to occur in pediatric patients and in individuals who experience secretory or infectious diarrhea.

Hypokalemia

Diarrhea, no matter what its cause, can be associated with excessive stool losses of potassium and result in hypokalemia. A clinically significant depletion of total body potassium is likely only when severe chronic diarrhea is present. Profound potassium depletion can occur in patients with colonic villous adenomas that secrete a profuse amount of potassium-rich, watery mucus.

Hypomagnesemia

Magnesium deficit can occur with prolonged diarrhea, particularly if magnesium is not adequately replaced. Most routine electrolyte solutions do not contain magnesium (e.g., lactated Ringer's solution and isotonic saline have none).

Sodium Imbalances

When the sodium content of the diarrheal fluid is similar to that of plasma, its loss causes an isotonic FVD (with no change in the plasma sodium level). This is often the case with diarrheal conditions classified as secretory diarrhea. In contrast, diarrhea caused by osmotic conditions tends to be associated with relatively greater losses of water than sodium, resulting in a tendency toward an elevated plasma sodium concentration. Hypernatremic dehydration due to watery diarrhea is most often seen in children younger than 2 years of age. In some types of diarrhea, sodium is lost in excess of water, causing a tendency toward hyponatremia. See Chapter 24 for a discussion of diarrhea in children. Of course, extraneous factors also affect the plasma sodium concentration; among these are the amount of water intake (oral or IV) and the presence of fever or hyperventilation (the latter occurs as a compensatory measure for metabolic acidosis).

Management of Diarrhea

Most acute diarrheal episodes of viral or bacterial origin are self-limited and do not require specific therapy. If diarrhea is due to accumulation of poorly absorbed solutes in the intestine (osmotic diarrhea), it usually subsides with fasting. In contrast, the diarrhea will usually persist despite fasting if it is a form of secretory diarrhea.

Oral rehydration with glucose and electrolytes in infantile diarrhea is described in Chapter 24. For adults with mild dehydration who are not vomiting, rehydration can usually be accomplished by the ingestion of juices and clear soups or a commercially available oral glucose-based rehydration solution.[6] The major purpose of the added glucose is to facilitate transport of electrolytes across the intestinal mucosa. If oral fluids are not tolerated, an intravenous solution (such as Lactated Ringer's) may be administered.[7] Attention must be paid to the serum potassium concentration to assure that adequate potassium is also provided.

IMBALANCES ASSOCIATED WITH LAXATIVES AND ENEMAS

Laxatives and enemas are frequently used to treat constipation and to cleanse the colon before diagnostic radiological studies and abdominal surgical procedures. Whenever possible, constipation should be treated by nonpharmacological means, such as increased dietary fiber and fluid intake. When these measures are not feasible or are ineffective, occasional use of laxatives or enemas may be indicated. In such scenarios, the fluid and electrolyte problems that may accompany their injudicious use must be considered. These fluid and electrolyte problems vary according to the nature of the laxative or enema solution used.

Laxatives

Magnesium-Containing Products

Among the most common magnesium-containing laxatives are milk of magnesia, magnesium citrate, and magnesium sulfate. In addition, magnesium is present in many over-the-counter antacids commonly used to self-manage indigestion. Taking in too much magnesium can cause a variety of toxic effects. Recall that magnesium is a natural calcium-channel blocker; thus its toxic effects are largely related to its antagonistic effect on calcium. The most pronounced of these toxic effects are those hindering neuromuscular, respiratory, and cardiac function.

Magnesium-containing agents are dangerous in patients with poor renal function because their kidneys are less able to excrete excess amounts of magnesium.[8] Hypermagnesemia may even occur in patients with *normal* renal function when large doses of magnesium sulfate are given. For example, a recent case was reported in which a 76-year-old woman with no preexisting renal dysfunction consumed a large quantity of magnesium citrate for treatment of constipation.[9] The next day she developed lethargy and hypotension, and her serum magnesium concentration was measured at 16.6 mg/dL (normal range, 1.6 to 2.5 mg/dL).

A study of elderly patients with congestive heart failure found that those with hypermagnesemia had a higher mortality rate than those without this condition; the authors concluded that caregivers should pay more attention to the abuse of magnesium-containing laxatives and antacids.[10]

Sodium Phosphate Liquid or Tablets

Because sodium phosphate is primarily administered for bowel cleansing prior to colonoscopy or other diagnostic procedures, it is discussed later in the chapter in the section titled "Bowel Preparation for Diagnostic Procedures or Surgery."

Enemas

Tap Water Enemas

While occasional tap water enemas may be well tolerated, repeated tap water enemas can result in excessive water absorption by the colon and, therefore, dilutional hyponatremia. Excessive water absorption from the colon has been observed in states of chronic constipation and megacolon. Especially at risk of this complication are young children. Also at increased risk are adults with congestive heart failure, acquired immune deficiency syndrome (AIDS), and malignancy.

A case of severe hyponatremia and irreversible brain damage associated with tap water enemas in a patient with spinal cord injury was reported.[11] Before receiving five tap water enemas of 1.5 to 3 L each over a 10-day period, the patient (a 65-year-old man with C6 quadriplegia) had mild symptomless hyponatremia and a baseline glomerular filtration rate (GFR) of 82 mL/min. During the fifth enema, the patient became confused and developed seizures. Despite treatment with hypertonic saline, the patient remained comatose. The authors of this case report emphasize that the colonic mucosa can absorb life-threatening amounts of water and cause hyponatremia in patients with ineffective renal water clearance ability.

Another situation was described in which a 42-year-old Chinese woman used a colonic irrigation with water as a form of an alternative medicine to promote health.[12] Afterward, she presented to the hospital with transient confusion and memory loss due to acute water intoxicational hyponatremia; as in the previous case, this report provides evidence that a substantial amount of water can be absorbed by the colon.

Sodium Phosphate Enemas

Sodium phosphate enemas are available in a variety of sizes (see Table 8-3). Because these enemas are composed of a hypertonic sodium phosphate solution, they cause an osmotic shift of fluid into the colon, thereby distending the colon and causing peristalsis to become more vigorous and produce defecation. Sodium phosphate enemas are widely used and most patients tolerate them without difficulty, provided they adhere to the manufacturer guidelines. However, severe toxicity may occur when the hypertonic sodium phosphate enema is retained in the colon and is absorbed. The probability of such adverse outcomes is greater in patients with a decreased glomerular filtration rate and in those who are very young or very old. For example, a recent systematic literature review found that most reports of side effects from sodium phosphate enemas involved patients younger than 18 years (66%) and older than 65 years (25%).[13] Further, the literature review found that the major risk factors for side effects from sodium phosphate enemas are gastrointestinal motility dis-

orders, renal failure, and cardiovascular conditions. Other risk factors include chronic inflammatory bowel disease (which may cause increased absorption of the enema solution), dehydration, colostomy, megacolon, and preexisting electrolyte imbalances.

Toxicity occurs when the sodium phosphate solution is absorbed by the colon (due to inability of the patient to expel the solution from the rectum), which results in a series of electrolyte problems (primarily hyperphosphatemia, hypernatremia, and hypocalcemia). The hyperphosphatemia and hypernatremia are caused by direct absorption of these electrolytes from the enema solution; hypocalcemia is a reciprocal response to hyperphosphatemia. There have been reports of hyperphosphatemia, hypernatremia, and hypocalcemia after the use of sodium phosphate enemas in patients with GI disorders that interfere with prompt elimination of the enema solution (such as megacolon or fecal impaction).[14, 15] Given this relationship, these enemas are not recommended for patients with conditions that would predispose them to retention of the enema solution (e.g., atonic colon, imperforate anus, or colostomy).

Risks in Children. Many published reports of adverse effects from sodium phosphate enemas involve small children. Reviewing some of these cases will help healthcare providers fully grasp the potential seriousness of the use of sodium phosphate enemas in young children. Some of the cases were reported several decades ago; others have been reported within the past few years. Often the case reports involve the use of adult-size sodium phosphate enemas in children, usually for the relief of constipation or for bowel cleansing before surgery or diagnostic procedures. Some examples are provided here:

- Hypocalcemia and severe hyperphosphatemia occurred in a 4-year-old boy who received adult-size sodium phosphate enemas for the treatment of constipation.[16] The child presented with a phosphate level of 17.5 mg/dL and a calcium level of 5.2 mg/dL. Due to tetany from hypocalcemia, the child's extremities were stiff and could not be actively or passively moved. After treatment with IV calcium gluconate and oral calcium supplements, in addition to hydration to promote diuresis, the child's condition improved.
- A similar case was described in which a previously healthy 5-month-old child suffered severe hyperphosphatemia, hypocalcemia, acidosis, and shock after

administration of an adult-size sodium phosphate enema for the treatment of constipation.[17]

- Four adult-size sodium phosphate enemas were administered to an 11-month-old boy admitted for surgical correction of an imperforate anus.[18] Two adult-size enemas were given in each barrel of a double-barreled colostomy that had been constructed shortly after the child's birth. Approximately 2.5 hours after the enemas were administered, cardiac arrest occurred. Despite extensive resuscitative efforts with IV calcium, phosphate-binding resins per ostomy, and peritoneal dialysis, the child died.

- A 28-month old child was admitted for an elective colostomy closure; he received five adult Fleet enemas as bowel preparation for the procedure.[19] Ninety minutes later, he became lethargic and developed tetany. Laboratory evaluation revealed an extremely high serum phosphate level (51.7 mg/dL) and an associated hypocalcemia. The child developed respiratory failure and required mechanical ventilation. With further treatment, the child eventually recovered fully.

Not all cases of serious electrolyte disturbances in children occurring after administration of sodium phosphate enemas involve the use of adult-size enemas. Some examples of cases in which pediatric-size enemas resulted in problems are highlighted here:

- A situation was reported in which two sodium phosphate *pediatric* enemas were administered to a 30-month-old girl in preparation for a radiographic procedure.[20] (The manufacturer guidelines recommend that no more than one-half of a pediatric enema be given to a child between the ages of 2 and 5 years.) The child developed coma, tetany, dehydration, hypotension, tachycardia, and hyperpyrexia. Laboratory results indicated that the child was suffering from severe hyperphosphatemia, hypocalcemia, hypernatremia, and acidosis. Apparently about one-third of the administered enema solution was absorbed systemically.

- Another case was reported in which a 13-year-old developmentally delayed boy with chronic constipation received four phosphate-containing pediatric enemas.[21] Within 24 hrs, he developed severe hyperphosphatemia, hypernatremia, and hypocalcemia. With early intervention and treatment, the child survived without sequelae. Children with developmental delays often display bowel dysfunction and chronic

constipation and, therefore, should be considered high-risk patients.

Although electrolyte disturbances associated with sodium phosphate enemas are more likely in high-risk patients (such as those with renal failure), they may occur in patients with no obvious underlying disease process. It is important to follow the manufacturer's guidelines when using hypertonic sodium phosphate enemas (see Table 8-3).[22]

Parent Education. Because sodium phosphate enemas can be purchased on an over-the-counter basis, parents should be made aware that both adult and pediatric sizes are available and that strict adherence to the product guidelines issued by the manufacturer is necessary to avoid serious problems. Nurses should take an active part in educating parents about the dangers of nonjudicious use of enemas. Parents should also be made aware that other treatments for constipation in their children are available.[23] For example, prune juice or other carbohydrate-containing juices may soften the stool. Also, merely increasing the dietary fiber intake may be helpful, as is assuring that the child has an adequate fluid intake. Mineral oil may be helpful in relieving a fecal impaction. Bulk-forming laxatives are available and cause an increase in stool water and bulk, thereby stimulating peristalsis. A mild irritant laxative, such as senna or bisacodyl, may be beneficial for short-term use; however, long-term use of these products should be avoided. Some authors recommend the use of polyethylene glycol 3350 to treat pediatric constipation and report it to be an effective and well-tolerated treatment (especially when used as an adjunct to education and behavioral training).[24]

Risks in the Elderly. The elderly are also at increased risk for electrolyte disturbances associated with sodium phosphate enemas, particularly if they have atonic colons or renal failure.[25] Several case reports involving adverse results in the elderly are summarized here:

- A case report of a 77-year-old woman who developed severe hyperphosphatemia and hypocalcemia after the administration of multiple sodium phosphate enemas to relieve fecal impaction indicates the potential problem in elderly patients.[26] The investigators cautioned against the over-aggressive use of sodium phosphate enemas in elderly patients with fecal impactions because of the potential for prolonged retention of the enema solution; they further recommended that isotonic enemas be used instead whenever possible.

- A more recent report described an elderly patient who died as a result of severe hypocalcaemia and hyperphosphatemia after treatment with a sodium phosphate enema; the authors cautioned that physicians should be aware of the risk of such imbalances when using these enemas, even in normal doses.[27]
- An unusual case involved an 83-year-old man who received a sodium phosphate enema that perforated through his colostomy; the patient subsequently died of fecal and chemical peritonitis.[28] However, there was also evidence that the sodium phosphate enema solution was absorbed from the peritoneal cavity. For example, laboratory analysis showed a low plasma calcium level [4.5 mg/dL], and a high sodium level [164 mEq/L]; the plasma phosphorus level was not measured.

In conclusion, it has been recommended that caregivers be aware of the risk of using sodium phosphate enemas in elderly patients, even when signs of renal failure are not present.[29]

Epsom Salts Enema

Years ago, Epsom salts (magnesium sulfate) enemas were advocated by some physicians. Although use of such enemas is considered an outdated method of treating constipation, a case was reported in 2005 in which a 7-year-old child was given an Epsom salts enema by his family for this purpose.[30] While the child initially felt better, he subsequently developed lethargy and was difficult to arouse. Despite intensive treatment (including intubation) in an emergency setting, the child did not recover. Near the time of his death, his serum magnesium level was found to be 41.2 mg/dL (normal range, 1.6 to 2.5 mg/dl). This case again demonstrates the ability of the colon to absorb substances administered via enema. Also, this case shows that folk remedies (such as the use of Epsom salts) persist in some populations.

BOWEL PREPARATION FOR DIAGNOSTIC PROCEDURES OR SURGERY

Bowel cleansing procedures for diagnostic tests and surgery vary from institution to institution, and sometimes even within institutions (according to individual physician preference). The best bowel preparation is one that does not disrupt fluid and electrolyte balance, adequately cleanses the colon, and encourages patient compliance. As indicated in the preceding discussion, the kinds of electrolyte imbalances likely to be associated with cathartics depend on the cathartic itself. There is no clear consensus as to which bowel cleansing method is "best"; however, most clinicians agree that individual patient characteristics should play a major role in the decision as to which bowel preparation procedure should be used.

Polyethylene Glycol Solution

One method commonly used to cleanse the colon prior to colonoscopy consists of the oral ingestion of either a 2-L or 4-L electrolyte polyethylene glycol (PEG) solution. Approximately 1.5 L of a PEG lavage solution is ingested per hour in adults until the rectal effluent is clear or up to 4 L is consumed. Large volumes may be administered without significant changes in fluid and electrolyte balance because the osmotic activity of the PEG lavage results in virtually no net absorption or excretion of ions or water. Although these solutions are advantageous in terms of electrolyte balance, patients often have difficulty consuming the required fluid volume in a relatively short period of time; thus adequate cleansing of the bowel may not occur. Although PEG solutions may be given to patients at risk for fluid and electrolyte problems, they should be avoided in patients with gastric retention, ileus, severe colitis, bowel perforation, or gastrointestinal obstruction.[31]

Aspiration of the fluid into the lung has been reported following the oral ingestion of a PEG solution. A case was also reported in which a PEG solution was introduced through a nasogastric tube inadvertently inserted into an 11-year-old child's respiratory tract, causing life-threatening respiratory failure.[32] Even when administered into the stomach via a nasogastric tube, aspiration can occur if the fluid administration rate exceeds the rate of gastric emptying.

For example, a case was reported in which an 86-year-old man had a nasogastric tube placed for the administration of four liters of a PEG solution; the patient complained of nausea after the administration of two liters of the solution over a 3-hour period.[33] Vomiting occurred and the flow of the PEG solution was stopped. Two hours later, the patient became dyspneic and was treated for aspiration. Another case was reported in which an 8-year-old girl had a nasogastric tube placed for the administration of a PEG solution.[34] Following infusion of the solution the patient vomited several times and subsequently experienced signs of aspiration. Similar cases have been reported by other authors.[35]

Some of the commercially available PEG solutions include GoLYTELY and NuLYTELY (Braintree Laboratories, Braintree, Massachusetts), and Colyte and NuLYTELY (sulfate free) (Schwartz Pharma, Milwaukee, Wisconsin).

Oral Sodium Phosphate

Sodium phosphate oral solution is sometimes prescribed as part of a bowel cleansing regimen in preparation for colonoscopy or bowel surgery. It acts by osmotically drawing fluid into the bowel to promote evacuation. Adverse effects of too large a dose of sodium phosphate solution include serious electrolyte disturbances (e.g., hyperphosphatemia, hypocalcemia, hypernatremia, metabolic acidosis) that may lead to renal failure and even death. The potential for acute phosphate nephropathy associated with acute renal failure exists with the administration of sodium phosphate tablets as well as with the liquid product. For example, Mackey et al recently reported 10 cases of acute phosphate nephropathy following the administration of sodium phosphate tablets for bowel preparation before colonoscopy.[36] Risk for acute phosphate nephropathy following the use of oral sodium phosphate include older age, hypertension, chronic kidney disease, female gender, and treatment with diuretics and angiotensin converting enzyme inhibitors.[37] Prevention of acute phosphate nephropathy includes avoiding oral sodium phosphate bowel purgatives in high risk patients, and aggressive hydration before, during and after the administration of oral sodium phosphate preparations.[38]

At present, although there are recognized risks associated with sodium phosphate, it remains an option for bowel preparation procedures; however, healthcare providers should recognize that patient selection and appropriate administration of this substance are key to ensuring patients' safety.[39]

LOSS OF FLUID THROUGH FISTULAS

A gastrointestinal fistula is defined as a tract between two epithelialized surfaces, such as the bowel or stomach and the skin. Fistulas may be classified as spontaneous or postoperative. They usually reflect the existence of either diseased bowel extending to surrounding structures or an anastomotic breakdown.[40]

Spontaneous fistulas are likely to occur in patients with cancer or those receiving radiation, or in persons with diverticular disease or perforated ulcer disease.[41] Approximately three-fourths of all enterocutaneous fistulas occur postoperatively, such as following procedures performed for malignancy, inflammatory bowel disease, or adhesions.[42] The major complications associated with small bowel fistulas include fluid and electrolyte disturbances, sepsis, and malnutrition.

Loss of fluids from fistulas can produce serious fluid and electrolyte disturbances. In general, the more proximal the fistula, the greater the fluid loss. For example, a fistula from the proximal small bowel (duodenum or jejunum) may be responsible for as much as 3 L of drainage per day.[43] Any fistula that drains 500 mL or more in 24 hours is considered to be a high-output fistula.[44] Failure to adequately replace large fistulous losses can lead to FVD, hypoperfusion, and eventually multi-organ failure. The electrolytes lost in fistulous drainage depend on the exact site of the fistula. An educated guess regarding imbalances likely to accompany a specific fluid's loss can be made by reviewing the usual electrolyte content of fluid in the region of the fistula (see Table 13-1). When doubt about the fistula's origin exists, sending a sample of the drainage fluid to the laboratory for analysis of pH and electrolyte composition can aid in determining the appropriate replacement therapy. Intestinal fluids, including pancreatic and biliary secretions, are relatively alkaline because of their high bicarbonate content. Thus loss of these fluids would likely lead to metabolic acidosis. In contrast, loss of chloride-rich gastric fluid predisposes patients to metabolic alkalosis.

Although fluid and electrolyte problems are possible with any fistula, they are most likely to be substantial in patients with pancreatic, duodenal stump, and gastro-jejunal anastomotic fistulas. Biliary and pancreatic fistulous drainage contains sizable amounts of sodium and bicarbonate; hence patients with such fistulas are vulnerable to fluid volume deficit and metabolic acidosis. Hyponatremia can easily occur if the fluid replacement therapy contains more free water than needed.

Drainage from external fistulas can often be collected with a well-fixed stoma appliance. The volume of drainage collected in this device should be measured and recorded on the intake and output record. If the drainage cannot be obtained and directly measured, an estimate should be made of the volume absorbed by dressings and bed linens. Of course, skin care is essential to guard against the effects of autodigestion by GI enzymes. Various skin barrier films and other preparations are available for this purpose.

Medical management of enterocutaneous fistulas initially focuses on correction of fluid and electrolyte imbalances, drainage of fluid collections, treatment of sepsis, and control of fistula output.[45] A crystalloid solution (such as isotonic saline or lactated Ringer's solution) may be used to replace the lost fluid volume. Electrolytes are replaced based on laboratory data and clinical signs. As stated previously, the type of electrolyte imbalance associated with a fistula depends on the origin of the fluid lost from the fistula. When replacing fluids, care must be taken to avoid overloading the circulatory system in patients at risk for pulmonary or cardiac dysfunction.[46] Antibiotics are administered when infections are present. A combination of parenteral and enteral nutrition may be needed to supply adequate calories until the GI tract becomes fully functional. (When enteral feedings are used, they are introduced below the level of the fistula to allow for absorption of the infused nutrients.) Unless the patient has an extremely high-output fistula, electrolytes can be replaced via the enteral and/or parenteral formula.[47]

Ideally, the fistula will close spontaneously following nutritional support; if not, surgical close is an alternative.[48]

IMBALANCES ASSOCIATED WITH ANOREXIA NERVOSA

Anorexia nervosa is a life-threatening disease with a higher incidence in teenagers than in other groups. According to the literature, approximately one-third of all deaths associated with this disease are due to cardiac complications.[49] Electrolyte imbalances, especially hypokalemia, play a major role in adverse cardiac outcomes in this group of patients. Before discussing the relationship between electrolytes and anorexia nervosa, it is helpful to review a few facts about the disease.

Anorexia nervosa can be subdivided into the "restricting" form, in which the patient loses weight by self-induced starvation and perhaps compulsive exercising, and the "bulimic" form, in which there is a combination of marked dietary restriction and episodes of binge eating, vomiting, and diuretic/laxative abuse. Serious, even life-threatening, fluid and electrolyte problems are understandably possible in patients with eating disorders. The prognosis for patients with severe bulimia nervosa is less favorable than that for patients with uncomplicated anorexia nervosa.

One study of 168 patients with bulimia or related eating disorders found nearly 50% had some sort of electrolyte abnormality.[50] The types of electrolyte abnormalities observed in anorectic patients depend on whether self-induced vomiting is the predominant behavior or whether laxative or diuretic abuse is dominant. A careful history is needed to determine which methods are used by the patient to lose weight. Among the more frequent fluid and electrolyte problems observed in patients with eating disorders are fluid volume deficit, hypokalemia, hypomagnesemia, hypophosphatemia, hyponatremia, hypocalcemia, and either metabolic alkalosis or metabolic acidosis.

Fluid Volume Deficit

Fluid volume deficit is most likely to occur in patients who take large doses of diuretics and laxatives. Clinically, hypotension (less than 90/60 mm Hg) and postural dizziness or syncope may be present. Also, the BUN is elevated out of proportion to the serum creatinine level. Skin turgor may appear normal despite FVD in adolescents or young adults, who characteristically have good skin elasticity.

Fluid volume deficit causes hemoconcentration and can mask anemia and hypoalbuminemia. For example, in a study of fluid balance in 14 young anorexic women, it was found that their hematocrit, hemoglobin, and plasma albumin were within normal range on admission to a treatment center.[51] Following intravenous fluid supplementation, however, their mean values of hemoglobin, hematocrit, and albumin decreased significantly. Upon discharge, although nutrition had improved the values, they did not reach the corresponding values observed on admission.

Hypokalemia

Hypokalemia is possible due to excessive losses from vomiting and laxative abuse, coupled with poor dietary intake. If the patient has access to potassium-losing diuretics, such as furosemide or hydrochlorothiazide, the likelihood of hypokalemia is even greater.

Hypokalemia is a particularly dangerous imbalance for patients with eating disorders because of the possibility of cardiac arrhythmias. While the QT interval is usually normal in anorexic patients, QT prolongation and ventricular arrhythmias may occur in those with severe hypokalemia, exposing them to the risk of a sudden cardiac event.[52] Very low serum potassium levels (such as less than 2.5 mEq/L) require hospitalization for monitoring and treatment. Fortunately, cardiac abnormalities may be reversible in adolescents with anorexia as they regain weight.[53]

Hypomagnesemia

Like hypokalemia, hypomagnesemia is possible because of excessive losses from vomiting and diuretic or laxative abuse, coupled with poor dietary intake. Hypomagnesemia is a common imbalance in patients with anorexia nervosa and is often associated with refractory hypokalemia and hypocalcemia that may not resolve unless the hypomagnesemia is corrected simultaneously.

Hypophosphatemia

Hypophosphatemia is an ominous sign in patients with eating disorders. The etiology of this imbalance is not clear, but it is most likely the result of inadequate oral intake and absorption of phosphorus. This deficiency is most problematic during aggressive refeeding, when rapid glucose-rich hyperalimentation causes extracellular phosphorus to shift into the cells, further lowering the serum phosphorus levels. This effect may result in myocardial dysfunction and neurological complications, such as convulsions. Thus plasma phosphorus levels should be monitored closely in any malnourished patient during refeeding and supplements administered as indicated.

Hypocalcemia

Hypocalcemia can result from poor dietary intake and diminished bone stores of calcium after prolonged malnutrition. Ionized levels of calcium are decreased in patients with metabolic alkalosis, a common imbalance in persons who engage in vomiting and potassium-losing diuretic abuse.

Hyponatremia

Hyponatremia may result from excessive sodium losses attributable to diuretic and laxative abuse, from self-induced vomiting, or from excessive water intake. Several cases have been reported in which patients affected by anorexia nervosa presented with seizures secondary to self-induced water intoxication. One of these was a 17-year-old girl who ingested an average water intake of 7 to 8 L/day.[54] Her history did not include abuse of laxatives or diuretics. On her admission to the hospital with a generalized tonic–clonic seizure, this patient's serum sodium level was 116 mEq/L.

Acid–Base Imbalances

In a study of 168 bulimic patients, metabolic alkalosis was the most frequent acid–base imbalance.[55] This condition is commonly associated with loss of gastric fluid from vomiting and with abuse of potassium-losing diuretics. Metabolic acidosis (due to the loss of alkaline intestinal fluid) may be the predominant acid–base disturbance if the patient is a heavy abuser of laxatives. Most commonly taken are stimulant-type laxatives that are available over the counter.

Summary

Patients with eating disorders must be observed closely for life-threatening electrolyte abnormalities. Cardiac action potential is affected by changes in extracellular potassium, calcium, and magnesium with electrocardiographic changes that vary from subtle to marked abnormalities.[56] As pointed out by Hofland and Dardia, bulimia is a psychiatric disorder, but morbidity and mortality can occur because of the physical problems associated with it.[57]

IMBALANCES ASSOCIATED WITH INTESTINAL OBSTRUCTION

Intestinal obstruction causes interference with the normal progression of intestinal contents and may be termed either complete or incomplete. A mechanical obstruction is defined as an actual physical barrier (e.g., adhesions, hernia, tumor, or diverticula) that blocks the normal passage of intestinal contents. A mechanical obstruction is termed *simple* when the vascular supply is not compromised; it is termed *strangulated* when the vascular supply is inhibited. A functional obstruction is sometimes referred to as *paralytic ileus,* or an *adynamic* or *neurogenic ileus.* As the name implies, this type of obstruction is caused by ineffective or nonpropulsive peristalsis. Although motor activity is slowed, it is not completely absent in such cases. Causes of paralytic ileus can include intra-abdominal conditions such as peritonitis, appendicitis, cholecystitis, and pancreatitis. Other causes involve trauma and systemic conditions such as hypokalemia, uremia, and septicemia.

Simple mechanical obstruction results in a striking accumulation of intestinal fluid and gas above the obstruction. Most of the gas is due to swallowed air, although some results from bacterial fermentation within the gut. Because of distention, large quantities of water and electrolytes are secreted into the bowel lumen, even in the absence of oral intake. Fluid also accumulates within the bowel wall. The edematous bowel wall is not able to absorb the large volume of intestinal secretions; therefore, distention becomes progressively greater, leading to isotonic contraction of the ECF compartment as fluid is sequestered in the bowel (third-space effect). During the course of an intestinal obstruction or ileus, several liters of extracellular fluid may become sequestered in the intestine.[58] Loss of fluid also occurs with vomiting (common in patients with bowel obstruction) and when nasogastric suctioning is necessary.

In adynamic ileus, decreased propulsive motility can affect the small intestine and the colon (separately or together). As in mechanical obstruction, gas accumulates in the involved intestine, producing marked distention. Fluid also accumulates in the intestine because of decreased absorption. Although third-space fluid loss may be significant, it is not likely to be as great as in mechanical obstruction.

Plasma concentrations of electrolytes are initially preserved in intestinal obstruction because the fluid lost is primarily isotonic; however, if the patient becomes thirsty and drinks only water, hyponatremia may develop. Contributing to hyponatremia is the endogenous release of water produced by oxidation. Sodium and other electrolytes (such as potassium and magnesium) are also lost by vomiting or as a result of GI suction after treatment is initiated. If the lost electrolytes are not replaced, deficits will eventually result.

The type of acid–base imbalance likely to be encountered is largely determined by the site of the obstruction. Metabolic alkalosis is common with pyloric or high small intestinal obstruction in which copious vomiting produces loss of acidic gastric juice. Sometimes in upper small intestinal obstruction, the patient will vomit roughly equal volumes of gastric and intestinal juice, thus preventing serious disturbances in pH levels. If the obstruction occurs in a distal segment of the small intestine, the patient may vomit larger quantities of alkaline fluids than of acid fluids. If the obstruction lies below the proximal colon, most of the GI fluids will be absorbed before reaching the point of obstruction, so acid–base balance may remain intact. In this situation, solid fecal matter accumulates until symptoms of discomfort develop. Respiratory acidosis can develop in patients with abdominal distention because respirations are compromised by upward pressure on the diaphragm, resulting in carbon dioxide retention. Impairment of renal function due to severe hypovolemia can lead to metabolic acidosis, as can starvation with subsequent ketoacidosis.

CASE STUDIES

Case Study 13-1

A 16-year-old high school student was brought to the emergency room after experiencing a seizure within a few minutes of complaints of dizziness and faintness. According to her parents, she had a history of restrictive dietary intake (interspersed with brief periods of binge eating), self-induced vomiting, and heavy abuse of laxatives. At the time of admission, her body weight was 79 lb (height, 63 in.). Lying flat, her blood pressure (BP) was 88/54 mm Hg and her pulse rate was 98/min; on standing, her BP dropped to 64/46 mm Hg and her pulse rate increased to 130/min. Abnormal laboratory results included hyponatremia (Na = 128 mEq/L), hypokalemia (K = 2.5 mEq/L), and mild metabolic alkalosis ("CO_2 content" = 29 mEq/L). The serum phosphorus level was 2.6 mg/dL (barely within normal limits). The serum Cr was 1.2 mg/dL and the BUN was 30 mg/dL. Fluid volume deficit was evident by a high BUN:Cr ratio (25:1). The patient was treated with intravenous 0.9% NaCl with added KCl. After stabilization, she was cautiously started on total parenteral nutrition (TPN). Several days after treatment was initiated, the patient experienced fluid retention (as evidenced by mild puffiness and bloating).

Commentary. This patient's seizure was probably caused by fluid volume deficit, which resulted in reduced cerebral perfusion, and hyponatremia, which predisposed her to a reduced seizure threshold because of mild brain swelling. Note that several typical indicators of fluid volume deficit were present in this patient—for example, postural hypotension, tachycardia, and a BUN elevated out of proportion to the serum creatinine level.

Isotonic saline was effective in expanding the patient's ECF volume, and also helped correct the lower than normal serum sodium and chloride levels. Both the FVD and hyponatremia were probably due to self-induced vomiting, laxative abuse, and poor dietary intake. The low serum potassium level (2.5 mEq/L) was quite serious and required admission to an intensive care unit for cardiac monitoring until corrected.

It is not uncommon for patients with anorexia nervosa who have chronic FVD to develop a compensatory increased production of aldosterone, which causes the kidneys to conserve sodium and water. This compensatory renal mechanism begins slowly but, once initiated, persists after fluid volume deficit is corrected, resulting in temporary fluid retention during purge-free periods. Patients with eating disorders usually find this phenomenon highly distressing and often renew their pattern of vomiting and laxative/diuretic abuse to relieve bloating.

Case Study 13-2

An 80-year-old woman was admitted to the hospital with a history of diarrhea (average of six watery stools per day) over a period of several weeks. The following abnormal laboratory results were found: hypokalemia (K = 3.0 mEq/L), and metabolic acidosis (manifested by an arterial pH of 7.25 and a low bicarbonate concentration, 12 mEq/L). An attempt by the lungs to compensate for the metabolic acidosis was evident in that the patient's $PaCO_2$ level was 28 mm Hg (normal range, 35–45 mm Hg). Her serum sodium concentration was in the lower range of normal (135 mEq/L). Recall that elderly individuals often have low normal sodium concentrations as a result of changes associated with normal aging (see Chapter 25).

Commentary. The metabolic acidosis in this patient was due to excessive bicarbonate loss in the diarrheal fluid. This condition is termed "normal anion gap" acidosis: Na − (HCO_3 + Cl) = 12 mEq/L (135 − [12 +111] = 12). As mentioned earlier, the $PaCO_2$ was appropriately reduced as a compensatory change.

Case Study 13-3

A 40-year-old woman was admitted with a 5-day history of nausea and episodic vomiting. She complained of feeling lightheaded on standing. Lying flat, her BP was 102/68 mm Hg and her pulse rate was 92/min; standing up, her BP fell 92/60 mm Hg and her pulse rate rose to 110/min. The following abnormal laboratory data were observed: hypokalemia (K = 2.9 mEq/L), hypochloremia (Cl = 85 mEq/L), metabolic alkalosis (pH = 7.53 and bicarbonate = 36 mEq/L), and a $PaCO_2$ of 47 mm Hg. The patient's serum sodium concentration was in the upper range of normal (143 mEq/L).

Commentary. This patient had fluid volume deficit, as evidenced by the postural changes in BP and pulse rate. Her metabolic alkalosis occurred secondary to the loss of chloride and hydrogen ions from vomiting. The $PaCO_2$ was elevated as a compensatory mechanism to help correct the pH imbalance. The low serum potassium was related to loss of potassium in vomitus and in the urine as well as to the presence of metabolic alkalosis. See Chapter 9 for a discussion of the relationship between pH and potassium balance.

Case Study 13-4

A 68-year-old woman with a prior history of jejunoileal bypass surgery was admitted to the emergency department with complaints of difficulty walking as well as numbness and tingling in all four extremities.[59] She had ingested 45 mL of Fleet's Phospho-Soda in preparation for a routine colonoscopy. Although she was scheduled to take an additional dose on the day of the procedure, her symptoms prevented her from doing so. On physical examination, the patient was found to have tetany in her toes and fingers and a positive Trousseau's sign (elicited in the right arm on inflation of a blood pressure cuff). Abnormal laboratory results included hypocalcemia (total calcium = 6.5 mg/dL; normal range, 8.4 to 10.2 mg/dL), hyperphosphatemia (phosphorus = 8.8 mg/dL; normal range, 2.5 to 4.5 mg/dL), and hypomagnesemia (magnesium = 1.1 mg/dL; normal range, 1.7 to 2.2 mg/dL). The serum albumin concentration (3.9 g/dL) was within the normal range (3.5 to 5.5 g/dL).

Following treatment over the next 24 hours, the patient's symptoms improved dramatically. A review of her medical history revealed that she had a similar episode almost a year earlier. In that situation, she also had ingested 45 mL of Fleet's Phospho-Soda in preparation for colonoscopy. She subsequently developed numbness in her arms and face and was evaluated in the emergency department and discharged with no diagnosis. Laboratory work at the time revealed low serum calcium (7.3 mg/dL), normal serum albumin, and high serum phosphorus (8.7 mg/dL). In retrospect, it was recognized that these abnormal values were related to the ingestion of the Fleet's Phospho-Soda.

Commentary. The ingestion of a high phosphorus load causes a reciprocal drop in the serum calcium level. The low serum calcium level in this case was accentuated by the patient's poor intestinal absorption of calcium due to her jejunoileal bypass. The chronic hypomagnesemia, secondary to malabsorption, may have also contributed to the development of hypocalcemia because magnesium deficiency can block parathyroid hormone secretion. In normal situations, when the serum calcium level drops below normal, secretion of parathyroid hormone is increased to cause release of calcium from the bone into the bloodstream. The fact that the patient had a normal serum albumin level means that the low total serum calcium level reflected a true hypocalcemia.

Case Study 13-5

An 88-year-old woman was admitted to the hospital after a sudden onset of acute confusion. Her husband reported that she had been her usual self before going to the bathroom to irrigate her colostomy.[60] Two hours later, she emerged talking "gibberish" and was unable to identify her family members. It was later learned that she had used 4 L of tap water (instead of the usual 1 L) to irrigate her colostomy because of difficulty with bowel elimination. On physical examination, her vital signs were essentially within their usual range; her body weight was 90 lb. A mental state examination confirmed her disorientation to time, place, and person and inappropriate noncontextual responses. Abnormal laboratory results included severe hyponatremia (Na = 118 mEq/L) and hypochloremia (Cl = 87 mEq/L). Her serum creatinine level (1.0 mg/dL) indicated adequate renal function. Her blood glucose concentration (94 mg/dL) was within normal range.

Commentary. This patient's acute confusional state occurred secondary to hyponatremia. After treatment with a hypertonic saline infusion, her sodium level improved; as it did so, she became more alert and responsive. Two days after her emergency admission, her mental status had returned to normal. This case report demonstrates that hyponatremia can result from over-enthusiastic lavage of a colostomy with water. Moreover, it illustrates that rapidly developing hyponatremia may present as an acute confusional state, especially in an elderly person who already has mild cerebral changes.

Case Study 13-6

A case was recently reported in which a young woman experienced nausea, vomiting, diarrhea, abdominal pain, distention, and a weight loss of 20 lb over the past month.[61] In preparation for a colonoscopy, the patient was given 90 mL of phosphosoda. Approximately 12 hours later, she developed Chvostek's sign, Trousseau's sign, numbness of the extremities, and circumoral paresthesia. A laboratory test showed a total serum calcium concentration of 6.4 mg (normal range in the reporting laboratory was 8.6 to 10.6 mg/dL) and a serum phosphorus level of 9.1 mg/dL (normal range, 2.6 to 4.5 mg/dL).

Commentary. Repeated doses of calcium gluconate were administered to this patient, and her clinical signs improved. The electrolyte levels normalized over the next two days following parenteral calcium gluconate supplementation. A diagnosis of celiac disease was made.

Case Study 13-7

A case was reported in which a 69-year-old woman was admitted to the hospital with lethargy and decreased mus-

cle strength.[62] At that time, her BUN was 40 mg/dL and her creatinine concentration was 1.7 mg/dL. An ECG showed a first-degree atrioventricular block and prolonged QRS and QT intervals. Quadriplegia developed over the next 12 hours, and the patient became comatose. A consulting neurologist diagnosed a brain stem infarct. Based on these findings, the family decided on a "do not resuscitate" approach. However, upon review of a routine laboratory screen ordered the day before, it was found that the patient's serum magnesium concentration was markedly elevated at 16.2 mg/dL (normal range for the reporting laboratory was 1.8 to 3.0 mg/dL). Upon treatment with vigorous intravenous fluids and furosemide, the magnesium level decreased to 7.4 mg/dL and the patient's clinical condition improved. The ECG results and renal function returned to normal, and she recovered without further sequelae. Upon regaining consciousness, the patient revealed that she had consumed two large bottles of magnesium-containing antacids daily to treat symptoms of indigestion and constipation.

Commentary. The hypermagnesemic symptoms in this patient included muscle weakness, hypoactive reflexes, drowsiness, and confusion—all of which may be easily mistaken for symptoms of an acute neurological event. Fortunately, the routine laboratory test included a magnesium level, allowing the physicians to diagnose the patient's real problem—unintentional overdose of magnesium.

Case Study 13-8

A case was reported in which a 69-year-old man was admitted to the hospital with nausea, vomiting, abdominal pain, hypoxia, areflexia, hypotension, and bradycardia.[63] He had a history of cardiac disease and chronic pulmonary obstructive disease. An x-ray showed air–fluid levels compatible with an ileus. Urine output and the estimated glomerular filtration rate were within normal limits. The patient was intubated and treated with intravenous fluids and inotropic medications. Prior to being taken to surgery for an exploratory laparotomy, an electrolyte panel was obtained and revealed a markedly elevated serum magnesium level (approximately 13.4 mg/dL). The patient's family reported that he had consumed a large quantity of a magnesium oxide–containing laxative for the past week. Further, he had frequently consumed an antacid that contained magnesium carbonate over the past year. The patient responded well to an infusion of isotonic saline, furosemide, and calcium gluconate. His paralytic ileus resolved within 12 hours and he was able to be extubated; the serum magnesium level normalized within a 2-day period.

Commentary. The authors of this case report emphasize the need for clinicians to consider hypermagnesemia in patients with lethargy, hyporeflexia, paralytic ileus, respiratory depression, hypotension, and bradycardia—even when renal function is normal, as it was with this patient.

Also see Case Studies 3-2, 6-6, 6-15, 7-3, 8-5, 11-2, 11-3, 12-2, and 12-4 for a discussion of other patients with gastrointestinal conditions associated with fluid and electrolyte problems.

Summary of Key Points

- Because as much as 9 L of fluid circulates through the GI tract each day in an adult, any abnormal route of loss—such as vomiting, diarrhea, or fistulas—can lead to serious fluid volume deficit.
- Major imbalances associated with gastric fluid loss include fluid volume deficit, metabolic alkalosis, and hypokalemia.
- Major imbalances associated with intestinal fluid loss include fluid volume deficit, metabolic acidosis, hypokalemia, and hypomagnesemia.
- Caregivers should be aware that electrolyte-containing laxatives and enemas may be associated with serious (and even life-threatening) effects. As such, they should be aware of safety rules regarding the use of these agents.
- Patients should be taught about the potential for serious electrolyte imbalances associated with use of over-the-counter laxatives, such as hypermagnesemia from magnesium-containing laxatives.
- Patients should be taught about the potential for serious electrolyte imbalances associated with enemas, especially those containing hypertonic sodium phosphate. They should be taught to follow safety guidelines for use of these agents.
- Patients with anorexia nervosa are at risk for serious (even life-threatening) electrolyte imbalances. A close watch for this condition is necessary because patients often will not disclose their problem to caregivers.

NOTES

1. Narins, R. (1994). *Clinical disorders of fluid and electrolyte metabolism* (5th ed.). New York: McGraw Hill, p. 947.
2. Pemberton, L., & Pemberton, D. (1994). *Treatment of water, electrolyte and acid–base disorders in the surgical patient.* New York: McGraw-Hill, p. 54.
3. Cooper, D. H., Krainik, A. J., Lubner, S. J., & Reno, H. E. (2007). *The Washington manual of medical therapeutics* (32nd ed.). Philadelphia: Lippincott Williams & Wilkins, p. 464.
4. Cooper et al., note 3, p. 464.
5. Narins, note 1, p. 1143.
6. McPhee, S. J., Papadakis, M. A., & Tierney, L. M. (2008). Current Medical Diagnosis & Treatment. New York: McGraw Hill Medical, p. 1118.
7. McPhee et al., note 6.
8. Schelling, J. R. (2000). Fatal hypermagnesemia. *Clinical Nephrology, 53*(1), 61–65.
9. Kontani, M., Hara, A., Ohta, S., & Iketa, T. (2005). Hypermagnesemia induced by massive cathartic ingestion in an elderly woman without pre-existing renal dysfunction. *Internal Medicine, 44,* 448–452.
10. Corbi, G., Acanfora, D., Iannuzzi, G. L., Longobardi, G., Cacciatore, F., Furgi, G., et al. (2008). Hypermagnesemia predicts mortality in elderly with congestive heart disease: Relationship with laxative and antacid use. *Rejuvenation Research, 11*(1), 129–138.
11. Chertow, G. M., & Brady, H .R. (1994). Hyponatremia from tap-water enema. *Lancet, 344*(8924), 748.
12. Norleta, S., Isham, C., & Khalid, B. (2004). Colonic irrigation-induced hyponatremia. *Malaysian Journal of Pathology, 26*(2), 117–118.
13. Mendoza, J., Legido, J. Rubio, S., & Giasbert, J. P. (2007). Systematic review: The adverse effects of sodium phosphate enema. *Alimentary Pharmacology & Therapeutics, 26,* 9–20.
14. Moseley, P., & Segar, W. (1968). Fluid and serum electrolyte disturbances as a complication of enemas in Hirchsprung's disease. *American Journal of Diseases of Children, 115,* 714.
15. Korzets, A., Dicker, D., Chaimoff, C, & Zevin, D. (1992). Life-threatening hyperphosphatemia and hypocalcemic tetany following the use of fleet enemas. *Journal of the American Geriatric Society, 40*(6), 210–221.
16. Edmondson, S., & Almquist, T. D. (1990). Iatrogenic hypocalcemic tetany. *Annals Emergency Medicine, 19,* 938–940.
17. Wason, S., Tiller, T., & Cunha, C. (1989). Severe hyperphosphatemia, hypocalcemia, acidosis, and shock in a 5-month old child following the administration of an adult: Fleet enema. *Annals of Emergency Medicine, 18,* 696–700.
18. Martin, R. R., Lisenhora, G. R., Braxton, M., & Barcia, P. J. (1987). Fatal poisoning from sodium phosphate enema: Case report and experimental study. *JAMA, 257*(16), 2190–2192.
19. Everman, D. B., Nitu, M. E., & Jacobs, B. R. (2003). Respiratory failure requiring extracorporeal membrane oxygenation after

sodium phosphate enema intoxication. *European Journal of Pediatrics, 162*(7–8), 517–519.

20. Sotos, J. F., Cutler, E. A., Finkel, M. A., & Doody, D. I. (1977). Hypocalcemic coma following two pediatric phosphate enemas. *Pediatrics, 60*, 305–307.

21. Biebl, A., Grillenberger, A., & Schmitt, K. (2009). Enema-induced severe hyperphosphatemia in children. *European Journal of Pediatrics, 168*(1), 111–112.

22. PDR Staff and Physicians. *Physician's desk reference* (64th ed.). (2010). Montvale, NJ: Thomson Reuters, p. 1143.

23. Bulloch, B., & Tenenbein, M. (2002). Constipation: Diagnosis and management in the pediatric emergency department. *Pediatric Emergency Care, 18*(4), 254–258.

24. Bell, E. A., & Wall, G. C. (2004). Pediatric constipation therapy using guidelines and polyethylene glycol 3350. *Annals of Pharmacotherapy, 38*(4), 686–693.

25. Grosskopf, I., Graff, E., Charach, G., Binyamin, G., Spinrad, S., & Blum, I. (1991). Hyperphosphatemia and hypocalcemia induced by hypertonic phosphate enema: An experimental study and review of the literature. *Human and Experimental Toxicology, 10*, 351–355.

26. Kosseifi, S., Nassour, D., Byrd, R.P., & Roy, T. M. (2008). Fatal iatrogenic hyperphosphatemia. *Journal of the Kentucky Medical Association, 106*(9), 431–434.

27. Farah, R. (2005). Fatal acute sodium phosphate enemas intoxication. *Acta Gastroenterologica Belgica, 68*(3), 392–393.

28. Viel, G., Cecchetto, G., Fabbri, L. D., Furlan, C., Ferrara, S. D., & Montisci, M. (2009). Forensic application of ESEM and XRF-EDS techniques to a fatal case of sodium phosphate enema intoxication. *International Journal of Legal Medicine. 123*(4), 345–350.

29. Grosskopf et al., note 25.

30. Tofil, N. M., Benner, K. W., & Winkler, M. K. (2005). Fatal hypermagnesemia caused by an Epsom salt enema: A case illustration. *Southern Medical Journal, 98*(2), 253–256.

31. Lichtenstein, G. (2009). Bowel preparations for colonoscopy: A review. *American Journal of Health-System Pharmacy, 66*, 27.

32. Narsinghani, U., Chadha, M., Farrar, H. C., & Anand, K. S. (2001). Life-threatening respiratory failure following accidental infusion of polyethylene glycol electrolyte solution into the lung. *Journal of Toxicology-Clinical Toxicology, 39*(1), 105–107.

33. De Graaf, P., Slagt, C., DeGraaf, J. L., & Loffeld, R. J. (2006). Fatal aspiration of polyethylene glycon solution. *Netherlands Journal of Medicine, 64*(6), 196–198.

34. Liangthanasarn, P., Nemet, D., Sufi, R., & Nussbaum, E. (2003). Case report: therapy for pulmonary aspiration of an ethylene glycol solution. *Journal of Pediatric Gastroenterology and Nutrition, 37*, 192–194.

35. Marschall, H. U., & Bartels, F. (1998). Life-threatening complications of nasogastric administration of polyethylene glycol–electrolyte solutions (Golytely) for bowel cleansing. *Gastrointestinal Endoscopy, 47*(5), 408–410.

36. Mackey, A. C., Green, L., St. Amand, K., & Avigan, M. (2009). Sodium phosphate tablets and acute phosphate nephropathy. *American Journal of Gastroenterology, 104*, 1903–1906.

37. Markowitz, G. S., & Perazella, M. A. (2009). Acute phosphate nephropathy. *Kidney International, 76*(10), 1027–1034.

38. Markowitz & Perazella, note 37.

39. Robertson, D. J. (2009). Risk vs. reward: Is it time to purge sodium phosphate from your prep portfolio? *American Journal of Gastroenterology, 104*, 1907–1908.

40. Evenson, A. R., & Fischer, J. E. (2006). Current management of enterocutaneous fistula. *Journal of Gastrointestinal Surgery, 10*, 455–464.

41. Evenson & Fischer, note 40.

42. Evenson & Fischer, note 40.

43. Klingensmith, M. E., Chen, L. I., Glasgow, S. C., Goers, T. A., & Melby, S. J. (2008). *The Washington Manual of Surgery* (5th ed.). Philadelphia: Lippincott Williams & Wilkins, p. 188.

44. Klingensmith et al., note 43.

45. Lloyd, D. A., Gabe, S. M., & Windsor, A. C. (2006). Nutrition and management of enterocutaneous fistula. *British Journal of Surgery, 93*(9), 1045–1055.

46. Evenson & Fischer, note 40.

47. Evenson & Fischer, note 40.

48. Lloyd et al., note 45.

49. Neumarker, K. J. (1997). Mortality and sudden death in anorexia nervosa. *International Journal of Eating Disorders, 21*, 205–212.

50. Mitchell, J. E., Pyle, R.L., Eclert, E. D., Hatsukami, D., & Lentz, R. (1983). Electrolyte and other physiological abnormalities in patients with bulimia. *Psychological Medicine, 13*, 273–278.

51. Caregaro, L., DiPascoli, L., Favaro, A., Nardi, M., & Santonastaso, P. (2005). Sodium depletion and hemoconcentration: Overlooked complications in patients with anorexia nervosa? *Nutrition, 21*, 438–445.

52. Facchini, M., Sala, L., Malfatto, G., Bragato, R., Redaelli, G., & Invitti, C. (2006). Low-K dependent QT prolongation and risk for ventricular arrhythmia in anorexia nervosa. *International Journal of Cardiology, 106*, 170–176.

53. Mont, L., Castro, J., Herreros, B., Pare, C., Azqueta, M., Magrina, J., et al. (2003). Reversibility of cardiac abnormalities in adolescents with anorexia nervosa after weight recovery. *Journal of the American Academy of Child and Adolescent Psychiatry, 42*(7), 808–812.

54. Cuesta, M. J., Juan, J. A, & Peralta, V. (1992). Secondary seizures from water intoxication in anorexia nervosa. *General Hospital Psychiatry, 14*, 212–213.

55. Mitchell et al., note 50.

56. Khan, M. U., Patel, A.G., Wilbur, S. L., & Khan, I. A. (2007). Electrocardiographic changes in combined electrolyte depletion. *International Journal of Cardiology, 116*(2), 276–278.

57. Hofland, S., & Dardia, P. (1992). Bulimia nervosa: Associated physical problems. *Journal of Psychosocial Nursing, 30*, 23.

58. Narins, note 1, p. 1147.

59. Ehrenpreis, E. D., Wieland, J. M., Cabral, J., Estevez, V, Zaitman, D., & Secrest, K. (1997). Symptomatic hypocalcemia, hypomagne-

colonoscopy preparation in a patient with a jejunoileal bypass. *Digestive Diseases and Sciences, 42,* 858–860.

60. Shiwach, R. (1996). Hyponatremia from colonic lavage presenting as an acute confusional state. *American Journal of Psychiatry, 153,* 10.

61. Oztas, E., Bektas, M., Kurt, M., Onal, I. K., & Ozden, A. (2009). Letter to editor: Oral Fleet Phospho-Soda laxative induced symptomatic hypocalcemia in an adult patient with celiac disease. *American Journal of Gastroenterology, 119.*

62. Fung, M. C., Weintraub, M., & Bowen, D. L. (1995). Hypermagnesemia: Elderly over-the-counter drug users at risk. *Archives of Family Medicine, 4,* 718.

63. Izdes, S., Kesimci, E., & Kanbak, O. (2008). Paralytic ileus as a complication of iatrogenic hypermagnesemia without renal dysfunction. *Anesthesia & Intensive Care, 36*(1), 124.

Chapter 14

Fluid Balance in the Surgical Patient

This chapter describes fluid and electrolyte imbalances that may be encountered in different phases of the perioperative period. Before surgery, potential perioperative problems should be identified by reviewing the patient's medical, surgical, and anesthesia history, and by examining laboratory results. This task is easier with hospitalized patients than with individuals who have "same-day" surgery in outpatient centers. Some ambulatory surgery centers require previsits for all patients (or at least those who will have general anesthesia); others rely on voluntary previsits. At times, the needed assessment is performed in the surgeon's office or clinic.

PREOPERATIVE PERIOD

Standard laboratory panels are often reviewed prior to surgery to identify specific problems that could affect the patient's outcome. (See Tables 2-3 and 2-4 for blood and urine tests useful in determining fluid and electrolyte status.) Any abnormalities should be called to the attention of the medical staff for early correction.

Fluid and Electrolyte Imbalances and Cancellation of Elective Surgeries

Because hypokalemia predisposes patients to cardiac arrhythmias, it is a frequent cause for cancellation of elective surgery (especially in patients with cardiac disease).[1] When hypokalemia is detected in a patient who is receiving potassium-losing diuretics, it is advisable to also screen the patient for hypomagnesemia, given that these two imbalances may occur together. Like hypokalemia, hypomagnesemia has arrhythmogenic capacity. In addition, it has the ability to worsen renal potassium wasting.[2] Correction of

potassium and magnesium deficiencies should be started only after adequate urine output has been established.

Avoiding Excessive "Nothing per Os" Time

Surgical patients are at risk for fluid volume deficit (FVD) for a number of reasons. For instance, fluid losses may have been incurred from the primary illness, and a prolonged period of "nothing per os" (NPO—"nothing by mouth") order may have been necessary for diagnostic tests (some of which may have required cathartics to empty the bowel or the use of contrast agents that produced osmotic diuresis). Also, a frequent contributor to fluid volume deficit is a prolonged NPO period in preparation for surgery.

A "nothing by mouth" status in the immediate preoperative period is necessary to reduce the risk of aspiration of gastric contents during surgery. In most surgical patients, an 8-hour restriction of oral fluids is sufficient. However, regardless of the scheduled surgical time, it is common practice to place all patients on NPO status at midnight. While this is acceptable for a patient scheduled for surgery at 8 AM, it is not reasonable for a patient scheduled for surgery much later in the day.

For patients who are not believed to be at high risk for aspiration of gastric contents, the physician may permit solid food up to 6 hours before surgery and may allow clear liquids up to 2 hours before surgery.[3, 4] Patients with conditions that may be associated with delayed gastric emptying (such as diabetes, ileus, or bowel obstruction) or those with esophageal reflux disease might require longer periods of oral fluid restriction.[5]

Before surgery, sufficient intravenous fluid must be given to stabilize the blood pressure and pulse and to increase hourly urine volume to an acceptable level (preferably 50

209

mL/hr in an adult). The rate of fluid administration varies considerably, depending on severity and type of fluid disturbances, presence of continuing losses, and cardiac status.

OPERATIVE PERIOD

Possible Need for Corticosteroid Replacement

In normal situations, the usual cortisol output is approximately 8–10 mg in 24 hours.[6] By comparison, the cortisol output may increase to 50 mg/day during a minor surgical procedure and up to 75–100 mg/day during a major abdominal or orthopedic procedure.[7] Cortisol output may be even greater (100–500 mg/day) during the stress of sepsis or shock.[8] Cortisol output during stress generally peaks in 6 hours and returns to baseline in 24 hours unless the stress continues.[9] After long-term treatment with glucocorticoids, the adrenal glands may undergo atrophy, causing them to be unable to make the expected adrenal cortical response to stress.[10] For this reason, part of the preoperative assessment includes determining if the patient has received long-term corticosteroid therapy (e.g., for rheumatoid arthritis, Crohn's disease, or asthma). If so, an evaluation is done to determine if additional steroids are required during the perioperative period. Some patients may get by with their usual daily corticosteroid dosage during the perioperative period, while others may require larger dosages. The latter individuals are likely to be those with primary disease of the hypothalamic–pituitary–adrenal axis.[11]

A suppressed response from atrophied adrenal glands may manifest as hypovolemia or circulatory shock.[12] Other symptoms may include nausea, vomiting, weakness, and fever. Hyponatremia may occur due to increased excretion of sodium by the kidney; also, hyperkalemia may occur due to renal potassium retention.[13]

Problems Associated with Poor Nutrition

The reasonably well-nourished and otherwise healthy individual undergoing an uncomplicated major surgical procedure has sufficient body fuel reserves to withstand the catabolic insult and partial starvation associated with such surgery for as long as 10 days.[14] In contrast, the nutritionally depleted patient undergoes surgery with a serious handicap, resulting in increased morbidity and mortality.[15] Atrophy of the mucous membrane linings of the respiratory and gastrointestinal (GI) tracts predisposes patients to infection, as does diminished ability to form antibodies. As a consequence, pneumonia, sepsis, and wound infections are more likely in severely malnourished patients. Hypoproteinemia follows prolonged negative nitrogen balance and increases susceptibility to shock. Diminished supplies of protein and vitamin C retard wound healing.

Those persons at greatest risk during surgery are moderately or severely malnourished patients. A moderately malnourished patient may be classified as having a 10% to 20% weight loss and a preoperative serum albumin in the range of 2.5 to 3.2 g/dL; a severely malnourished patient may be classified as having a more than 20% weight loss and a preoperative serum albumin less than 2.5 g/dL.[16] Other useful indicators of malnutrition are physical problems that interfere with eating, loss of appetite for more than 5 days, and being maintained for more than a week on "routine" intravenous fluids. Recall that one liter of intravenous fluid with 5% dextrose contains 170 calories, all from carbohydrates (electrolyte solutions without dextrose have essentially no calories). Unfortunately, a number of patients who must undergo surgery have nutritional problems. For example, one study found that 38% of patients undergoing abdominal operations for benign disease had protein-energy malnutrition.[17]

Because malnutrition greatly increases perioperative risk, the malnourished patient should be identified early so that appropriate interventions can be undertaken. Starting nutritional support early provides essential nutrients for maintenance of gut integrity, prevention of bacterial translocation, and preservation of organ function, wound healing, and immune function.[18] The parenteral route (in the form of total parenteral nutrition) or the enteral route (in the form of tube feeding) may be used for nutritional support; the choice is based on individual patient characteristics. When possible, the enteral route is preferred.

Blood Loss During Surgery

Albumin synthesis and erythropoiesis can compensate for minor blood losses. When a crystalloid (such as lactated Ringer's solution) is used to replace lost blood, it is customary to administer approximately 3 mL of crystalloid for each 1 mL of blood loss. If a colloid or blood is used, the replacement volume should equal the volume of blood lost.[19] Because of the hazards of infectious diseases and complications associated with blood transfusions, many surgical centers are now focused on the reduction of perioperative blood transfusions. Options include preoperative autologous donation of 1 to 3 units of packed red blood cells; these units are then reinfused as needed in the intraoperative and postoperative periods. A second option is auto-transfusion of shed blood during surgery and in the immediate postoperative period. Autotransfusion is used most commonly with cardiovascular, orthopedic, and vascular surgeries.

Third-Space Fluid Shifts During Surgery

In trauma and postoperative patients, large volumes of fluid may seep from the vascular space into a third-space (such as the surgical site or a generalized interstitial space due to decreased plasma oncotic pressure after albumin loss). These fluid shifts cannot be measured directly, so the amount of fluid needed for replacement may not be known with certainty. It has been estimated that minor incisions (such as that made during an inguinal hernia repair) may result in a third-space loss equivalent to 1 to 3 mL/kg/hr. By comparison, with medium-sized incisions (such as that made during an uncomplicated sigmoidectomy), the loss may be about 3 to 7 mL/kg/hr; in large operative procedures with major tissue dissection (such as pancreaticduodenectomy), the loss may be equivalent to 9 to 11 mL/kg/hr.[20]

The length of the surgical procedure can affect fluid balance. In one study, investigators used a mathematical model to try to determine the desired rate of crystalloid fluid administration during abdominal surgical procedures to maintain plasma volume without producing excessive interstitial edema at the surgical site; the model predicted that restrictive fluid management is indicated in abdominal surgeries that last more than 6 hours to avoid excessive interstitial edema.[21]

Effect of Irrigating Solutions During Surgery

Irrigation solutions are used during a variety of surgical procedures and have the potential to disrupt fluid and electrolyte balance. Two of these procedures are briefly discussed here: transurethral prostatectomy and transcervical resection of the endometrium. With some types of procedures, use of an electrolyte solution is not possible because it conducts an electric current. In these scenarios, a nonconductive solution is needed, such as glycine, sorbitol, or mannitol.

Transurethral Prostatectomy

Although a variety of transurethral methods are available to surgically treat benign prostatic hypertrophy, the older, well-established method of transurethral resection of the prostate (TURP) is considered the gold standard.[22, 23] One

form of this surgery uses a wire loop to cut away the tissue and an electric current to seal the blood vessels. This procedure requires the administration of a large quantity of electrolyte-free fluid (such as 1.5% glycine, a mannitol–sorbitol solution, or sterile water). The safety of water as an irrigating solution is controversial; glycine 1.5% is generally the most popular irrigating fluid.[24] During transurethral prostatectomy, the prostatic veins are opened and the irrigant solution—which is used to distend the urethra and clear fragments and blood from the operative field—can be absorbed. The amount of fluid that is absorbed varies with the surgical procedure and the length of the operation. For example, during a 45-minute transurethral prostatectomy procedure, the average amount of fluid used is 15 L.[25] Absorption of enough fluid to produce symptoms leads to a condition called TURP syndrome.

The fundamental pathology in TURP syndrome is volume overload and dilutional hyponatremia. The severity and rapidity of the hyponatremia are proportional to the volume of the absorbed irrigant. While hyponatremia follows the excessive absorption of an irrigant fluid such as glycine, sorbitol, or mannitol, the plasma osmolality may be near normal due to absorption of the osmotically active bladder irrigant.[26] In this situation, the hyponatremia is deemed "isotonic hyponatremia" and helps prevent cerebral edema. Conversely, if the absorbed fluid is water, the condition is deemed "hypotonic hyponatremia" and cerebral edema is likely to occur if the serum sodium is markedly low.

Risk factors for TURP syndrome include preoperative hyponatremia, chronic obstructive pulmonary disease, and congestive heart failure. Measures that can be taken to prevent this syndrome include using low-pressure irrigation and limiting the surgical procedure to less than 1 hour to decrease the degree of volume overload. Use of epidural or spinal anesthesia also allows for earlier symptom recognition. Hypertonic saline, perhaps in combination with furosemide, may be required to treat a patient with symptomatic hyponatremia.[27]

Alternatives to the TURP method include transurethral vapor resection of the prostate and holmium laser enucleation of the prostate; one of the aims of these procedures is to reduce complications associated with TURP (such as irrigant absorption).[28]

Transcervical Resection of the Endometrium

A variety of methods are available for the transcervical removal or desiccation of intrauterine tissue.[29] When the diathermy method is used, a hypotonic irrigating solution is infused into the uterine cavity to wash away operative debris.[30] Approximately 9 L of an irrigant fluid may be used during a 45-minute transcervical resection of the endometrium.[31] Because uterine veins are opened during this procedure, there is the possibility for intravenous absorption of substantial quantities of fluid, leading to hyponatremia. Hyponatremia is especially problematic in women of childbearing age because this group is most susceptible to hyponatremic encephalopathy.[32–34] See Chapter 4 for a discussion of hyponatremic encephalopathy.

While hyponatremia associated with transcerbical resection of the endometrium is not common, there are case reports in which it has occurred. For example, a case was reported in which a 44-year-old woman underwent hysteroscopy for a myoma under general anesthesia; following the absorption of a large volume of the fluid, she developed a serum sodium concentration of 106 mEq/L.[35] In another report, a 41-year-old woman developed a serum sodium concentration of 88 mEq/L following a lengthy procedure to remove uterine fibroids; during the procedure, the uterus was irrigated with 1.5% glycine.[36] Arieff and Ayus described four patients with hyponatremia due to endometrial ablation.[37] Hyponatremia in three of the women was detected early and treated (mean sodium levels were corrected from 102 to 123 mEq/L within the first 24 hours); all three recovered completely. Unfortunately, the fourth patient suffered respiratory arrest before therapy could be initiated; she never regained consciousness and died several days later. Autopsy revealed cerebral edema with tonsillar herniation.

The endogenous production of antidiuretic hormone (ADH) that accompanies surgical stress worsens the hyponatremia by causing water retention. The presence of symptoms suggesting hyponatremia should lead to immediate testing of the plasma sodium level; if it is below normal, early and appropriate therapy for the hyponatremia should be instituted before respiratory arrest occurs. In patients with general anesthesia during endometrial ablation, the possibility of hyponatremia should be suspected if the patient has a drop in body temperature, shows decreased oxygen saturation, or displays tremulousness or dilated pupils.[38] Because it is easier to detect developing hyponatremia when the patient is awake, some anesthetists favor regional anesthesia over general anesthesia during hysteroscopic surgical procedures.[39] Another suggestion to minimize risks for bad outcomes during hysteroscopy is to use an accurate system to measure the volume and weight of the fluid drained from the operative area during the surgical procedure.[40]

The influence of syndrome of inappropriate secretion of antidiuretic hormone (SIADH) should not be overlooked in young women undergoing a surgical procedure such as described in this section, even when these procedures are generally considered to qualify as "minor."[41] A significant decline in serum sodium concentration can even occur in women who undergo hysteroscopy with use of isotonic saline or lactated Ringer's solution as intravenous replacement fluid.[42]

POSTOPERATIVE PERIOD

The stress response described earlier remains during the early postoperative period. Cortisol and ACTH levels generally remain elevated for 2 to 4 days after surgery; however, with extensive trauma or the complications of sepsis or shock, the levels may remain elevated for weeks.[43] Antidiuretic hormone also remains elevated, and increases are likely to be especially pronounced in patients who experience a lot of pain or nausea.

Fluid Replacement

The volume of fluid required in the postoperative period is highly variable. For example, in addition to routine maintenance needs, the patient may be experiencing third-space fluid shifts or insensible fluid losses (such as from an open abdomen). In the initial postoperative period, an isotonic solution, such as 0.9% sodium chloride, is generally recommended; after the initial 24 to 48 hours, fluids can be changed to 0.45% sodium chloride.[44] Potassium is added when urine output is adequate, provided renal function is normal. The volume of fluid to be administered is guided by clinical signs, such as urine output and vital signs. Measurement of fluid intake and output and body weight are also helpful in determining parenteral fluid needs. The excessive use of hypotonic fluids in the immediate preoperative period predisposes patients to hyponatremia because of high output of antidiuretic hormone for the first few days postperatively. Other electrolytes are replaced as indicated by individual need.

Positive Versus Negative Fluid Balance

Positive fluid balance refers to a fluid intake that exceeds fluid output; conversely, negative fluid balance refers to a fluid output that exceeds fluid intake. Sometimes the differences are relatively small, such as several hundred milliliters. In general, the type of surgery often dictates whether negative or positive fluid balance might improve patient outcomes. For example, "triple-H therapy" (hypertensive, hypervolemic, and hemodilution therapy) is generally accepted as a treatment for cerebral vasospasm following subarachnoid hemorrhage.[45] In the setting of abdominal surgery, however, a patient at increased risk for abdominal compartment syndrome (ACS) may benefit from a slightly negative fluid balance. In general, there does not appear to be agreement as to whether a positive fluid balance or a slightly negative fluid balance produces the best outcomes in patients who have undergone abdominal surgery.[46–49]

Abdominal Compartment Syndrome

Abdominal compartment syndrome is characterized by a sustained intra-abdominal pressure above 20 mm Hg followed by organ dysfunction.[50] Massive fluid resuscitation with crystalloid solutions, such as isotonic saline or lactated Ringer's solution, may play a role in the development of ACS. For example, a recent study of 77 patients with major abdominal surgery found that intra-abdominal hypertension occurred more commonly in patients with a positive 24-hour fluid balance.[51] Other authors have reported that a treatment strategy to produce a negative fluid balance may result in a dramatic decrease in intra-abdominal pressure.[52]

Postoperative Fluid and Electrolyte Imbalances

Hyponatremia

Excessive secretion of ADH in the immediate postoperative period, associated with anesthesia and the stress of surgery, predisposes to the development of hyponatremia. Pain also enhances the release of ADH by direct stimulation of the hypothalamus. Nausea, which is frequently present in postoperative patients, can increaseADH release as much as 1000-fold; the nausea does not have to be associated with vomiting.[53] In one study, hyponatremia was present in 4.4% of postoperative patients within 1 week of surgery.[54]

Because of the tendency for hyponatremia in new postoperative patients, the excessive administration of electrolyte-free solutions during the first 2 to 4 postoperative days should be avoided. In fact, because elevated plasma levels of ADH are essentially a universal postoperative occurrence in the first few days after surgery, some authors state that it may be important to avoid hypotonic intravenous solutions altogether in the immediate postoperative period. Even isotonic fluids should be given only as needed, according to a

patient's size, to maintain hemodynamic stability in the postoperative period, because the kidney can also generate electrolyte-free water from a large sodium excretion in the urine.[55]

A serum sodium level of 130 to 135 mEq/L warrants attention in a postoperative patient; the simple act of restricting free water may be sufficient to avoid the full-blown syndrome of water intoxication (severe dilutional hyponatremia).[56] Cases of permanent brain damage related to profound hyponatremia have been reported in postoperative patients receiving excessive free water.[57] Refer to Case Study 4-4 and the section on postoperative hyponatremia in menstruant women, and to the section on endometrial ablation earlier in this chapter.

Fluid Volume Deficit

The most common fluid disorder in the postoperative patient is extracellular fluid volume deficit. Contributing factors to postoperative FVD include loss of GI fluids, third-space fluid shifts, fever, overzealous blood sampling for repeated chemical determinations, hyperventilation, injudicious administration of diuretics, and an unhumidified tracheostomy with hyperventilation. Among the indicators of FVD are decreased urine output, postural hypotension and tachycardia, diminished skin turgor, decreased capillary refill time, and blood urea nitrogen (BUN) elevated out of proportion to the serum creatinine (see Chapter 3). If fluids are directly lost from the body (as from vomiting or diuresis), body weight will decrease acutely as well.

As described earlier, third-spacing is a special kind of FVD in which fluid shifts from the vascular space to another space in the body. Third-spacing of fluids from surgical trauma is not limited to the operative period; indeed, it may continue slowly for a few hours or more during the first day of injury. If FVD is due to third-spacing, decreased body weight does not occur because the fluid "lost" from the vascular space pools in another part of the body (such as the surgical site or bowel due to adynamic ileus). Actually, as parenteral fluids are administered to correct the vascular volume deficiency, the patient will gain weight. Intake and output (I & O) measurements are mandatory when FVD is suspected; in general, in the adult an acceptable hourly urine volume is in the range of 30 to 50 mL.

Unrecognized deficits of extracellular fluid volume during the early postoperative period may be manifested as circulatory instability. Decreased urine volume coupled with tachycardia and decreased blood pressure should cause one to suspect a FVD of several liters. After a period of time, as the third-spacing resolves and fluid shifts back into the intravascular space, diuresis and weight loss will occur. In patients with cardiac or renal dysfunction, the shift of fluid back into the vascular bed may result in congestive heart failure or pulmonary edema.

Urine Output. A decreased urine output is often an indication of fluid volume deficit. As noted earlier, urinary output should be at least 30 to 50 mL/hr in adults; an hourly urinary output of less than 30 mL should be investigated. Factors associated with decreased urinary volume in the postoperative patient may include the following conditions:

- Inadequate preoperative fluid replacement
- Hypovolemia resulting from fluid loss incurred during surgery—either direct loss or subtle third-space accumulation at the surgical site or intestinal ileus
- Disturbance in myocardial function causing decreased blood flow to the kidneys and, therefore, decreased urine formation
- Renal failure (a serious cause of postoperative oliguria)

Postoperative Renal Failure. Postoperative renal failure occurs most often in elderly patients undergoing cardiac surgery or aortic aneurysm repair. Although oliguric renal failure may occur postoperatively in the patient who has suffered poor renal perfusion during surgery, high-output renal failure is actually the more frequent complication. High-output renal failure is characterized by uremia accompanied by a daily urine volume greater than 1000 to 1500 mL. It probably represents the renal response to a less severe episode of renal injury than is required to cause the classic oliguric renal failure. Although high-output renal failure is usually easier to manage than oliguric renal failure, it is more difficult to recognize. Typically, the urine volume is normal or greater than normal and the BUN level is increased. A danger of hyperkalemia exists when potassium is administered to a patient with unrecognized high-output failure.

Fluid Volume Excess

In the surgical patient with normal renal function, the most common cause of intravascular volume excess is overload with isotonic saline (which contains 154 mEq/L of sodium and 154 mEq/L of chloride). Among the earliest signs is weight gain during the catabolic period, when the patient is expected to lose ¼ to ½ lb/day.[58] Although volume overload can occur at any time in the postoperative period, it is more common soon after surgery.

Another possible cause of fluid volume excess in the postoperative patient is continuing to administer intravenous fluids during the period in which third-spaced fluid is in the process of shifting back into the bloodstream. This usually occurs several days after the event that produced the third-space fluid shift—although it might not occur until much later, depending on the type of injury. When the fluid is shifting back into the bloodstream, healthcare providers might see increased urine output and increased blood pressure.

Potassium Imbalances

Provided renal function is adequate, potassium is administered daily following surgery to replace urinary and GI potassium losses. Generally, a daily supplementation of 60 to 100 mEq is required postoperatively.[59] The needed potassium should be distributed evenly in the total daily maintenance fluids. For example, if 2 L of fluid is prescribed over 24 hours and 80 mEq KCl is the required daily potassium supplement, 40 mEq KCl is generally added to each liter of solution. This makes far more sense than routinely administering "K-runs" to meet maintenance potassium needs. (See the discussion of IV potassium replacement in Chapter 5.) For patients at risk for renal failure due to hypotensive episodes during the surgical procedure, even small potassium supplements can be detrimental.

Hyperkalemia is rare in the postoperative patient, except in the presence of renal failure, rhabdomyolysis, massive hemolysis, or tissue necrosis. If hyperkalemia occurs at any time during the postoperative period, the possibility of impaired renal function—manifested by rising serum creatinine in the presence of low, normal, or high urine output—should be explored. Release of cellular potassium following crushing injuries and electrical injuries, plus acute renal failure, can lead to lethal hyperkalemia within hours.

Hypocalcemia Following Parathyroid, Thyroid, or Neck Surgery

Postsurgical hypocalcemia may accompany parathyroidectomy, thyroidectomy, or radical neck dissection. In a study of 162 patients who underwent thyroidectomy, it was found that 69 (43%) had temporary hypocalcemia and 9 (5%) had permanent hypocalcemia; the latter condition was defined as requiring calcium supplementation at 6 months postoperatively.[60] A below-normal serum calcium level was more common in patients who had a total thyroidectomy. Although hypocalcemia occurred in almost half of the patients, it was symptomatic in only 24%.

Various causative mechanisms have been proposed to explain this imbalance. For example, the inadvertent removal of (or injury to) parathyroid tissue at the time of surgery may lead to hypocalcemia. If permanent parathyroid damage has not occurred, parathyroid insufficiency resolves as edema at the surgical site lessens and revascularization occurs. Others have postulated that the release of calcitonin secondary to the manipulation of the thyroid gland during surgery may be the culprit; recall that calcitonin lowers the serum calcium level.[61] Still others have postulated that a phenomenon known as the "hungry bone syndrome" is responsible; in this condition, an abrupt postoperative uptake of calcium occurs in patients who have preexisting osteodystrophy.[62] One likely mechanism for hypocalcemia after radical neck dissection is reduced blood flow to the parathyroid glands after dissection and hemostatic maneuvers.

Most patients who develop hypocalcemia after neck surgery are asymptomatic; however, some may develop paresthesia, laryngeal spasm, or tetany. Ionized calcium may be checked every 12 hours after neck surgery—and more frequently if symptoms of hypocalcemia are present—until the concentration begins to elevate, indicating recovery of the parathyroid glands. The most critical period for calcium level monitoring is thought to be the first 24 to 96 hours after surgery. Some authors advocate checking serum calcium levels 6 hours after surgery and on the first postoperative day to predict which patients will develop hypocalcemia.[63] Still other authors advocate direct measurement of parathyroid hormone following thyroid surgery.[64, 65] For example, a recent study suggested that a 1-hour postoperative PTH level of 2.5 pmol/L or less can identify individuals at risk for developing symptomatic hypocalcemia.[66] It is possible that postoperative hypoparathyroidism may manifest itself months to years after neck surgery; therefore, serum ionized calcium levels should be serially monitored in patients at risk. Moreover, stress may potentially induce hypocalcemia in these individuals, which is why critically ill patients with a history of neck surgery should have a serum calcium test performed.

Permanent hypocalcemia (i.e., hypocalcemia lasting 2 months or longer) associated with thyroid surgery may be due to accidental removal of the parathyroid glands or to vascular necrosis.[67] Fortunately, permanent postsurgical hypoparathyroidism occurs in only a small percentage of patients; the frequency of this complication is partially dependent on the technical skill of the surgeon.[68] Indeed, surgeons performing thyroidectomies and parathyroidectomies strive to preserve the blood supply to the parathyroid glands. Extensive neck surgeries—as in radical neck dissection for cancer—are more likely to be associated with permanent hypoparathyroidism than are less involved surgical maneuvers.

Of course, symptomatic patients should receive supplemental calcium to increase their serum calcium levels to the low normal range. One study suggested that some patients, such as those older than 50 years and those with low preoperative serum 25-hydroxy vitamin D levels, should be placed on calcium or vitamin D supplementation after total thyroidectomy to avoid postoperative hypocalcemia.[69]

Acid–Base Disorders

Surgical patients may have normal pH or develop virtually any acid–base abnormality, depending on their individual circumstances. Respiratory acidosis may result from shallow respirations related to anesthesia, narcotics, abdominal distention, pain, or large cumbersome dressings. On assessment, decreased respirations and decreased breath sounds may be noted. Measures to increase gas exchange—such as encouraging frequent coughing and deep breathing, suctioning of tracheobronchial secretions, avoidance of oversedation, and turning and ambulating the patient—will decrease the likelihood of respiratory acidosis.

Subclinical respiratory alkalosis is common in surgical patients. Among the causes of this imbalance are hyperventilation due to pain, hypoxia, central nervous system injury, and assisted ventilation. Respiratory alkalosis is disturbing in the presence of metabolic alkalosis, for which hypoventilation with subsequent carbon dioxide retention is needed for compensatory purposes.

The most common causes of metabolic alkalosis in the surgical patient are loss of gastric acid due to nasogastric drainage or vomiting and therapy with potassium-losing diuretics. The most common causes of metabolic acidosis in surgical patients include ketoacidosis, renal failure, lactic acidosis associated with shock, and loss of alkali from biliary and pancreatic drainage.

Acute Respiratory Disease Syndrome

Acute respiratory distress syndrome (ARDS) and acute lung injury (ALI) are possible complications in surgical patients.[70] To date, no consensus has been reached regarding what constitutes the ideal fluid and hemodynamic management for these patients. Keeping fluid administration to the lowest effective volume is advantageous in minimizing risk for pulmonary edema. Recall that critically ill patients with ARDS or ALI have increased capillary permeability, which can result in pulmonary edema and alveolar collapse. This condition worsens in the presence of intravascular hydrostatic pressure.[71] In a post hoc analysis of 1000 patients enrolled in a study titled the ARDS Clinical Trials Network Fluid and Catheter Treatment Trial (FACTT), investigators concluded that a conservative fluid-administration strategy and monitoring with a central venous catheter resulted in a major reduction in net fluid balance and fewer ICU days; they further concluded that conservative fluid administration did not result in more renal failure.[72] Nevertheless, these authors stated that their conclusions should be cautiously interpreted because the original trial did not prospectively plan a surgical subgroup analysis.

CASE STUDIES

Case Study 14-1

A 60-year-old man underwent surgical repair of an abdominal aortic aneurysm and was brought to the surgical intensive care unit for follow-up care. He was mechanically ventilated with an inspired gas mixture containing 40% oxygen; tidal volume was set at 950 mL and breathing rate at 12 breaths per minute. A nasogastric tube was connected to suction. The patient received 2 L 5% dextrose in 0.11% NaCl solution every 24 hours for the first 2 postoperative days. In addition, he received 20 mg furosemide IV twice daily. On the morning of the third postoperative day, the following abnormal laboratory results were found: hyponatremia (Na = 128 mEq/L), hypokalemia (K = 3.3 mEq/L), respiratory alkalosis (arterial pH = 7.62 and $PaCO_2$ = 26 mm Hg; normal range, 35–45 mm Hg), and hypoxemia (PaO_2 = 74 mm Hg), and metabolic alkalosis (elevated HCO_3 of 28 mEq/L).

Commentary. Furosemide, a powerful diuretic, causes sodium loss in the urine. In addition, some sodium was lost in nasogastric suction. However, very little sodium was replaced via the IV route (5% dextrose in 0.11% NaCl solution contains only 19 mEq of sodium per liter of fluid). In addition, pain and surgical stress stimulate production of ADH, which causes water retention—thus diluting the serum sodium level, especially when hypotonic fluid is supplied IV.

Two primary pH abnormalities were present in this case: respiratory alkalosis and metabolic alkalosis. Possible causes

of metabolic alkalosis in this patient included loss of acidic gastric fluid via suction and use of a potassium-losing diuretic. Because the patient was mechanically ventilated at a fixed volume and rate, he was unable to make the usual compensatory respiratory change (hypoventilation) seen when metabolic alkalosis exists. In fact, the high minute volume set by mechanical ventilation caused *hyper*ventilation and, therefore, respiratory alkalosis.

Case Study 14-2

A 32-year-old woman presented with hypercalcemia and was diagnosed with primary hyperparathyroidism. On neck exploration, the surgeon found four enlarged parathyroid glands and removed three. On the first postoperative day, the patient's total serum calcium was 8.6 mg/dL; it decreased to 6.8 mg/dL by the third postoperative day. At that time, the patient complained of feeling lightheaded and having paresthesias of the mouth, fingers, and toes. On examination, she was found to have a positive Chvostek's sign. Later, she developed twitching of the facial muscles. She was treated with 10 mL 10% calcium gluconate IV over 10 minutes.

Commentary. The hypocalcemia was caused by surgical hypoparathyroidism (after the removal of three of the four parathyroid glands). A potential serious consequence that could have occurred with this degree of hypocalcemia was laryngeal spasm, which compromises the airway.

Case Study 14-3

A 66-year-old woman with a history of coronary artery disease and manic–depressive disorder underwent a coronary artery bypass graft. She was started back on her preoperative dose of lithium on the first postoperative day; at that time, her serum sodium level was 142 mEq/L. After the second dose of lithium, her urine output increased to more than 400 mL/hr for 4 consecutive hours. After that time, her output ranged from 250 to 300 mL/hr for the next 24 hours. Her only source of fluid intake was by the oral route; her appetite was described as poor. No intravenous fluids were infused. By the morning of the second postoperative day, the patient's serum sodium level was 153 mEq/L; it reached a high of 170 mEq/L on postoperative day 3. At that time, her serum osmolality was 351 mOsm/kg and her urine osmolality was 228 mOsm/kg. A review of her I & O record for the postoperative period revealed that her fluid output exceeded her fluid intake by 11,000 mL. A toxic lithium level was revealed by laboratory analysis. She had mental status changes and required reintubation on the evening of postoperative day 2. Intravenous water replacement therapy with D_5W was initiated on postoperative day 3. Frequent measurements of the serum sodium level were made to ensure that the serum sodium level was not dropped too quickly—a situation that is more likely to occur when hypernatremia is corrected with a sodium-free fluid as opposed to a low-sodium fluid, such as 0.22% sodium chloride.

Commentary. A reduced intake of fluid and sodium can accelerate lithium retention with resultant toxicity. Further, a toxic lithium level can lead to a large output of dilute urine. Fluid retention typically follows bypass surgery; thus the staff should have been alerted to the abnormal nature of this case. More attention should have been paid to the far greater fluid output than fluid intake as well as to the elevated serum sodium level. Once the hypernatremia was detected, healthcare providers recognized that gradual correction of the imbalance was indicated to avoid causing adverse neurological changes. Too rapid a correction of hypernatremia can result in cerebral edema, seizures, permanent neurological damage, and death (see Chapter 4 for a more thorough discussion of the treatment of hypernatremia).

Case Study 14-4

A 43-year-old woman was admitted for an elective endometrial ablation for the treatment of menorrhagia.[73] The medical history was unremarkable except for migraine-type headaches and irritable bowel syndrome. The patient's preoperative serum sodium level was 139 mEq/L. She underwent hysteroscopic endometrial ablation using 3% sorbitol solution for irrigation. Because she had heavy bleeding, a laparoscopy was performed to rule out perforation. Eight liters of 3% sorbitol irrigation fluid was instilled; in contrast, the measured affluent was only 4100 mL. During the procedure, the patient also received 3800 mL of lactated Ringer's solution. The blood loss was estimated at approximately 300 mL. The procedure was well tolerated and the patient was moved to the recovery room. There she complained of headache and was noted to be drowsy but easily arousable. Facial puffiness was noted and her rectal temperature was found to be 92°F. A positive Babinski sign was noted on the right side. Laboratory tests revealed a serum sodium concentration of 112 mEq/L. Once the hyponatremia was recognized, the patient was moved to an ICU and treated with 3% NaCl solution; her serum sodium was slowly corrected to129 mEq/L over the next 12 hours. The next day, the patient was substantially improved and was transferred out of the ICU.

Commentary. The condition described in this case has been labeled the "female TURP syndrome." The fact that this patient's perioperative fluid intake greatly exceeded the recorded output supports excessive absorption of hypotonic fluid as at least one reason for the rapid decline in the serum sodium level. It is likely that the elevated ADH level commonly observed in surgical patients contributed to the hyponatremia. The sudden decline in the serum sodium concentration likely caused brain swelling, accounting for the neurological symptoms. The authors correctly concluded that a hypertonic sodium chloride was needed because the fatality rate for hyponatremia is quite high once cerebral edema develops. This relationship is especially strong in menstruant women; see Chapter 4 for a more thorough discussion of this topic.

Measures to help prevent complications from fluid overload revolve around three principles: (1) avoiding excess fluid absorption during the procedure, (2) recognizing and treating the fluid overload early should it occur, and (3) using the distending medium least likely to cause serious complications should it be absorbed in excess. An accurate account of fluid intake and output throughout the procedure is important to detect excess fluid absorption. Also, use of regional anesthesia (when possible) would help detect neurological symptoms early.

Case Study 14-5

A case was recently reported in which a 46-year-old woman who had undergone weight reduction (Roux-en-Y) surgery 8 months earlier was admitted for a near-total thyroidectomy to remove a possibly malignant nodule.[74] Roux-en-Y surgery creates a small gastric pouch that holds only a few ounces of food or liquid; the jejunum is connected directly to the pouch, thereby bypassing the duodenum. The bulk of orally consumed calcium is absorbed in the duodenum and proximal jejunum. In this case, because of the patient's gastric bypass operation, the length of small bowel available to absorb food and other substances consumed orally was significantly reduced.

The patient initially did well in the immediate postoperative period and was started on calcium carbonate 1000 mg three times per day and a synthetic form of a natural thyroid hormone two times per day. On the first postoperative day, her serum calcium decreased to 7.4 mg/dL and she complained of tingling in her right hand. As a result, she was given 2 g of calcium gluconate IV during the day and started on calcitriol 0.5 mcg twice daily. On the second postoperative day, her total serum calcium declined further to 7.0 mg/dL and her parathyroid (PTH) level was less than 3 pg/mL (normal is approximately 10–55 pg/mL). To correct these problems, she was given an additional gram of intravenous calcium gluconate. On the third postoperative day, her serum calcium was 6.7 mg/dL and a Chvostek's sign became apparent (a carpopedal spasm of the hand when blood flow to the area is restricted, as by an inflated blood pressure cuff). At this point, the patient's oral calcium intake was increased to 5 g per day (by a combination of calcium carbonate and milk). In addition, she received 5 g of IV magnesium sulfate over the course of the day to treat a low serum magnesium level (1.6 mg/dL; normal range for reporting laboratory was 1.6 to 2.6 mg/dL). Her condition became worse on postoperative day 4, when the patient developed hand cramping and worsening paresthesia. The dosage of calcium was increased and more calcium was administered intravenously (as was more IV magnesium sulfate). Tests revealed that no significant absorption of calcium was occurring from the small bowel, likely as a result of gastric bypass surgery. With intravenous calcium and magnesium replacement, the patient improved and became asymptomatic (serum calcium rose to 8.6 mg/dL on postoperative day 5). It was found that the patient did not recover parathyroid function following her thyroidectomy.

Commentary. In this case, the patient had two reasons for developing hypocalcemia. First, her gastric bypass limited the amount of small bowel available for absorption of orally consumed calcium. Second, her thyroid surgery resulted in permanent hypoparathyroidism. Thus she developed permanent hypoparathyroidism and required long-term use of very high doses of calcium, vitamin D, and calcitriol to prevent symptomatic hypocalcemia. The problem of hypocalcemia was not present prior to the thyroidectomy because (at that time) she had a normal PTH level.

Also see Case Studies 4-3, 4-4, 4-8, 4-9, 13-8, 15-1, 17-5, and 19-3 for reports of electrolyte problems in surgical patients.

Summary of Key Points

- Hypokalemia is a common reason for cancelling elective surgery, as this type of electrolyte imbalance increases the risk for cardiac dysrhythmias.
- Antidiuretic hormone is greatly elevated in the first 24 to 48 hours postoperatively as part of the stress response. ADH production is also stimulated by pain and nausea. As such, the postoperative patient is at increased risk for hyponatremia.
- Use of excessive volumes of hypotonic fluids in the postoperative period can lead to life-threatening hyponatremia, a condition that is most serious in women of menstruant age.
- The type of surgical procedure performed has a major influence on risk for electrolyte imbalances. For example, hypocalcemia is prominent in head and neck surgery, while hyponatremia is prominent in surgeries that require the use of hypotonic irrigating solutions.
- Third-space fluid shifts are common in patients who have undergone major abdominal surgical procedures; abdominal compartment syndrome should be carefully observed for in these individuals.
- Intake and output measurements are important to determine when positive or negative fluid balance is present.
- Frequent monitoring of serum electrolytes during the postoperative period will allow the detection of problems before they become life-threatening.
- Preexisting conditions, such as renal or heart disease, greatly influence the type of fluid and electrolyte problems expected during the perioperative period.

NOTES

1. Narins, R. (Ed.). (1994). *Clinical disorders of fluid and electrolyte metabolism* (5th ed.). New York: McGraw-Hill, p. 1412.

2. Narins, note 1, p. 1412.

3. Practice guidelines for preoperative fasting and the use of pharmacologic agents to reduce the risk of pulmonary aspiration: Application to healthy patients undergoing elective procedures: A report by the American Society of Anesthesiologist Task Force on Preoperative Fasting. (1999). *Anesthesiology, 90*(3), 896–905.

4. Klingensmith, M. E., Chen, L. E., Glasgow, S. C., Goers, T. A., & Melby, S. J. (2008) . *The Washington manual of surgery* (5th ed.). Philadelphia: Wolters Kluwer Lippincott Williams & Wilkins, p. 56.

5. Practice guidelines, note 3.

6. Fleager, K., & Yao, J. (2010). Perioperative steroid dosing in patients receiving chronic oral steroids, undergoing outpatient hand surgery. *Journal of Hand Surgery-American Volume, 35*(2), 316–318.

7. Salem, M., Tannish, R. E. Jr., Bronberg, J., Loriaux, D. L., & Chernow, B. (1994). Preoperative glucocorticoid coverage: A reassess-

ment 42 years after emergence of a problem. *Annals of Surgery, 219,* 416–425.

8. Salem et al., note 7.

9. Klingensmith et al., note 4, p. 12.

10. Jabbour, S. A. (2001). Steroids and the surgical patient. *Medical Clinics of North America, 85*(5), 1311–1317.

11. Marik, P. E., & Varon, J. (2008). Requirement of perioperative stress doses of corticosteroids. *Archives of Surgery, 143*(12), 1222–1226.

12. Wakin, J. H., & Sledge, K. C. (2006). Anesthetic implications for patients receiving exogenous corticosteroids. *AANA Journal, 74*(2), 133–139.

13. Brunicardi, F. C., Andersen, D., Billiar, T. R., Dunn, D. L., Hunter, J. G., & Pollock, R. E. (eds.). (2005). *Schwartz's principles of surgery* (8th ed.). New York: McGraw-Hill Medical Publishing Division, p. 6.

14. Merritt, R. (2005). *The A.S.P.E.N. nutrition support practice manual* (2nd ed.). Silver Spring, MD: American Society for Parenteral and Enteral Nutrition, p. 260.

15. DeLegge, M. H. (2008). *Nutrition and gastrointestinal disease.* Totowa, NJ: Humana Press, p. 47.

16. Merritt, note 14, p. 259.

17. Dannhauser, A., Van Zyl, J. M., & Nel, C. J. (1995). Preoperative nutritional status and prognostic nutritional index in patients with benign disease undergoing abdominal operations: Part I. *Journal of the American College of Nutrition, 14,* 80–95.

18. Merritt, note 14, p. 259.

19. Klingensmith et al., note 4, p. 86.

20. Klingensmith et al., note 4, p. 86.

21. Tatara, T., Nagao, Y., & Tashiro, C. (2009). The effect of duration of surgery on fluid balance during abdominal surgery: A mathematical model. *Anesthesia & Analgesia, 109*(1), 211.

22. Hoffman, R. M., MacDonald, R., Monga, M., & Wilt, T. J. (2004). Transurethral microwave thermotherapy vs transurethral resection for treating benign prostatic hyperplasia: A systematic review. *BJU International. 94*(7), 1031–1036.

23. Gupta, N. P., & Anand, A. (2009). Comparison of TURP, TUVRP and HoLEP. *Current Urology Reports, 10,* 276–278.

24. Moharari, R. S., Khajavi, M. R., Khademhosseini, P., Hosseini, S. R., & Najafi, A. (2008). Sterile water as an irrigating fluid for transurethral resection of the prostate: Anesthetical view of the records of 1600 cases. *Southern Medical Journal, 101*(4), 373–375.

25. Hahn, R. G., Prough, D. S., & Svenson, C. H. (2007). *Perioperative fluid therapy.* New York/London: Informa Healthcare, p. 477.

26. Rothenberg, D. M. (2009). Letter. Proper diagnosis and treatment of transurethral resection of prostate syndrome requires more than transesophageal Doppler. *Anesthesia & Analgesia, 108*(3), 1048–1049.

27. Haggstrom, J., Hedlund, M., & Hahn, R. G. (2001). Subacute hyponatremia after transurethral resection of the prostate. *Scandinavian Journal of Urology and Nephrology, 35,* 250–251.

28. Gupta & Anand, note 23.

29. Mushambi, M. C., & Williamson, K. (2002). Anaesthetic considerations for hysteroscopic surgery. *Best Practice & Research Clinical Anesthesiology, 16*(1), 35–52.

30. Arieff, A., & Ayus, C. (1993). Endometrial ablation complicated by fatal hyponatremic encephalopathy. *Journal of the American Medical Association, 3*(279), 1230.

31. Hahn et al., note 25, p. 477.

32. Ayus, C., Wheeler, J., & Arieff, A. (1992). Postoperative hyponatremic encephalopathy in menstruant women. *Annals of Internal Medicine, 117,* 891.

33. Ayus, C., & Arieff, A. (1996). Brain damage and postoperative hyponatremia: The role of gender. *Neurology, 45,* 323.

34. Steele, A., Gowrishankar, M., Abrahamson, S., Mazer, C. D., Feldman, R. D., & Halperin, M. L. (1997). Postoperative hyponatremia despite near-isotonic saline infusion: A phenomenon of desalination. *Annals of Internal Medicine, 126,* 20–25.

35. Serocki, G., Hanss, R., Bauer, M., Scholz, J., & Bein, B. (2009). The gynecological TURP syndrome: Severe hyponatremia and pulmonary edema during hysteroscopy. *Anaesthetist, 58*(1), 30–34.

36. Shah, V. R., Parikh, P., & Bhosale, G. (2002). Central pontine myelinolysis: Sequel of hyponatremia during transcervical resection of endometrium. *Acta Anaesthesiologica Scandinavica, 46,* 914–916.

37. Arieff & Ayus, note 30.

38. Goodnough, L. T., Grishaber, J. E., Monk, T. G. & Catalona, W. J. (1994). Acute preoperative hemodilution in patients undergoing radical prostatectomy: A case study analysis of efficacy. *Anesthesia & Analgesia, 78,* 932–937.

39. Mushambi & Williamson, note 29.

40. Nezhat, C. H., Fisher, D. T., & Datta, S. (2007). Investigation of often reported ten percent hysteroscopy fluid overfill: Is this accurate? *Journal of Minimally Invasive Gynecology, 14*(4), 489–493.

41. Cooper, B., & Murray, C. (2006). Syndrome of inappropriate antidiuretic hormone in a healthy woman after diagnostic laparoscopy and hysteroscopy: A case report. *Journal of Reproductive Medicine, 51*(3), 199–201.

42. Steele et al., note 34.

43. Kokko, J., & Tannen, R. (1996). *Fluids and electrolytes* (3rd ed.). Philadelphia: W. B. Saunders, p. 731.

44. Brunicardi et al., note 13, p. 56.

45. Muench, E., Horn, P., Bauhuf, C., Roth, H., Phillipps, M., & Hermann, P. (2007). Effects of hypervolemia and hypertension on regional cerebral blood flow, intracranial pressure, and brain tissue oxygenation after subarachnoic hemorrhage. *Critical Care Medicine, 35*(8), 1844–1851.

46. Bellamy, M. C. (2006). Wet, dry or something else? *British Journal of Anaesthesia, 97,* 755–757.

47. Hahn, R. G. (2007). Fluid therapy might be more difficult than you think. *Anesthesia and Analgesia, 105,* 304–305.

48. Kleespies, A., Thiel, M., Jauch, K. W. & Hartl, W. H. (2009). Perioperative fluid retention and clinical outcome in elective, high-risk colorectal surgery. *International Journal of Colorectal Disease, 24,* 699–709.

49. Walsh, S. R., Tang, T. Y., Farooq, N., Coveney, E. C., & Gaunt, M. E. (2008). Perioperative fluid restriction reduces complications after major gastrointestinal surgery. *Surgery, 143*(4), 466–468.

50. Kula, R., Szturz, P., Sklienka, P., & Neiser, J. (2008). Negative fluid balance in patients with abdominal compartment syndrome: Case reports. *Acta Chirurgica Belgica, 108*(3), 346–349.

51. Serpytis, M., & Ivaskevicius, J. (2008). The influence of fluid balance on intra-abdominal pressure after major abdominal surgery. *Medicina, 44*(6), 421–427.

52. Kula et al., note 50.

53. Narins, note 1, p. 599.

54. Chung, H. (1986). Postoperative hyponatremia. *Archives of Internal Medicine, 146,* 333.

55. Gowrishankar, M., Lin, S. H., Mallie, J. P., Oh, M. S., & Halperin, M. L. (1998). Acute hyponatremia in the perioperative period: Insights into its pathophysiology and recommendations for management. *Clinical Nephrology, 50,* 352–360.

56. Kokko & Tannen, note 43, p. 744.

57. Arieff & Ayus, note 30.

58. Brunicardi, note 13.

59. Kokko & Tannen, note 43, p. 744,

60. Pfeiderer, A. G., Ahmad, N., Draper, M. R., Vrotsou, K., & Smith, W. K. (2009). The timing of calcium measurements in helping to predict temporary and permanent hypocalcaemia in patients having completion and total thyroidectomies. *Annals of the Royal College of Surgeons of England, 91*(2), 140–146.

61. Narins, note 1, p. 1025.

62. See, A., & Soo, K. (1997). Hypocalcemia following thyroidectomy for thyrotoxicosis. *British Journal of Surgery, 84,* 95.

63. Pfeiderer et al., note 56.

64. Lim, J. P, Irvine, R., Bugis, S., Holmes, D., & Wiseman, S. M. (2009). Intact parathyroid hormone measurement 1 hour after thyroid surgery identifies individuals at high risk for the development of symptomatic hypocalcemia. *American Journal of Surgery, 197*(5), 648–653.

65. Asari, R., Passler, C., Kaczirek, K., Scheuba, C., & Niederle, B. (2008). Hypoparathyroidism after total thyroidectomy: A prospective study. *Archives of Surgery, 143*(2), 132–137.

66. Lim et al., note 64.

67. Bourrel, C., Uzzan, B., Tison, P., Despreaux, G., Frachet, B., Modigliani, E., et al. (1993). Transient hypocalcemia after thyroidectomy. *Annals of Otology, Rhinology, and Laryngology, 102,* 496–501.

68. Narins, note 1, p. 1025.

69. Erbil, Y., Barbaros, U., Temel, B., Turkoglu, U., Issever, H., Bozbora, A., et al. (2009). The impact of age, vitamin D(3) level, and incidental parathyroidectomy on postoperative hypocalcemia after total or near total thyroidectomy. *American Journal of Surgery, 197*(4), 439–446.

70. Stewart, R. M., Park, P. K., Hunt, J .P., McIntyre, R. C. Jr., McCarthy, J., Zarzabal, L, A., et al. (2009). Less is more: Improved outcomes in surgical patients with conservative fluid administration and central venous catheter monitoring. *Journal of the American College of Surgeons, 208,* 725–737.

71. Sibbald, W. J., Short, A. K., Warshawski, F. J., Cunningham, D. G., & Cheung, H. (1985). Thermal dye measurements of extravascular lung water in critically ill patients: Intravascular Starling forces and extravascular lung water in the adult respiratory distress syndrome. *Chest, 87,* 585–592.

72. Stewart et al., note 70.

73. Agraharkar, M., & Agraharkar, A. (1997). Posthysteroscopic hyponatremia: Evidence for a multifactorial cause. *American Journal of Kidney Diseases, 30,* 717.

74. Pietras, S. M., & Holick, M. F. (2009). Refractory hypocalcemia following near-total thyroidectomy in a patient with a prior Roux-en-Y gastric bypass. *Obesity Surgery, 19,* 524–526.

Chapter 15

Hypovolemic Shock in Trauma and Postoperative Patients

Management of the patient experiencing hypovolemic shock as a result of traumatic injury or surgical procedures is the focus of this chapter. Death in trauma patients has a trimodal pattern, with the first peak occurring within seconds to minutes after injury. The second peak occurs within minutes to a few hours after injury, in which case death is usually due to epidural or subdural hematoma, hemopneumothorax, ruptured spleen, liver laceration, pelvic fracture, or any injuries associated with significant blood loss. The third peak of deaths occurs several days or weeks after the initial injury; mortality in such cases is primarily due to complications of shock including sepsis, acute respiratory distress syndrome (ARDS), and multiple system organ failure (MSOF).

Treatment should be initiated early because prolonged shock leads to cellular swelling and damage, compounding the overall impact of blood loss and hypoperfusion. The overall goal of therapy is to reestablish adequate tissue perfusion and, therefore, oxygen delivery to metabolically active cells. Care focuses on restoring cellular perfusion rather than simply restoring the patient's blood pressure and pulse rate. Of course, active bleeding must be controlled by whatever means necessary.

DEFINITION AND PATHOPHYSIOLOGY OF SHOCK

Shock has been defined as an abnormality of the circulatory system that results in inadequate organ perfusion and tissue oxygenation. It starts when oxygen delivery to the cells is inadequate to meet metabolic demands.

The most common form in the injured patient is *hypovolemic shock* occurring after acute blood loss, either externally or internally. External blood loss can result from lacerations, amputations, open fractures, or stab or gunshot wounds. Blood is also frequently lost internally at the injury site, especially after major closed fractures. Depending on the injury site, a significant volume of blood may be sequestered into body cavities such as the thorax, intraperitoneal space, and retroperitoneal space. Examples of lethal internal spaces for exsanguination include the abdominal cavity/retroperitoneum (4000 mL) and hemithorax (2500 mL).[1] Losses of fluids other than blood also occur as a result of tissue injury; this obligatory edema adds to the deficit in the intravascular volume.

In *cardiogenic shock,* failure of the heart as a pump causes a decrease in tissue perfusion. In the trauma patient, cardiogenic shock may occur if compensatory mechanisms have failed or if cardiac tamponade, tension peumothorax, air embolus, or cardiac contusion is present.

Neurogenic shock results from the loss of vasomotor tone, which causes vasodilation in much of the peripheral vascular system. As a consequence, the blood volume becomes abnormally distributed in the peripheral vessels. Direct injury to the medullary vasomotor center or interruption of sympathetic innervation due to cervical or high thoracic spinal cord injury causes such a loss of vasomotor control. The classic picture of neurogenic shock is hypotension without tachycardia or cutaneous vasoconstriction. Intracranial injuries alone do not produce circulatory inadequacy until the brain stem and its reticular activating system are profoundly involved. Therefore, the presence of shock in a patient with a head injury indicates a search for another cause, such as internal bleeding from an abdominal injury.

For trauma patients who survive the first 3 days after injury, sepsis is the principal cause of death. *Septic shock* is uncommon immediately after a traumatic insult. How the patient presents with septic shock depends partly on his or her volume status. For example, septic patients who are also hypovolemic are difficult to distinguish clinically from those in hypovolemic shock. In contrast, in the normovolemic septic patient, an elevated cardiac output, tachycardia, low systemic vascular resistance, and warm, flushed extremities may be evidence of septic shock.

Classes of Shock

The initial assessment and resuscitation of trauma patients categorizes each patient into one of four classes of hypovolemic shock based on the amount of blood lost (**Table 15-1**). The classes are related to physiological responses and can be helpful in understanding the clinical manifestations.

Compensatory Mechanisms

During hypovolemic shock, circulatory reflexes and fluid shifts occur to compensate for the diminished blood volume. Circulatory reflexes trigger a response from the sympathetic nervous system when there is a blood loss greater than 10% of the total blood volume. The result is an increased heart rate as well as constriction of arterioles and veins in the peripheral circulation. Fortunately, sympathetic stimulation does not cause significant constriction of either the cerebral or cardiac vessels, although blood flow in many areas of the body is markedly diminished. Thus blood flow through the heart and brain is maintained at essentially normal levels until the mean arterial pressure falls below 60 mm Hg. Another compensatory mechanism that occurs over a number of hours is a fluid shift from the interstitial space to the vascular space, thereby increasing blood volume. Still another mechanism triggered by hypovolemia is increased release of the hormones aldosterone and antidiuretic hormone (ADH). Aldosterone increases renal sodium reabsorption and conserves intravascular water. ADH functions to increase water reabsorption in the kidney.

ADMINISTERING INTRAVENOUS FLUIDS

Initiating an Intravenous Line

In the presence of severe hypovolemia, the aim of fluid resuscitation is to quickly infuse large volumes of fluid so as to restore organ perfusion. To help accomplish this goal, two large-bore peripheral intravenous lines (minimum of 16 gauge) should be placed. Recall that flow of intravenous fluids depends directly on the internal diameter of the administration device and inversely on its length. Of course, other factors also influence fluid flow rate, such as the pressure under which the fluid is administered, the use of filters, and the size of the intravenous tubing. General principles to consider when intravenous fluids need to be infused rapidly are summarized here:

- Use the largest-diameter intravenous device available.
  - A large-diameter device offers less resistance to fluid flow. For example, in a laboratory setting, it was demonstrated that the flow rate via gravity through a 14-gauge device was much faster than

Table 15-1 Clinical Classes of Severity of Hypovolemic Shock After Hemorrhage

	Class I	Class II	Class III	Class IV
Blood loss (mL)	Up to 750	750–1500	1500–2000	> 2000
Blood loss (%)	Up to 15%	15–30%	30–40%	> 40%
Heart rate (beat per min)	< 100	> 100	> 120	> 140
Systolic blood pressure	Normal	Normal	Decreased	Decreased
Pulse pressure	Normal	Decreased	Decreased	Decreased
Respiratory rate	14–20	20–30	30–40	> 35
Capillary refill	Delayed	Delayed	Delayed	Delayed
Urine output (mL/hr)	> 30	20–30	5–15	Minimal
Mental status	Slightly anxious	Anxious	Confused	Confused and lethargic

Source: This table was published in Parillo JE & Dellinger RP. *Critical Care Medicine: Principles and Management in the Adult*, 3rd edition, p. 499. Copyright Elsevier, 2008.

that through an 18-gauge device (147 mL/min versus 87 mL/min).[2]
- Use the shortest intravenous device available.
  - The flow rate slows significantly as the length of the intravenous device increases.[3]
- Use the largest-diameter IV tubing set available.
  - Large-diameter tubing offers less resistance to flow rate. For example, the flow rate of a crystalloid solution via a 14-gauge device with large tubing is substantially faster than the flow of the solution via a 14-gauge device with regular-size tubing (417 mL/min versus 268 mL/min).[4]
- Select the most desirable infusion site.
  - Either a peripheral vein or a central vein may be used to administer intravenous fluids to a hypovolemic patient. In some patients, the intraosseous site is preferred (see the discussion later in this chapter). The site that will allow the quickest route for fluid resuscitation is the most desirable in most situations.

Site Selection

Peripheral Vein. It is possible to achieve high flow rates with a peripheral line; this is fortunate because peripheral veins are often easily accessible in emergency situations. Percutaneous access in the upper extremities is preferred, primarily in the forearms and antecubital veins. Extremities that show evidence of proximal injury should not be used because of the potential for venous extravasation and fluid loss.

Central Vein. When a peripheral site is not available, cannulation of the subclavian vein with a central line introducer (usually 8 Fr) may also be considered. Central sites for rapid fluid resuscitation include the subclavian, femoral, or internal jugular veins. These sites, when cannulated with large-diameter devices, can accept rapid flow rates. A standard 8.5 Fr short introducer sheath is commonly used. Later, this same device can be used as an introducer for a hemodynamic monitoring catheter.

Typical central venous catheters are not well suited for rapid fluid replacement because of their relatively small diameter and long length, which produces resistance to rapid flow rate. A wide variety of central venous catheters are in use. While most vary in length from 6 to 12 inches, those that are inserted by the peripheral route into a central vein are longer. Although some catheters have single lumens, most have two or more lumens. The gauge of the lumen and length of the catheter influence the maximal flow rate

through that particular IV line. For example, some catheters have triple lumens (two 18-gauge lumens and one 16-gauge lumen; in that event, the 16-gauge lumen would facilitate flow rate more quickly than either of the 18-gauge ports).

Intraosseous Site. Blood vessels in the intraosseous space connect to the central circulation, thus allowing the intraosseous space to be used for fluid administration. Although this route is primarily used in pediatric patients, its use in adults is becoming more common in military settings and occasionally in civilian prehospital settings. The intraosseous route is especially advantageous for blood administration in emergency settings when intravenous cannulation cannot be rapidly achieved. For example, in a population of emergency room patients, investigators found that proximal humerus intraosseous catheter placement was significantly faster than either peripheral intravenous or central venous catheter placement.[5] Medications may also be given via the intraosseous route.

The most commonly used site is the upper tibial end, approximately 2 to 3 cm medial and inferior to the tibial tuberosity.[6] For adults, a sternal intraosseous cannula system is available for use during shock and trauma. Contraindications for using an intraosseous device include fractures in the same extremity or previous surgery involving the target site; pain may be a concern in a conscious patient.[7]

Intraosseous infusion is viewed as a temporary emergency measure. According to the Infusion Nursing Society, the dwell time for an intraosseous device should be no more than 24 hours.[8] Complications that have been reported include extravasation of resuscitation fluids and medications[9] and compartment syndrome.[10]

Selection of Fluids

Crystalloids

Warmed isotonic sodium-containing fluids, such as lactated Ringer's (LR) solution and normal saline (NS; 0.9% sodium chloride), are used for initial resuscitation; both of these fluids are referred to as crystalloids. (Heating these solutions to 102.2°F helps prevent or reverse hypothermia in a trauma patient).[11] Lactated Ringer's solution is preferred in many settings, whereas normal saline is the second choice. Although NS is a satisfactory fluid, it has the potential to cause hyperchloremic acidosis, especially if renal function is impaired. Recall that NS contains 154 mEq of chloride per liter, whereas the plasma chloride concentration is close to 100 mEq/L. However, several situations in trauma patients could favor NS over LR. For example, for patients in renal failure, the small amount of potassium in LR may be a concern. Also, the slightly higher osmolality of NS might be better for patients with a closed head injury, where cerebral edema is a potential problem.[12] Recall that a hypotonic solution predisposes to brain swelling. Although LR is generally considered an isotonic solution, it has a lower osmolality than NS (274 mOsm/L compared to 308 mOsm/L).

For trauma victims, fluid resuscitation with isotonic electrolyte solutions is usually initiated in the field by medics. An initial fluid bolus of 1 to 2 L of an isotonic electrolyte solution is given as rapidly as possible for an adult; a dose of 20 mL/kg is used for a pediatric patient. (A pumping device or manual pumping is used to administer the fluid rapidly.) For children, the dose of 20 mL/kg can be repeated once; if there is no response to these two fluid boluses, blood transfusion and ongoing crystalloid infusion and perhaps blood transfusion are required. The patient's response to initial fluid administration must be observed and further action taken as needed. If the shock state fails to show signs of resolution after aggressive fluid replacement, the healthcare provider should suspect continued blood loss or inadequate fluid delivery.

It is possible that quickly elevating the blood pressure of a bleeding patient may make the bleeding worse. Thus, in addition to fluid replacement, the source of the bleeding needs to be identified and corrected.

Colloids

Colloids are solutions that rely on their high molecular weight to draw fluid from the extravascular space into the bloodstream. Because they tend to remain in the intravascular space longer than crystalloids, smaller volumes of colloids are needed to restore the circulating blood volume. Although smaller volumes are needed, colloids are significantly more expensive than crystalloids.[13] Among the available colloids are albumin, hydroxyethyl starches (such as Hespan and Voluven), dextran 40 and dextran 70, and gelatins. Chapter 10 describes these products in more depth. The next section compares the efficacy of colloids and crystalloids in hypovolemic trauma and surgical patients.

Crystalloids Versus Colloids. After administration of the first few liters of a crystalloid, a question arises as to when (or if) colloids should be added to the regimen. The main factors considered when deciding between crystalloids and colloids are the hemodynamic and pulmonary effects of the fluids. Some theorize that the greater volume of crystalloid solution (three to seven times that of a colloid) needed to attain adequate volume replacement predisposes patients to accumulation of fluid in the pulmonary interstitium. Others argue that colloids may also extravasate into the interstitial space if capillaries are damaged (endothelial leakiness), leading to ARDS and organ failure. It is likely that both the overall volume used and the presence or absence of sepsis affect pulmonary function to a far greater extent than does the type of resuscitation fluid used. In a review of randomized controlled trials that compared crystalloid resuscitation with a variety of colloids, the authors concluded that there is no evidence that resuscitation with colloids reduces risk of death, compared to resuscitation with crystalloids in postoperative or trauma patients.[14] They further concluded that because colloids are more expensive than crystalloids, it is difficult to justify their use outside the context of randomized controlled trials.

An interesting finding in a recent report was a significant correlation between a low ionized calcium concentration and the amount of colloid infused in a group of patients with severe trauma.[15] Among the suggested causative factors for this relationship were colloid-induced hemodilution, calcium binding to lactate and colloid solution, and severe shock. A similar association was not found between ionized calcium concentration and the amount of infused crystalloids.

Hypertonic Saline

Small-volume resuscitation of trauma victims with hypertonic saline (such as 7.5% NaCl with dextran or hetastarch) is of interest to the military and some segments of the civilian community.[16] Hypertonic sodium chloride solutions contain large concentrations of sodium, ranging from 250 to 1200 mEq/L; as a consequence, they are capable of expanding the plasma volume by pulling fluid from the interstitial and intracellular spaces into the intravascular space. Thus much smaller volumes of hypertonic saline (as compared to isotonic sodium solutions) are needed to increase the intravascular fluid volume. However, the efficacy of hypertonic saline in improving patient outcomes remains controversial.

Proponents of hypertonic saline suggest that this fluid is effective in providing for volume resuscitation in cases of combined hemorrhagic shock and head injury. For example, in a recent literature review, Strandvik indicated that hypertonic saline solutions are effective for blood pressure restoration in hemorrhagic shock and for reducing intracranial pressure in conditions that cause acute intracranial hypertension.[17] Nevertheless, some reports describe rebound increases in intracranial pressure after discontinuation of hypertonic saline in patients with brain injuries.[18] Others point out that cerebral dehydration could develop rapidly with subsequent bleeding, as could central pontine myelinolysis due to rapid variations in serum sodium levels.

Another consideration is that resuscitation with hypertonic saline can lead to hypernatremia and hyperosmolarity. An animal study suggested that hypertonic saline resuscitation after hemorrhagic shock may help protect against the development of lung injury, presumably by suppressing neutrophil activation.[19] However, no difference in ARDS-free overall survival was found when a comparison was made between a group of 110 trauma patients who received 250 mL of 7.5% hypertonic saline/6% dextran (HSD) and 99 trauma patients who received lactated Ringer's solution.[20] In the same study, a small subset of patients who required 10 units or more of packed red blood cells benefited from the HSD solution. The investigators suggested that the use of HSD may offer maximal benefit in patients at highest risk for ARDS.

The osmolality of hypertonic saline is such that it can damage the endothelium near the catheter insertion site if administered in a peripheral vein, resulting in severe thrombophlebitis. Thus administration via a central vein is recommended.[21] A study that compared the peripheral and central infusion of 7.5% NaCl/6% dextran 70 over a 2-minute period in a group of unanesthetized sheep found no damage at the injection sites either by gross inspection or by histologic examination.[22] However, the ability to extrapolate these findings to humans is questionable. Thus, if a central vein is not accessible, caution is needed to protect the infusion site. It has been suggested that concurrently infusing an isotonic crystalloid at the peripheral injection site may help prevent damage to the vein.[23] While care should be taken to avoid infiltration of all intravenous fluids into the local tissues, this consideration is especially important when hypertonic saline is being infused.

Blood

Current practice calls for keeping donor blood transfusions to a minimum because of their potential to decrease immune status as well as to stimulate an acute inflammatory response.[24] Nevertheless, blood replacement therapy is generally needed in patients with blood loss greater than 20% (see **Table 15-2**). The most highly preferred option is cross-matched blood. Cross-matching requires about an hour in most blood banks, however; in contrast, type-specific blood can usually be provided in 10 minutes.[25] Blood can be heated in specialized blood warmers.

Table 15-2 Responses to Initial Fluid Resuscitation*

	Rapid Response	Transitory Response	Minimal or No Response
Vital signs	Return to normal	Transitory improvement, recurrence of decreased blood pressure and increased heart rate	Remain abnormal
Estimated blood loss	Minimal (10%–20%)	Moderate and ongoing (20%–40%) ·	Severe (>40%)
Need for more crystalloid	Low	High	High
Need for blood	Low	Moderate to high	Immediate
Blood preparation	Type and cross-match	Type specific	Emergency blood release
Need for operative intervention	Possibly	Likely	Highly likely
Early presence of surgeon	Yes	Yes	Yes

*2000 mL of isotonic solution in adults; 20 mL/kg bolus of Ringer's lactate solution in children.

Source: Courtesy of *Advanced Trauma Life Support Student Course Manual,* 8th edition. Chicago: American College of Surgeons, 2008.

Essentially, donated blood that has not been fractionalized into various components is no longer available.[26] Instead, packed red blood cells (PRBCs) are primarily used to replace blood loss. These are obtained by centrifuging a unit of whole blood and drawing off 200 to 225 mL plasma, leaving a product with a hematocrit of approximately 70% and a volume of approximately 200 mL. When PRBCs are preserved with AS-1 Adsol solution, the hematocrit is decreased to roughly 53% and the unit volume is approximately 350 mL.[27] Platelets are given when thrombocytopenia is present.[28]

Electrolyte Problems Associated with Blood Transfusion

Hyperkalemia. Due to the hypoxia that occurs during their storage, red blood cells leak potassium into the plasma. For example, the plasma potassium concentration in stored blood may increase to 10 to 25 mEq/L or higher after 21 days of storage. When the red blood cells are infused into a recipient, the cells are reoxygenated and take up the extracellular potassium. If the blood is administered rapidly, however, transient hyperkalemia can occur before the cellular uptake of potassium has time to take place.

For example, 16 cases of cardiac arrest associated with hyperkalemia during red blood cell transfusion were reported in a group of 11 adults and 5 children during the perioperative period.[29] The mean serum potassium level during cardiac arrest was 7.2 mEq/L (range, 5.9 to 9.2 mEq/L). At the time of cardiac arrest, most of the patients had acidosis, hypocalcemia, and hypothermia. The number of units of red blood cells given before cardiac arrest ranged from 1 unit in a 2.7-kg neonate to 54 units in an adult. Fourteen of the patients received the blood via a central vein; the blood was delivered under pressure (by either infusion pump, pressure bag, or syringe). Interestingly, the investigators found that a 14-day-old unit of packed red blood cells had a serum potassium concentration of 77 mEq/L.

When possible, fresh blood should be used for patients with end-stage renal failure or other patients at high risk for hyperkalemia during transfusions.

Hypocalcemia. The citrate in preservatives added to blood products can combine with the patient's ionized calcium level and produce a deficit of ionized calcium. This outcome is most likely to occur in a patient who has received large volumes of fresh, frozen plasma or platelets.[30] A patient with good hepatic function is less likely to suffer from hypocalcemia because the liver converts the adminis-

tered citrate to bicarbonate. Another mechanism to protect against hypocalcemia is mobilization of calcium from the bone.

Hemodynamic parameters remain stable in most patients with transfusion-related hypocalcemia. However, hypocalcemic patients with underlying cardiac disease are at increased risk for hypotension and heart failure; these individuals may require calcium replacement therapy. Any patient whose ionized calcium level falls to 50% of the lower limit of normal range should receive calcium supplementation.[31]

pH Imbalances. The pH of 2-week-old bank blood is approximately 6.5, due to leakage of lactate and pyruvate into the plasma as a result of red blood cell hypoxia; thus metabolic acidosis is expected after massive blood transfusions. As a rule, metabolic acidosis is already present in patients who require large volumes of blood due their poor tissue perfusion. Metabolic alkalosis may eventually result during rapid transfusion because the citrate in the blood is metabolized into bicarbonate by the liver.

Artificial Blood

Artificial blood products that mimic human blood's oxygen transport ability have been evaluated in clinical trials. Among such products are polymerized hemoglobin solutions, also called hemoglobin-based oxygen carriers (HBOCs).[32] A meta-analysis of 16 randomized controlled trials of five different blood substitutes revealed that patients who received these products were at significantly increased risk for death and myocardial infarction compared to patients in control groups.[33]

Evaluating the Response to Fluid Resuscitation

It is extremely important to monitor a patient's response to fluid resuscitation because it is easy to give too little or too much fluid. Too little fluid predisposes patients to prolonged hypovolemia and decreased perfusion of major organs. Too much fluid can overwhelm the circulation and perhaps cause pulmonary edema. Volume overload is common in patients with shock during aggressive fluid resuscitation, because their compensatory mechanisms—that is, increased secretion of aldosterone and ADH—make it difficult for them to excrete fluid via the renal route. Even when the intravascular volume is not excessive, it is common for skin, muscles, and subcutaneous tissue to become edematous after massive volume resuscitation. This change occurs because approximately 75% of every liter of balanced salt solution shifts into the interstitial space within 1 hour after administration. Problems associated with the resulting soft-tissue edema include a decreased rate of wound healing and an increased propensity to develop pressure sores.

Some patients (usually those who have lost less than 20% of their blood volume) respond rapidly to the initial fluid bolus and remain stable when the infusion is slowed. No further fluid bolus or immediate blood administration is indicated for this group of patients, although cross-matched blood should be made available. Other patients respond to the initial fluid bolus but show signs of deterioration when the rate of fluid administration slows; most of these patients have lost 20% to 40% of their blood volume, or are still bleeding and require continued crystalloid administration as well as blood transfusion and surgical intervention. Little or no response to fluid resuscitation is seen in a small but significant percentage of injured patients. For most of these individuals, failure to respond to adequate crystalloid and blood administration indicates the need for unlimited blood and fluid resuscitation and immediate surgical intervention to control hemorrhage.

When active bleeding is taking place, an attempt may be made to give enough fluids to maintain organ perfusion without raising the patient's blood pressure to normal. Rapid elevation of blood pressure may make bleeding worse. It is important to remember that fluid resuscitation is a bridge to—but not a substitute for—control of bleeding.[34]

Noninvasive Clinical Signs

Traditionally, a patient's response to resuscitation therapy has been determined by a variety of noninvasive clinical indicators:

- Systolic blood pressure
- Heart rate
- Level of consciousness
- Urine output
- Pulse pressure

See Table 15-2 for a classification of responses to initial fluid resuscitation.

In an adult, an adequate urine output following resuscitation is approximately 0.5 mL/kg/hr; in a child, an adequate urine output is 1 mL/kg/hr.[35] For a child younger than the age of 1 year, an output of 2 mL/kg/hr should be maintained.[36] Although urine output is one of the primary indicators of response to fluid resuscitation, it can be affected by variables other than adequate fluid replace-

ment. For example, diuretics or vasopressors can increase urinary flow rate despite underlying tissue perfusion problems.

Hypoperfusion, and thus poor cellular oxygen delivery, can persist even when the conventional signs return to a normal range. For some patients, a pulmonary artery catheter is required to monitor fluid status. Other parameters to assess include hematocrit, blood pH, and lactate levels, which are discussed in the following sections.

Laboratory Studies

Hematocrit and Hemoglobin as Predictors of Need for Blood Replacement. Although a very low hematocrit suggests significant blood loss or preexisting anemia, an early near-normal hematocrit does not rule out significant blood loss (see Case Study 15-1). Thus reliance on hemoglobin and hematocrit values alone is unreliable in initially estimating the degree of blood loss because up to 4 hours may elapse before any significant changes are evident.

After fluid shifts from the extravascular space into the bloodstream have occurred, a hematocrit less than 30% or a hemoglobin concentration less than 10 g/dL are sometimes viewed as triggers for the administration of packed red blood cells to provide oxygen-carrying capacity to the tissues. However, the hemoglobin concentration at which blood transfusion should be initiated is controversial.[37]

Theoretically, in a 70-kg person, a unit of blood will increase the hematocrit by 3% and the hemoglobin concentration by 1 g/dL. However, this assumption has been challenged by findings from a retrospective study of 61 transfusions in 48 patients with pelvic fractures.[38]

Lactate Levels to Assess Tissue Oxygenation. Serum lactate determinations have been used to assess the adequacy of tissue oxygenation in critically ill patients. When intracellular oxygen is not available, energy is produced by anaerobic metabolic pathways, resulting in increased lactate production. Thus an elevated serum lactate level is an indirect measure of oxygen deficiency and can be used to approximate the magnitude and duration of the severity of shock.[39]

A blood lactate level in a critically ill patient is generally considered to be abnormal if it is greater than 2.0 mmol/L; a level greater than 4.0 mmol/L is considered to be significantly elevated and a sign of poor tissue perfusion.[40] Blood lactate levels can be measured in arterial, central venous, or peripherally obtained specimens; apparently there is good correlation between results from samples acquired from different locations.[41] When peripherally drawn blood is used for lactate measurement, it is preferred that a tourniquet not be used (since the prolonged use of a tourniquet may cause a falsely elevated reading).[42]

Blood lactate measurement is an important adjunct in determining shock severity; for example, in a large study of trauma patients admitted to a level I trauma center, researchers reported that blood lactate levels were a better predictor of the need for significant transfusions than were systolic blood pressure readings.[43] Fortunately, point-of-care devices are available for the measurement of blood lactate in pre-hospital settings.

Factors to consider include the admission lactate level, the highest lactate level, and the time interval to normalization of the serum lactate level.[44] For example, a prospective study was reported in which 76 consecutive patients with multiple trauma had serum lactate levels measured on ICU admission and again at 8, 16, 24, 36, and 48 hours after admission.[45] All of the patients whose lactate levels normalized in 24 hours survived. In contrast, the survival rate fell to 75% in patients whose lactate levels normalized between 24 and 48 hours. Only 3 of the 22 patients whose lactate levels remained elevated at 48 hours survived.

Base Deficit to Assess Tissue Oxygenation. Base deficit is usually measured during arterial blood gas analysis and is an assessment of the degree of metabolic acidosis present. Base deficit can be categorized as mild (3–5 mmol/L), moderate (6–14 mmol/L) or severe ($\geq$ 15 mmol/L).[46] An elevated base deficit in the trauma patient may indicate ongoing bleeding.

Acid–Base and Electrolyte Changes. The majority of acid–base abnormalities that develop in shock improve spontaneously once adequate ventilation and perfusion are achieved. Early in hypovolemic shock, respiratory alkalosis occurs due to tachypnea; it is followed by a mild metabolic acidosis. Patients with severe traumatic injury and hemorrhagic shock become acidotic as a result of loss of oxygen-carrying capacity and decreased cardiac output. As lactate and hydrogen ions accumulate during shock, a high anion gap metabolic acidosis develops. Respiratory acidosis will also develop as the number of functional pulmonary capillaries decreases, causing carbon dioxide (CO_2) retention. In the final stages of shock, a combination of metabolic and respiratory acidosis results in an increase in the arterial carbon dioxide tension ($PaCO_2$), a low bicarbonate level, and a very low pH.

Hemodynamic Parameters

Central Venous Pressure. The response of the central venous pressure (CVP) to fluid administration (when properly interpreted) helps evaluate the adequacy of volume replacement. Some points to remember about CVP measurements are summarized here:

1. CVP is an indirect measure of volume.
2. Normal CVP is in the range of 0 to 7 mm Hg when a transducer system is used; it is in the range of 1 to 10 cm H_2O when a water manometer is used.
3. CVP is often low in hypovolemic shock because of inadequate filling of the right side of the heart.
4. The initial CVP and actual blood volume are not necessarily related.
5. A high CVP may be observed even with a volume deficit. For example, patients with generalized vasoconstriction and fluid replacement may show a high pressure related to the application of pneumatic anti-shock garment or inappropriate use of vasopressors.
6. A minimal rise in the initial, low CVP with fluid therapy suggests the need for further volume expansion.
7. A decrease in CVP suggests an ongoing fluid loss.
8. An abrupt or persistent elevation in CVP suggests that volume replacement has been adequate or is too rapid
9. CVP is best monitored in terms of trends, especially in response to fluid therapy.

Pulmonary Capillary Wedge Pressure. The pulmonary capillary wedge pressure (PCWP) is a measure of preload, which reflects left ventricular end-diastolic volume; this measure is easily obtained at the bedside from the pulmonary artery catheter. Although CVP and PCWP do not reflect blood volume accurately in all patients, they are useful measures when healthcare providers are trying to prevent acute volume overload during rapid fluid restoration and fluid challenges. In critically ill patients, a PCWP in the range of 15 to 18 mm Hg is the goal to increase cardiac output.[47]

Shock Index. In a retrospective study of more than 16,000 patients, a group of investigators concluded that the shock index (SI) may help clinicians measure hemodynamic stability in patients at risk for hemorrhagic shock better than using heart rate or systolic blood pressure alone.[48] The shock index is calculated as heart rate divided by systolic blood pressure. The normal range for the shock index is 0.5–0.7; a value greater than 1.0 is associated with increased mortality.[49]

CASE STUDIES

Case Study 15-1

After undergoing a sigmoid colectomy and splenectomy, a 47-year-old man was returned to the postoperative recovery room at noon in good condition. At that time, he was receiving lactated Ringer's solution through an 18-gauge port of a triple-lumen central venous catheter (CVC). His vital signs were normal, as was perfusion of the kidneys and brain, as evidenced by an adequate level of consciousness and urinary output. Approximately 4 hours later, he developed seizure-type activity and became unresponsive. At that time, the following vital signs were obtained:

- Blood pressure: 44/20 mm Hg
- Heart rate: 136 beats/min
- CVP: 0 cm H_2O
- Rapid gasping respirations

Blood work was drawn and showed a hemoglobin of 11 g/dL and a hematocrit of 36%. No bleeding was noted from the abdominal incision. The physician was notified. The IV line was immediately turned to "wide open" through the 18-gauge port of the CVC, and 2 units of PRBCs were given through the 16-gauge port of the CVC (with the assistance of a pressure cuff). Despite this intervention, the patient's vital signs remained extremely poor, urine output was almost nil, and full consciousness was never regained. His hemoglobin dropped to 6 g/dL and the hematocrit to 19%.

The patient was returned to surgery, where a short 14-gauge catheter was inserted in the external jugular vein; warmed blood and crystalloids were pumped in through this device. An exploratory laparotomy revealed that a ligature had slipped from the splenic artery and the patient's abdomen was filled with blood. Despite aggressive fluid resuscitation in the operating room and control of bleeding, the patient did not survive.

Commentary. Because a major compensatory shift of fluid from the extravascular extracellular space into the vascular space (to help replace the diminished blood supply) had not had time to occur, the patient's hemoglobin and hematocrit values were close to normal at the time of the hemorrhagic event. Later, hemodilution from this process became more obvious (hemoglobin, 6 g/dL; hematocrit, 19%). The patient's clinical status did not improve despite IV fluid given "wide open" because the fluids were administered via gravity with the flow control

clamp wide open. Because a small port (18 gauge) of a long, narrow CVC was used, the fluid met resistance as it attempted to flow through the catheter. (One could equate this scenario to using a long, narrow ordinary garden hose to apply water to a major fire; ideally, one would use a wide short hose for this purpose, preferably with the water delivered under pressure). Failure of the patient to respond to the inadequate fluid regimen described in the case was an indication that more aggressive fluid resuscitation (along with more rapid surgical intervention) was urgently needed.

A lack of visible incisional bleeding is insufficient to rule out hemorrhagic shock after abdominal surgery. In this instance, the patient was bleeding internally. All other clinical signs pointed to hemorrhagic shock; unfortunately, they went unrecognized.

Although placement of a pulmonary catheter is often helpful in the early diagnosis of hypovolemic shock and to allow titration of fluids during resuscitation to achieve a satisfactory outcome, this patient could have been managed without a pulmonary artery catheter. The blood pressure, heart rate, and CVP should have guided treatment to more aggressive fluid resuscitation along with more rapid surgical intervention. Clinical indicators of hypovolemic shock were obvious, as was the inadequate clinical response to too little fluid resuscitation.

Case Study 15-2

A 56-year-old man was trapped between two railroad cars in a mining accident. He was hypotensive at the scene of the accident and was resuscitated with 3000 mL lactated Ringer's solution before being transported to a trauma center. On arrival, he was anxious and confused. His vital signs were as follows:

- Blood pressure: 98/60 mm Hg
- Pulse rate: 120/min
- Respiratory rate: 40/min
- Estimated blood loss at this time: 2000 mL

The patient was given an additional 3000 mL of lactated Ringer's solution before being rushed to surgery. During surgery, he was found to have the following injuries: right diaphragmatic hernia, herniation of kidney and liver into the thoracic cavity, liver laceration, avulsion of the right ureter from the renal pelvis, injury to the lumbar vessels, crush injury to the head of the pancreas, and serosal tears of the duodenum. The surgical procedure consisted of an exploratory laparotomy with ligation of bleeding lumber vessels, a repair of the right renal vein, a right nephrectomy, repair of the diaphragm, drainage of the pancreatic injury, and repair of the duodenal serosal tears. During surgery, the patient received the following fluids:

- 5% albumin: 500 mL
- Fresh frozen plasma: 785 mL
- Hetastarch: 500 mL
- Platelets: 200 mL
- PRBCs: 12 units
- 0.9% NaCl: 1000 mL

Urinary output from the time of admission through the end of the surgical procedure was 2,000 mL. The total estimated blood loss from the time of injury was 5000 mL. Because of the need for rapid fluid resuscitation, fluids were warmed and administered under pressure with a fluid infusion warming system.

Vital signs and other data available from the time of admission through the first 24 hours were as shown in Table A. Arterial lactate levels and hematocrit levels were as shown in Table B.

Total intake from the time of injury through the first 24 hours was 20,035 mL; urine output during this time was 6900 mL. During this same period, the patient sustained an estimated blood loss of 5000 mL.

Commentary. This patient was experiencing class III shock (see Table 15-1) at the time of his admission to the trauma center (based on estimated blood loss, vital signs, and mental status). His condition worsened during the surgical procedure. (Note the increased heart rate and lowered blood pressure at the third surgical hour.) See Table A.

On admission, the patient had a combination of metabolic acidosis and respiratory acidosis. For example, the bicarbonate level was below normal (18 mEq/L). The *expected* $PaCO_2$ in this situation would be calculated as follows (using Winter's formula; see Chapter 9): 1.5 (18) + 8 $\pm$ 2 = 33–37 mm Hg. In reality, it was 44 mm Hg, indicating an excess of $PaCO_2$.

Adding the urinary output to the estimated blood loss, the patient lost a total of approximately 12 L of fluid; during the same period, he gained about 20 L by the IV route. The discrepancy of about 8 L can partially be explained by third-

Table A

	Hour 1 (ER)	Hour 3 (OR)	Hour 5 (OR)	Hour 10 (ICU)	Hour 16 (ICU)	Hour 22 (ICU)	Hour 24 (ICU)
Heart rate (beats/min)	120	130	118	98	110	118	113
Blood pressure (mm Hg)	98/60	< 60	110/70	166/90	138/78	136/76	140/80
CVP (mm Hg)	—	—	—	6	2	5	13
PCWP (mm Hg)	—	—	—	3	2	6	12

Table B

	Hr 1 (ER)	Hr 12 (ICU)	Hr 18 (ICU)	Hr 24 (ICU)
Lactate (mmol/L)	—	5.8	3.6	1.8
Hematocrit (%)	26	—	—	33

spacing caused by the initial trauma as well as trauma sustained during the surgical procedures. The third-spacing resulted in hypovolemia as fluid shifted from the vascular space into the injured tissues. Fluid was administered in sufficient quantities to keep the vital signs and other parameters within normal limits.

The serum lactate level may be used to assess adequacy of fluid resuscitation. Note how these readings improved from hour 12 to hour 24. Other parameters that improved with resuscitation were vital signs (blood pressure and pulse), hemodynamic readings (CVP and PCWP), hematocrit values, and arterial blood gas values.

Case Study 15-3

A case was reported in which a 39-year-old man sustained a life-threatening injury due to stabbing of the abdomen.[50] While in transit to the emergency department, he received 2100 mL of lactated Ringer's solution via a large-bore catheter. Upon admission, his heart rate was 156 and the patient was pale with delayed capillary refill in all extremities. His body temperature was 92.9°F. A Thermister Foley catheter was placed to monitor the core body temperature. Laboratory results revealed a hematocrit of 29.8% and a hemoglobin of 9.9 g/dL. Arterial blood gases revealed metabolic acidosis (pH, 7.24;, HCO_3, 15 mEq/L; $PaCO_2$, 35.4 mm Hg). An abdominal ultrasound revealed hemoperitoneum. The Glasgow Coma Score was 7, and blood toxicology screening revealed the presence of alcohol and cocaine.

Upon arrival to the emergency department, the patient received an additional 300 mL of warmed LR. The patient's blood pressure fell to 61/31 mm Hg. Within 16 minutes of admission to the emergency department, the patient was taken to the operating room with an infusion of LR "wide open." In the OR, the patient's hematocrit level decreased to 19% and he consequently received 8 units of packed red blood cells in addition to large volumes of LR. According to the surgeon, the patient had lost 5 L of blood (equivalent to his entire blood volume). During the first 10 days of hospitalization, the patient received a total of 24 units of packed red blood cells in addition to 11 units of fresh, frozen plasma and 8 units of platelets.

Commentary. This patient displayed classic symptoms of hypovolemic shock. As is typical for hypovolemic shock, the patient was hypothermic (necessitating the placement of warmed blankets and a warming light). The profoundly low

hemoglobin and hematocrit levels clearly indicated the need for multiple units of packed red blood cells; in addition, crystalloids in the form of lactated Ringer's solution were administered, all in an attempt to maintain the patient's blood volume. The metabolic acidosis was caused by poor tissue perfusion secondary to hypovolemia. Surgical correction of the bleeding site was life-saving, as were the multiple blood transfusions and other therapies.

Summary of Key Points

- Although any type of shock is possible in a patient with trauma or a recent surgical procedure, hypovolemic shock from hemorrhage is most likely.
- When rapid fluid resuscitation is needed in an adult, two large-bore peripheral intravenous lines (minimum of 16 gauge) should be placed. If this is not possible, the intraosseous route should be considered.
- The best type of fluid to use for resuscitation varies with the specific situation, but by far the most commonly used is an isotonic electrolyte solution—either lactated Ringer's solution or isotonic saline (0.9% sodium chloride). Also available are hypertonic saline, colloids, and blood.
- The extent of hemorrhage often cannot be determined visually; thus a variety of methods are used to assess the degree of hypovolemic shock. (See Table 15-1.)
- Observation of vital signs is helpful in determining whether the patient is responding adequately to fluid resuscitation. (See Table 15-2.)

NOTES

1. Sheridan, R. L. (2004). *The trauma handbook of the Massachusetts General Hospital.* Philadelphia: Lippincott Williams & Wilkins, p. 81.
2. Dutky, P. A., Stevens, S. L., & Maull, K .I. (1989). Factors affecting rapid fluid resuscitation with large-bore introducer catheters. *Journal of Trauma, 29,* 856–860.
3. Landow, L., & Shahnarian, A. (1990). Efficacy of large bore intravenous fluid administration sets designed for rapid volume resuscitation. *Critical Care Medicine, 18,* 540–543.
4. Dutky et al., note 2.
5. Paxton, J. H., Knuth, T. E., & Klausner, H. A. (2009). Proximal humerus intraosseous infusion: A preferred emergency venous access. *Journal of Trauma, Injury, Infection and Critical Care, 67*(3), 606–611.
6. Tareq, A. A. (2008). Gangrene of the leg following intraosseous infusion. *Annals of Saudi Medicine, 28,* 456–457.

7. Infusion Nurses Society. (2009). The role of the registered nurse in the insertion of intraosseous access devices. *Journal of Infusion Nursing, 32*(4), 187–188.

8. Infusion Nurses Society, note 7.

9. Tareq, note 6.

10. Moen, T. C., & Sarwark, J. F. (2008). Compartment syndrome following intraosseous infusion. *Orthopedics, 31*(8), 815.

11. *Advanced trauma life support student course manual* (8th ed.). (2008). Chicago: American College of Surgeons, p. 65.

12. Sheridan, note 1, p. 185.

13. Bongard, F. S., Sue, D. Y., & Vintch, J. R. (2008). *Current diagnosis and treatment: Critical care* (3rd ed.). New York: McGraw-Hill/Lange.

14. Perel, P., & Roberts, I. (2007). Colloids versus crystalloids for fluid resuscitation in critical ill patients. *Cochrane Database of Systematic Reviews, 4*, CD000567.

15. Vivien, B., Langeron, O., Morell, E., Devilliers, C., Carli, P. A., Coriat, P., et al. (2005). Early hypocalcemia in severe trauma. *Critical Care Medicine, 33*(9), 1946–1952.

16. Dubick, M. A., Bruttig, S. P., & Wade, C. E. (2006). Issues of concern regarding the use of hypertonic/hyperoncotic fluid resuscitation of hemorrhagic hypotension. *Shock, 25*(4), 321–328.

17. Strandvik, G. F. (2009). Hypertonic saline in critical care: A review of the literature and guidelines for use in hypotensive states and raised intracranial pressure. *Anaesthesia, 64*, 999–1003.

18. Doyle, J. A., Davis, D. P, & Hoyt, D. B. (2001). The use of hypertonic saline in the treatment of traumatic brain injury. *Journal of Trauma Injury Infection & Critical Care, 50*, 367–383.

19. Angle, N., Hoyt, D. B., Coimbra, R., Liu, F., Herdon-Remelius, C., Loomis, W., et al. (1998). Hypertonic saline resuscitation diminishes lung injury by suppressing neutrophil activation after hemorrhage. *Shock, 9*, 164–170.

20. Bulger, E. M., Jurkovich, G. J., Nathens, A. G., Copass, M. K., Hanson, S., Cooper, C., et al. (2008). Hypertonic resuscitation of hypovolemic shock after blunt trauma. *Archives of Surgery, 143*(2), 139–148.

21. Zubkov, A. Y., & Wijdicks, E. F. (2009). Reversal of transtentorial herniation with hypertonic saline. *Neurology, 72*, 200–201.

22. Hands, R., Holcroft, J. W., Perron, P. R., & Kramer, G. C. (1988). Comparison of peripheral and central infusions of 7.5% NaCl/6% dextran 70. *Surgery, 103*, 684–689.

23. Johnson, A. L., & Criddle, L. M. (2004). Pass the salt: Indications for and implications of using hypertonic saline. *Critical Care Nurse, 24*, 36–46.

24. Malone, D. L., Dunne, J., Tracy, J. K., Putnam, A. T., Scalea, T. M., & Napolitano, L. M. (2003). Blood transfusion, independent of shock severity, is associated with worse outcome in trauma. *Journal of Trauma-Injury Infection & Critical Care, 54*, 898–907.

25. *Advanced trauma life support student course manual*, note 11, p. 66.

26. Sheridan, note 1, p. 133.

27. Sheridan, note 1, p. 133.

28. Muhlberg, A. H., & Ruth-Sahd, L. (2004). Holistic care: Treatment and interventions for hypovolemic shock secondary to hemorrhage. *Dimensions in Critical Care Nursing, 23*(2), 55–59.

29. Smith, H. M., Farrow, S. J., Ackerman, J. D., Stubbs, J. R., & Sprung, J. (2008). Cardiac arrests associated with hyperkalemia during red blood cell transfusion: A case series. *Anesthesia & Analgesia, 106*(4), 1062–1069.

30. Sheridan, note 1, p. 143.

31. Sheridan, note 1, p. 144.

32. Santry, H. P., & Alam, H. B. (2010). Fluid resuscitation: past, present, and the future. Shock. *33*(3), 229–241.

33. Natanson, C., Kern, S. J., Lurie, P., Banks, S. M., & Wolfe, S. M. (2008). Cell-free hemoglobin based blood substitutes and risk of myocardial infarction and death: A meta-analysis. *Journal of the American Medical Association, 299*(19), 2304–2312.

34. *Advanced trauma life support student course manual*, note 11, p. 64.

35. *Advanced trauma life support student course manual*, note 11, p. 64.

36. *Advanced trauma life support student course manual*, note 11, p. 64.

37. Bongard et al., note 13, p. 230.

38. Elzik, M. E., Dirschi, D. R., & Dahners, L. E. (2006). Correlation of transfusion volume to change in hematocrit. *American Journal of Hematology, 81*, 145–146.

39. Kruse, J. A., & Carlson, R. W. (1987). Lactate metabolism. *Critical Care Clinics. 3(4)* 725–746.

40. Strehlow, M. C. (2010). Early identification of shock in critically ill patients. *Emergency Medical Clinics of North America, 28*, 57–66.

41. Weil, M. H., Michaels, S., & Rackow, E. C. (1987). Comparison of blood lactate concentrations in central venous, pulmonary artery, and arterial blood. *Critical Care Medicine. 15*, 489.

42. Strehlow, note 40.

43. Vandromme, M. J., Griffin, R. L., Weinberg, J. A., Rue, L. W., & Kerby, J. D. (2010). Lactate is a better predictor than systolic blood pressure for determining blood requirement and mortality: Could prehospital measures improve trauma triage? *Journal of American College of Surgeons, 210*, 861–869.

44. Brunicardi, F. C., Andersen, D., Billiar, T. R., Dunn, D. L., Hunger, J. G., & Pollock, R. E. (2005). *Schwartz's principles of surgery.* (8th ed.). New York: McGraw-Hill Medical Publishing Division, p. 103.

45. Abramson, D., Scalea, T. M., Hitchcock, R., Trooskin, S. Z., Henry, S. M., & Greenspan, J. (1993). Lactate clearance and survival following injury. *Journal of Trauma-Injury Infection & Critical Care, 35*(4), 584–589.

46. Brunicardi et al., note 44, p. 103.

47. Packman, M. I., & Rackow, E. C. (1983). Optimum left heart filling pressure during fluid resuscitation of patients with hypovolemic and septic shock. *Critical Care Medicine, 11*, 165–169.

48. Zarzaur, B. L., Croce, M. A., Fischer, P. E., Magnotti, L. J., & Fabian, T. C. (2008). New vitals after injury: Shock index for the young and age x shock index for the old. *Journal of Surgical Research, 147*, 229–236.

49. Oh, J. M., Cline, D. M., Tintinalli, J. E., Kelen, G. D., & Stapczynski, J. S. (2004). *Emergency medicine manual* (6th ed.). New York: McGraw Hill.

50. Muhlberg & Ruth-Sahd, note 28.

Chapter 16

Congestive Heart Failure: Fluid and Electrolyte Problems

Congestive heart failure (CHF) is a condition in which the heart is unable to pump sufficient blood to the kidneys and other organs, producing a variety of symptoms (**Table 16-1**). Fluid and electrolyte imbalances associated with CHF (**Table 16-2**) are due to the disease process itself as well as to side effects of some of the medications used to treat this condition. Descriptions of these imbalances are provided in this chapter.

FLUID VOLUME EXCESS

Shunting of blood away from the kidneys following decreased cardiac output stimulates the renin-angiotensin II-aldosterone (RAA) system. Angiotensin II is a strong arterial vasoconstrictor that helps to support arterial blood pressure. While RAA stimulation is critical in maintaining arterial pressure, the associated renal vasoconstriction results in renal sodium and water retention. Prolonged poor renal perfusion can lead to renal dysfunction in patients with advanced CHF; in this instance, even a modest increase in serum creatinine is associated with greater risk for cardiovascular morbidity and mortality.[1] Because excessive aldosterone secretion causes sodium and water retention, the patient with CHF typically presents with an expanded extracellular fluid (ECF) volume, evidenced by swollen legs, engorged neck veins, congested liver, and pulmonary crackles.

Stretching of the cardiac wall in CHF patients increases the synthesis and release of atrial and brain natriuretic peptides, substances that help to offset excessive peripheral vascular vasoconstriction. Brain natriuretic peptide (BNP) has several physiological effects, including vasodilatation and increase in excretion of sodium (natriuresis) and fluid (diuresis).[2] Brain natriuretic peptide (BNP) and N-terminal proBNP are used as specific markers in patients with suspected congestive heart failure, especially in emergency departments.[3]

Clinical Signs

Weight Gain

Weight gain usually occurs initially with CHF because of abnormal retention of fluid. A simple, yet effective method for monitoring fluid volume status is to measure daily body weights. For accuracy, it is best to use the same scale and perform the procedure at the same time each day. Any change in daily weight of more than 0.25 kg (0.5 lb) can be assumed to have resulted from changes in total body fluid; thus these measures can be used to monitor the effectiveness of therapy with diuretics and other medications. Early in the therapeutic period, a baseline body weight should be obtained to compare with subsequent weight measurements so as to monitor response to treatment. Daily weight measurements provide valuable information for both hospitalized and home patients. Home-care patients may be taught to chart their weight and to consult a healthcare provider if a rapid gain of more than 1 kg (2.2 lb) occurs. If fluid intake is being monitored, it will be noted that fluid intake exceeds fluid output in case of rapid weight gain.

Weight Loss

As CHF becomes chronic, unintentional weight loss with muscle wasting (cardiac cachexia) may occur. Dietary caloric supplementation may be helpful in stemming this loss; however, anabolic steroids are not recommended because of risk for fluid retention.[4]

Table 16-1 Signs and Symptoms Associated with Congestive Heart Failure

Symptom or Sign	Possible Cause(s)
Dyspnea on exertion, later at rest	Cardiac output inadequate to provide for the increased oxygen required by exertion (results in increased breathing effort).
	Pulmonary congestion with accumulation of interstitial or intra-alveolar fluid.
	Respiratory muscle fatigue.
Edema (initially in dependent parts, later generalized)	Hydrostatic pressure is greatest in dependent parts of the body. Eventually, progressive heart failure causes a substantial increase in hydrostatic pressure in all parts of the body.
Orthopnea	Redistribution of fluid from the splanchnic circulation and lower extremities into the central circulation during recumbency with increased pulmonary capillary pressure.
Cough	Elevated pulmonary capillary pressure causes transudation of serum into the alveoli, which causes pulmonary congestion and diminished oxygen–carbon dioxide exchange.
Paroxysmal nocturnal dyspnea in left-sided heart failure	When recumbent, edema fluid from dependent parts of the body returns to the bloodstream, increasing preload. Increased pressure in bronchial arteries leads to airway compression and interstitial pulmonary edema.
Decreased urinary output	Decreased cardiac output and renal perfusion results in secondary hyperaldosteronism, which causes sodium and water retention. Increased antidiuretic hormone (arginine vasopressin) causes water retention.
Nocturia	While resting at night, deficit in cardiac output in relation to oxygen demands is reduced, leading to decreased renal vasoconstriction and increased glomerular filtration rate.
Tachycardia, various dysrhythmias	Effort to compensate for decreased cardiac output; arrhythmias may be stimulated by hypoxia, digitalis toxicity, hypokalemia, or hypomagnesemia.
Anorexia, nausea, and vomiting	Edema of bowel wall and liver.
	Impulses arising from the dilated myocardium in acute heart failure.
	Digitalis toxicity.
Confusion, mood disturbances	Reduced cerebral perfusion—most likely in elderly patients with cerebral arteriosclerosis.

Peripheral Edema

The patient should be taught to monitor for fluid retention by noting tight shoes or tight clothing as the day progresses. Clinicians can assess serial changes in edema by measuring extremities with a millimeter tape. Pitting edema can be assessed for by compressing the tissues over a bone (such as the tibia).

Management

Diuretics

Diuretics are a valuable aid in the symptomatic treatment of CHF. Their primary purpose is to promote sodium and water excretion via the kidney, thereby lowering intravascular volume. Data obtained from daily weight measurements and fluid intake and output (I & O) records are invaluable in regulating diuretic dosage and dietary sodium restriction.

Because orally administered diuretics (such as furosemide) may be poorly absorbed by the GI tract due to congested abdominal organs, it is sometimes necessary to administer diuretics by the IV route to achieve positive therapeutic results. The relationship between diuretics and potassium balance is discussed later in this chapter.

Poor response to diuretic therapy may be due to lack of compliance with the drug regimen, or to progression of the underlying heart failure. In severe cases of fluid retention that do not respond to diuretic therapy, ultrafiltration and dialysis may be used.[5]

Dietary Sodium/Fluid Restriction

Restriction of dietary sodium is a valuable aid in the management of CHF (see Chapter 4 for a discussion of low-sodium diets). In general, a decrease in sodium intake results in a decrease in fluid volume. Authorities generally recommend a sodium intake of no more than 2–3 g/day.[6,7]

Table 16-2 Fluid and Electrolyte Disturbances Associated with Congestive Heart Failure

Disturbance	Etiology
Fluid volume excess	Secondary hyperaldosteronism results from decreased renal blood flow associated with decreased cardiac output.
	Excessive aldosterone causes excessive sodium and water retention.
Hyponatremia	Although the total body sodium content is above normal, excessive secretion of antidiuretic hormone (ADH) causes relatively greater retention of water, thereby diluting the serum sodium concentration.
	Contributors to hyponatremia may include vomiting, diarrhea, and large doses of diuretics.
Hypokalemia	Excessive aldosterone levels predispose patients to potassium excretion.
	Excessive use of potassium-losing diuretics may lead to hypokalemia.
	Contributors to hypokalemia include diarrhea and vomiting.
Hypomagnesemia	Similar mechanisms to those described for hypokalemia.
	Most likely to be problematic in patients with moderately severe to severe congestive heart failure who are receiving long-term or aggressive thiazides or loop diuretic therapy.
Hyperkalemia	Caused by excessive use of potassium-sparing diuretics, potassium supplements, or angiotensin-converting enzyme inhibitors in patients with renal dysfunction.
Metabolic (lactic) acidosis	Increased liberation of lactic acid from anoxic tissues occurs, and the body fails to metabolize it rapidly.
	Slowing of circulation interferes with the excretion of metabolic acids.
Respiratory acidosis	Pulmonary congestion interferes with elimination of CO_2 from the lungs.

For recently hospitalized or unstable patients, an intake much lower than 2–3 g/day may be appropriate. Aggressive attempts to lower sodium intake might not be warranted in stable patients on a complicated medical regimen who have become acclimated to a higher sodium intake.[8]

The degree of sodium restriction necessary to control edema varies with the degree of rest, dosage, and type of diuretic. For example, an ambulatory patient requires more extensive sodium restriction than a patient on bedrest because rest in itself encourages diuresis. A patient receiving potent diuretics has less need for severe sodium restriction than one not receiving diuretics. Indeed, a drastic reduction of sodium intake can be dangerous to the patient who is taking a potent diuretic, particularly during bouts of abnormal sodium loss, such as occurs with vomiting or diarrhea.

Control of Fluid Intake

Reduction of fluid intake (such as to less than 2000 mL in 24 hours) may be necessary for CHF patients who experience recurrent fluid retention despite sodium restriction and use of diuretics.[9,10] The degree of fluid restriction should not be so severe that it allows the patient to become volume depleted because volume depletion further impairs cardiac output by decreasing the preload's stimulation of cardiac contractility. Patients who are receiving care at home must understand the precise fluid regimen best suited for their condition and recognize those situations that can complicate this regimen (such as increased fluid loss in vomiting and diarrhea).

Hemodynamic monitoring offers a means to determine the appropriate fluid replacement therapy in seriously ill patients with CHF. Frequent checks of central venous pressure and pulmonary capillary wedge pressures during fluid administration can give an early warning of circulatory overload or underload and guide the safe administration of needed water and electrolytes.

Avoidance of NSAIDs

Use of nonsteroidal anti-inflammatory drugs (NSAIDs) can markedly decrease renal blood flow in individuals with heart failure and predispose these patients to fluid retention. Thus heart failure patients who are unexplainably resistant to diuretics should be questioned about NSAID use. Treatment with selective COX-2 inhibitors and nonselective NSAIDs has been shown to be associated with increased mortality in patients with chronic heart failure.[11] In a study involving more than 39,000 patients with heart failure, rofecoxib was associated with the highest risk and showed a dose-dependent increase in risk.[12] A recent recommendation from the American Heart Association is to avoid COX-2 inhibitors in patients with established or increased risk for cardiovascular disease; another recommendation is to consider alternative pain medications for these patients before selecting NSAIDS.[13]

PULMONARY EDEMA

Patients with cardiogenic pulmonary edema usually have an identifiable cause of acute left ventricular failure, such as an arrhythmia or ischemia/infarction.[14] Cardiogenic pulmonary edema presents an emergency situation and results from an excessive accumulation of water in the lungs due to left ventricular failure. To deal with it, the patient should be quickly placed in a high Fowler's position with legs dangling from the side of the bed to reduce venous pressure and preload. This position facilitates better ventilation and decreased work of breathing. Humidified oxygen is best delivered by a face mask. In extreme cases, endotracheal intubation and mechanical ventilation may be needed. Positive end-expiratory pressure (PEEP) may be used, albeit with caution because an excessive increase in intrathoracic pressure compromises cardiac output.

A variety of medications are indicated in patients with pulmonary edema. Furosemide (a loop diuretic) is the diuretic of choice in most situations. It acts as a venodilator and can reduce preload rapidly, prior to any diuretic effect becoming apparent.[15] Sublingual nitroglycerin, a vasodilator, is considered first-line therapy for acute cardiogenic pulmonary edema.[16] Morphine is a transient venodilator that relieves dyspnea and anxiety while also reducing preload. Angiotensin-converting enzyme (ACE) inhibitors may be used in hypertensive patients.[17]

Patients with acute pulmonary edema may develop severe acid–base problems—namely, respiratory acidosis and metabolic (lactic) acidosis. Reversal of the pulmonary edema is usually effective in restoring acid–base balance by improving gas exchange and allowing metabolism of excess lactate into bicarbonate.

HYPONATREMIA

Hyponatremia in a CHF patient correlates with both the severity of the disease and its ultimate outcome.[18] Reduction in cardiac output in severe CHF is the most crucial factor in the development of hyponatremia. Thus, with the exception of patients with hyponatremia due to overdiuresis (combined with hypotonic fluid replacement), hyponatremia in CHF usually indicates a severe clinical stage. Most patients with CHF who have hyponatremia have a disease categorized as New York Heart Association (NYHA) functional Class IV and exhibit volume overload.[19] In one study, a serum sodium level less than 130 mEq/L was found in 5% of heart failure patients at the time of clinical presentation.[20] Hyponatremia is independently associated with adverse outcomes in CHF patients.[21–23]

In a patient with CHF, hyponatremia is primarily due to increased activity of arginine vasopressin (AVP; also called antidiuretic hormone [ADH]), a substance that is often elevated in patients with heart failure.[24] This hormone acts on the distal tubules to cause water retention; thus hyponatremia in patients with CHF is primarily due to a limited ability of the kidneys to excrete water. More precisely, AVP binds to V_2 receptors in the renal collecting duct and promotes water retention.[25] The lowered serum sodium concentration in a CHF patient does not represent a decrease of total body sodium, but rather is a dilution of the actual excessive amount of total body sodium. CHF patients with hyponatremia are volume overloaded and may be clinically compromised to the extent that they are unable to carry on any physical activity without discomfort.

Treatment

Restricted Water Intake

Fluid restriction is a cornerstone treatment for hyponatremia in CHF patients who are euvolemic or hypervolemic. When necessary, fluid intake is limited to such a degree that a negative balance state arises relative to free water intake. This strategy is easier to implement in the long-term management of hypervolemic forms of hyponatremia than in acutely ill hospitalized patients who require relatively large volumes of intravenous fluid-diluted medications. Water intake may not be restricted in the long-term management of CHF unless the serum sodium becomes diluted to less than 130 mEq/L.

ACE Inhibitors

ACE inhibitors are helpful in treating mild hyponatremia (such as 131–135 mEq/L) in a CHF patient; these agents work by increasing renal water excretion.[26] The beneficial effect of ACE inhibitor therapy in treating hyponatremia is seen as long as cardiac output remains adequate for renal perfusion.[27]

Aquaretics

As stated earlier, ADH (also called vasopressin) acts via V_2 receptors in the kidneys to regulate water balance. An above normal ADH level in the CHF patient promotes renal water retention. A class of drugs referred to as "aquaretics" act to antagonize the V_2 receptors in the kidney, thereby promoting solute-free water clearance to help correct hyponatremia. Among the drugs classified as aquaretics are tolvaptan, conivaptan, and lixivaptan. In several clinical trials, patients with CHF who were treated with conivaptan had greater increases in serum sodium levels than did patients who received placebos.[28–32]

Vasopressin antagonists appear to be generally well tolerated.[33] Some reports note an increase in thirst and dry mouth in patients treated with vasopressin antagonists compared to those treated with placebos. As pointed out by Goldsmith in a recent review of treatment options for hyponatremia in heart failure, the V_2- and dual V_{1A}/V_2-receptor antagonists offer a physiologically based method for treating dilutional hyponatremia.[34] Other authors concur, stating that all information to date indicates that the AVP antagonists are effective in producing safe aquaresis and thus increasing serum sodium concentrations in hyponatremic patients with CHF.[35]

ASSOCIATION BETWEEN POTASSIUM BALANCE AND HEART FAILURE

Potassium homeostasis is essential for normal heart function. When this homeostasis is not maintained, the patient with heart failure is subject to increased risk for morbidity and mortality.

Hypokalemia

A low serum potassium level is poorly tolerated by patients with heart failure and can cause fatal arrhythmias. Most laboratories classify a serum potassium level less than 3.5 mEq/L as hypokalemia. However, it has been suggested that a higher level be used to classify patients with heart failure as hypokalemic (such as less than 4.0 mEq/L) because patients with cardiac disease, compared with individuals with no cardiac disease, are more vulnerable to cardiac dysrhythmias when the serum potassium concentration is low. In a study of 6845 patients with chronic, mild to moderate heart failure, researchers found that 1189 had serum potassium levels less than 4 mEq/L.[36] When compared to patients with normal serum potassium levels, these individuals had higher mortality and trended toward increased hospitalization. Some clinicians favor maintaining the serum potassium concentration in a range of 4.5 to 5.0 mEq/L in the CHF patient to minimize the potential for hypokalemic-associated dysrhythmias.[37,38]

Whereas CHF patients have an inherent propensity for developing hypokalemia due to increased aldosterone production, potassium-losing diuretics further increase this risk for hypokalemia. Among the diuretics that predispose patients to hypokalemia are loop diuretics (such as furosemide) and thiazides (such as hydrochlorothiazide). For example, hypokalemia may occur in 5% to 30% of patients receiving hydrochlorothiazides and in 5% to 20% of patients receiving loop diuretics.[39,40]

The severity of heart disease is considered when diuretics are prescribed for heart failure patients. For example, patients with NYHA Class III and IV symptoms may be treated with an aldosterone-blocking agent (such as spironolactone or eplerenone) to treat edema without causing hypokalemia.[41] A Class III patient is defined as one whose cardiac disease has resulted in marked limitation of physical activity, being comfortable only at rest; a Class IV patient is defined as one whose cardiac disease has resulted in inability to carry on any physical activity without discomfort.[42]

As indicated previously, hypokalemia poses a serious threat in the setting of cardiac disease because it increases the risk for arrhythmias and sudden death, especially in patients with CHF. For example, in a retrospective study of more than 6000 patients enrolled in the Studies of Left Ventricular Dysfunction (SOLVD) project, researchers found that the use of non-potassium-sparing diuretics was associated with an increased risk of arrhythmic death; in contrast, use of a potassium-sparing diuretic, whether alone or in combination with a non-potassium-sparing diuretic, was not independently associated with increased risk for death from arrhythmia.[43]

Regardless of the serum potassium level, patients with CHF (who have good renal function) tend to have reduced total *body* potassium levels. Therefore, almost all patients with CHF should receive some medication to maintain normal potassium balance (such as a potassium-sparing diuretic or an ACE inhibitor).[44]

In the presence of serious dysrhythmias, intravenous administration of potassium chloride is the best course of action. When hypokalemia does not respond to potassium replacement, it may be necessary to administer magnesium concurrently.

Hyperkalemia

Hyperkalemia has been reported to occur in 1.2% to 4.9% of CHF patients.[45,46] The risk for hyperkalemia is increased in heart failure patients with renal insufficiency, especially when they are receiving drugs that predispose them to developing this imbalance. (**Table 16-3**).

Table 16-3 Association Between Electrolytes and Selected Medications Used in Patients with Heart Failure

Drugs with Potential to Increase Serum Potassium Concentration

- Spironolactone
- Epleronone
- Amiloride
- Triamterene
- Angiotensin-converting enzyme (ACE) inhibitors
- Angiotensin-receptor blockers (ARBs)
- Beta blockers
- Heparin

Drugs with Potential to Decrease Serum Potassium Concentration

- Loop diuretics
- Thiazide diuretics

Drugs with Potential to Increase Serum Calcium Concentration

- Thiazide diuretics

Because CHF patients have a tendency to develop a total body deficit of potassium (due to the secondary hyperaldosteronism associated with this condition), they may be treated with potassium-conserving or potassium-containing agents. Among the potassium-conserving diuretics that predispose individuals to hyperkalemia are triamterene and amiloride. Other drugs that predispose to hyperkalemia include the aldosterone-blocking agents (such as spironolactone [Aldactone] or epleronone [Inspra]), which are often used to treat a patient with the secondary hyperaldosteronism associated with advanced CHF. In the Randomized Aldactone Evaluation Study (RALES), the rate of hyperkalemia in patients taking Aldactone was 2%; and, the rate was 5.5% in patients taking epleronone in the Eplerenone Post-Acute Myocardial Infarction Heart Failure Efficacy and Survival Study (EPHESUS).[47,48]

Other medications associated with potassium retention are also frequently prescribed for patients with CHF; among these are ACE inhibitors. ACE inhibitors can cause hyperkalemia even in patients without overt renal disease.[49] For example, these agents are reportedly used in 10% to 38% of patients who end up hospitalized with hyperkalemia.[50] Given this risk, it is important to check potassium levels carefully when initiating or maintaining therapy with these agents. Angiotensin-receptor blockers (ARBs) have effects similar to ACE inhibitors and may be substituted for them

when the unpleasant symptoms associated with the latter agents occur. Notably, ACE inhibitors may be associated with severe hypotension when started in patients with hypovolemia.

Despite their hyperkalemic effects, ACE inhibitors and ARBs have been shown to decrease the mortality rates associated with heart failure.[51–54] Because of the efficacy of these drugs in improving mortality, efforts are made to implement or continue their use when at all possible.[55] Dietary changes, including restriction of potassium intake, may be implemented preemptively, especially if a combination of two blockers of the renin–angiotensin–aldosterone system is used. Also, patients receiving these agents should be questioned about their use of salt substitutes as seasoning agents, as most of the salt substitutes contain potassium chloride.

To help reduce the risk for hyperkalemia associated with the use of potassium-conserving diuretics, a combination of a potassium-losing and potassium-conserving diuretic may be helpful. In addition, a combination diuretic acts in different locations in the kidney and increases diuresis. Several examples of combinations of potassium-losing and potassium-conserving diuretics are listed here:

- Spironolactone plus hydrochlorothiazide (Aldactazide)
- Triamterene plus hydrochlorothiazide (Dyazide)
- Amiloride plus hydrochlorothiazide (Moduretic)

ASSOCIATION BETWEEN MAGNESIUM BALANCE AND HEART FAILURE

Hypomagnesemia occurs infrequently in well-compensated ambulatory patients with CHF; however, it is prevalent in more severely ill patients. In a study of 404 consecutive CHF patients admitted for treatment, 50 (12.3%) were found to be hypomagnesemic; further, these patients had a significantly shorter survival than did patients with normal magnesium concentrations.[56] Magnesium deficiency is most likely to occur in patients with severe CHF who are receiving chronic or aggressive therapy with loop or thiazide diuretics. Most of the causes of magnesium deficiency parallel those described earlier for the development of hypokalemia. For example, the secondary hyperaldosteronism that predisposes patients to renal potassium wasting also predisposes these persons to renal magnesium wasting. Thus aldosterone antagonists protect against hypokalemia and hypomagnesemia; they also reduce the risk for dysrhythmias associated with these imbalances.[57]

It is difficult to correct hypokalemia in a patient who also has hypomagnesemia. Presumably magnesium provides the necessary cofactor required for normal potassium utilization. Thus magnesium administration is important in the management of hypokalemia that does not respond to simple potassium replacement.

Serum magnesium levels may be normal in patients with heart disease despite evidence of low magnesium concentrations in cardiac tissue.[58] Therefore, supplemental magnesium or other magnesium-retaining agents (e.g., potassium-sparing diuretics or ACE inhibitors) should be considered for patients with moderately severe to severe CHF.[59] Hypomagnesemia and whole-body magnesium depletion in CHF patients are thought to be arrhythmogenic and probably increase these patients' risk of morbidity and mortality, especially in the presence of digitalis toxicity or acute myocardial infarction and after surgery. Routine magnesium supplementation is probably unnecessary for patients with mild CHF who are normokalemic and who are receiving an ACE inhibitor or a potassium-sparing diuretic. In contrast, patients with advanced CHF who require aggressive thiazide or loop diuretic therapy and those with uncomplicated hypomagnesemia should be considered as candidates for long-term orally administered magnesium.[60]

It has been suggested that oral magnesium supplementation to heart failure patients may attenuate blood levels of C-reactive protein (CRP), a biomarker of inflammation.[61] A small study reported in 2006 suggested that oral magnesium supplementation may improve endothelial function in symptomatic heart failure patients.[62] Certainly, supplementation should be considered for patients with risk factors for deficiency and should be instituted for patients showing symptoms of deficiency.[63]

A recent study found that hypermagnesemia was significantly associated with mortality in elderly patients with CHF.[64] Patients with hypermagnesemia reported higher antacid and laxative use; the authors suggested that clinicians should pay more attention to abuse of magnesium-containing over-the-counter drugs.

ELECTROLYTES AND DIGOXIN

A therapeutic digoxin level is generally defined as ranging between 0.8 and 2.0 ng/mL; unfortunately, this level overlaps with the range in which toxic results may be seen.[65] Hypokalemia and hypomagnesemia sensitize the heart to the toxic effects of digoxin, even in the presence of therapeutic digoxin levels.[66] For this reason, both hypokalemia and hypomagnesemia should be avoided in patients receiving digitalis preparations. When digoxin toxicity is mild, the patient may develop symptoms such as visual disturbances and nausea. When digoxin toxicity is severe, the Na^+/K^+ pump is poisoned, allowing potassium to move from the cells into the blood stream, producing hyperkalemia and increased risk for cardiac arrest.

Hypocalcemia decreases the heart's sensitivity to digoxin, whereas hypercalcemia increases the sensitivity. Thus administering digoxin to a hypercalcemic patient can be dangerous. Moreover, administration of calcium to a digitalized patient should be done with caution.

ELECTROLYTES AND CARDIOPULMONARY RESUSCITATION

In the past, sodium bicarbonate was routinely used during cardiopulmonary resuscitation. Its administration was intended to counteract the lactic acidosis associated with hypoxia, poor perfusion, and anaerobic metabolism.[67] Today, however, the routine use of sodium bicarbonate is no longer recommended because there is no proof that it improves outcomes during CPR.[68,69] In fact, sodium bicarbonate may cause complications such as metabolic alkalosis, hypernatremia, and hyperosmolarity.[70,71] Situations in which sodium bicarbonate may be used include preexisting metabolic acidosis, hyperkalemia, or tricyclic or phenobarbital drug overdoses.[72]

Because there is no evidence that calcium improves outcomes during CPR, its routine use is not recommended.[73] In fact, it has been suggested that calcium use during pediatric CPR may be associated with decreased survival to hospital discharge and unfavorable neurologic outcome.[74] Situations in which this agent may be used include the presence of hypocalcemia or hyperkalemia or overdose of calcium-channel blockers.[75]

Magnesium may be given to manage recurrent ventricular tachycardia or ventricular fibrillation when hypomagnesemia is suspected.[76] In a recent literature review, investigators were unable to identify enough information to allow them to recommend for or against the use of magnesium during resuscitation.[77]

CASE STUDIES

Case Study 16-1

A 60-year-old woman with a history of hypertension and myocardial infarction was admitted to the hospital with complaints of dyspnea and increased pitting edema of the lower extremities. She reported that she had not adhered to her sodium-restricted diet for several weeks and that she had recently increased in weight from her usual 55 kg to 68 kg. At the time of her last physician visit, her serum sodium level was 135 mEq/L and her serum creatinine was 1.3 mg/dL. Abnormal laboratory results present on admission included hyponatremia (Na = 128 mEq/L), elevated blood urea nitrogen (BUN =75 mg/dL; normal range = 10–20 mg/dL), and an elevated serum creatinine level (2.0 mg/dL).

Commentary. Fluid volume overload was evidenced by pitting edema, an acute weight gain, and increasing dyspnea. Both the fluid volume excess and the hyponatremia were due to the patient's worsening CHF. The increased BUN and creatinine levels reflected a reduced glomular filtration rate (GFR) secondary to a decreased cardiac output. The symptoms that caused the patient to seek medical attention were dyspnea and edema, both of which are associated with worsening cardiac failure. No symptoms related to hyponatremia were present. The patient was treated with furosemide, an ACE inhibitor, and a low-sodium diet. Water intake was restricted until her serum sodium level normalized. Following her treatment in the hospital, the patient's serum sodium level returned to the lower limit of normal, the excess body fluid was eliminated, and her renal function returned to baseline level. Discharge instructions included information about her new medications (furosemide and an ACE inhibitor) and the need to adhere to her sodium-restricted diet.

Case Study 16-2

A 60-year-old man was admitted to the hospital with acute pulmonary edema secondary to a myocardial infarction. At the time of admission, his BUN was 10 mg/dL and his serum creatinine was 1 mg/dL (both values indicated good renal function). A 20-mg dose of furosemide was given intravenously, followed by an oral dose of 40 mg/day. Within a short period of time, the patient's pulmonary edema resolved. By the eighth day of hospitalization, it was noted that the patient had lost 6 kg (roughly equivalent to 13 lb) of body weight. In addition, his skin turgor was poor. At this time, the following abnormal laboratory results were noted: BUN of 100 mg/dL (markedly elevated), and serum creatinine of 4 mg/dL (also markedly elevated). The BUN/Cr ratio was 25:1, indicating reduced renal perfusion. The urine sodium concentration was 2 mEq/L, indicating a healthy renal response to the markedly reduced fluid volume. A urine osmolality of 500 mOsm/kg also indicated a healthy renal response to fluid volume deficit.

Commentary. All of these signs pointed to prerenal azotemia—a condition that occurs when blood supply to the kidneys is compromised by decreased renal perfusion secondary to fluid volume depletion. This was actually fortunate, given that the alternative could have been acute tubular necrosis (ATN) due to profound fluid volume depletion. In differentiating between prerenal azotemia and ATN, it is necessary to consider the BUN/Cr ratio as well as urine osmolality and sodium content. The table at the bottom of the page distinguishes between prerenal azotemia and ATN.

In this case, diuretics were temporarily discontinued and an increase in dietary sodium intake was begun while the

Differentiation Between Prerenal Azotemia and Acute Tubular Necrosis (ATN)

Laboratory Finding	Prerenal Azotemia	Acute Tubular Necrosis
BUN/Cr ratio	> 20:1	10:1
Urine sodium (mEq/L)	< 20	> 40
Urine osmolality (mOsm/kg)	> 500	< 350

patient was being closely observed. The BUN and creatinine levels returned to normal and the patient was started on a lower daily dose of diuretics; his body weight and laboratory values were closely monitored until the right balance between diuretic use and sodium intake was achieved.

Case Study 16-3

A 65-year-old woman with congestive heart failure and generalized edema plus pulmonary edema was admitted to the hospital for treatment. At the time of admission, her BUN was 20 mg/dL and her serum creatinine was 1.2 mg/dL (BUN:Cr ratio 16.7 to1). Following 4 days of diuretic therapy, she was found to have sustained a 5-kg (11-lb) weight loss. While her peripheral edema had resolved, she still had a mild degree of pulmonary edema. Further, her laboratory results showed increased BUN and serum Cr levels (BUN, 90 mg/dL; Cr, 3.0 mg/dL). The BUN:Cr ratio was now 30 to 1, indicating renal hypoperfusion caused by excessive diuresis.

Commentary. The patient's CHF severity was such that diuresis alone was insufficient to relieve her pulmonary edema (even when diuretics were used in high dosages). Therapy was then directed toward improving her cardiac output with other medications.

Case Study 16-4

A 70-year-old woman with cardiomyopathy was admitted with severe peripheral edema. In addition to CHF, her history included diabetes mellitus and osteoarthritis. Among her current medications were an ACE inhibitor, furosemide 40 mg/day, and aspirin. Due to worsening of her osteoarthritis pain, the patient started taking large daily doses of ibuprofen (an NSAID). In addition, she admitted to eating more high-sodium snacks. Upon examination, sparse pulmonary crackles and decreased breath sounds were noted in both lung bases. A chest film showed small bilateral pleural effusions; an echocardiogram found no significant changes from a previous study 6 months earlier. A mild elevation in her serum creatinine was noted (changed from 1.3 mg/dL 6 months earlier to 1.9 mg/dL at the time of admission).

Commentary. The patient's worsened clinical condition was attributed to the use of NSAIDs and failure to adhere to a sodium-restricted diet. In addition, the increased serum creatinine indicated worsened renal function.

Also see Case Studies 12-1, 17-1, 17-2, and 17-11 regarding fluid and electrolyte problems in patients with heart conditions.

Summary of Key Points

- Most patients with congestive heart failure who have hyponatremia are clinically compromised, have disease categorized as New York Heart Association functional Class IV, and are experiencing volume overload.
- Diuretics are commonly used in patients with congestive heart failure to treat fluid volume overload; depending on their type, these agents may predispose individuals to potassium imbalances. Commonly used potassium-losing diuretics include furosemide and hydrochlorothiazide. Commonly used potassium-sparing diuretics include spironolactone and amiloride.
- A low serum potassium level is poorly tolerated by patients with heart failure and can cause fatal arrhythmias. Some clinicians favor maintaining the serum potassium level in cardiac patients in the mid- to high-normal range to minimize these individuals' risk of developing dysrhythmias.
- Hypokalemia and hypomagnesemia sensitize the heart to the toxic effects of digoxin, even in the presence of therapeutic digoxin levels.
- The risk of hyperkalemia is increased in patients with both heart failure and renal insufficiency, especially when they are taking drugs that predispose individuals to hyperkalemia (see Table 16-3).
- Patients with CHF should be cautioned to consult their healthcare providers before taking over-the-counter drugs (for example, NSAIDs predispose patients to fluid retention).
- A relatively new class of drugs—the arginine vasopressin antagonists—shows promise in treating hyponatremia associated with congestive heart failure.
- Reduction of fluid intake (such as less than 2000 mL in 24 hours) may be necessary for CHF patients who experience recurrent fluid retention despite sodium restriction and use of diuretics.
- The routine use of sodium bicarbonate is no longer recommended during cardiopulmonary resuscitation because there is no proof that this treatment improves outcomes.

NOTES

1. Schrier, R. W., Masoumi, A., & Elhassan, E. (2009). Role of vasopressin and vasopressin receptor antagonists in type I cardiorenal syndrome. *Blood Purification, 27*(1), 28–32.

2. Woodard, G. E., & Rosado, J. A. (2008). Natriuretic peptides in vascular physiology and pathology. *International Review of Cell and Molecular Biology, 268,* 59–93.

3. Gruson, D., Rousseau, M. F., Ahn, S., Van Linden, F., Thys, F., Ketelslegers, J. M., et al. (2008). Accuracy of N-terminal-pro-atrial natriuretic peptide in patients admitted to emergency department. *The Scandinavian Journal of Clinical & Laboratory Investigation, 68*(5), 410–414.

4. Mann, D. L. (2008). Heart failure and cor pulmonale. In A. S. Fauci, E. Braunwald, D. L. Kasper, et al. (Eds.), *Harrison's internal medicine* (17th ed.). New York: McGraw-Hill, p. 1448.

5. Mann, note 4, p. 1449.

6. Riegel, B., Moser, D. K., Anker, S. D., Appel, L. J., Dunbar, S. B., Grady, K. L., et al. (2009). State of the science: Promoting self-care in persons with heart failure: A scientific statement from the American Heart Association. *Circulation, 120*(12), 1141–1163.

7. Mann, note 4, p. 1448.

8. Riegel et al., note 6.

9. Riegel et al., note 6.

10. Mann, note 4, p. 1448.

11. Gislason, G. H., Rasmussen, J. N., Abildstrom, S .Z., Schramm, T. K., Hansen, M. L., Fosbol, E. L., et al. (2009). Increased mortality and cardiovascular morbidity associated with use of nonsteroidal anti-inflammatory drugs in chronic heart failure. *Archives of Internal Medicine, 169*(2), 141–149.

12. Gislason et al., note 11.

13. Antman, E. M., Elliott, M., Bennett, J. S., Daugherty, A., Furberg, C., Roberts, H., et al., American Heart Association. (2007). Use of nonsteroidal anti-inflammatory drugs: An update for clinicians: A scientific statement from the American Heart Association. *Circulation, 115*(12), 1634–1642.

14. Hochman, J. S., & Ingbar, D. H. (2008). Cardiogenic shock and pulmonary edema. In A. S. Fauci, E. Braunwald, D. L. Kasper, et al. (Eds.), *Harrison's internal medicine* (17th ed.). New York: McGraw-Hill, p. 1706.

15. Hochman & Ingbar, note 14.

16. Hochman & Ingbar, note 14.

17. Hochman & Ingbar, note 14.

18. Leier, C. V., Dei Cas, L., & Metra, M. (1994). Clinical relevance and management of the major electrolyte abnormalities in congestive heart failure. *American Heart Journal, 128(3),* 564–567.

19. Leier et al., note 18.

20. Kumar, S. K., & Mather, P. J. (2009). AVP receptor antagonists in patients with CHF. *Heart Failure Reviews, 14*(2), 83–86.

21. Goldsmith, S. R. (2009). Treatment options for hyponatremia in heart failure. *Heart Failure Reviews, 14*(2), 65–73.

22. Klein, L., O'Connor, C. M., Leimberger, J. D., Gattis-Stough, W., Pina, I. L., Felker, G. M., et al. (2005). Lower serum sodium is associated with increased short-term mortality in hospitalized patients with worsening heart failure: Results from the Outcomes of a Prospective Trial of Intravenous Milrinone for Exacerbations of Chronic Heart Failure (OPTIME-CHF) study. *Circulation, 111,* 2454–2460.

23. Oren, R. M. (2005). Hyponatremia in congestive heart failure. *American Journal of Cardiology, 95*(9A), 2B–7B.

24. Hoque, M. Z., Arumugham, P., Huda, N., Verma, N., Afiniwala, M., & Karia, D. H. (2009). Conivaptan: Promise of treatment in heart failure. *Expert Opinion on Pharmacotherapy, 10*(13), 2161–2169.

25. Hoque et al., note 24.

26. Elisaf, M., Theodorou, J., Pappas, C. & Siamopoulos, K. (1995). Successful treatment of hyponatremia with angiotensin-converting enzyme inhibitors in patients with congestive heart failure. *Cardiology, 86*(6), 477–80.

27. Sica, D. A. (2006). Hyponatremia and heart failure – Treatment considerations. *Congestive Heart Failure, 12*(1), 55–60.

28. Zeltser, D., Rosansky, S., Van Rensburg, H., Verbalis, J. G., & Smith, N. (2007). Assessment of the efficacy and safety of intravenous conivaptan in euvolemic and hypervolemic hyponatremia. *American Journal of Nephrology, 27*(5), 447–457.

29. Annane, D., Decaux, G., Smith, N., & Conivaptan Study Group. (2009). Efficacy and safety of oral conivaptan, a vasopressin-receptor antagonist, evaluated in a randomized, controlled trial in patients with euvolemic or hypervolemic hyponatremia. *American Journal of the Medical Sciences, 337*(1), 28–36.

30. Ghali, J. K., Koren, M. J., Taylor, J. R., Brooks-Asplund, E., Fan, K., Long, W. A., et al. (2006). Efficacy and safety or oral conivaptan: A V_{1A}/V_2 vasopressin receptor antagonist, assessed in a randomized, placebo-controlled trial in patients with euvolemic or hypervolemic hyponatremia. *Journal of Clinical Endocrinology & Metabolism, 91*(6), 2145–2152.

31. Verbalis, J. G., Zeltser, D., Smith, N., Barve, A., & Andoh, M. (2008). Assessment of the efficacy and safety of intravenous conivaptan in patients with euvolemic hyponatremia: Subgroup analysis of a randomized, controlled study. *Clinical Endocrinology, 69,* 159–168.

32. Verbalis et al., note 31.

33. Finley, J. J., Konstam, M. A., & Udelson, J. E. (2008). Arginine vasopressin antagonists for the treatment of heart failure and hyponatremia. *Circulation, 118,* 410–421.

34. Goldsmith, note 21.

35. Kumar & Mather, note 20.

36. Ahmed, A., Zannad, F., Love, T. E., Tallaj, J., Gheorghiade, M., Ekundayo, O. J., et al. (2007). A propensity-matched study of the association of low serum potassium levels and mortality in chronic heart failure. *European Heart Journal, 28,* 1334–1343.

37. Leier et al., note 18.

38. Macdonald, J. E., & Struthers, A. D. (2004). What is the optimal serum potassium level in cardiovascular patients? *Journal of the American College of Cardiology, 43,* 155–161.

39. Dursun, I., & Sahin, M. (2006). Difficulties in maintaining potassium homeostasis in patients with heart failure. *Clinical Cardiology, 29*(9), 388–392.

40. Khan, M. G. (2003). *Cardiac drug therapy* (6th ed.). Philadelphia: W. B. Saunders.

41. Ahmed et al., note 36.

42. Criteria Committee of the New York Heart Association. (1994). *Nomenclature and criteria for diagnosis of diseases of the heart and great vessels* (9th ed.). Boston: Little, Brown & Company, pp. 253–256.

43. Cooper, H. A., Dries, D. L., Davis, C. E., Shen, Y. L., & Domanski, M. J. (1999). Diuretics and risk of arrhythmic death in patients with left ventricular dysfunction. *Circulation, 100*(12), 1311–1315.

44. Leier et al., note 18.

45. Kostis, J. B., Shelton, B., Gosselin, G., Goulet, C., Hood, W. B., Kohn, R. M., et al. (1996). Adverse effects of enalapril in the Studies of Left Ventricular Dysfunction (SOLVD). *American Heart Journal, 131*(2), 350–355.

46. Kober, L., Torp-Pedersen, C., Carlsen, J. E., Bagger, H., Eliasen, P., Lyngborg, K., et al. (1995) A clinical trial of the angiotensin-converting enzyme inhibitor trandolapril in patients with left ventricular dysfunction after myocardial infarction: Trandolapril Cardiac Evaluation (TRACE) Study Group. *New England Journal of Medicine, 333*(25), 1670–1676.

47. Pitt, B., Zannad, F., Remme, W. J., Cody, R., Castaigne, A., Perez, A., et al. (1999). The effect of spironolactone on morbidity and mortality in patients with severe heart failure: Randomized Aldactone Evaluation Study Investigators. *New England Journal of Medicine, 341*(10), 709–717.

48. Pitt, B., Remme, W., Zannad, F., Neaton, J., Martinez, F., Roniker, B., et al. (2003). Eplerenone, a selective aldosterone blocker, in patients with left ventricular dysfunction after myocardial infarction: Eplerenone Post-Acute Myocardial Infarction Heart Failure Efficacy and Survival Study Investigators. *New England Journal of Medicine, 348*(14), 1309–1321.

49. Bongard, F. S., Sue, D. Y., & Vintch, J. R. (2008). Current Diagnosis & Treatment Critical Care. (3rd ed.). New York: McGraw Hill Medical, p. 397.

50. Palmer, B. F. (2004). Managing hyperkalemia caused by inhibitors of the renin–angiotensin–aldosterone system. *New England Journal of Medicine, 351*, 585–592.

51. Pfeffer, M. A., Swedberg, K., Granger, C. B., Held, P., McMurray, J. J., Michelson, E. L., et al. (2003). Effects of candesartan on mortality and morbidity in patients with chronic heart failure: The CHARM-Overall programme. *Lancet, 362*, 759–766.

52. Dickstein, K., Kjekshus, J., & OPTIMALL Steering Committee of the OPTIMALL Study Group. (2002). Effects of losartan and captopril on mortality and morbidity in high-risk patients after acute myocardial infarction: The OPTIMAAL randomised trial. *Lancet, 360*(9335), 752–760.

53. Cohn, J. N., Tognoni, G., Valsartan Heart Failure Investigators. (2001). A randomized trial of the angiotensin-receptor blocker valsartan in chronic heart failure. *New England Journal of Medicine, 345*(23), 1667–1675.

54. Pitt, B., Segal, R., Martinze, F. A., Meurers, G., Cowley, A. J., Thomas, I., et al. (1997). Randomized trial of losartan versus captopril in patients over 65 with heart failure: Evaluation of losartan in elderly study (ELITE). *Lancet, 349*(9054), 747–752.

55. Segura, J., & Ruilope, L. M. (2008). Hyperkalemia risk and treatment of heart failure. *Heart Failure Clinics, 4*(4), 455–464.

56. Cohen, N., Almoznino-Sarafian, D., Zaidenstein, R., Alon, I., Gorelik, O., Shteinshnaider, M., et al. (2003). Serum magnesium aberrations in furosemide treated patients with congestive heart failure: Pathophysiological correlates and prognostic evaluation. *Heart, 89*, 411–416.

57. Gao, X., Peng. L., Adhikari, C. M., Lin, J., & Zuo, Z. (2007). Spironolactone reduced arrhythmia and maintained magnesium homeostasis in patients with congestive heart failure. *Journal of Cardiac Failure, 13*(3), 170–177.

58. Haigney, M. C., Silver, B., Tanglao E., Silverman, H. S., Hill, J. D., Shapiro, E., et al. (1995). Noninvasive measurement of tissue magnesium and correlation with cardiac levels. *Circulation, 92*(8), 2190–2197.

59. Leier et al., note 18.

60. Leier et al., note 18.

61. Almoznino-Sarafian, D., Berman, S., Mor, A., Shteinshnaider, M., Gorelik, O., Tzur, I., et al. (2007). Magnesium and C-reactive protein in heart failure: an anti-inflammatory effect of magnesium administration? *European Journal of Nutrition, 46*(4), 230–237.

62. Fuentes, J. C., Salmon, A. A., & Silver, M. A. (2006). Acute and chronic oral magnesium supplementation: effects on endothelial function, exercise capacity, and quality of life in patients with symptomatic heart failure. *Congestive Heart Failure, 12*(1), 9–13.

63. Gums, J. G. (2004). Magnesium in cardiovascular and other disorders. *American Journal of Health-System Pharmacy, 61*(15), 1569–76.

64. Corbi, G, Acanfora, D., Iannuzzi G. L., Longobardi, G., Cacciatore, F., Furgi, G., et al. (2008). Hypermagnesemia predicts mortality in elderly with congestive heart disease: Relationship with laxative and antacid use. *Rejuvenation Research, 11*(1), 129–138.

65. Bongard et al., note 49, p. 495.

66. Opie, L. H., & Gersh, B. J. (2009). *Drugs for the heart* (7th ed.). Philadelphia: Saunders Elsevier, p. 187.

67. Geraci, M. J., Klipa, D., Heckman, M. G., & Persoff, J. (2009). Prevalence of sodium bicarbonate–induced alkalemia in cardiopulmonary arrest patients. *Annals of Pharmacotherapy, 43*(7), 1245–1250.

68. Parillo, J. E., & Dellinger, R. P. (2008). *Critical care medicine: Principles of diagnosis and management in the adult* (3rd ed.). Philadelphia: Mosby Elsevier, p. 9.

69. Aschner, J. L., & Poland, R. L. (2008). Sodium bicarbonate: Basically useless therapy. *Pediatrics, 122*(4), 831–835.

70. Bishop, R. L., & Weisfeldt, M. L. (1976). Sodium bicarbonate administration during cardiac arrest: Effect on arterial pH, PCO_2 and osmolarity. *Journal of the American Medical Association, 235*, 506–509.

71. Mattar, J. A., Weil, M. H., Shubin, H., & Stein, L. (1974). Cardiac arrest in the critically ill. II. Hyperosmolar states following cardiac arrest. *American Journal of Medicine, 56*, 162–168.

72. Parillo & Dellinger, note 68, p. 9.

73. Parillo & Dellinger, note 68, p. 9.

74. Srinivasan, V., Morris, M. C. Helfaer, M. A., Berg, R. A., Nad-karni, V. M., & American Heart Association National Registry of CPR Investigators. (2008). Calcium use during in-hospital pediatric cardiopulmonary resuscitation: A report from the National Registry of Cardiopulmonary Resuscitation. *Pediatrics, 121*(5), e1144–e1151.

75. Parillo & Dellinger, note 68, p. 9.

76. Parillo & Dellinger, note 68, p. 9.

77. Reis, A. G., Ferreira de Paiva, E., Schvartsman, C., & Zaritsky, A. L. (2008). Magnesium in cardiopulmonary resuscitation: Critical review. *Resuscitation, 77*(1), 21–25.

Chapter 17

Renal Failure

Among their numerous functions, the kidneys excrete water, electrolytes, and organic materials after conserving whatever amounts of these substances the body requires. They act both autonomously and in response to blood-borne messengers, such as the mineralocorticoids and antidiuretic hormone (ADH). They excrete the breakdown products of protein metabolism, drugs, and toxins; produce the hormone erythropoietin (which is essential for red blood cell production); and convert an unusable form of vitamin D to a substance (calcitriol) that the body can use. Not surprisingly, then, failure of renal function causes a variety of water and electrolyte disturbances and other metabolic derangements (**Figure 17-1**). Topics covered in this chapter include fluid and electrolyte disorders associated with acute and chronic renal failure.

Acute renal failure (ARF), also called acute kidney injury (AKI),[1] refers to a sudden (hours or days) steep decrease in kidney function. *Chronic renal failure* (CRF) refers to a gradual, progressive decrease over months or years, allowing time for the development of partial adaptation to the condition. To some degree, both types of renal failure are characterized by the accumulation of nitrogenous waste products (urea and creatinine) and an inability to regulate fluid and electrolyte homeostasis. *Prerenal azotemia* is a condition in which renal blood flow is decreased (usually due to hypovolemia), causing the BUN to become elevated while the serum creatinine level remains essentially unchanged (indicating a healthy renal response to reduced renal blood flow). *Kidney damage* is defined as pathologic abnormalities in the kidney or

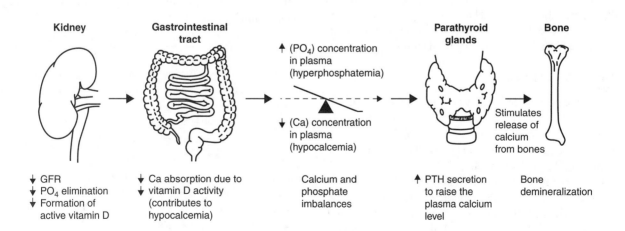

Figure 17-1 Metabolic derangements in renal failure.

markers of damage that include abnormal blood tests, urine tests, or imaging studies.[2]

Because the clinical presentation and management of ARF and CRF are somewhat different, it is helpful to consider these conditions separately. In addition, prior to addressing the various fluid and electrolyte problems associated with ARF and CRF, it is helpful to review several laboratory tests used to determine if renal failure is present.

LABORATORY TESTS FOR RENAL FUNCTION

Serum Creatinine

Creatinine (Cr) is generated from muscle metabolism and is produced from creatine. Normal serum creatinine levels vary slightly according to the reporting laboratory; however, typical normal values range between 0.8 and 1.4 mg/dL. Women have a lower creatinine level than men because they have less muscle mass than men. Muscular individuals produce more creatinine and, therefore, may have higher serum creatinine levels, especially when they consume a high-protein diet. Individuals who consume only a vegetarian diet may have reduced serum creatinine levels due to low protein intake. From the circulation, creatinine is excreted by the kidneys.

The glomerular filtration rate must decrease by approximately half before the serum creatinine concentration changes appreciably (more than 1 mg/dL).[3] Thus serum creatinine may grossly underestimate the prevalence and severity of chronic kidney disease.[4] Indeed, some patients with a serum creatinine level within the "normal" range may have significantly reduced renal function.[5]

The serum creatinine level may elevate by 1 to 2 mg/dL during periods of acute renal failure.[6] Serum creatinine levels are considered in relation to hourly urine output in the classification of the stage of acute renal failure.

Blood Urea Nitrogen

Urea is the primary end-product of protein metabolism and is primarily excreted via the kidneys. Normal values for BUN vary slightly according to the reporting laboratory, but generally range between 10 and 20 mg/dL. In normal situations, 35% to 50% of the urea filtered by the kidneys is reabsorbed in the tubules.[7] When renal blood flow is decreased, however, much more urea is reabsorbed, resulting in an elevated BUN concentration. Another factor that can elevate the BUN level is a high dietary protein intake, because approximately 6 g of protein yields 1 g of urea nitrogen.[8] Bleeding into the gastrointestinal tract causes an increased BUN due to digestion of the protein-rich blood. One unit of whole blood contains approximately 200 g of protein.[9]

BUN:Creatinine Ratio

The normal ratio between BUN and Cr is 10:1. A ratio greater than 20:1 is an indicator of reduced renal blood flow, such as occurs in fluid volume deficit or reduced cardiac output. In the presence of reduced renal blood flow, the rate of urea reabsorption is much higher than that of creatinine. The BUN:Cr ratio is used frequently in clinical situations to help distinguish between prerenal azotemia and acute tubular necrosis. (See Case Studies 16-2 and 17-1.)

Glomerular Filtration Rate

Glomerular filtration rate (GFR) describes the flow rate of filtered fluid through the kidney. It varies according to age, sex, and body size, and declines with age. The normal GFR is greater than 90 mL/min per 1.73 m^2 body surface area. This rate is commonly used to determine the degree of chronic renal insufficiency and help determine doses of drugs that are primarily excreted via the kidney. In addition, the level of GFR helps determine when specific electrolyte imbalances will occur. Because the serum creatinine concentration is not a sensitive indicator of modest decreases in renal function, it is helpful to determine a patient's GRF. As shown in **Table 17-1**, the GRF is used to classify levels of chronic kidney disease.[10] The Cockcroft-Gault formula is commonly used to estimate the GFR and classify kidney function:[11]

$$GFR = \frac{[140 - age]\,[weight\,(kg)]}{72 \times serum\,Cr\,(mg/dL)}$$

Example 1. Assume a 70-year-old man who weighs 80 kg has a serum Cr level of 1.4 mg/dL. The equation shows that he has a GRF of 55.6 mL/min. A review of Table 17-1 indicates that this patient has a moderately decreased GRF.

$$GFR = \frac{[140 - 70]\,[80]}{72 \times 1.4} = \frac{5600}{100.8} = 55.6\ mL/min$$

Example 2. Now assume the same values as in Example 1 for a woman. The final value is multiplied by 0.85 because women have less creatinine than men. According to Table 17-1, this patient also has a moderately decreased GFR.

$$GFR = \frac{[140 - 70]\,[80]}{72 \times 1.4} = \frac{5600}{100.8} = 55.6\ mL/min \times .85 = 47.3\ mL/min$$

Table 17-1 Stages of Chronic Kidney Disease

Stage	Description	Glomerular Filtration Rate (mL/min/1.73m²)
1	Kidney damage with normal or elevated GFR	≥ 90
2	Kidney damage with mild decrease in GFR	60 to 89
3	Moderate decrease in GFR	30 to 59
4	Severe decrease in GFR	15 to 29
5	Kidney failure	< 15 (or dialysis)

Chronic kidney disease is defined as either kidney damage or GFR < 60 mL/min/1.73 m² for 3 months or longer. Kidney damage is defined as pathologic abnormalities or markers of damage, including abnormalities in blood or urine tests or imaging studies.

Source: Reprinted from National Kidney Foundation. K/DOQI clinical practice guidelines for chronic kidney disease: evaluation, classification, and stratification. *American Journal of Kidney Diseases, 39*(2 suppl 1), S46, 2002. Reprinted with permission from the National Kidney Foundation and Elsevier.

Urine Sodium and Osmolality

Urinary sodium and osmolality are helpful tests to distinguish between prerenal azotemia and acute tubular necrosis (ATN). Despite the reduced renal blood flow in prerenal azotemia, the kidneys are still able to conserve needed sodium; thus the affected individual excretes urine with low sodium content, such as less than 20 mEq/L. Also, in prerenal azotemia, the kidneys are still able to excrete wastes and produce urine with a fairly high osmolality, such as greater than 500 mOsm/kg. In contrast, when the tubules are damaged (as in ATN), the kidneys are unable to conserve sodium; thus the person excretes urine with a high sodium content, such as greater than 40 mEq/L. In addition, the impaired kidneys are no longer able to concentrate urine, so the urine osmolality is closer to that of the plasma (such as less than 350 mOsm/kg).

ACUTE RENAL FAILURE

Among patient characteristics strongly associated with ARF are older age, male gender, and black race.[12] ARF is particularly likely to occur after cardiac surgery. Mortality in patients with ARF depends on the cause of the condition; it is generally higher in surgical and post-traumatic patients than in medical patients. Most deaths occur in the first week following the onset of ARF and are primarily related to the underlying cause of failure.

Anatomic Site of Involvement

Acute renal failure is often classified according to its anatomical site of involvement, such as prerenal, intrarenal, or postrenal:

- *Prerenal* refers to hypoperfusion of the kidney that leads to azotemia (accumulation of urea nitrogen and other nitrogenous products in the blood) without actual damage to renal tissue. In this condition, the renal tubules remain intact and avidly conserve needed salt and water (an appropriate physiologic response). Prerenal azotemia accounts for 40% to 80% of the cases of acute renal failure (depending on the population studied).[13] When renal blood flow is restored, renal function returns to normal. In contrast, if hypoperfusion persists, the renal tubules will become damaged.
- *Intrarenal* refers to actual kidney tissue damage and may be subdivided into primary vascular, glomerular, interstitial, or tubular injury. This form of renal failure accounts for approximately 50% of all ARF cases.[14]
- *Postrenal* refers to an obstruction in the renal system that arises distal to the site of urine formation (such as the ureter or bladder neck). Correction of the obstruction is mandatory if renal damage is to be averted. This is the least common form of acute renal failure, accounting for 5% to 10% of the cases; because it is reversible, it is important to detect this condition early.[15]

Acute Tubular Necrosis

Acute renal failure has many causes; however, by far the most common is acute tubular necrosis (**Table 17-2**). This condition involves damage to the renal tubules and usually complicates a systemic insult such as shock, trauma (particularly involving skeletal muscle), sepsis, or exposure to nephrotoxic agents. Conditions associated with renal hypoperfusion at first result in decreased urine output and prerenal azotemia; if left untreated, acute tubular necrosis can develop—that is, the renal tubules undergo histological changes.

ATN Versus Prerenal Azotemia

To prevent prerenal azotemia from advancing to ATN, it is important to make an early distinction between these two conditions. **Table 17-3** compares a variety of laboratory

Table 17-2 Causes of Acute Tubular Necrosis

Ischemic of Kidneys Due to Prolonged Hypovolemia

- Loss of gastrointestinal fluids
- Third-spacing of fluid
- Hemorrhage
- Diuretic abuse

Nephrotoxic Drugs

- Aminoglycosides (e.g., tobramycin, gentamicin, amikacin)
- Amphotericin B
- Radiocontrast agents
- Cisplatin
- Nonsteroidal anti-inflammatory drugs

Intra-tubular Obstruction

- Myoglobin (rhabdomyolysis: trauma, muscle disease, seizures, severe exercise)
- Hemoglobin (as in intravascular hemolysis, transfusion reactions, toxic hemolysis)

Exogenous Nephrotoxins

- Mercury
- Arsenic
- Carbon tetrachloride
- Toluene
- Ethylene glycol
- Oxalic acid

tests that are helpful in distinguishing between prerenal azotemia and ATN. Also see Case Studies 16-2 and 17-1 for examples.

ARF Due to Contrast Media

A leading cause of acute renal failure in hospitalized patients is contrast medium-induced nephropathy (CIN).[16]

Table 17-3 Approximate Values to Differentiate Between Prerenal Azotemia and Acute Tubular Necrosis

Laboratory Finding	Prerenal Azotemia	Acute Tubular Necrosis
BUN/Cr ratio	> 20:1	10:1
Urine Na (mEq/L)	< 20	> 40
Urine osmolality (mOsm/kg)	> 500	< 350
Urine/plasma osmolality	> 1.5	< 1.1

Expanded use of contrast-enhanced imaging is exposing an increasing number of patients to this renal toxin.[17] Although the pathogenesis of CIN is unclear, the contrast medium apparently has direct cytotoxic effects on renal structures.[18] The typical definition of CIN is an increase in serum creatinine by 25% or more over baseline within the first 2 to 3 days following administration of the contrast agent.[19] Fortunately, most patients with CIN recover renal function within 3 to 7 days.[20]

Persons most at risk for CIN are those with preexisting renal disease (serum creatinine greater than 2 mg/dL), advanced age, diabetes mellitus, volume depletion, congestive heart failure, and recent exposure to nephrotoxic agents, such as NSAIDs and ACE inhibitors.[21] The prevalence of CIN is greater than 30% in patients whose estimated GFR is less than 60 mL/min per 1.73 m². [22] For this reason, preventive treatment may be recommended for those individuals with a GFR less than 60 mL/min.[23]

The best way to prevent CIN is to provide adequate periprocedureal hydration to patients at risk of developing this condition.[24] The cornerstone of care in preventing CIN is the administration of intravenous fluids beginning 12 to 24 hours before the contrast study and ending 12 hours after the study.[25] Most often recommended fluids are isotonic saline or half-strength saline.[26,27] Also, sodium bicarbonate may be administered to alkalinize the urine. A drug sometimes administered prior to use of the contrast medium is *N*-acetylcysteine (NAC), an agent that promotes renal vasodilation. Some studies have suggested that adding *N*-acetylcysteine to the regimen is more renoprotective than hydration alone.[28,29] For this reason, *N*-acetylcysteine prophylaxis is often recommended (especially in high-risk patients) to protect against CIN.[30] Other agents shown to be helpful in decreasing the risk of CIN include theophylline, bicarbonate, and ascorbic acid.[31]

ARF Due to Rhabdomyolysis

Rhabdomyolysis is the breakdown of skeletal muscle, resulting in the release of myoglobin into the systemic circulation. It can result from conditions such as traumatic crush injury, acute muscle ischemia, prolonged seizure activity, excessive exercise, heatstroke, a viral illness, or selected medications (such as statin drugs). The hallmark of rhabdomyolysis is an elevated serum creatine kinase (CK) level. Normal values for serum CK range between 55 and 170 units/L for males and between 30 and 135 units/L for females.[32] Generally, the diagnosis of rhabdomyolysis is based on elevated serum CK levels of more than 1000 units/L.[33] The serum creatine kinase level may reach extremely high levels in patients with rhabdomyolysis (such as more than 600,000 units/L).[34] More than half of all patients with acute renal failure associated with rhabdomyolysis have serum CK levels exceeding 16,000 units/L.[35]

Depending on the amount of myoglobin in the urine, the urine's appearance can range from tea colored to cola colored in a person with rhabdomyolysis. Renal damage results from obstruction of the tubules with myoglobin precipitation; acute renal failure develops in as many as 15% of patients with rhabdomyolysis and is associated with high mortality.[36]

In adults, provided persistent oliguria is not present, treatment consists of the intravenous infusion of 0.9% sodium chloride at a rate to maintain an hourly urine output of 300 mL/hr until myoglobinuria has ceased and the serum CK concentration decreases to or falls below 1000 units/L.[37] If sufficient urine flow can be established, sodium bicarbonate may be used to elevate urine pH to a level greater than 6.5 to increase solubility of myoglobin.[38]

Reversible Versus Irreversible Renal Failure

Acute renal failure may be classified as either irreversible or reversible. In *irreversible renal failure,* kidney function does not return and uremia progresses, requiring the patient to undergo lifetime dialysis or receive a kidney transplant. *Reversible renal failure* can be divided into two phases—oliguria and diuresis.

Phases of Reversible Acute Renal Failure

Oliguric Phase

The oliguric (maintenance) phase usually lasts 1 to 2 weeks and is followed by the diuresis (recovery) phase, after which normal renal function often returns. However, the oliguric phase may be absent or permanent or may last 2 to 6 weeks or longer. Acute renal failure may occur in the presence of low, normal, or even high urine output. Total anuria is defined as zero urine output, anuria as less than 50 to 100 mL/day, and oliguria as less than 400 mL/day; non-oliguric renal failure may be associated with a urine output greater than 1 to 2 L/day.[39]

More important than the volume of urine is the ability of the kidney to excrete solutes. A convenient indicator of ARF is an abrupt twofold increase in the plasma creatinine concentration.

Anuria is generally thought to be a poor prognostic indicator and is more likely to require renal replacement therapy (defined as some form of dialysis). In contrast, non-oliguric ARF represents a less severe injury and usually results in fewer complications and a quicker recovery.

Fluid Replacement. Usually 0.45% sodium chloride is used to replace fluids in a volume equal to insensible fluid loss (approximately 500 mL in a fever-free adult) plus urinary and other drainage losses.[40] Accurate daily weights provide a check of the patient's overall fluid balance status and give an indication of the adequacy of fluid therapy; during the oliguric phase of ARF, the patient should lose 0.2 to 0.5 kg body weight per day.[41] To help safeguard against fluid overload, it is important to eliminate all unnecessary infusions (such as "keep vein open" fluids) and to administer IV medications in the smallest possible volume of fluid.

Diuretic Phase

During the diuretic phase of ARF, the kidneys usually excrete hypotonic urine that has a sodium content of approximately 50 mEq/L.[42] The actual amount of urine excreted is largely determined by how well fluid balance was maintained during the oliguric phase; the urine volume is expected to be greater in patients who gained an excess of salt and water than in those who did not. To achieve appropriate fluid and electrolyte replacement during this phase, healthcare providers must carefully measure the urine output and consider its electrolyte content. Although a weight loss of several pounds is generally expected during this phase, it is not unusual to see a gradual improvement in renal function without a large diuresis in a patient who was well maintained during the oliguric phase.

Fluid and Electrolyte Problems in Acute Renal Failure

Fluid, electrolyte, acid–base, and other derangements commonly encountered in the patient with ARF are summarized in **Table 17-4** and discussed in the following subsections.

Fluid Volume Overload

It is common for acutely ill patients with diminishing urine output to undergo vigorous intravenous fluid replacement (usually with an isotonic saline solution) to attempt to prevent ARF and rule out prerenal causes for oliguria. If oliguric renal failure ensues despite this action, the patient invariably becomes fluid overloaded. Loop diuretics are

Table 17-4 Summary of Fluid, Electrolyte, and Acid–Base Problems Commonly Associated with Renal Failure

Imbalance	Pathophysiology
Fluid volume excess	• As the GFR decreases, the kidneys lose their ability to regulate sodium excretion in response to sodium intake and changes in the ECF volume.
Hyperkalemia	• Potassium retention occurs when renal function is seriously impaired.
	• Metabolic acidosis adds to the hyperkalemia by driving cellular potassium into the extracellular space.
	• Increased endogenous release of potassium from the cellular breakdown (catabolism) of infected or necrotic tissue occurs.
	• High intake of protein causes the serum potassium level to elevate.
	• Certain medications (such as cyclosporine following renal transplantation) predispose patients to hyperkalemia.
Hyperphosphatemia	• Renal phosphate retention is inevitable when the GFR is significantly reduced.
Hypocalcemia	• Hypocalcemia is invariably present during the oliguric phase of ARF; a decrease occurs within the first 2–4 days and concentrations may fall as low as 5–7.5 mg/dL.
	• Hyperphosphatemia chelates calcium and causes hypocalcemia.
	• Reduced absorption of dietary calcium occurs in the setting of a deficiency of active vitamin D.
	• Prolonged hypocalcemia in CRF leads to bone demineralization.
Hypermagnesemia	• Renal magnesium retention occurs when the GFR is significantly reduced.
	• Usually hypermagnesemia is only mild to moderate unless the patient is inadvertently given medications containing magnesium. In general, there are no symptoms unless the serum magnesium level exceeds 4–5 mg/dL; most patients with CRF do not exceed this range.
Metabolic acidosis	• Damaged kidneys are unable to excrete acids produced during metabolism.
	• Usually the bicarbonate stabilizes at 12–18 mEq/L and the arterial pH at 7.25–7.30; however, hypercatabolic conditions cause acidosis to become much worse (sometimes with arterial pH values dropping below 7.0).
	• Typically, a high anion gap acidosis (owing to the accumulation of sulfate, phosphate, and a variety of organic acids) occurs. The anion gap in ARF is almost invariably less than 30 mEq/L, whereas it is usually less than 20 mEq/L in CRF.
Hyponatremia	• This imbalance is relatively common and occurs because of excessive water intake when the kidneys are unable to excrete the excess water.

sometimes administered to patients with fluid overload in an attempt to convert oliguric failure to polyuric failure; however, a substantial proportion of patients do not respond to this regimen. In these cases, renal replacement therapy is usually necessary. Untreated fluid overload can ultimately lead to pulmonary edema with infiltrates; if severe enough to cause hypoxemia, the patient may require mechanical ventilation (an ominous sign).[43]

Because fluid balance is precarious in patients with ARF, meticulous attention must be paid to maintaining salt and water intake. To plan appropriate fluid replacement therapy, a reliable assessment of all fluid losses and gains must be maintained. This can be done by keeping accurate intake and output records and by weighing the patient daily.

Hyperkalemia

Hyperkalemia is a major cause of death during the oliguric phase of ARF. Because elimination of potassium occurs almost exclusively through the kidneys, it is not surprising that hyperkalemia is a common imbalance in oliguric patients. However, this imbalance does not generally occur unless renal function is significantly decreased (GFR < 50–60 mL/min/1.73 m^2).[44]

Although an increase in the serum potassium concentration is primarily due to the inability of the injured kidneys to excrete potassium, another cause is a release of cellular potassium into the bloodstream (as may occur in prolonged fasting). The cells contain large concentrations of potassium (close to 150 mEq/L) as opposed to the relatively low concentrations of this ion (only 4 mEq/L) found in the blood-stream. Therefore, release of cellular potassium into the vascular space during even normal tissue breakdown (catabolism) is an important consideration when considering potassium balance. For example, the serum potassium concentration may increase as much as 1 to 2 mEq/L within a few hours when the patient is extremely catabolic.[45] Metabolic acidosis aggravates hyperkalemia by driving potassium out of the cells and into the extracellular fluid.

Because of the danger of hyperkalemia during the oliguric phase of ARF, it is important to minimize the endogenous production of potassium by treating infections, debriding necrotic tissue, draining accumulations of blood, and providing non-protein calories in the form of glucose and fat. It is also important to avoid administering exogenous potassium in the form of medications (such as potassium penicillin).

Although clinical signs of hyperkalemia include paresthesias, muscle weakness, and paralysis, cardiac abnormalities predominate and are the most life-threatening problems in this scenario. The untoward effects of hyperkalemia on the heart are exacerbated by the presence of hyponatremia, hypocalcemia, and acidosis. For example, a serum potassium concentration of 8.5 mEq/L when the serum sodium concentration is 140 mEq/L may be less detrimental than a serum potassium concentration of 7 mEq/L when the serum sodium concentration is 120 mEq/L.[46] When death occurs from hyperkalemia, it is usually attributable to ventricular fibrillation. Electrocardiographic (ECG) changes associated with hyperkalemia follow definite patterns that are most apparent in the precordial leads.

In addition to the extent of hyperkalemia, the rate of its development is important. For example, death from hyperkalemia is less likely in patients with CRF because of adaptive changes that occur over time in these individuals. Because non-oliguric ARF is associated with less renal damage than is oliguric renal failure, it tends to pose a lesser problem in regard to the development of hyperkalemia. If severe hyperkalemia develops, potassium redistribution or removal, or both, must be achieved.

Emergent Management of Hyperkalemia. The serum potassium concentration should be measured frequently (such as twice daily) in patients with ARF. When this level reaches 6 mEq/L or greater, frequent ECGs should also be obtained, especially if the trend in the concentration is rising.[47] The ECG is especially helpful in monitoring for this imbalance because it represents a summation of the influences of potassium as well as various other extracellular electrolytes on cardiac function. The presence of life-threatening cardiac abnormalities is an indication to institute emergency measures to protect the heart and lower the serum concentration. **Table 17-5** summarizes the emergent management of hyperkalemia.

Calcium. The IV administration of calcium does not change the serum potassium concentration but it does rapidly decrease myocardial membrane sensitivity. If needed, 10 mL of a 10% calcium gluconate solution can be given IV over 2 to 3 minutes with cardiac monitoring.[48] The onset of action begins in a few minutes and the effect lasts for 30 to 60 minutes.[49]

Insulin. Administration of insulin with a glucose solution promotes movement of serum potassium into the cells, thereby temporarily reducing the serum potassium concentration. A common preparation consists of 10–20 units of regular insulin and 25–50 g of glucose.[50] If the patient has a serum glucose concentration greater than 360 mg/dL, insulin is given alone.[51] The onset of action for insulin occurs in approximately 15 minutes, and the peak effect is reached in 60 minutes; the effects last for 4 to 6 hours.[52] The decrease in serum potassium is in the range of 0.5 to 1.0 mEq/L in 15 to 30 minutes, and this effect may last for several hours.[53] The magnitude of reduction is dose dependent; that is, 20 units of insulin produces a greater drop is serum potassium than does 10 units of insulin.

Sodium Bicarbonate. Bicarbonate therapy can also cause potassium to shift into the cells. For example, 150 mEq of sodium bicarbonate may be added to 1 L of 5% dextrose to treat hyperkalemic patients who also have metabolic acidosis.[54] However, it is important to note that patients in end-stage renal failure may not be able to tolerate the sodium load and volume expansion imposed by the administration of sodium bicarbonate.[55] Moreover, sodium bicarbonate is thought to have poor efficacy as a potassium-lowering agent when used alone.[56]

Albuterol. Albuterol, a β2-adrenergic agonist, causes a shift of potassium into the cells; for that reason, it is sometimes used to treat hyperkalemia. This agent can be administered via mask nebulization (10–20 mg in 4 mL of saline).[57] The onset of action occurs in approximately 30 minutes, and the effect lasts 2 to 4 hours.[58] The reduction in serum potassium ranges from 0.4 to 1.5 mEq/L.[59] In one study, a group of

Table 17-5 Examples of Measures to Treat Hyperkalemia

Approach	Method	Benefits/Potential Complications
Antagonize cardiac conduction abnormalities associated with life-threatening hyperkalemia	Calcium salt (such as 10 mL of 10% calcium gluconate IV)	Onset of action is 1–5 minutes; effect lasts 30–60 minutes; may exacerbate digitalis toxicity.
Shift potassium into cells temporarily when life-threatening hyperkalemia present	Regular insulin and glucose (such as 10–20 units regular insulin with 25–50 g glucose IV)	Onset of action is 15 minutes; peak occurs in 60 minutes; effect lasts 4–6 hours; potential for hypoglycemia.
	Sodium bicarbonate (such as 150 mEq of NaHCO$_3$ added to 1 L of 5% dextrose solution IV) for patients who also have metabolic acidosis	Onset of action is 15–30 minutes; effects last 1–2 hours; possibility for fluid overload due to sodium infusion; also possibility that symptoms of hypocalcemia will be exacerbated if acidosis is over-corrected.
	Nebulized albuterol (such as 10–20 mg albuterol in 4 mL normal saline inhaled over 10 minutes)	Onset of action is 30 minutes; effect last 2–4 hours; may cause tachycardia.
	Decrease dietary potassium intake according to level of renal function	Contributes to decreased plasma potassium concentration.
Lower total body concentration	Increase fecal excretion of potassium by administering a cation exchange resin (such as Kayexalate) orally or by enema.	Reduces serum potassium concentration by about 1 mEq/L in 24 hours in a normally catabolic patient with ARF. When sodium polystyrene resin is used, adds sodium to the body and increases potential for fluid volume overload.
	Increase renal excretion of potassium by the administration of a loop diuretic (such as furosemide 40–160 mg IV or orally)	Amount of potassium removed depends on level of remaining renal function; potential for hypovolemia and hypotension if diuresis is excessive.
	Hemodialysis or peritoneal dialysis	

hemodialysis patients who received a 10-minute nebulizer treatment consisting of 10 mg albuterol had a 0.6 mEq/L decrease in the plasma potassium concentration; a greater decrease (1.0 mEq/L) was observed in patients who received a 20-mg dose.[60]

The emergency measures described above allow time to initiate treatments to remove potassium from the body (cation exchange resins or dialysis).

Cation Exchange Resins

Sodium polystyrene (Kayexalate) is a resin that exchanges sodium for potassium; sulfonate resin (Calcium Resonium) is a resin that exchanges calcium for potassium.[61] These resins can be given orally or rectally, although the oral route tends to be more effective because of the longer transit time involved. For oral consumption, the resin is mixed with an osmotic laxative (such as sorbitol or lactulose) to increase stool excretion of potassium. For rectal administration, the resins can be dissolved in water and administered via enema; the solution should be retained for 30 to 45 minutes for maximum benefit. Cation resins are rather slow in reducing serum potassium concentrations, and usually the dose needs to be repeated several times. These agents are best used to prevent a modestly elevated serum potassium concentration from advancing to a severely elevated level.

Recall that the bowel's ability to excrete potassium is increased in a patient with chronic renal failure. This is one way in which the body attempts to compensate for the kidneys' diminished ability to excrete potassium. In fact, stool excretion of potassium is as much as three times higher in patients with chronic renal failure and end-stage disease than in individuals with normal renal function.[62]

Dialysis

Hemodialysis is the treatment of choice for reducing the serum potassium concentration quickly, but it has the attendant risks of rapid electrolyte shifts and complications associated with obtaining venous access. Because conventional intermittent hemodialysis is not well tolerated by hemodynamically unstable patients with ARF, a variety of alternative therapies may be considered. When peritoneal dialysis is not feasible, one of the slow continuous ultrafiltration methods may be used, such as continuous venovenous hemofiltration (CVVH). Slow continuous therapies allow large volume and solute removal with minimal effect on blood pressure, heart rate, and cardiac output.

Hyperphosphatemia

Renal phosphate retention is inevitable when the GFR is abruptly reduced to less than 25% of normal.[63] Serum phosphate levels become elevated early in the course of ARF and parallel inversely the development of hypocalcemia. Although patients with CRF and hyperphosphatemia are often treated with phosphate-binding antacids, those with ARF and hyperphosphatemia usually are not. This difference arises because patients with ARF are usually confined to bed and are more prone to constipation or obstipation; the negative effects of severe constipation (such as anorexia and hyperkalemia) outweigh the risks of transient mild to moderate hyperphosphatemia. However, when the serum phosphorus concentration is greater than 8 mg/dL, it may be necessary to administer a phosphate-binding agent.

Hypocalcemia

Hypocalcemia is invariably present during the oliguric phase of ARF. A decrease in the total serum calcium occurs within the first 2 to 4 days, and concentrations may fall as low as 7.5 to 5 mg/dL. The hypocalcemia is partially due to an elevated phosphate level (recall the inverse relationship between these two electrolytes). Another cause of hypocalcemia is a deficiency in the amount of active vitamin D available to promote intestinal absorption of dietary calcium. (The kidneys are the site of conversion of 25-hydroxyvitamin D to its active form, 1,25-dihydroxyvitamin D; with decreased functional renal cells, the amount of active vitamin D formed is diminished.) Yet another reason for hypocalcemia is the resistance of bone to the attempts of parathyroid hormone to stimulate calcium release from bone stores.

Symptoms associated with the hypocalcemia are infrequent because patients with renal failure have a concurrent metabolic acidosis, which increases calcium ionization. Probably the most significant feature of hypocalcemia is its potential to worsen the adverse cardiac effects of hyperkalemia.

Hypermagnesemia

Because the kidneys are the major site of magnesium excretion, it is understandable why there is a tendency toward hypermagnesemia when the GFR is reduced. This imbalance is usually not a major problem unless the patient consumes an exogenous source of magnesium (such as magnesium-containing laxatives or antacids). If this occurs, magnesium intoxication is possible: It is characterized by central nervous system depression, muscular weakness, and, when extreme (8–10 mEq/L), circulatory collapse.[64] Management of magnesium intoxication includes the administration of calcium gluconate to antagonize the effects of magnesium as well as dialysis against a magnesium-free dialysate to reduce the serum magnesium concentration. Magnesium levels usually return to normal during recovery from acute renal failure.

Metabolic Acidosis

Because the kidneys are the primary route for eliminating acids generated from the body each day, it not surprising that patients with ARF typically develop metabolic acidosis. The degree of acidosis they experience depends on the cause of the failure, the rate of endogenous acid production, and the rate of recovery of residual renal function. In general, the rate of development of metabolic acidosis is greater in patients with oliguric failure than in those with nonoliguric failure.

Patients with ARF typically have a high anion gap (AG) metabolic acidosis due to the retention of strong acids and accompanying anions not routinely measured by the standard laboratory tests; these include sulfate, phosphate, and a variety of organic acids. In the absence of hypercatabolic states, the high AG metabolic acidosis of ARF is usually relatively mild (less than 20 mEq/L) and is not progressive. The mild nature of the metabolic acidosis seen in ARF rarely requires therapy.[65] Approximately 20% of all patients with ARF develop a bicarbonate concentration of less than 15 mEq/L.[66]

Hyponatremia

Hyponatremia is a relatively common imbalance because patients with renal failure typically receive an excess of free water (as in hypotonic intravenous solutions) that the kidneys are unable to excrete normally. To help prevent hyponatremia, it is wise to limit water intake to less than 500 mL/day in oliguric euvolemic patients who are not undergoing ultra-filtration.[67] The usual treatment for hyponatremia in patients with ARF is fluid restriction rather than sodium replacement; sometimes, however, sodium replacement is indicated. When symptomatic hyponatremia is present, the condition may be corrected by dialysis.

Uncommon Imbalances

Hypernatremia

Hypernatremia is uncommon in patients with ARF. When it occurs, its emergence is usually in the diuretic phase, when urine tends to contain relatively more water than sodium. Probably the best way to prevent hypernatremia is to measure the volume and electrolyte content of the urine and to replace the losses with oral or IV fluids of similar tonicity. If urinary electrolyte content cannot be measured, the urine volume may be replaced with 0.45% saline (milliliter for milliliter).[68]

Hypokalemia

Hypokalemia is another uncommon imbalance in patients with ARF. In a hospital setting, the most common causes of hypokalemic ARF are aminoglycoside nephrotoxicity and overzealous use of diuretics.[69]

Other Common Problems

Anemia

Anemia may develop within 48 hours after the onset of ARF. In this condition, the red blood cells are normal in color (normochromic) and shape (normocytic) but are decreased in number. The hematocrit usually stabilizes at a level of 30% to 35%.[70] Fewer red blood cells are produced due to a deficiency in erythropoietin. Further contributing to anemia is the reduced life span of red blood cells associated with uremia.

Clinically significant bleeding may occur in 10% to 30% of patients with ARF.[71] Severe bleeding may occur into the gastrointestinal tract, lungs, or brain. The cause of the bleeding tendency in uremic patients may be partially related to a defect in platelets.[72]

Increased Susceptibility to Infection

Patients with renal failure are highly susceptible to infection,(which is a common cause of death in this population). Approximately half to three-fourths of critically ill patients with ARF develop at least one infectious complication.[73] Simple measures to prevent pneumonia (such as incentive spirometry) and urinary tract infection (such as the removal of indwelling urinary catheters as soon as feasible) plus the scrupulous care of wounds and IV devices are important to prevent hospital-acquired infections.

CHRONIC RENAL FAILURE

Chronic renal failure generally refers to kidney damage that lasts longer than 3 months.[74] The most frequent causes of CRF include diabetes mellitus and hypertension. Table 17-1 lists the five stages of chronic renal failure, based on decreased glomerular filtration rates. Fluid and electrolyte disturbances observed in patients with CRF are similar to those found in patients with ARF. A major difference between the two forms of renal failure is the frequent development of renal osteodystrophy in patients with advanced CRF. **Table 17-6** summarizes the effects of renal failure on the major body systems.

Fluid Volume Excess

As the GFR decreases in patients with CRF, the kidneys lose their ability to adjust sodium excretion in response to dietary sodium intake. As a result, fluid retention is common and is manifested by peripheral edema, pulmonary edema, and hypertension. A moderate limitation in sodium intake may be needed. In contrast, euvolemic, normotensive patients need not limit their salt intake. Diuretics are sometimes used to produce natriuresis. Thiazide diuretics are ineffective when the GFR is less than 20 mL/min and necessitate the use of the more potent loop diuretics. The use of potassium-sparing diuretics is strongly discouraged in moderate to severe CRF because of the danger of life-threatening hyperkalemia.

When fluid volume excess and other imbalances become too severe to manage by medical therapies, dialysis becomes necessary. During this therapy, fluid removal is usually

Table 17-6 Summary of Effects of Renal Failure on the Major Body Systems

System	Effects
Integumentary	• Itchy, dry, scaly skin; due to calcium and phosphate disturbances
	• Yellow color to skin due to excretion of urochrome pigment through sweat glands
	• Pale skin possible due to anemia
	• Purpura and ecchymoses due to platelet dysfunction
	• Uremic frost in very late stages (urea crystals excreted through sweat glands—heaviest on nose, forehead, and neck)
Gastrointestinal	• Anorexia, nausea, vomiting, and ileus due to uremic toxins on GI mucosa
	• GI bleeding due to platelet dysfunction
	• Unpleasant metallic taste in mouth
	• Ammonia odor to the breath
Pulmonary	• Pulmonary edema related to fluid volume excess
	• Pneumonia due to poor resistance to infection
	• Increased rate and depth of respiration as compensation for metabolic acidosis
Cardiac	• Congestive heart failure (contributed to by the combination of fluid overload, hypertension, anemia, and acidosis)
Neurological	• Gradual diminution of mental acuity, due to uremic toxins and acidosis
	• Peripheral neuropathy (numbness, pain, and burning sensations in the legs and arms—may progress to motor weakness and paralysis)
Skeletal	• Over a sustained period, hyperphosphatemia and hypocalcemia lead to osteodystrophy
Hematologic	• Anemia related to a combination of decreased erythropoietin, decreased red cell survival time, and bleeding
	• Platelet dysfunction leads to elevated bleeding time and to clinically important bleeding
Endocrine	• Defects in granulocyte and chemotaxis and phagocytic activity predispose to infection
Reproductive	• Decreased libido; impotence in men, decreased ovulation in women

achieved by ultra-filtration to achieve a clinically derived value for "dry weight." In most dialysis centers, dry weight reflects the lowest weight a patient can tolerate without developing intradialytic symptoms and hypotension.

Patients on hemodialysis usually gain both sodium and water between the end of one dialysis treatment and the beginning of the next. In a compliant patient, this weight gain may be in the range of 1 to 2 kg. In a noncompliant patient, it may be 5 kg or greater.

Metabolic Acidosis

When the serum creatinine exceeds 4 mg/dL, metabolic acidosis with a modest elevation in anion gap may be observed. Most patients with stage 4 or 5 chronic failure have a serum bicarbonate concentration of 12 to 18 mEq/L with a blood pH of 7.3 or greater; as a rule, the mild meta-bolic acidosis seen in chronic renal failure rarely needs alkalinization therapy.[75]

Hyperkalemia

Owing to the gradual onset of chronic renal failure, the body has time to make adaptive changes that augment potassium excretion. For example, the fraction of dietary potassium eliminated in feces can rise from 12% in patients with normal renal function to 35% in patients with CRF.[76] For this reason, it is especially desirable to prevent constipation in these patients. Unfortunately, constipation is a common problem in this population because of the use of large doses of phosphate binders to lower the serum phosphate level.

Despite the development of certain protective mechanisms, it is important to remember that potentially fatal hyperkalemia remains a threat in patients with CRF and renders the regulation of serum potassium concentration very important. Especially at risk are patients whose disease conditions involve the use of drugs known to increase serum potassium levels, such as angiotensin-converting enzyme (ACE) inhibitors, angiotensin-receptor blockers (ARBs), and spironolactone. According to a recent study, the risk of hyperkalemia is small if the GFR is higher than 40 mL/min/1.73 m² in nondiabetic, hypertensive patients with chronic kidney disease treated with ACE inhibitors.[77] In the same study, a body mass index (BMI) of 25 or less was associated with a significantly higher risk of hyperkalemia compared with a BMI greater than 25.

Reliance on serum creatinine levels rather than the glomerular filtration rate to determine whether it is safe to administer medications that have the potential to elevate serum potassium levels may be problematic, especially in elderly patients with a low muscle mass. See Case Study 17-11.

Rapid treatment of severe hyperkalemia was described earlier in this chapter and in Table 17-5. To manage hyperkalemia in patients undergoing hemodialysis, the potassium concentration in the dialysate is lowered to a level that is less than the serum potassium concentration. The typical dialysate potassium concentrations are in the range of 0 to 3 mEq/L (with 1 or 2 mEq/L considered standard).[78] The total amount of potassium removed during a typical dialysis treatment is in the range of 50 to 80 mEq.[79] Potassium shifts during dialysis predispose patients to arrhythmias, especially those with cardiovascular disease. For this reason, the potassium content in the dialysate is adjusted as needed on an individual basis.

In dialysis patients, as well as those not requiring this treatment, prevention of severe hyperkalemia requires dietary compliance and avoidance of medications that may promote hyperkalemia. Also, prolonged fasting should be avoided in that it provokes tissue breakdown and subsequent hyperkalemia.[80]

Hypermagnesemia

Magnesium excretion is diminished in patients with CRF; however, hypermagnesemia is rarely dangerous unless the patient also receives magnesium through exogenous sources. To minimize their risk of hypermagnesemia, patients with severe chronic kidney disease should avoid over-the-counter antacids that contain magnesium and aluminum (such as Maalox and Mylanta).[81] Further, cathartic agents that contain magnesium should be avoided, as their indiscriminate use can lead to severe hypermagnesemia.[82]

Hyperphosphatemia and Hypocalcemia

The major complications of abnormalities of phosphate and calcium metabolism in patients with renal failure occur in the skeleton and vascular bed, with occasional severe involvement of extraosseous soft tissues.[83] The clinical consequences of severe hyperphosphatemia are primarily due to the formation of widespread calcium phosphate precipitates. When plasma concentrations of calcium and phosphate are normal, their product—calcium times phosphate—is in the range of 30 to 40. A high concentration of both electrolytes will produce a much higher product; when this value exceeds 60 to 70, the probability of calcium–phosphate precipitate formation is greatly increased. Metastatic calcification with calcium–phosphate precipitates may occur in the skin (causing pruritus), the eyes (causing band keratopathy and conjunctival irritation), the heart (causing conduction abnormality), the lungs (causing pleural scarring), and the blood vessels (causing occlusive disease). In patients with end-stage renal failure, a serum phosphorus level greater than 5.5 mg/dL is associated with a 20% to 40% increase in mortality.[84]

The initial treatment for hyperphosphatemia consists of dietary restriction of high-phosphorus foods (such as dried beans, cheese, meats, and cola beverages); however, this therapy is rarely effective alone, especially in dialysis patients. It is difficult to limit phosphorus intake when most commercially available foods are rich in phosphorus-containing food additives, which are widely used to improve foods' flavor and enhance their stability. Thus phosphate binders are the mainstay of treatment for hyperphosphatemia. Calcium-free phosphate binders are effective in slowing the progression of coronary and aortic calcifications.[85]

Other Problems

Anemia

The classic normochromic/normocytic anemia of chronic renal failure has multiple causes and is largely related to a relative deficiency of erythropoietin.[86] Among other causes are decreased survival of red blood cells and iron deficiency (the latter contributed to by GI bleeding and repeated laboratory testing).[87] The recommended hematocrit concentration for patients with stages 4 and 5 chronic renal failure is 11 to 12 g/dL.[88] In recent years, the availability of erythropoietin (EPO) and modified EPO products has significantly reduced the need for blood transfusions in patients with severe anemia.[89]

Cardiopulmonary Changes

Hypertension due to salt and water retention becomes increasingly common as CRF progresses in severity. Congestive heart failure is common in this setting, caused by fluid volume overload, hypertension, and anemia. Thus salt intake needs to be curtailed in this population, and diuretics may be of benefit. Thiazide diuretics are less effective than loop diuretics when the GFR is low.

CASE STUDIES

Case Study 17-1

A 50-year-old man was admitted with acute pulmonary edema secondary to a myocardial infarction. On admission, he was given furosemide intravenously and then was continued on an oral dose of furosemide, 40 mL/day. The pulmonary edema resolved and the patient was having an uneventful recovery when on the ninth day it was noted that his BUN had risen from 10 mg/dL on admission to 110 mg/dL and his plasma creatinine (Cr) had increased from 1 mg/dL to 4.5 mg/dL. An acute weight loss of 6 kg was also noted. His skin turgor was poor and his neck veins were flat. A review of laboratory data also revealed a BUN:Cr ratio greater than 24:1, a urine sodium of 2 mEq/L, and a urine osmolality of 550 mOsm/kg.

Commentary. As shown in the table at the top of the page, all of this patient's signs pointed to prerenal failure secondary to fluid volume depletion following the excessive diuresis. The low urine sodium concentration indicated renal conservation of sodium—a normal renal response to fluid volume depletion. The urine osmolality was high as the kidneys attempted to retain needed fluid. The elevated BUN:Cr ratio strongly indicated fluid volume depletion.

Case Study 17-2

A 70-year-old woman with congestive heart failure was admitted with distended neck veins and pedal edema. On admission, her BUN was 20 mg/dL and her serum creatinine was 1.2 mg/dL. A 5-kg weight loss occurred after 3 days of diuretic therapy; although a marked improvement was noted in her clinical status, a mild degree of pulmonary edema persisted. The BUN had increased to 90 mg/dL and the serum creatinine increased to 3.0 mg/dL.

Differentiation Between Prerenal Azotemia and Acute Tubular Necrosis (ATN)

Laboratory Finding	Prerenal Azotemia	Acute Tubular Necrosis
BUN/Cr ratio	>20:1	10:1
Urine Na (mEq/L)	< 20	> 40
Urine osmolality (mOsm/kg)	> 500	< 350

Commentary. The elevated BUN and serum creatinine levels (BUN/Cr ratio = 30:1) were the result of renal hypoperfusion secondary to excessive diuresis. This patient's heart disease was so severe that she could not simultaneously be edema-free and have a normal plasma creatinine concentration. Therapy was initiated to improve her cardiac output.

Case Study 17-3

A 25-year-old woman with a 10-year history of progressive renal failure was admitted with mild hypertension. Laboratory data included a normal serum sodium level (139 mEq/L) and mild hyperkalemia (K 5.9 mEq/L). The BUN was elevated (80 mg/dL) and the bicarbonate was low (14 mEq/L).

Commentary. The low bicarbonate level indicated metabolic acidosis (the expected acid–base imbalance in a patient with CRF). In renal insufficiency, metabolic acidosis is due to the inability of the kidneys to excrete the large daily hydrogen load. The anion gap (AG) is calculated by subtracting the sum of the serum bicarbonate and chloride levels from the serum sodium level.

$$AG = Na - (HCO_3 + Cl)$$

$$AG = 139 - (14 + 105) = 20 \text{ mEq/L}$$

This patient's AG of 20 mEq/L was high; the normal range is approximately 12 ± 2 mEq/L. This high AG acidosis reflected the retention of phosphate, sulfate, and other organic anions.

The patient's serum potassium level was above normal because renal failure causes poor renal excretion of potassium; further, metabolic acidosis favors shifting of cellular potassium into the plasma. Oral bicarbonate replacement may be prescribed to keep the serum bicarbonate at approximately 20 mEq/L.

Case Study 17-4

A young man with multiple contusions was found unconscious and admitted to the emergency room. His urine was brown and tested positive for blood. Abnormal laboratory findings revealed hyperkalemia (K = 7.5 mEq/L), a markedly elevated serum creatinine (17 mg/dL), a markedly elevated blood urea nitrogen level (125 mg/dL), mild hypernatremia (Na = 150 mEq/L), and acidosis (pH 7.30). The plasma chloride concentration was mildly elevated (Cl = 113 mEq/L). The patient was diagnosed as having ARF secondary to rhabdomyolysis (a condition in which myoglobin is released into the bloodstream from injured muscles). The subsequent attempt of the kidneys to excrete the myoglobin resulted in acute tubular necrosis and accounted for the heme-positive urine.

Commentary. The plasma potassium concentration of 7.5 mEq/L was life-threatening and required immediate treatment. It occurred because large amounts of potassium were released from the injured muscle cells into the bloodstream; the presence of metabolic acidosis added to the hyperkalemia by fostering a shift of potassium from the cells into the extracellular space. Using the formula AG = Na − (Cl + HCO$_3$), it was noted that a high AG metabolic acidosis was present; this is characteristic in ARF. The BUN/Cr ratio was close to 10:1.

Case Study 17-5

A 35-year-old woman underwent a kidney transplant. In the course of this procedure, she received 1 L of lactated Ringer's solution, 1 L of 0.9% NaCl, and 20 g mannitol.[90] The surgery was uneventful, and urine output appeared promptly. Postoperatively, the patient's urine output averaged 1000 mL/hr due to a temporary acute tubular dysfunction. She then received 0.45% NaCl intravenously at a rate to match her hourly urine output. Two boluses of 0.9% NaCl were required to keep her blood pressure in the normal range. Fifteen hours postoperatively, the patient suffered a generalized seizure; she was drowsy but arousable. Blood work revealed hyponatremia (Na 120 mEq/L), mild hypokalemia (K 3.4 mEq/L), and a low total calcium level (7.0 mg/dL).

Commentary. The most likely basis for the patient's seizure was acute hyponatremia, brought about by the excessive infusion of a hypotonic saline solution. During a period of 14 hours, she had received a total of 1009 mEq Na (13.1 L of 0.45% NaCl, which contains 77 mEq of sodium per liter. However, her urinary loss of sodium during the same time was calculated at 1441 mEq. Therefore, she had a total sodium deficit of 432 mEq during this period. In other words, hyponatremia in this patient represented the outcome of the administration of large amounts of IV fluid that were hypotonic to her polyuric losses. The patient subsequently recovered following treatment. A lesson to be learned from this case is that plasma and urine electrolytes should be monitored frequently (such as every 2 to 4 hours) when polyuria occurs after transplantation and the urine should be replaced with IV therapy appropriate for both volume and tonicity.

Case Study 17-6

A 63-year-old man with diabetes mellitus whose renal function had worsened over the last few years noticed that his urine output had been decreasing, as had the number of voids per day. On a visit to his physician, the following symptoms were noted: body weight 88 kg (normal 83 kg), shortness of breath, wet breath sounds, muscle weakness (especially in his legs), low urine output (less than 180 mL/24 hours), increased thirst, and a decreased level of consciousness. Laboratory results included hyperkalemia (K = 6.2 mEq/L), mild hyponatremia (Na = 132 mEq/L), an elevated serum creatinine level (5.5 mg/dL) and an elevated blood urea nitrogen level (42 mg/dL).

It was concluded that the patient's condition had progressed to end-stage renal disease and that hemodialysis was indicated. A subclavian double-lumen central venous catheter was inserted the next morning and the patient was scheduled to have an arteriovenous access inserted in his left forearm. A hemodialysis treatment was performed that afternoon after the subclavian catheter was inserted. Following this treatment, the patient's dry weight was 84 kg and the following laboratory values were obtained: serum sodium increased from 132 mEq/L to 142 mEq/L (within normal range), serum potassium decreased from 6.2 mEq/L to 4.7 mEq/L (within normal range), and BUN decreased from 42 mg/dL to 15 mg/dL (within normal range). Serum creatinine decreased from 5.5 mg/dL to 3.5 mg/dL (improved but still elevated). Clinically, the patient appeared much improved. His shortness of breath and wet breath sounds disappeared. Although he was still weak, his level of consciousness was significantly improved.

Commentary. The hemodialysis treatment was effective in reducing the patient's fluid volume overload, hyperkalemia, high BUN, and serum creatinine. The patient was scheduled to receive hemodialysis three times per week. Without this treatment, serious fluid volume overload and hyperkalemia, as well as other uremic abnormalities, would develop. It is not unusual for patients to feel exhausted after a hemodialysis treatment, largely due to the shifting of fluids and particles from the patient to the dialysate over a short period of time. Note that this patient lost 4 kg of weight during the hemodialysis treatment: It is important to monitor for hypotension and excessive fluid loss during hemodialysis.

Case Study 17-7

A 48-year-old woman who had been on hemodialysis for 3 years was apparently doing well but wished to switch to peritoneal dialysis so that she could be more independent. She discussed her wishes with her physician, who agreed to the change in treatment. A Tenchkhoff peritoneal catheter was placed in her abdomen and her incision healed without complication. The patient remained on hemodialysis while she trained for peritoneal dialysis at home. Following her training classes, her vital signs were within normal limits, her lungs were clear, her catheter exit site was clean, and her dry weight was 55 kg. Her laboratory values included normal serum sodium (Na = 142 mEq/L), normal serum potassium (K = 4.1 mEq/L), normal blood urea nitrogen (BUN = 10 mg/dL), and mildly elevated serum creatinine (Cr = 2.1 mg/dL).

The patient was started on five 2-L dialysate exchanges daily. After the first month of peritoneal dialysis, her weight had increased to 62 kg and she had dependent edema and wet breath sounds. Her laboratory values were hyperkalemia (K = 6.2 mEq/L), normal serum sodium (Na = 138 mEq/L), elevated blood urea nitrogen (BUN = 60 mg/dL), and markedly elevated serum creatinine (Cr = 19 mg/dL). It was discovered that the patient had not been leaving her peritoneal dialysate fluid in as long as prescribed; also, she had used only three exchanges per day (not the prescribed five exchanges). As a consequence, fluid and wastes were inadequately removed. The patient indicated she had developed progressively greater difficulty in remembering how many exchanges she had performed.

A peritoneal dialysis treatment was administered while the patient was seen at the clinic. She returned home with her peritoneal dialysis prescription reinforced to accomplish five exchanges daily. The patient's in-clinic dialysis laboratory values were improved and included normal serum potassium (K = 5.0 mEq/L), normal serum sodium (Na = 142 mEq/L), elevated blood urea nitrogen (BUN = 33 mg/dL), and elevated, but much improved, serum creatinine (Cr = 9.0 mg/dL).

Commentary. The patient's serum potassium, BUN, and Cr levels became markedly elevated when she switched from hemodialysis to the improperly performed peritoneal dialysis treatment. By comparison, the patient's laboratory values improved significantly following a properly performed in-clinic dialysis. Although patients on peritoneal dialysis have more flexibility than those on hemodialysis, healthcare providers must emphasize to them as part of patient education that interruptions in the peritoneal fluid and dialysate exchanges can lead to progressive changes in laboratory values and clinical status.

Case Study 17-8

A 23-year-old man with acute myelogenous leukemia had a bone marrow transplant; his weight following this procedure was 78 kg. Two weeks later, he developed graft-versus-host disease (GVHD) and his BUN, creatinine, and bilirubin levels began to progressively increase. For the next 2 weeks, his urine output remained greater than 30 mL/hr. However, during the third week following his bone marrow transplant, his urine output dropped to less than 10 mL/hr, the patient gained 5 kg (weight = 83 kg), and his level of consciousness decreased. Laboratory values were: hyperkalemia (K = 6.5 mEq/L), hyponatremia (Na = 123 mEq/L), markedly elevated blood urea nitrogen (BUN = 222 mg/dL), and markedly elevated serum creatinine (Cr = 50 mg/dL). His output was only 6 mL/hr. Vital signs included temperature 101.4°F, heart rate 120 beats per minute, and BP 86/40 mm Hg.

Because he was fluid volume overloaded and in acute renal failure, the patient was transferred to the intensive care unit and placed on continuous venovenous hemodialysis (CVVH). After 17 hours, his laboratory values had significantly improved: normal serum potassium (K = 4.1

mEq/L), normal serum sodium (Na = 142 mEq/L), and a still elevated, but much improved blood urea nitrogen (BUN = 100 mg/dL). Similarly, his creatinine was still elevated but much improved (Cr = 20 mg/dL). The patient's vital signs were also improved: blood pressure, 118/72; pulse, 92; and temperature, 99.6°F. His body weight decreased from 83 kg to 80 kg.

Commentary. With the initiation of CVVH, the critical care team was able to correct the patient's fluid volume overload and hyperkalemia. There were significant improvements in the BUN and serum creatinine levels. The patient remained on CVVH for 5 days, during which time his GVHD worsened. This condition stimulated the generation of large amounts of BUN and creatinine, causing the patient's condition to progressively degenerate. He ultimately suffered cardiac arrest and died.

Case Study 17-9

A 50-year-old man with liver failure caused by chronic alcohol abuse developed hepato-renal failure. His baseline body weight was 90 kg. The patient's serum albumin level had remained close to 3.0 g/dL for the previous year. His food intake was essentially limited to snack foods and alcohol. Over a period of approximately a year, his abdominal girth progressively increased while he continued to lose weight. When he was seen in a clinic, the following laboratory values were observed: hyponatremia (Na = 130 mEq/L), normal serum potassium (K = 5.1 mEq/L), a markedly elevated blood urea nitrogen (BUN = 200 mg/dL) and a markedly elevated serum creatinine (Cr = 30 mg/dL). In addition, his liver enzymes were elevated. The patient's body weight was 78 kg and his vital signs included a blood pressure of 72/56 mm Hg and pulse of 112. Due to his worsening BUN and serum creatinine (as well as elevated liver enzymes), the patient was admitted to the hospital for hemodialysis treatments and close monitoring. Because he was hypotensive, it was decided that continuous venovenous hemofiltration was more appropriate than hemodialysis. After he was on CVVH for 24 hours, the patient's laboratory values improved. The blood urea nitrogen decreased from 200 mg/dL to 120 mg/dL, and his serum creatinine decreased from 30 mg/dL to 10 mg/dL. The serum sodium level increased from 130 mEq/L to 140 mEq/L, and his potassium level decreased from 5.1 mEq/L to 4.4 mEq/L. The patient's weight was maintained at 78 kg

but his vital signs improved: blood pressure increased from 72/56 mm Hg to 112/70 mm Hg, and his pulse rate decreased from 112 to 96.

Commentary. Patients with advancing liver failure often present with signs and symptoms of fluid volume overload, increased abdominal girth, low serum albumin levels, elevated BUN levels, and elevated liver enzyme levels. These patients may be admitted to critical care units and placed on continuous renal replacement therapy until they are stable enough for a liver transplant.

Case Study 17-10

A 76-year-old woman with type 1 diabetes mellitus and a double above-the-knee amputation had been maintained on hemodialysis for 5 years. She was dialyzed 3 times per week, on a Monday–Wednesday–Friday schedule. During her years on hemodialysis, she had varying weight gains between dialysis treatments. Her most current set of laboratory values were normal serum sodium (Na = 139 mEq/L), hyperkalemia (K = 6.6 mEq/L), elevated blood urea nitrogen (BUN = 38 mg/dL), and elevated serum creatinine level (Cr = 12 mg/dL). Her weight was 79.6 kg, her blood pressure was 112/76 mm Hg, and her pulse rate was 88.

While attending a family reunion on a Sunday afternoon, the patient ate large quantities of strawberries and watermelon. (One cup of raw strawberries contains 6.5 mEq of potassium; 1 cup of watermelon contains 5 mEq of potassium.) When she came to the hemodialysis unit on Monday morning, she was listless, confused, and not her usual self. Although her goal dry weight was 73 kg, her weight at this time was 83 kg. Stat laboratory data revealed hyperkalemia (K = 10.2 mEq/L), hyponatremia (Na = 132 mEq/L), elevated blood urea nitrogen (BUN = 75 mg/dL), and a markedly elevated serum creatinine level (Cr = 30 mg/dL). Her pulse rate was 44 and her blood pressure was 90/40 mm Hg. Hemodialysis was initiated with a zero-mEq potassium concentration in the dialysate. During dialysis, the patient's heart rate dropped to 30 beats/min and she become hypotensive and lost consciousness. A temporary pacemaker was inserted while she was in the dialysis unit. Following the hemodialysis treatment, her weight was 78 kg. She was admitted to the coronary care unit and was found to have a third-degree heart block. While in the coronary unit, a permanent pacemaker was inserted and paced at 72 beats/min. Her laboratory values following the hemodialysis showed improvement in hyperkalemia (decreased from

10.2 mEq/L to 6.8 mEq/L), improvement in serum sodium concentration (increased from 132 mEq/L to 140 mEq/L), improvement in BUN level (decreased from 75 mg/dL to 36 mg/dL), and improvement in Cr level (decreased from 30 mg/dL to 10 mg/dL).

Commentary. Although changes in fluid and electrolyte levels are common between dialysis treatments, this patient's fluctuations were intensified by her high consumption of potassium-containing foods. It was necessary to carefully reduce her weight and serum potassium level because her history of cardiovascular disease increased her likelihood of developing complications if rapid shifts were achieved. Dietary counseling was provided to prevent a recurrence of this unfortunate set of circumstances.

Case Study 17-11

A 67-year-old man with a history of chronic renal failure, congestive heart failure, diabetes mellitus, hypertension, and coronary artery disease was admitted to the hospital with increased severity of his congestive heart failure.[91] His home medications included spironolactone (Aldactone) 25 mg and enalapril (Vasotec) 20 mg. Baseline laboratory values included mildly elevated serum creatinine (1.7 mg/dL) and mild hyper-

kalemia (5.4 mEq/L). The patient's glomerular filtration rate (GFR) was 28 mL/min, indicating stage 4 chronic renal failure. On admission to the hospital, the patient's serum creatinine was found to be further elevated (2.1 mg/dL) and a significant increase in his serum potassium level was noted (7.4 mEq/L). The patient developed cardiac arrest and died.

Commentary. Severely impaired baseline renal function was present, as evidenced by a GFR of 28 mL/min. While spironolactone (a potassium-conserving agent) is commonly used to treat patients with heart failure, it should have been avoided in this patient because of his severe renal disease. Adding to his problem was decreased renal perfusion secondary to his worsening congestive heart failure and use of an ACE inhibitor (enalapril—a drug that predisposes individuals to hyperkalemia). A potassium-sparing drug (such as spironolactone) should generally not be used in patients with heart failure who are receiving enalapril. The authors of this case report pointed out that the serum creatinine level in this patient was misleading, and estimation of the GFR was a more reliable indicator of his renal function.

Also see Case Studies 4-6, 4-9, 5-9, 5-10, 7-5, 7-6, 8-6, 16-2, and 16-3 regarding fluid and electrolyte problems in patients with renal conditions.

Summary of Key Points

- Glomerular filtration rate (GFR) describes the flow rate of filtered fluid through the kidneys. It varies according to age, sex, and body size, and declines with age. The normal GFR is more than 90 mL/min per 1.73 m^2 body surface area.

- The glomerular filtration rate must decrease by approximately half before the serum creatinine concentration changes appreciably (more than 1 mg/dL). Thus serum creatinine may grossly underestimate the prevalence and severity of chronic kidney disease.

- Factors that can increase the blood urea nitrogen (BUN) include reduced renal blood flow, high dietary protein intake, and bleeding into the GI tract.

- Prerenal failure (also called prerenal azotemia) refers to hypoperfusion of the kidney (such as occurs in fluid volume deficit or reduced cardiac output) that leads to azotemia without actual damage to renal tissue. It is often characterized by a BUN to creatinine ratio that exceeds 20:1.

- The most common cause of acute renal failure is acute tubular necrosis (ATN). To prevent prerenal azotemia from advancing to ATN, it is important to make an early distinction between these two conditions.

- A major cause of acute renal failure in hospitalized patients is contrast medium-induced nephropathy (CIN). To help prevent CIN, intravenous fluids are started 12 to 24 hours before the contrast study begins and continued up to 12 hours after the study ends.

- Fluid balance is precarious in patients with acute renal failure. To plan appropriate fluid replacement therapy, all fluid losses and gains must be assessed and monitored on an ongoing basis.

- Hyperkalemia is a major cause of death during the oliguric phase of acute renal failure; it does not generally occur unless the GFR is less than 50–60 mL/min/1.73 m^2.

- The IV administration of calcium to treat hyperkalemia does not change the serum potassium concentration, but does rapidly decrease myocardial membrane sensitivity and reduces the ill effects of hyperkalemia on the heart.

- Administration of insulin with a glucose solution promotes movement of serum potassium into the cells, thereby temporarily reducing an elevated serum potassium concentration.

- Cation resins are rather slow in reducing serum potassium concentrations and usually the dose needs to be repeated several times. These agents are best used to prevent a modestly elevated serum potassium concentration from advancing to a severely elevated level.

- In the presence of renal failure, the body adapts by increasing potassium excretion via the bowel. Thus it is important to prevent constipation in patients with renal failure.

- Serum phosphate levels become elevated early in the course of acute renal failure, and have an inverse parallel relationship with the development of hypocalcemia.

- Hypermagnesemia is usually not a major problem unless the patient with renal failure consumes an exogenous source of magnesium (such as magnesium-containing laxatives or antacids).

- Patients with acute renal failure typically have a high anion gap (AG) metabolic acidosis due to the retention of strong acids and accompanying anions not routinely measured by the laboratory; these include sulfate, phosphate, and a variety of organic acids.

- Patients with chronic renal failure may develop hypertension and congestive heart failure as a result of fluid volume overload.

NOTES

1. Josephs, S. A., & Thakar, C. V. (2009). Perioperative risk assessment, prevention, and treatment of acute kidney injury. *International Anesthesiology Clinics, 47*(4), 89–105.

2. American Kidney Foundation. (2002). K/DOQI Clinical practice guidelines for chronic kidney disease: Evaluation, classification, and stratification. *American Journal of Kidney Diseases, 39*(2 suppl 1), S1–S266.

3. Bongard, F. S., Sue, D. Y., & Vintch, J. R. (2008). *Current diagnosis and treatment, critical care* (3rd ed.). New York: McGraw-Hill/Lange, p. 314.

4. Acquarone, N., Castello, C., Antonucci, G., Lione, S., & Bellotti, P. (2009). Pharmacologic therapy in patients with chronic heart failure and chronic kidney disease. *Journal of Cardiovascular Medicine, 10,* 13–21.

5. Paige, N. M., & Nagami, G. T. (2009). The top 10 things nephrologists wish every primary care physician knew. *Mayo Clinic Proceedings, 84*(2), 180–186.

6. Bongard et al., note 3, p. 314.

7. Bongard et al., note 3, p. 315.

8. Bongard et al., note 3, p. 316.

9. Bongard et al., note 3, p. 316.

10. American Kidney Foundation, note 2.

11. Cockroft, D. W., & Gault, M. H. (1976). Prediction of creatinine clearance from serum creatinine. *Nephron, 16*(1), 31–41.

12. Xue, J. L., Daniels, F., Star, R. A., Kimmel, P. L., Eggers, P. W., Molitoris, B. A., et al. (2006). Incidence and mortality of acute renal failure in Medicare beneficiaries, 1992 to 2001. *Journal of the American Society of Nephrology, 17,* 1135–1142.

13. McPhee, S. J., Papadakis, M. A., & Tierney, M. L. (2008). *Current medical diagnosis and treatment.* New York: McGraw-Hill/Lange, p. 789.

14. McPhee et al., note 13, p. 789.

15. McPhee et al., note 13, p. 789.

16. Massicotte, A. (2008). Contrast medium-induced nephropathy: Strategies for prevention. *Pharmacotherapy, 28*(9), 1140–1150.

17. Sinert, R., & Doty, C. I. (2007). Prevention of contrast-induced nephropathy in the emergency department. *Annals of Emergency Medicine, 50,* 335–345.

18. Pucelikova, T., Dangas, G., & Mehran, R. (2008). Contrast-induced nephropathy. *Catheterization & Cardiovascular Interventions, 71*(1), 62–72.

19. Pucelikova et al., note 18.

20. Sinert & Doty, note 17.

21. McPhee et al., note 13, p. 790.

22. Sinert & Doty, note 17.

23. Benko, A., Fraser-Hill, M., Magner, P., Capusten, B., Barrett, B., Myers, A., et al. (2007). Canadian Association of Radiologists: Consensus guidelines for the prevention of contrast-induced nephropathy. *Canadian Association of Radiologists Journal, 58*(2), 79–87.

24. Pucelikova et al., note 18.

25. Cooper, D. H., Krainik, A. J., Lubner, S. M., & Reno, H. E. (Eds.). (2007). *The Washington manual of medical therapeutics* (32nd ed.). Philadelphia: Wolters Kluwer/Lippincott Williams & Wilkins, p. 320.

26. Asif, A., Garces, G., Preston, R. A., & Roth, D. (2005). Current trials of interventions to prevent radiocontrast-induced nephropathy. *American Journal of Therapeutics, 12*(2), 127–132.

27. Marenzi, G., & Bartorelli, A. L. (2004). Recent advances in the prevention of radiocontrast-induced nephropathy. *Current Opinion in Critical Care, 10*(6), 505–509.

28. Al-Ghonaim, M., & Pannu, N. (2006). Prevention and treatment of contrast-induced nephropathy. *Techniques in Vascular & Interventional Radiology, 9*(2), 42–49.

29. Alonso, A., Lau, J., Jaber, B. L., Weintraub, A., & Sarnak, M. J. (2004). Prevention of radiocontrast nephropathy with *N*-acetyl-

cysteine in patients with chronic kidney disease: A meta-analysis of randomized, controlled trials. *American Journal of Kidney Diseases, 43*(1), 1–9.

30. Kelly, A. M., Dwamena, B., Cronin, P., Bernstein, S. J., & Carlos, R. C. (2008). Meta-analysis: Effectiveness of drugs for preventing contrast-induced nephropathy. *Annals of Internal Medicine, 148*(4), 284–294.

31. Sinert & Doty, note 17.

32. Ward, M. M. (1988). Factors predictive of acute renal failure in rhabdomyolysis. *Archives of Internal Medicine, 148,* 1553–1557.

33. Melli, G., Chaudry, V., & Cornblath, D. R. (2005). Rhabdomyolysis: An evaluation of 475 hospitalized patients. *Medicine, 84*(6), 377–385.

34. Nauss, M. D., Schmidt, E. L., & Pancioli, A. M. (2009). Viral myositis leading to rhabdomyolysis: A case report and literature review. *American Journal of Emergency Medicine, 27*(3), 372–375.

35. McPhee et al., note 13, p. 780.

36. Sauret, J. M., Marinides, G., & Wang, G. K. (2002). Rhabdomyolysis. *American Family Physician, 65,* 907–912.

37. Sauret et al., note 36.

38. Sauret et al., note 36.

39. Narins, R. (1994). *Maxwell & Kleeman's clinical disorders of fluid and electrolyte metabolism* (5th ed.). New York: McGraw-Hill, p. 1177.

40. Cooper et al., note 25, p. 321.

41. Narins, note 39, p. 1183.

42. Narins, note 39, p. 1184.

43. Arieff, A., & De Fronzo, R. (1995). *Fluid, electrolyte, and acid–base disorders* (2nd ed.). New York: Churchill Livingstone, p. 643.

44. Takaichi, K., Takemoto, F., Ubara, Y., & Mori, Y. (2008). The clinically significant estimated glomerular filtration rate for hyperkalemia. *Internal Medicine, 47*(14), 1315–1323.

45. Arieff & De Fronzo, note 43, p. 665.

46. Narins, note 39, p. 1185.

47. Arieff & De Fronzo, note 43, p. 665.

48. Singer, G. G., & Brenner, B. M. (2008). Fluid and electrolyte disturbances. In A. S. Fauci et al. (Eds.), *Harrison's principles of internal medicine* (17th ed.). New York: McGraw-Hill Medical, p. 284.

49. Singer & Brenner, note 48, p. 284.

50. Singer & Brenner, note 48, p. 284.

51. Sood, M. M., Sood, A. R., & Richardson, R. R. (2007). Emergency management and commonly encountered outpatient scenarios in patients with hyperkalemia. *Mayo Clinic Proceedings, 82*(12), 1553–1561.

52. Sood et al., note 51.

53. Singer & Brenner, note 48, p. 284.

54. Cooper et al., note 25, p. 77.

55. Singer & Brenner, note 48, p. 284.

56. Kim, H. J., & Han, S. W. (2002). Therapeutic approach to hyperkalemia. *Nephron, 92*(suppl 1), 33–40.

57. Sood et al., note 51.

58. Cooper et al., note 25, p. 77.

59. Sood et al., note 51, p. 77.

60. Allon, M. (1995). Hyperkalemia in end-stage renal disease: Mechanism and management. *Journal of the American Society of Nephrology, 6*(4), 1134–1142.

61. Sood et al., note 51, p. 77.

62. Mathialahan, T., Maclennan K. A, Sandle, L. N., Verbeke, C., & Sandle, G. I. (2005). Enhanced large intestinal potassium permeability in end-stage renal disease. *Journal of Pathology, 206*(1), 46–51.

63. Narins, note 38, p. 1189.

64. Arieff & De Fronzo, note 43, p. 557.

65. Parillo, J. E., & Dellinger, R. P. (2008). *Critical care medicine: Principles of diagnosis and management in the adult* (3rd ed.). Philadelphia: Mosby Elsevier, p. 1179.

66. Arieff & De Fronzo, note 43, p. 663.

67. Arieff & De Fronzo, note 43, p. 663.

68. Arieff & De Fronzo, note 43, p. 663.

69. Arieff & De Fronzo, note 43, p. 537.

70. Parillo & Dellinger, note 65, p. 1179.

71. Parillo & Dellinger, note 65, p. 1179.

72. Parillo & Dellinger, note 65, p. 1179.

73. Parillo & Dellinger, note 65, p. 1179.

74. Parillo & Dellinger, note 65, p. 1198.

75. Parillo & Dellinger, note 65, p. 1196.

76. Narins, note 39, p. 1204.

77. Weinberg, J. M., Appel, L. J., Bakris, G., Gassman, J. J., Greene, T., Kendrick, C. A., et al. (2009). African American Study of Hypertension and Kidney Disease Collaborative Research Group: Risk of hyperkalemia in nondiabetic patients with chronic kidney disease receiving antihypertensive therapy. *Archives of Internal Medicine, 169*(17), 1587–1594.

78. Arieff & De Fronzo, note 43, p. 805.

79. Arieff & De Fronzo, note 43, p. 806.

80. Putcha, N. & Allon, M. (2007). Management of hyperkalemia in dialysis patients. *Seminars in Dialysis, 20*(5), 431–439.

81. Paige & Nagami, note 5.

82. Paige & Nagami, note 5.

83. Bargman, J. M., & Skorecki, K. (2008). Chronic kidney disease. In A. S. Fauci et al. (Eds.), *Harrison's internal medicine* (17th ed.). New York: McGraw-Hill Medical.

84. Sullivan, C., Sayre, S. S., Leon, J. B., Machekano, R., Love, T. E., Porter, D., et al. (2009). Effect of food additives on hyperphosphatemia among patients with end-stage renal disease: A randomized controlled trial. *Journal of the American Medical Association, 301*(6), 629–635.

85. Connor, A. (2009). Novel therapeutic agents and strategies for the management of chronic kidney disease mineral and bone disorder. *Postgraduate Medical Journal, 85,* 274–279.

86. Parillo & Dellinger, note 65, p. 1196.

87. Parillo & Dellinger, note 65, p. 1196.

88. Parillo & Dellinger, note 65, p. 1196.

89. Bargman & Skorecki, note 83, p. 1767.

90. Zaltzman, J. S. (1996). Post-renal transplantation hyponatremia. *American Journal of Kidney Disease, 27*(4), 599–602.

91. Blaustein, D. A., Babu, K., Reddy, A., Schwenk, M. H., & Avram, M. M. (2002). Estimation of glomerular filtration rate to prevent life-threatening hyperkalemia due to combined therapy with spironolactone and angiotensin-converting enzyme inhibition or angiotensin receptor blockade. *American Journal of Cardiology, 90*(6), 662–663.

Chapter 18

Diabetic Ketoacidosis and Hyperglycemic Hyperosmolar State

DIFFERENTIATION BETWEEN DKA AND HHS

Diabetic ketoacidosis (DKA) and hyperglycemic hyperosmolar state (HHS) are metabolic complications of an absolute or relative lack of insulin and an excess of glucose-elevating hormones. The major characteristics of DKA are severe hyperglycemia, metabolic acidosis, and ketosis (**Table 18-1**). In contrast, HHS is characterized by severe hyperglycemia, hyperosmolality, and dehydration in the absence of significant ketoacidosis.[1] Most patients with DKA have autoimmune type 1 diabetes, whereas most patients with HHS have type 2 diabetes. Nevertheless, some crossover occurs between these conditions such that individuals with type 2 diabetes

may also experience DKA when they are subjected to acute illness or stress. Also, HHS—a condition typically associated with older individuals—is being increasingly reported in young diabetics.[2,3] Because childhood obesity has become a pandemic healthcare problem, more cases of type 2 diabetes are occurring in children; incidence in this group has increased 10-fold in the past 20 years.[4]

Precipitating Factors

A variety of factors can predispose individuals to the development of DKA and HHS (**Table 18-2**). Probably the most common precipitating factor in DKA is infection, with

Table 18-1 Diagnostic Criteria for DKA and HHS

	DKA			HHS
	Mild	Moderate	Severe	
Plasma glucose (mg/dL)	> 250	> 250	> 250	> 600
Arterial pH	7.25–7.30	7.00 to < 7.24	< 7.00	> 7.30
Serum bicarbonate (mEq/L)	15–18	10 to < 15	< 10	> 18
Urine ketones[a]	Positive	Positive	Positive	Small
Serum ketones[a]	Positive	Positive	Positive	Small
Effective serum osmolality (mOsm/kg)[b]	Variable	Variable	Variable	> 320
Anion gap[c]	> 10	> 12	> 12	Variable
Mental status	Alert	Alert/drowsy	Stupor/coma	Stupor/coma

  a. Nitroprusside reaction method.

  b. Calculation: 2 [measured Na (mEq/L)] + glucose (mg/dL)/18.

  c. Calculation: (Na) – (Cl + HCO_3) (mEq/L).

Table 18-2 Examples of Factors That May Predispose to DKA or HHS

Infections (especially pneumonia and urinary tract infections)

Deliberate omission of insulin

Failure of insulin delivery systems

Eating disorders in young persons with type 1 diabetes

Alcohol abuse

Illicit drugs (such as cocaine)

Surgery

Trauma

Dehydration

Psychological stress

Second-generation antipsychotic agents

Diuretics (especially thiazides)

Corticosteroids

Total parenteral nutrition or enteral feedings

Pancreatitis

Myocardial infarction

Cerebrovascular accidents

---

pneumonia and urinary tract infections being responsible for 30% to 50% of all cases.[5] In patients with HHS, the problem is often an underlying medical illness that provokes the release of counter-regulatory hormones.[6]

Clinical Signs

The clinical presentations of patients with DKA and HHS are similar in many respects. Both demonstrate a history of polyuria, polydipsia, fatigue, weight loss, dehydration, and mental status changes. However, the conditions usually differ in time of onset. For example, DKA typically develops quickly (over a period less than 24 hours), whereas HHS usually emerges over a period of several days to weeks. HHS is characterized by severe hyperglycemia and dehydration with mental status changes in the absence of significant acidosis. The patient with HHS has sufficient insulin to prevent lipolysis and subsequent ketogenesis, but not enough to prevent hyperglycemia.[7]

Emesis in patients with DKA is common and may have a coffee-ground appearance (likely due to hemorrhagic gastritis).[8] Abdominal pain is also common in patients with DKA and may be related to acidosis or reduced mesenteric perfusion.[9] If the abdominal pain does not subside following correction of acidosis, a search for abdominal pathology should be initiated, including measurement of serum amy-

lase and lipase along with an ultrasound of the abdomen.[10] Patients with HHS are less likely to experience vomiting and abdominal pain than are patients with DKA.

A patient with DKA typically has deep air-hunger respirations (Kussmaul respirations), while the HHS patient does not (because the latter individual does not have acidosis). Recall that hyperventilation is a compensatory action by the lungs to reduce the $PaCO_2$ in an attempt to more closely match the decreased bicarbonate concentration. Another marker for DKA may be a fruity odor to the breath, indicating the presence of exhaled acetone (**Table 18-3**).

Leukocytosis in the range of 10,000 to 15,000 m^3 is a common finding in patients with DKA and HHS and may be due to the stress response rather than resulting from an infectious process.[11] In any event, a count of 25,000 m^3 requires further evaluation.

The normal serum osmolality ranges between 285 and 295 mOsm/kg. When the effective serum osmolality is 330 mOsm/kg or greater, the majority of patients will be severely obtunded or comatose. If mental status changes are observed in a patient without a significantly elevated serum osmolality, a search should be initiated for a neurological event, such as a cerebrovascular accident.

In some patients, DKA or HHS is the presenting indicator of diabetes mellitus. For example, new-onset diabetes accounts for as many as 30% of patients presenting with DKA.[12]

Laboratory Evaluations

While clinical observations are important, laboratory evaluations are crucial in distinguishing between DKA and HHS, in determining the severity of the conditions, and in analyzing the response to treatment (Table 18-1). Although point-of-care testing is helpful in emergency situations, analyses performed in a laboratory are more accurate.[13] In addition to glucose, the most important laboratory tests are serum and urinary ketones, serum creatinine, blood urea nitrogen (BUN), and an electrolyte panel that includes potassium, sodium, phosphorus, calcium, and magnesium. A complete blood count (CBC) with a differential is also performed to determine if infection is present. Arterial blood gas (ABG) evaluations are needed in acutely ill patients to monitor the severity of acidosis and determine their oxygenation status. Until the patient has been stabilized, serum glucose levels are checked hourly, and serum electrolytes are checked every 2 to 4 hours. A standardized flow sheet to monitor laboratory results is commonly used in acute care facilities to monitor the status of seriously ill patients with DKA and

Table 18-3 Clinical Signs of DKA and Their Probable Causes

Clinical Signs	Probable Causes
Hyperglycemia: Normal blood glucose is in the range of 80–120 mg/dL. Elevations associated with DKA may be as high as 4000 mg/dL.	Faulty glucose metabolism causes glucose to accumulate in the bloodstream: The lack of insulin decreases glucose uptake by most cells and increases gluconeogenesis in the liver.
Glucosuria	The blood glucose level exceeds the renal threshold (normally 180 mg/dL, but higher in elderly persons), causing glucose to spill into the urine.
Polyuria (initially) with high specific gravity	Osmotic diuretic effect of hyperglycemia; high renal solute load.
Polydipsia	Thirst due to cellular dehydration: Cells become dehydrated when water is drawn from them by the hypertonic ECF.
Anorexia, nausea, and vomiting	Follow onset of DKA; interfere with fluid intake, hastening the development of fluid volume deficit.
Poor skin turgor, dry mucous membranes, and poor tongue turgor	Fluid volume deficit.
Acute weight loss	Parallels acute loss of body fluids.
Ketonemia and ketonuria	Excessive accumulation of ketones in the bloodstream causes them to spill out into the urine.
Deep "air hunger" respirations (Kussmaul respirations)	Compensatory mechanism that seeks to increase plasma pH by eliminating large amounts of carbon dioxide.
Acetone odor to breath—similar to that of overripe apples	Acetone, a volatile ketone, is vaporized in the expired air. This odor may sometimes be obscured by the odor of vomitus.
Abdominal pain: can simulate acute appendicitis, pancreatitis, or other acute abdominal problems	Apparently due to the DKA. Anorexia, nausea, and vomiting precede the abdominal pain when it is due to DKA; this is in contrast to most surgical emergencies, in which the pain usually occurs first.
Postural hypotension	Fluid volume deficit; eventually the person is hypotensive even when supine.
Fatigue and muscular weakness	Lack of carbohydrate utilization; hypokalemia.
Hypothermia or normal temperature	Fever is present only when there is a concurrent illness associated with fever.
Oliguria and anuria (late)	Fluid volume deficit causes a decreased renal blood flow and a decreased glomerular filtration rate.
Depressed sensorium, ranging from somnolence to coma	The level of consciousness correlates best with the level of hyperglycemia and plasma osmolality.
Elevated serum osmolality: Normal is in the range of 280–295 mOsm/kg	High glucose level; high BUN from fluid volume deficit.
Potassium variations	Serum potassium concentration usually elevated before treatment; later, however, it may drop to seriously low levels.
Hypophosphatemia	Phosphate excretion increases during osmotic diuresis.
Increased blood urea nitrogen: Normal is in the range of 10–20 mg/dL	Fluid volume deficit leads to decreased GFR and urinary retention of urea waste products.
Decreased serum bicarbonate (HCO_3)	Excessive ketonic anions in the bloodstream cause a compensatory drop in bicarbonate.
Decreased arterial pH: usually less than 7.25, but may be as low as 6.8 in severe cases. Normal is in the range of 7.35–7.45	Metabolic acidosis due to excessive ketones.
High anion gap (AG) acidosis: Normal AG < 12–15 mEq/L	Excessive ketones in the bloodstream.
Leukocytosis	Fluid volume deficit; acidosis; adrenocortical stimulation.
Increased hemoglobin, hematocrit, and total protein	Fluid volume deficit causes concentration of formed elements in the blood: Amounts are not actually increased, just suspended in a smaller volume of plasma.

HHS. For long-term follow-up of the patient's glycemic control after DKA and HHS have been corrected, glycosylated hemoglobin (HbA1c) is monitored (**Table 18-4**).

Variations Within Specific Populations

Children

DKA is an especially serious problem in children and adolescents with diabetes. The most dreaded complication in this population is cerebral edema, a condition that reportedly occurs in conjunction with 0.3% to 1.0% of DKA episodes in children.[14] The mortality rate associated with this condition ranges from 20% to 40% and is responsible for the majority of DKA-related deaths in children.[15] Risk factors for cerebral edema include younger age, high initial BUN (demonstrating a prolonged period of fluid volume deficit), severe acidosis, and hypocapnia (after adjusting for the degree of acidosis).[16–18] Cerebral edema associated with DKA is reported to be rare in individuals older than 20 years of age.[19] Symptoms include headache, gradually diminishing level of consciousness, seizures, pupillary changes, bradycardia, elevated blood pressure, and respiratory arrest.[20]

The cause of cerebral edema in children with DKA is not clear. One possible mechanism is a rapid shift in extracellular and intracellular fluids, which results in changes in osmolality.[21] Nevertheless, cerebral edema in DKA may be due as much to individual variance as to the severity of the metabolic derangements or treatment factors.[22] Prevention might involve avoidance of excessive fluid administration and avoidance of rapid reduction in plasma osmolality. Among the treatment options for cerebral edema associated with DKA are elevation of the head of the bed, mannitol infusion, and mechanical ventilation.[23,24] Obviously, the best way to prevent cerebral edema in a diabetic patient is to prevent DKA.[25]

Elderly

With advancing age, a decrease in insulin secretion and sensitivity to insulin occurs.[26] Further, elderly individuals do not experience normal thirst and tend to drink too little fluid; thus they are especially vulnerable to hyperglycemia and dehydration (usually in the form of HHS). The mortality rate for diabetic emergencies is much higher in HHS than in DKA, primarily because HHS is more likely to occur in elderly patients with significant comorbidities.[27]

Pregnant Women

DKA in pregnancy is considered a medical emergency that compromises both the mother and the fetus. In fact, once this condition is diagnosed in a pregnant woman, she will likely be directly admitted to an ICU.[28] Triggers for DKA in pregnancy are similar to those in nonpregnant patients—primarily, cessation of insulin therapy and development of infection. Approximately one-third of pregnant women who develop DKA have previously undiagnosed diabetes.[29] There have been reports in which pregnant women developed DKA at a lower blood glucose level than nonpregnant women.[30]

While HHS is usually associated with older adults, a case was recently reported in a 29-year-old pregnant African American woman.[31] The patient, a known diabetic, had been noncompliant with her diet and had missed her evening insulin dosage prior to admission to the hospital in labor. At that time, her blood glucose was 869 mg/dL; serum and urine ketones were negative. The patient delivered a baby with an Apgar score of 0 at 1 minute; the child died on the second day after birth.

Individuals Using Antipsychotic Drugs

Antipsychotic medications, as well as the agents used to treat schizophrenia, are known to be associated with increased risk for diabetes.[32] Recently, five cases of DKA associated with aripiprazole use were reported in the literature.[33–35] Four of these cases occurred in previously nondia-

Table 18-4 Estimated Average Glucose

NGSP HbA1$_c$ (%)	mg/dL	mmol/L
5	97 (76–120)	5.4 (4.2–6.7)
6	126 (100–152)	7.0 (5.5–8.5)
7	154 (123–185)	8.6 (6.8–10.3)
8	183 (147–217)	10.2 (8.1–12.1)
9	212 (170–249)	11.8 (9.3–13.9)
10	240 (193–282)	13.4 (10.7–15.7)
11	269 (217–314)	14.9 (12.0–17.5)
12	298 (240–347)	16.5 (13.3–19.3)

NGSP: National Glycohemoglobin Standardization Program.

Data in parentheses represent the 95% confidence interval for ranges in glucose levels.

Source: From Lai, LC. (2008). Review: Global standardisation of HbA1$_c$. *Malaysian Journal of Pathology.* 30(2), 67–71. Used with permission.

betic patients. Screening of all patients on antipsychotic treatment regimens for symptoms of new-onset diabetes has been recommended.[36]

PATHOPHYSIOLOGY

Hyperglycemic and Hyperosmolality

The underlying defects in DKA and HHS are decreased insulin secretion (DKA) or ineffective action of insulin (HHS). Most cells are relatively impermeable to glucose in the absence of insulin.

Both DKA and HHS are characterized by elevated levels of the counter-regulatory hormones: glucagon, catecholamines, cortisol, and growth hormone. Glucagon appears to be the primary hormone responsible for stimulation of hepatic gluconeogenesis and the direct activation of glycogen breakdown. Because of these processes, the blood glucose concentration rises markedly and increases plasma osmolality. As indicated in Table 18-1, HHS is typically associated with greater hyperglycemia and hyperosmolality than is DKA. Osmotic diuresis causes increased water loss and can lead to a high serum osmolality. As indicated earlier, a positive linear relationship exists between serum osmolality and mental changes.

Calculation of Plasma Osmolality

The following formula is the most commonly recommended way to calculate plasma osmolality in a patient with DKA or HHS: [37]

$$pOsm = 2(Na) + Glucose (mg/dL)/18$$

Example :. A patient with hyperglycemia has Na = 140 mEq/L and serum glucose = 1800 mg/dL.

$$2(140) + 1800/18 = 380 \ mOsm/kg$$

This elevated osmolality of extracellular fluid (ECF) produces cellular dehydration as water shifts from the cells to the ECF.

Another equation used to calculate osmolality includes blood urea nitrogen (BUN). However, clinicians caring for patients with DKA and HHS may choose to omit the urea component because urea diffuses freely across cell membranes and does not create an osmotic gradient between the intracellular and extracellular spaces.

Osmotic Diuresis and Fluid Volume Deficit

When the blood glucose level exceeds the renal threshold (normal is 180 mg/dL), glucose spills into the urine, taking water and electrolytes with it and increasing urine volume.

Osmotic diuresis resulting from hyperglycemia promotes the loss of sodium, potassium, magnesium, phosphate, calcium, and chloride. Replacement of these lost electrolytes may take days or weeks to achieve. The polyuria eventually leads to fluid volume deficit (FVD). As the FVD worsens and fluid volume is not replaced, glomerular filtration rate (GFR) decreases, as does renal blood flow, causing the patient to become oliguric or even anuric despite marked hyperglycemia. Thus FVD presents a danger of potential renal tubular damage with its resultant acute renal failure.

Ketosis

While the pathogenesis of DKA and HHS is similar, the two conditions differ in that in HHS there is sufficient insulin to prevent lipolysis. It takes one-tenth as much insulin to suppress lipolysis as it does to stimulate glucose use.[38] Thus, it is understandable why the severe insulin deficiency associated with type 1 diabetes causes excessive hydrolysis of triglycerides (from peripheral fat stores), yielding a greater release of free fatty acids and glycerol. The excess fatty acids are converted by the liver to ketones, resulting in ketosis. The insulin deficiency also interferes with uptake of the ketones by peripheral tissues, further increasing the buildup of ketones in the bloodstream. The ketones (ketoacids) present in DKA are β-hydroxybutyrate and acetoacetate. Because ketones are acids, with one hydrogen ion being created with each ion of β-hydroxybutyrate and acetoacetate, this overproduction and impaired metabolism soon overload the body's buffers, resulting in metabolic acidosis. In the process, the anionic charge of bicarbonate is replaced by the negatively charged ketones.

The type of metabolic acidosis that occurs in DKA is manifested by a decrease in bicarbonate with a reciprocal increase in the anion gap (AG) as large amounts of unmeasured anions (primarily ketones) are produced. In a patient with HHS, the anion gap is near normal unless another condition commonly associated with a high anion gap is present, such as lactic acidosis associated with heart failure.

Calculation of the Anion Gap

$$AG = Na - (HCO_3 + Cl) = 12 - 15 \ mEq/L$$

Example: A patient with ketoacidosis has the following lab findings: Na = 131 mEq/L, Cl = 95 mEq/L, HCO_3 = 5 mEq/L.

$$AG = 131 - (5 + 95) = 31 \ mEq/L$$

Calculation of AG is important in the assessment of acid–base disturbances in DKA because other findings may be misleading. For example, the vomiting that frequently accompanies DKA can superimpose a metabolic alkalosis on the preexisting ketoacidosis, making the plasma pH appear nearly normal. Measurement of the AG, however, will reveal the abnormal levels of ketone ions that are disrupting metabolism.

Excessive ketosis leads to ketonuria and even excretion of volatile acetone from the lungs (resulting in the classic "fruity" odor of the breath associated with DKA). It is not unusual for the plasma pH to drop to 7.25 or less and for the bicarbonate level to drop to 12 mEq/L or less. Possibly the greatest risks of prolonged uncorrected acidosis are decreased cardiac function, arrhythmia, and impaired hepatic handling of lactate.

Measuring the Degree of Respiratory Compensatory for Ketoacidosis

The kidneys and lungs attempt to compensate for the metabolic acidosis associated with DKA. The kidneys excrete hydrogen ions and conserve bicarbonate ions, resulting in a more acidic urine. The lungs attempt to lighten the acid load by blowing off extra carbon dioxide, resulting in the deep, rapid breathing known as Kussmaul respirations. The expected decrease in arterial carbon dioxide pressure ($PaCO_2$) to compensate for metabolic acidosis can be calculated using the following formula:

$$\text{Expected } PaCO_2 \text{ (mm Hg)} = 1.5 \, (HCO_3) + 8 \pm 2$$

Example: The expected $PaCO_2$ in a patient with a bicarbonate level of 12 mEq/L would be between 24 and 28 mm Hg:

$$PaCO_2 = 1.5 \, (12) + 8 \pm 2 = 24 - 28 \text{ mm Hg}$$

A decrease below the calculated amount indicates a superimposed respiratory alkalosis; failure of the $PaCO_2$ to decrease to the expected level indicates a complicating respiratory acidosis (a dangerous combination).

Potassium Imbalances

Potassium imbalances are especially important in patients with DKA. Initially, acidosis in these patients causes serum potassium concentrations to become elevated due to a shift of potassium out of the cells into the ECF, thereby masking the total body deficit of potassium associated with DKA. A patient with a low normal or low serum potassium concentration upon admission, therefore, should be considered to have a severe total-body deficit of potassium and undergo careful cardiac monitoring. When treatment is initiated, insulin favors movement of the extracellular potassium into

the cells; in addition, intravenous fluids dilute the serum potassium concentration. Potassium is lost in the urine during osmotic diuresis in both DKA and HHS patients. Hypokalemia is likely to be observed at this time and requires careful monitoring and potassium replacement to prevent cardiac dysrhythmias.

Hypophosphatemia

Upon admission of patients with DKA to the hospital, the serum phosphate level is usually elevated and fails to reflect the actual total-body deficit of phosphate. The mechanisms at work in this imbalance are essentially the same as those described earlier for potassium. Following the initiation of treatment, hypophosphatemia almost invariably occurs in the patient with DKA, for the same reasons that hypokalemia occurs.

One potentially serious consequence of phosphorus deficiency is decreased erythrocyte 2,3-diphosphoglycerate (2,3-DPG); a low level of 2,3-DPG may result in decreased peripheral oxygen delivery. When the serum phosphate concentration decreases to less than 0.5 mg/dL, serious disturbances in metabolism and neurological abnormalities (both central and peripheral) may result. For instance, seizures, respiratory failure, impaired leukocyte and platelet function, abnormal skeletal muscle function, and gastrointestinal bleeding have been reported.

Sodium Imbalances

Accumulation of glucose in the ECF creates an osmotic gradient, causing water to be pulled out of the cells into the ECF and resulting in dilution of the plasma sodium level. To correct for this dilutional effect, the corrected serum sodium can be calculated by adding 1.6 mEq/L to the measured serum sodium level for every 100 mg/dL the glucose is above normal. A normal or increased serum sodium concentration in the presence of hyperglycemia may indicate a profound degree of free water loss.[39] Hypernatremia is not uncommon in patients with HHS because their condition is often associated with poor water intake or increased water loss.

TREATMENT

Goals of therapy for DKA and HHS patients are to improve the circulatory volume and tissue perfusion, gradually reduce the serum glucose and plasma osmolality, correct electrolyte imbalances, steadily resolve ketosis (if present), and identify and treat any precipitating cause.[40] Monitored closely during the treatment period are clinical signs and results from laboratory tests. A flow sheet should be used to record treatments until the acute phase of the illness is past. Serum glucose levels should be checked hourly, and serum electrolytes should be checked every 2 to 4 hours to determine the adequacy of treatment.[41]

Standardized protocols are helpful in guiding therapy. For example, a study of 241 consecutive nonpregnant patients older than 18 years of age was recently undertaken in a medical ICU where patients were treated for DKA between January 2000 and January 2005.[42] An intervention was developed in the form of a mandatory treatment protocol in 2003. Upon comparing outcomes in patients before and after the mandatory protocol was implemented, investigators found that those who received the intervention had shorter ICU and hospital stays, and achieved a normal anion gap and cleared ketones more quickly than those who did not receive the intervention. No significant difference in the number of hypoglycemic episodes was observed. The investigators emphasized that protocol-driven care can decrease lengths of stay and complications rates.

Fluid Replacement

Meticulous charting of fluid intake and output (I & O) is critical to adequate fluid replacement therapy. The purpose of fluid replacement is to restore the depleted intravascular volume and improve tissue perfusion. Fluids are given rapidly enough to achieve hemodynamic stability (considering the patient's cardiovascular and renal status) and then slowed to a rate adequate to replace the lost fluids over a period of 24 hours.[43] In patients who are hypotensive, aggressive fluid replacement with isotonic saline is needed until blood pressure is stabilized. In an adult, fluid replacement may consist of the administration of 1 to 2 L of isotonic saline (0.9% NaCl) infused at a rate of approximately 1 L/hr. Isotonic (normal) saline will expand the ECF and begin to correct the hyperosmolality. In patients with HHS and significant hypernatremia, half-strength saline (0.45% NaCl) may be used. It is important to monitor the patient's corrected serum sodium concentration during fluid replacement to determine the type of fluid required. When the corrected serum sodium is normal or elevated, 0.45% sodium chloride is appropriate; in contrast, when the corrected serum sodium is lower than normal, 0.9% sodium chloride is appropriate.[44]

When concern arises regarding the adequacy of the patient's cardiovascular status, central venous pressure or hemodynamic monitoring may be needed to gauge the most appropriate rate of fluid replacement. Patients with HHS may need larger amounts of fluids to correct the FVD. If the plasma glucose level falls below 250 mg/dL, a solution containing 5% dextrose should be used to prevent hypoglycemia and other complications that might occur as a result of a too-rapid decline in the blood glucose level.[45] If the serum glucose falls below 100 mg/dL, a 10% or 20% dextrose solution may be indicated. As soon as oral intake is adequate, IV fluids can be discontinued.

A danger exists that too much fluid may be administered as part of fluid replacement, especially in young children and elderly patients. To guard against this possibility, careful attention should be paid to lung sounds and oxygenation parameters. As mentioned earlier, the most feared problem in children with DKA is cerebral edema (see the discussion earlier in this chapter). While excessive administration of intravenous fluids has been implicated as a cause of cerebral edema, a recent review of three observational studies that included DKA patients younger than 18 years found a lack of consistent results implicating the rate or volume of fluid administration as a precipitant cause of cerebral edema.[46]

Insulin Administration

Administration of insulin is necessary to improve hyperglycemia in patients with DKA and HHS. It is also needed to improve ketosis and acidosis in patients with DKA. The intravenous route is best for the very ill patient because absorption of insulin from poorly perfused muscle and fat depots may be erratic, especially if the patient is hypotensive. Insulin therapy is provided secondary to intravenous fluid replacement and initially should be withheld in patients with hypokalemia and hypotension.[47] (Recall that insulin forces potassium into the cells, so it could worsen an existing serious hypokalemic state.) In hypotensive patients, the administration of insulin can lead to vascular collapse due to rapid fluid shifts into the intracellular space.[48] It is important to measure the serum potassium concentration before starting insulin therapy.[49] It has been recommended that insulin therapy not be initiated until the patient's serum potassium concentration is greater than 3.3 mEq/L.[50]

A standard insulin regimen consists of an intravenous drip of regular insulin at a rate of 0.1 unit per kilogram of body weight per hour.[51] Some clinicians also favor administering an IV bolus of insulin in the amount of 0.1 U/kg body weight, followed by an hourly rate of 0.1 U/kg body weight per hour.[52] For example, the insulin bolus in a 70-kg patient would be 7 units, and the hourly insulin rate would be 7 units as well.

The blood glucose level should be checked every hour, with a goal of decreasing the glucose by approximately 50 to 75 mg/dL per hour.[53] When the plasma glucose reaches 200 mg/dL in a patient with DKA or 300 mg/dL in a patient with HHS, it may be possible to reduce the insulin infusion rate to 0.02 to 0.05 unit per kilogram per hour.[54]

Of primary importance is individualization of the insulin dosage based on the response of the patient. A too-rapid drop in blood glucose level creates the risk of complications such as hypoglycemia and hypokalemia. A too rapid correction of hyperglycemia (at a rate > 100 mg/dL per hour) increases risk of osmotic encephalopathy.[55] Presumably, the risk for cerebral edema is increased by a rapid decline in blood glucose concentration because this change alters the osmotic gradient created between the brain and serum osmolality. As discussed earlier, cerebral edema is uncommon in adults, but can be fatal in children (or lead to developmental disabilities for years after resolution of the DKA episode).

Eventually, patients with DKA and HHS can be changed from IV administration of insulin to the subcutaneous route. Criteria that must be met for this switch in patients with DKA include a blood glucose concentration less than 200 mg/dL and two of the following: a serum bicarbonate concentration of 15 mEq/L or greater, a venous pH greater than 7.3, and a normal anion gap.[56] Criteria for switching to subcutaneous insulin administration in patients with HHS are normal plasma osmolality and return of normal mental status.[57] It may be best to make the transition from IV to subcutaneous insulin at the time of a meal.[58] If the patient cannot resume oral intake, intravenous insulin infusion and fluid replacement should be maintained.[59]

Although insulin replacement may be life-saving to patients with DKA and HHS, this therapy is also associated with risk for hypoglycemia. Fortunately, this risk has been substantially reduced by the advent of low-dose insulin replacement therapy. Regular assessment of blood glucose levels is needed to detect possible hypoglycemia during treatment because many patients with DKA do not experience the typical adrenergic manifestations of hyperinsulinism, such as sweating, nervousness, hunger, and tachycardia.[60]

Electrolyte Replacement

Potassium

Potassium is not added to the IV fluids until adequate urinary output has been established, unless serum potassium levels have already been shown to be below normal. That is, potassium replacement is initiated after the serum potassium concentration falls below the upper limit of normal.[61] The aim of treatment is to maintain the serum potassium within a normal range. Potassium replacement is usually accomplished by adding 20 to 30 mEq of potassium chloride or potassium phosphate to 1 L of fluid, infused at a rate appropriate to the status of the patient. Occasionally, larger amounts of potassium are needed if the hypokalemia is severe. Because the IV administration of potassium is associated with risk of hyperkalemia, it is wise to monitor the serum potassium level at 1- or 2-hour intervals and to review serial electrocardiogram (ECG) tracings. (Rules for safe potassium administration are discussed in Chapter 5.)

Phosphorus

Because phosphate is lost during the osmotic diuresis of DKA and HHS, some authorities favor replacing at least a part of the lost potassium with potassium phosphate. Phosphate replacement is definitely needed when the serum phosphate concentration is less than 1.0 mg/dL. It may also be needed when cardiac dysfunction, anemia, or respiratory depression is present. Phosphate replacement likely accelerates the recovery of reduced 2,3-DPG levels in red blood cells, thereby decreasing hemoglobin–oxygen affinity and improving tissue oxygenation. It is imperative, however, that significant renal failure be ruled out before phosphate is administered IV. Administering too much phosphate can induce hypocalcemia; therefore, calcium levels should also be monitored if phosphate is administered.

Bicarbonate

Use of bicarbonate in the treatment of DKA remains controversial. Severe metabolic acidosis is dangerous in that it can lead to impaired myocardial contractility, cerebral vasodilatation, and coma.[62] However, there is no clear evidence that administration of bicarbonate improves outcomes in patients with DKA. A current recommendation is that adult patients with a pH less than 6.9 receive bicarbonate replacement until the pH exceeds 7.0.[63] In a patient who has a pH greater than 7.0, insulin therapy inhibits lipolysis and corrects ketoacidosis without the use of bicarbonate.

According to some authors, it is almost never necessary to give bicarbonate to treat DKA unless the patient's renal function is permanently impaired.[64]

Sodium

Isotonic saline that is administered initially supplies enough sodium to correct sodium loss. Because the patient with DKA or HHS may lose proportionately more water than sodium, a hypotonic solution (such as 0.45% NaCl) will likely be prescribed after the administration of several liters of isotonic saline. Hypotonic solutions provide free water to correct cellular dehydration.

Other Electrolytes

Losses of calcium and magnesium may occur as a result of the osmotic diuresis. Often they are not considered of clinical consequence. In other cases, magnesium is replaced if renal function is adequate.

Sick Day Rules

Diabetics need to be provided with information about self-care and when to contact healthcare providers for help. **Table 18-5** provides examples of some simple rules that can be included in patient education.

Table 18-5 Example of Sick Day Instructions

1. When ill, always take your usual dose of insulin. **Never skip your insulin even if you are unable to eat**. People with type 2 diabetes may need to stop their oral medications when ill. If you are uncertain what to do and are taking oral diabetes medicines or the newer injectable diabetes medications Pramlintide, Exenatide, or Liraglutide, consult your doctor or diabetes health professional for specific guidelines during illness, as some of these drugs can induce or worsen nausea and vomiting.

2. Test blood glucose levels before and 2 hours after each meal. If you are unable to eat, check your blood glucose levels every 2 to 4 hours. It is essential that blood glucose levels be tested a **minimum** of 4 times per day when you are ill.

3. If you have type 1 diabetes and your blood glucose levels are greater than 240 mg/dL, test your urine for ketones. Ketone testing should always be done when nausea and vomiting are present. Patients with type 2 diabetes rarely have ketosis; however, positive nonfasting urine ketones in a patient with type 2 diabetes is a worrisome finding that requires further evaluation. If ketones are present along with high serum glucose levels, you will need extra insulin. Short-acting insulin such as regular insulin or rapid-acting insulins such as Lispro, Aspart, or Glulisine should be used. Consult your physician or diabetes health professional immediately to obtain guidelines for how much short- or rapid-acting insulin you should use and how often to take it; during most illnesses 10% of the total daily dose can be given safely as a supplemental dose of short- or rapid-acting insulin every 1 to 4 hours. Be sure to check the expiration date of the ketone strips; purchasing individually foil wrapped strips will help to keep your supply of ketone strips fresh.

4. Drink 8 ounces of caffeine-free and alcohol-free liquid every hour or take small sips every 10 to 15 minutes to prevent dehydration, fight the illness, and prevent complications. Fluids that are acceptable are water, caffeine-free tea, consommé, bouillon broth, and regular or diet sodas. If your blood glucose levels are less than 240 mg/dL and you are unable to eat, drink fluids with calories, such as regular soda, so that 15 grams of carbohydrate is taken every 1 to 2 hours. If your blood glucose levels are greater than 240 mg/dL, drink calorie-free liquids such as water and bouillon. If you are unable to take liquids because of nausea and vomiting, consult your doctor because a medication may be prescribed to stop the nausea and vomiting.

5. When ill with diabetes, maintain a meal plan that provides **at least** 150 grams of carbohydrate per day. You should eat or drink 45 to 50 grams of carbohydrate at least 3 times per day in addition to the frequent fluid intake necessary to avoid dehydration. If you are too nauseated to tolerate a large volume of liquid at a time, it is suggested that you "sip" carbohydrate-containing fluids (see below) so that you are taking in about 15 grams of carbohydrate every 1 to 2 hours to prevent hypoglycemia and ketosis. If you are unable to eat your usual diet, then try more easily tolerated foods such as those listed here.

Examples of Sick Day Foods and Corresponding Carbohydrate Content

Food Item	Grams of Carbohydrate
½ cup regular soda	15
½ cup diet soda	0
½ cup orange juice	15

continues

Table 18-5 Example of Sick Day Instructions—*continued*

½ cup apple, grape, or pineapple juice	15
1 cup milk	12
1 cup bouillon	0
½ cup regular gelatin	15
½ cup vanilla ice cream	15
½ cup orange sherbet	26
6 saltine crackers	15
½ cup sugar-free pudding	15
½ cup regular pudding	30
1 cup artificially sweetened yogurt	15
1 Popsicle	24
½ cup cooked cereal	15
1 cup soup made with water	15
1 cup soup made with milk	27

6. Contact your physician or diabetes health professional immediately if you have pain, fever greater than 101.5°F, blood glucose levels greater than 240 mg/dL that are not responsive to increased insulin, vomiting, persistent diarrhea, rapid labored breathing, moderate or large urine ketones, mental status changes, signs of dehydration (such as dry tongue), or if you are unable to eat food for more than 1 day. When you are ill, contact your physician or diabetes health professional any time you have a question or concern about your blood sugar level.

7. Be sure to read the labels of over-the-counter antihistamines/decongestants and cough syrups. Keep the sugar-free versions of these medications on hand in case of illness.

Source: Revised, March 2010. Mary Kay Macheca, RN, MSN(R), ANP-BC, CDE. Washington University Clinical Associates, St. Louis, MO. With permission.

CASE STUDIES

Case Study 18-1

A 35-year-old woman with insulin-dependent diabetes developed viral gastroenteritis with nausea and vomiting. Two days before admission, she skipped her insulin because she was not eating. Her husband brought her to the emergency department because she was becoming increasingly lethargic. On initial examination, she was found to have tachycardia (pulse rate, 140/min) and deep, rapid (Kussmaul) respirations. Her blood pressure when lying flat was 98/70 mm Hg. She was able to void only a few milliliters; the urinary glucose and ketone levels were both 4+. Her skin and mucous membranes were dry, and she had a fruity odor to her breath. Laboratory results revealed hyperglycemia (glucose = 940 mg/dL), hyponatremia (Na = 130 mEq/L), hyperkalemia (K = 6.8 mEq/L), elevated blood urea nitrogen (BUN = 45 mg/dL), elevated serum creatinine (Cr = 2.2 mg/dL), a low serum bicarbonate concentration (5 mEq/L), a low serum chloride level (90 mEq/L), and an extremely low arterial pH (7.07), indicating severe metabolic acidosis. The $PaCO_2$ was also low (13 mm Hg), indicating respiratory compensation by hyperventilation. On the basis of the examination and the laboratory findings, a diagnosis of DKA was made. The patient was then was treated with 0.9% sodium chloride IV to correct the FVD and with low-dose regular insulin (5 U/hr).

Commentary. DKA developed because the patient unwisely skipped her insulin during a time of increased need. The laboratory data indicate a severe high AG metabolic acidosis (pH = 7.07). The AG is calculated by subtracting the sum of the bicarbonate and chloride levels from the serum sodium level (130 − [5 + 90] = 35 mEq/L). The calculated AG in this patient was 35 mEq/L; the accepted normal range is 12 to 15 mEq/L. The high AG indicated flooding of the bloodstream with ketones (due to a lack of insulin). The deep rapid (Kussmaul) respirations were the body's attempt to compensate for the extremely low serum pH. Signs of FVD included hypotension, tachycardia, dry skin and mucous membranes, low urinary output, and a high BUN/creatinine ratio. The serum sodium concentration was low initially because of the high serum glucose concentration (which pulled water out of the cells, thereby diluting the serum sodium concentration). The serum potassium level was elevated initially due to the effect of starvation (release of potassium from the cells), acidosis (which facilitates movement of cellular potassium into the bloodstream), and decreased renal excretion of potassium (due to the poor renal perfusion associated with FVD).

Note how the abnormal parameters were corrected to normal (or were improved) during the course of the first 16 hours of treatment. This was accomplished solely by the combination of low-dose insulin and fluid volume replacement with isotonic saline. These treatments allowed the metabolic defects to be corrected. For example, the formation of ketones was stopped by the insulin. The metabolic acidosis corrected itself as this halt occurred; no bicarbonate was administered. As the patient's blood glucose level decreased, her serum sodium level increased. This correction of the dilutional hyponatremia occurred because water was no longer being pulled out of the cells and into the intravascular space. In addition, isotonic saline contains a sizable amount of sodium and helped correct any sodium losses from vomiting. The potentially dangerously high serum potassium level (6.8 mEq/L) decreased to normal as the starvation effect (due to a lack of insulin) and metabolic acidosis were corrected by treatment with insulin and fluid resuscitation. The gradual drop in the BUN and serum creatinine levels reflected improved renal perfusion secondary to fluid resuscitation.

Case Study 18-2

A case was reported in which a 15-year-old African American boy presented to the emergency department with an acute change in mental status and slurred speech.[65] During one of two visits to an emergency department for the same illness, the obese child (123 kg) complained of abdominal pain, for which a H_2-receptor antagonist was prescribed. At the current admission, the serum glucose concentration was found to be markedly elevated (1638 mg/dL). Despite fluid resuscitation and insulin administration, the patient died 14 hours from the time of his admission to the emergency department.

Commentary. The authors of this case report described 18 other case reports of HHS in children, in which 13 of the pediatric patients (72%) died.[66] They further emphasized that it is critical to recognize HHS early and start appropriate treatment. Unfortunately, the diagnosis in this patient was missed in previous admissions to emergency departments. Other authors have pointed out that diabetic complications may be missed in children because they can resemble other more common pediatric illnesses, such as gastroenteritis.[67] This was a mistake obviously made in the case reported here during the visit to the emergency department, where the child was prescribed a drug to reduce gastric acidity.

Case Study 18-3

A case was recently reported in which a 14-year-old girl with type 1 diabetes for 6 years was admitted to the hospital with DKA.[68] Following treatment, she recovered without incident. However, within a few weeks, she experienced two additional episodes of DKA and had a

Changing Laboratory Values for Case Study 18-1

Time	Blood Glucose (mg/dL)	Arterial pH	Sodium (mEq/L)	Potassium (mEq/L)	Bicarbonate (mEq/L)	Chloride (mEq/L)	BUN:Cr Ratio
5 PM	940	7.07	130	6.8	5	90	45:2.2
7 PM	520		132	6.6	7	100	43:1.9
9 PM	400	7.26	136	4.3	8	105	44:1.6
2 AM	325		140	4.5	16	115	30:1.4
9 AM	300		142	4.4	23	114	22:1.1

hemoglobin A1c level of 12.2%, indicating poor compliance with her treatment regimen. Following a third admission with DKA, the patient was visited by a diabetic specialist nurse, who found that the patient's insulin delivery device (a Novopen 3 injection device) was faulty; specifically, the plunger at the end of the piston rod was broken. The patient was given a new pen and her Hb$_{A1c}$ dropped to 9% with 6 weeks.

Commentary. This case demonstrates that poor diabetic control can be related to a faulty insulin delivery device. Fortunately, the diabetic nurse specialist took the time to review the integrity of the insulin delivery device. In short, the problem was "fixable" with a new pen.

Case Study 18-4

A case was reported in which a 48-year-old man with type 2 diabetes mellitus presented with large amounts of glucose and ketones in his urine and a serum glucose concentration of 379 mg/dL.[69] His venous blood CO_2 content—representative primarily of serum bicarbonate concentration—was below normal at 14 mEq/L, indicating metabolic acidosis. A high anion gap (22 mEq/L) was present and indicated the presence of ketones. (The normal anion gap is variably defined as 12 mEq/L or less.) Treatment included intravenous fluids and an insulin drip at a rate of 6 units per hour. By the second day of treatment, his serum glucose had decreased to 268 mg/dL; it was 154 mg/dL on day 7 of treatment.

Commentary. The authors of this case report emphasize that ketoacidosis is increasingly being found in persons with type 2 diabetes.[70] In the not too recent past, it was thought that patients with type 2 diabetes would develop only HHS if their diabetes were poorly controlled. A review of this patient's history revealed good diabetic control until a week prior to admission. There were no overt signs of infection. Six months after the patient's bout with DKA, his insulin therapy was discontinued. (This would not have been possible had the patient had type 1 diabetes.)

Case Study 18-5

A 27-year-old obese man with type 2 diabetes mellitus was admitted to the hospital with a 5-day history of nausea and vomiting, polyuria, and polydipsia. He complained of low back pain and said he had lost 10 lb of body weight over the past week. A review of his history found that he had been diagnosed several years earlier with similar symptoms. The patient was given a prescription for an oral hypoglycemic agent but did not continue taking the medication after his prescription ran out. At the time of his admission, the following laboratory values were observed: metabolic acidosis (pH = 7.1; bicarbonate = 5 mEq/L), hyperglycemia (glucose = 320 mg/dL), elevated anion gap (24 mEq/L), and an elevated white blood cell count. The patient's hemoglobin A1c was markedly elevated (13.5%, indicating poor diabetic control). The patient was diagnosed with DKA and treated with isotonic saline and IV insulin. Upon a medical workup, an epidural abscess was located and evacuated.

Commentary. Poor compliance was evident in this patient with type 2 diabetes. Adding to his problem was an acute infection in the form of an abscess. Although the patient had type 2 diabetes, he experienced metabolic acidosis during his acute infection.

Case Study 18-6

A 12-year-old girl with insulin-dependent diabetes was admitted to the emergency department in a state of altered consciousness. Her skin and mucous membranes were very dry, and Kussmaul respirations were evident. There was evidence of black-colored emesis (which tested positive for blood) in and around the patient's mouth. The child had been left unattended for approximately 24 hours. Laboratory results were as follows: hyperglycemia (glucose = 1400 mg/dL), strong ketones in the urine, and profound metabolic acidosis (arterial pH = 6.95; bicarbonate = 3 mEq/L). The PaCO$_2$ was also quite low (9 mm Hg), indicating an attempt by the lungs to compensate for the severe metabolic acidosis.

A urinalysis revealed a bladder infection. The child was treated with intravenous normal saline and an infusion of regular insulin at a rate of 8 units per hour. Also, an antibiotic was started, along with a gastric acid inhibitor.

Commentary. This child clearly had severe DKA secondary to an infectious process. Fortunately, following treatment, she made a full recovery.

Also see Case Studies 17-6 and 20-4 for a discussion of other diabetic patients with fluid and electrolyte problems.

Summary of Key Points

- The major characteristics of diabetic ketoacidosis (DKA) are severe hyperglycemia and ketotic metabolic acidosis. This condition usually develops quickly, over a period of less than 24 hours. Kussmaul respirations are usually present as the body's attempt to compensate for metabolic acidosis.

- Hyperglycemic hyperosmolar state (HHS) is also characterized by severe hyperglycemia, hyperosmolality, and dehydration, but it is not associated with acidosis. HHS usually develops slowly, over a period of several days to weeks.

- Most patients with DKA have autoimmune type 1 diabetes; most patients with HHS have type 2 diabetes. However, there is crossover between these conditions such that patients with type 2 diabetes may also experience DKA when they are subjected to acute illness or stress.

- Because childhood obesity has become a pandemic healthcare problem, more cases of type 2 diabetes are occurring in children; incidence in this population has increased 10-fold in the past 20 years.

- While clinical observations are important, laboratory evaluations are crucial in distinguishing between DKA and HHS.

- Initially, acidosis in patients with DKA causes serum potassium concentrations to become elevated as potassium shifts out of the cells, masking the total-body deficit of potassium associated with DKA. A normal or low serum potassium level upon admission likely signals a serious total-body potassium deficiency.

- The cornerstones of treatment for DKA and HHS are fluid replacement and insulin administration. A patient with DKA or HHS is markedly volume depleted as a result of the high serum glucose concentration.

- Insulin is given intravenously in the very ill patient with DKA or HHS, because absorption of insulin from poorly perfused muscle and fat depots may be erratic, especially if the patient is hypotensive.

- Because insulin forces potassium into the cells temporarily, it has been recommended that insulin therapy not be initiated until the patient's serum potassium concentration is greater than 3.3 mEq/L.

- During treatment of patients in the acute phases of DKA and HHS, the blood glucose level is usually checked hourly, with a goal of decreasing the glucose by approximately 50 to 75 mg/dL per hour. Low-dose insulin therapy often consists of administering 0.1 unit of regular insulin per kilogram of body weight per hour. For example, a 70-kg patient would receive 7 units per hour.

- When the plasma glucose reaches 200 mg/dL in a patient with DKA or 300 mg/dL in a patient with HHS, the rate of insulin administration is usually significantly slowed to avoid a too-rapid decrease in serum glucose level.

- The most dreaded complication of DKA in children is cerebral edema. Although the cause of this complication is not fully understood, its prevention might involve avoiding excessive fluid administration, thereby preventing a rapid reduction in plasma osmolality.

NOTES

1. Kitabchi, A. E., Umpierrez, G. E., Miles, J. M., & Fisher, J. N. (2009). Hyperglycemic crises in adult patients with diabetes. *Diabetes Care, 32*(7), 1335–1343.

2. Canarie, M. F., Bogue, C. W., Banasiak, K. J., Weinzimer, S. A., & Tamborlane, W. V. (2007). Decompensated hyperglycemic hyperosmolarity without significant ketoacidosis in the adolescent and young adult population. *Journal of Pediatric Endocrinology, 20*(10), 1115–1124.

3. Cochran, J. B., Walters, S., & Losek, J. D. (2006). Pediatric hyperglycemic hyperosmolar syndrome: Diagnostic difficulties and high mortality rate. *American Journal of Emergency Medicine, 24*(3), 297–301.

4. Cochran et al., note 3.

5. Charfen, M. A., & Fernandez-Frackelton, M. (2005). Diabetic ketoacidosis. *Emergency Medical Clinics of North America, 23*(3), 609–628.

6. Kitabchi et al., note 1.

7. Kitabchi, A. E., Umpierrez, G. E., Murphy, M. B., Barrett, E. J., Kreisberg, R. A., Malone, J. I., et al. (2001). Management of hyperglycemic crises in patients with diabetes. *Diabetes Care, 24*(1) 131–153.

8. Kitabchi, A. E., Umpierrez, G. E., Murphy, M. B., & Kreisberg, R. A. (2004). American Diabetes Association: Hyperglycemic crises in diabetes. *Diabetes Care, 27*(suppl 1), S94–S102.

9. Charfen & Fernandez-Frackelton, note 5.

10. Koul, P. B. (2009). Diabetic ketoacidosis: A current appraisal of pathophysiology and management. *Clinical Pediatrics, 48*(2), 135–144.

11. Kitabchi et al., note 1.

12. Charfen & Fernandez-Frackelton, note 5.

13. Blank, F. S., Miller, M., Nichols, J., Smithline, H., Crabb, G., & Pekow, P. (2009). Blood glucose measurement in patients with suspected diabetic ketoacidosis: A comparison of Abbott Medi-Sense PCx point-of-care meter values to reference laboratory values. *Journal of Emergency Nursing, 35*(2), 93–96.

14. Kitabchi et al., note 1.

15. Wolfsdorf, J., Glaser, N., & Sperling, M. A. (2006). Diabetic ketoacidosis in infants, children, and adolescents: A consensus statement from the American Diabetes Association. *Diabetes Care, 29*(5), 1150–1159.

16. Koul, note 10.

17. Tasker, R. C., Lutman, D., & Peters, M. J. (2005). Hyperventilation in severe diabetic ketoacidosis. *Pediatric Critical Care Medicine, 6*(4), 405–411.

18. Rosenbloom, A. L. (2007). Hyperglycemic crises and their complications in children. *Journal of Pediatric Endocrinology. 20*(1), 5–18.

19. Rosenbloom, A. L. (1990). Intracerebral crises during treatment of diabetic ketoacidosis. *Diabetes Care, 13*(1), 22–33.

20. Marcin, J. P., Glaser, N., Barnett, P., McCaslin, I., Nelson, D., Trainor, J., et al. (2002). Factors associated with adverse outcomes in children with diabetic ketoacidosis-related cerebral edema. *Journal of Pediatrics, 141*, 793–797.

21. Kitabchi et al., note 1.

22. Levin, D. L. (2008). Cerebral edema in diabetic ketoacidosis. *Pediatric Critical Care Medicine, 9*, 320–329.

23. Kitabchi et al., note 1.

24. Koul, note 10.

25. Levin, note 22.

26. Gaglia, J. L., Wyckoff, J., & Abrahamson, M. J. (2004). Acute hyperglycemic crisis in the elderly. *Medical Clinics of North America, 88*(4), 1063–1084.

27. MacIsaac, R. J., Lee, L. Y., McNeil, K. J., Tsalamandris, C., & Jerums, G. (2002). Influence of age on the presentation and outcome of acidotic and hyperosmolar diabetic emergencies. *Internal Medicine Journal, 32*(8), 379–385.

28. Carroll, M. A., & Yeomans, E. R. (2005). Diabetic ketoacidosis in pregnancy. *Critical Care Medicine, 33*(10 suppl), S347–S353.

29. Montoro, M. N., Myers, V. P., Mestman, J. H., Xu, Y., Anderson, B. G., & Golde, S. H. (1993). Outcome of pregnancy in diabetic ketoacidosis. *American Journal of Perinatology, 10*, 17–20.

30. Guo, R. X., Yang, L. Z., Li, L. X., & Zhao, X. P. (2008). Diabetic ketoacidosis in pregnancy tends to occur at lower blood glucose levels: Case-control study and a case report of euglycemic diabetic ketoacidosis in pregnancy. *Journal of Obstetrics & Gynecology, 34*(3), 324–330.

31. Nayak, S., Lippes, H. A., & Lee, R. V. (2005). Hyperglycemic hyperosmolar syndrome (HHS) during pregnancy. *Journal of Obstetrics & Gynecology, 25*(6), 599–601.

32. Cohen, D. & Correll, C. U. (2009). Second-generation antipsychotic-associated diabetes mellitus and diabetic ketoacidosis: Mechanisms, predictors, and screening need. *Journal of Clinical Psychiatry, 70*(5), 765–766.

33. Church, C. O., Stevens, D. L., & Fugate, S. E. (2005). Diabetic ketoacidosis associated with aripiprazole. *Diabetic Medicine, 22*(10), 1440–1443.

34. Logue, D. D., Gonzalez, N., Heligman, S. D., McLaughlin, J. V., & Belcher, H. M. (2007). Hyperglycemia in a 7-year-old child treated with aripiprazole. *American Journal of Psychiatry, 164*(1), 173.

35. Reddymasu, S., Bahta, E., Levine, S., Manas, K., & Slay, L. E. (2006). Elevated lipase and diabetic ketoacidosis associated with aripiprazole. *Journal of the Pancreas, 7*(3), 303–305.

36. Cohen & Correll, note 32.

37. Kitabchi et al., note 7.

38. Kitabchi, A. E., & Nyenwe, E. A. (2006). Hyperglycemic crises in diabetes mellitus: Diabetic ketoacidosis and hyperglycemic hyperosmolar state. *Endocrinology and Metabolism Clinics of North America, 35*(4), 725–751.

39. Kitabchi et al., note 1.

40. Kitabchi & Nyenwe, note 38.

41. Charfen & Fernandez-Frackelton, note 5.

42. Bull, S. V., Douglas, I. S., Foster, M., & Albert, R. K. (2007). Mandatory protocol for treating adult patients with diabetic ketoacidosis decreases intensive care unit and hospital lengths of stay: Results from a nonrandomized trial. *Critical Care Medicine, 35*(1), 41–46.

43. Charfen & Fernandez-Frackelton, note 5.

44. Kitabchi et al., note 1.

45. Kitabchi et al., note 1.

46. Hom, J. & Sinert, R. (2008). Is fluid therapy associated with cerebral edema in children with diabetic ketoacidosis? *Annals of Emergency Medicine, 52*(1), 69–75.

47. Charfen & Fernandez-Frackelton, note 5.

48. Charfen & Fernandez-Frackelton, note 5.

49. Eledrisi, M. S., Alshanti, M. S., Shah, M. F., Brolosy, B., & Jaha, N. (2006). Overview of the diagnosis and management of diabetic ketoacidosis. *American Journal of Medical Sciences, 331*(5), 243–251.

50. Kitabchi et al., note 8.

51. Charfen & Fernandez-Frackelton, note 5.

52. Kitabchi & Nyenwe, note 38.

53. Kitabchi et al., note 8.

54. Kitabchi et al., note 1.

55. Cooper, D. H., Krainik, A. J., Lubner, S. J., & Reno, H. E. (Eds.). (2007). The Washington Manual of Medical Therapeutics (32nd ed.). Philadelphia: Wolters Kluwer/Lippincott Williams & Wilkins. p 607

56. Kitabchi et al., note 1.

57. Kitabchi et al., note 1.

58. Cooke, D.W, & Plotnick, L. (2008). Management of diabetic ketoacidosis in children and adolescents. *Pediatrics in Review, 29*(12), 431–435.

59. Kitabchi et al., note 1.

60. Kitabchi et al., note 1.

61. Kitabchi et al., note 1.

62. Mitchell, J. H., Wildenthal, K., & Johnson, R. L. (1972). The effects of acid–base disturbances on cardiovascular and pulmonary function. *Kidney International, 1*(5), 375–389.

63. Kitabchi et al., note 1.

64. Sabatini, S., & Kurtzman, N. A. (2009). Bicarbonate therapy in severe metabolic acidosis. *Journal of the American Society of Nephrology, 20*(4), 692–695.

65. Cochran et al., note 3.

66. Cochran et al., note 3.

67. Sherry, N. A., & Levitsky, L. L. (2008). Management of diabetic ketoacidosis in children and adolescents. *Pediatric Drugs, 10*(4), 209–215.

68. Muralidharan, S., Datta, V., & Palanivel, V. (2009). Recurrent diabetic ketoacidosis in an adolescent. *Archives of Disease in Childhood, 94*(5), 365.

69. Hu, M. & Isaacson, J. H. (2009). A 48-year-old man with uncontrolled diabetes. *Cleveland Clinical Journal of Medicine, 76*(7), 413–416.

70. Hu & Isaacson, note 69.

Chapter 19

Brain Injuries

Traumatic brain injury (TBI) affects people of all ages and is a leading cause of death.[1] Like most serious conditions, TBI is associated with significant fluid and electrolyte problems. Because the central nervous system plays a major role in regulating sodium and water homeostasis, sodium imbalances are prominent in patients with head injuries.

CEREBRAL EDEMA AND INTRACRANIAL PRESSURE

Cerebral edema is common in brain-injured patients regardless of the pathophysiology behind the injury. By definition, *cerebral edema* is an increase in brain water content with resultant increased brain tissue volume. Untreated cerebral edema, regardless of the etiology, leads to elevated intracranial pressure (ICP). An elevated ICP, in turn, can lead to impaired cerebral microcirculation.[2]

Cerebral edema represents a disruption in the pressure and volume equilibrium within the intracranial compartments. These compartments, which are encased in the rigid cranial vault, contain brain tissue, blood, and cerebrospinal fluid (CSF). In adults, the pressure is maintained by an intracranial volume of approximately 1900 mL, of which 80% is brain volume, 10% is blood volume, and 10% is CSF volume.[3] When one compartment increases, there must be a compensatory change in one or both of the other compartments to maintain a constant total pressure, a relationship known as the Monro-Kellie doctrine:

$$V_{\text{cranial contents}} = V_{\text{brain tissue}} + V_{\text{blood}} + V_{\text{cerebrospinal fluid}}$$

For example, because the brain is relatively incompressible, compensation occurs through one or more mechanisms: (1) shunting of CSF into the spinal dural sac, (2) increased absorption of CSF, and (3) vasoconstriction to decrease the volume of blood in the brain. When the total volume of brain mass, blood, or CSF exceeds the compensatory capacity, any additional increase in brain mass causes an exponential increase in ICP. Once ICP is raised to the stage of decompensation, intracranial hypertension results and the risk of brain displacement with herniation through the foramen magnum occurs.

In approximately half of all patients who die after traumatic brain injury, elevated ICP is the primary cause of death.[4] An ICP value is most important in its relationship with cerebral perfusion pressure (CPP).

CEREBRAL PERFUSION PRESSURE

Cerebral perfusion pressure (CPP) is equal to the mean arterial pressure (MAP) minus the intracranial pressure (ICP). Obviously, a low MAP or a high ICP can cause the CPP to drop and lead to profound reductions in cerebral blood flow. Thus, to assure adequate cerebral perfusion, healthcare providers must pay attention to both the patient's blood pressure and intracranial pressure. It has been recommended that a systolic blood pressure less than 90 mm Hg be avoided, and that treatment should be initiated when ICP passes a threshold higher than 20 mm Hg.[5,6] Maintenance of CPP at a level of at 60 to 70 mm Hg is needed to maintain constant cerebral blood flow.[7] This is accomplished by administering sufficient fluids to maintain normal blood volume, by administering vasopressors when needed, and by instituting measures to keep the ICP less than 20 mm Hg.[8]

MEASURES TO CONTROL INTRACRANIAL PRESSURE

Maintenance of Adequate Ventilation

Decreased oxygenation (hypoxemia) and elevated levels of carbon dioxide (hypercapnea) are potent vasodilators and, therefore, contribute to a high ICP; for this reason, it is important to maintain adequate ventilation in patients with head injuries. For example, guidelines published in 2007 by the Brain Trauma Foundation recommend that hypoxia (PaO_2 less than 60 mm Hg or O_2 saturation less than 90%) and hypercapnea be avoided.[9] Maintaining an arterial $PaCO_2$ of approximately 35 mm Hg has been recommended to avoid cerebral vasoconstriction.[10] Although hypoxemia and hypercapnea usually occur together, hypercapnea alone will stimulate vasodilation. Many patients with severe brain injuries require endotracheal intubation and mechanical ventilation. While endotracheal suctioning is needed to alleviate airway obstruction by mucus, it must be remembered that endotracheal suctioning is associated with transitory increases in ICP.

Hyperventilation

When ICP becomes dangerously high, hyperventilation may be considered to temporarily reduce the $PaCO_2$ (such as to a level of 25–30 mm of Hg for 30 minutes).[11] With temporary hyperventilation, the desired effect is vasoconstriction of blood vessels with subsequent reduced brain volume. Unfortunately, it is accompanied by an undesired effect: reduced blood flow to brain tissues. As a consequence, hyperventilation should be used only briefly to lower ICP. It has been recommended that hyperventilation be avoided during the first 24 hours after brain injury when cerebral blood flow is often low.[12]

Osmotic Agents

Despite traumatic brain injury, usually a significant portion of uninjured brain tissue is present in the patient with a head injury. The intact blood–brain barrier in the uninjured tissue will allow fluid to be pulled out by osmotic agents. Mannitol is the agent most frequently used for this purpose. Hypertonic saline may also be used,[13] however, and is sometimes favored over mannitol to reduce elevated ICP.[14]

During the administration of mannitol, arterial hypotension (systolic blood pressure less than 90 mm Hg) should be avoided.[15] Mannitol immediately expands the plasma volume and reduces the hematocrit and blood viscosity. This agent's onset of action is delayed for 15 to 30 minutes, and its effects last for a variable period ranging from 90 minutes to 6 or more hours.[16] Compared to a continuous infusion of mannitol, a bolus is less likely to lead to extravasation of the drug into brain tissue.[17] A potential problem associated with mannitol use is a rebound increase in ICP. This rebound may result from retention of mannitol in the brain tissue as the blood level of the drug is dropping, which reverses the pressure gradient and allows water to diffuse back into the brain tissue, thereby increasing ICP.

Hypertonic saline acts by the osmotic mobilization of water across the intact blood–brain barrier. Other potential beneficial effects of hypertonic saline include plasma volume expansion with improved blood flow as well as a reduction in leukocyte adhesion in the traumatized brain.[18] Sometimes a combination of mannitol and hypertonic saline is used as hyperosmolar therapy for patients with TBI.

Measurement of fluid intake and output (I & O) is mandatory during the use of osmotic therapy. To facilitate accurate measurements, an indwelling urinary catheter is placed. The rate of intravenous (IV) fluid infusion is usually adjusted to maintain a urine flow of at least 30 to 50 mL/hr. A volume less than this amount—or another amount designated by the physician—may signal the need to stop the infusion so as to avoid fulminant fluid overload. (Recall that the kidneys must be able to excrete the fluid being pulled into the bloodstream.) Serum sodium levels should be monitored frequently during mannitol administration: Some sources recommend that the drug be discontinued if the serum sodium concentration rises above 160 mEq/L.[19,20]

Central pontine myelinolysis is a possible complication of hypertonic saline administration, especially when this fluid is given to a patient with a low serum sodium concentration. Recall that a rapid change in the serum sodium concentration is associated with a higher risk of brain damage. For this reason, the serum sodium level should be checked before an infusion is started and frequently thereafter. A second risk with hypertonic saline administration is fluid volume overload, which could induce or aggravate pulmonary edema in patients with underlying cardiac or pulmonary problems.[21]

Barbiturate-Induced Coma

Thiopental infusion to induce barbiturate coma is sometimes used to manage elevated ICP, primarily in patients who have not responded to more conventional therapeutic methods. Thiopental acts as a neuroprotectant in a number of ways; however, it may also be associated with severe potassium imbalances.[22–24] Potassium disturbances during thiopental infusion have a biphasic pattern: *Hypo*kalemia occurs in the first 48 hours, followed by *hyper*kalemia when the infusion is stopped.[25] The reason why potassium rebounds after a thiopental infusion is stopped is unclear. Regardless of the cause, it has been concluded that aggressive treatment of hypokalemia during barbiturate-induced coma should be avoided, and that a tapering dose should be used upon discontinuation of the drug to minimize a rebound elevation in the serum potassium concentration.[26]

Induced Hypothermia

Hypothermia is sometimes used to prevent or mitigate elevated ICP and reduce cerebral edema.[27] Despite its benefits, this approach can be associated with a variety of side effects, the most significant of which is increased risk for infection (usually of the respiratory tract).[28] Other side effects include increased urinary losses of potassium, magnesium, and phosphate,[29] which can predispose patients to arrhythmias. Hypophosphatemia increases the risk for infection by altering white blood cell function. Treatment is aimed at replacing potassium, magnesium, and phosphate to maintain their levels in the high-normal range during the hypothermic treatment.[30]

Upon rewarming, hyperkalemia becomes a threat as cellular potassium (originally sequestered into the cells during induction of hypothermia) is released into the extracellular fluid.[31] Hyperkalemia can be prevented by slow and controlled rewarming, thereby allowing the kidneys to excrete the excess potassium.[32] In patients with anuria or severe oliguria, renal replacement therapy may be started before the patient is rewarmed.

FLUID MANAGEMENT

Fluid management is a crucial component of care for patients with brain injuries, especially when other serious injuries are concurrently present (perhaps with associated hemorrhage or third-spacing of fluids into the injury site). Major considerations are the correct volume and type of fluid.

Volume of Fluid

Fluid management of the brain-injured patient must provide sufficient volume to prevent hypotension while also considering intracranial hemodynamics and ICP. Failure to maintain an adequate vascular volume (and thus arterial pressure) compromises CPP, as does an elevated ICP. In the past, fluid restriction was advocated for patients with trau-

matic brain injury, but it is now known that this practice can lead to a worsened neurological outcome. As indicated earlier, failure to maintain an adequate vascular volume interferes with CPP.

Type of Fluid

Normovolemia should be restored by the administration of isotonic saline, as needed, to achieve a central venous pressure of 7 to 12 cm H_2O.[33] Most clinicians agree that 0.9% sodium chloride solution is the best fluid to maintain normovolemia.[34,35] Lactated Ringer's solution is not the first choice because each liter of this fluid provides roughly 110 mL of free water, which could theoretically predispose patients to brain swelling if used in large quantities.[36] Hypotonic intravenous fluids should be avoided because they predispose patients to brain swelling. Packed red blood cells are administered when necessary to restore the hematocrit to at least 30%.[37]

Use of hypertonic saline to decrease ICP, while also treating hypotension, is advocated by some authors.[38] Because the infusion of hypertonic saline may lead to moderate or severe hypernatremia, it is important to monitor serum sodium levels closely when this fluid is administered.[39] While albumin has also been suggested as a resuscitation fluid, findings from the Saline Versus Albumin Fluid Evaluation study indicated that patients with TBI who were resuscitated with albumin had a higher mortality rate than those who were resuscitated with saline.[40]

Caloric Intake

Because nitrogen wasting is associated with severe TBI, the aim is to provide at least 140% of the daily basal metabolic caloric requirement by the third or fourth day after the injury occurs.[41] For long-term tube feedings, a jejunostomy is preferred to minimize the risk for aspiration.

SODIUM IMBALANCES ASSOCIATED WITH BRAIN INJURY

Sodium imbalances (either hyponatremia or hypernatremia) are common in brain-injured patients, in part because the central nervous system plays a major role in the regulation of sodium and water homeostasis.[42] The two conditions most commonly associated with hyponatremia are syndrome of inappropriate antidiuretic hormone (SIADH) and cerebral salt wasting (CSW). Regardless of its cause, hyponatremia promotes cerebral edema and neurological worsening.[43] A recent study suggests that head-injured females younger than 50 years of age have a significantly greater mortality rate than head-injured males in the same age group.[44]

The patient with brain injury is also at risk for serious hypernatremia when central diabetes insipidus occurs. For example, in a study of 102 consecutive patients who suffered severe or moderate TBI, investigators found that 22 (21.6%) developed diabetes insipidus in the immediately postoperative period.[45] Permanent diabetes insipidus was present in 6.9% of those who survived their traumatic brain injuries.

Syndrome of Inappropriate Antidiuretic Hormone

When hyponatremia occurs with neurological injury, SIADH is often suspected, although other causes of hyponatremia, such as cerebral salt wasting, also need to be considered. A variety of central nervous system disorders may produce SIADH, presumably by increasing production of antidiuretic hormone (ADH). Among these are head injury, encephalitis, meningitis, and brain tumors. SIADH can cause cerebral edema due to cellular swelling (cytotoxic edema). For the most part, this syndrome is self-limiting and subsides as the brain tissue heals; however, it can last for weeks or even months or show up months later.[46, 47]

Clinical Signs

The clinical criteria for SIADH include hyponatremia, a relatively high urine sodium concentration (greater than 20 mEq/L), and a urine osmolality that exceeds serum osmolality. **Table 19-1** compares the clinical presentation of SIADH to other conditions associated with sodium imbalances in patients with neurological injuries.

Management

As is the case with all causes of SIADH, restriction of electrolyte-free water intake is indicated. Adequate free water restriction

Table 19-1 Comparison of Pathophysiology, Clinical Signs, and Treatment of SIADH, CSW, and CDI

Clinical Problem	Pathophysiology	Typical Clinical Findings	Usual Laboratory Findings	Usual Treatment
Syndrome of inappropriate antidiuretic hormone secretion (SIADH)	High secretion of ADH, causing the kidneys to retain water	Fluid intake exceeds urine output Increased body weight No change in CVP	Hyponatremia Urine Na > 20 mEq/L No change in BUN/Cr ratio Serum osmolality < urine osmolality	Fluid restriction 3% or 5% NaCl, if needed
Cerebral salt wasting (CSW)	Sodium loss into urine, results in extracellular fluid volume deficit	Decreased body weight Fluid intake less than fluid output Decreased CVP Perhaps dry skin and mucous membranes	Hyponatremia Urine Na > 20 mEq/L BUN/Cr ratio increased Serum osmolality < urine osmolality	Fluid replacement with sodium-containing fluid (such as 0.9% NaCl) to expand the ECF
Central diabetes insipidus (CDI)	Low secretion of ADH, causing increased loss of water by the kidneys	Polyuria Polydipsia (if alert) Decreased body weight	Hypernatremia Dilute urine (SG often < 1.010) Serum osmolality > urine osmolality	Fluid replacement Vasopressin

ADH = antidiuretic hormone; BUN = blood urea nitrogen; Cr = creatinine; CVP = central venous pressure; ECF = extracellular fluid; SG = specific gravity.
Source: Adapted from Zafonte R, Watanabe T, Mann N, Ko D. Psychogenic polydipsia after traumatic brain injury: A case report. *Am J PhysMed Rehabil* 1997;75:246, and Harrigan M. Cerebral salt wasting syndrome: A review. *Neurosurgery* 1996; 38:152. ADH, antidiuretic hormone; BUN, blood urea nitrogen; Cr, creatinine; CVP, central venous pressure; ECF, extracellular fluid; SG, specific gravity.

will eventually increase the serum sodium concentration. In non-edematous patients, extra salt is sometimes given in the diet (or in the form of salt tablets) in combination with mild fluid restriction. If severe symptoms are present, it may be necessary to cautiously infuse a hypertonic saline solution, such as 3% or 5% NaCl. As discussed in Chapter 4, these solutions are extremely dangerous and should be handled with care. Hypertonic saline should be administered only in intensive care units under close observation. A danger of too-rapid correction of the serum sodium level is myelinolysis.

A new treatment has recently become available to treat patients with SIADH. Conivaptan, a vasopressin-receptor antagonist, promotes free water excretion. In a recent trial in which this drug was administered to 19 hyponatremic patients in a neurointensive setting, serum sodium levels rose by 5.8 ± 3.2 mEq/L within 12 hours.[48]

Cerebral Salt Wasting

Cerebral salt wasting is a syndrome characterized by hyponatremia, renal sodium loss, and extracellular volume contraction. It is most often seen in patients with subarachnoid hemorrhage, but it also occurs in patients with head trauma and brain tumors. Although the mechanism by which the renal salt wasting associated with CSW occurs is not fully understood, atrial natriuretic peptide (ANP) appears to be involved.[49] In the presence of increased levels of ANP, salt loss in the urine increases. Although most reports of this condition have involved adults, some case reports document its occurrence in young children.[50, 51]

Clinical Signs

The hyponatremia seen in CSW is attributed to true sodium loss; in contrast, the hyponatremia of SIADH is due to water retention. Therefore, careful assessment of the patient's fluid volume status is the most helpful way to distinguish between these two entities. To do so, it is necessary to obtain highly accurate daily weights and measurements of fluid I & O, along with daily urinary sodium measurements. As noted in Table 19-1, patients with CSW who are not adequately hydrated will lose weight and show other signs of extracellular fluid deficit, such as decreased central venous pressure. In contrast, patients with SIADH do not have signs of extracellular fluid deficit. A weight loss of more than 1 kg/day (or other signs of decreased fluid volume) in the presence of worsening hyponatremia favors the diagnosis of CSW.

Management

Although hyponatremia is present in both CSW and SIADH, opposite treatment strategies are recommended (see Table 19-1). Whereas SIADH requires fluid restriction to allow water loss to exceed fluid intake, CSW requires intravascular volume resuscitation and sodium replacement.[52] Isotonic sodium solutions such as 0.9% NaCl or possibly 3% NaCl may be used; for patients who are able to swallow, salt tablets are sometimes used to replace sodium.

When CSW presents in patients with subarachnoid hemorrhage, there is an increased risk of brain infarction due to cerebral vasospasm. A protocol referred to as "hypervolemic, hypertensive therapy" is considered the cornerstone of treatment for patients with symptomatic vasospasm. In a group of patients with acute symptomatic vasospasm, researchers separately evaluated the effects of volume expansion and hypertension induced by IV pressors on neurological examinations during the first two hours following each intervention.[53] First, volume expansion with normal saline and/or 5% albumin solution was used. If deemed necessary, this was followed by IV pressors to maintain an elevated systolic BP (target range 180–220 mm Hg). Volume expansion was used in 89 patients, 43% of whom had a positive clinical response within a 2-hour time frame. Pressors were used in 81 patients, 68% of whom had a positive clinical response within a 2-hour time frame.

Central Diabetes Insipidus

Central diabetes insipidus (CDI) can occur when the injured brain is unable to release sufficient ADH (vasopressin). Recall that ADH is synthesized in the hypothalamus, stored in the posterior lobe of the pituitary gland, and released in response to many stimuli—the most important of which is increased plasma osmolality. Unfortunately, after head trauma, ADH deficiency can occur. Inadequate ADH production permits the excretion of a large volume of dilute urine; left untreated, this imbalance can lead to hypernatremia, hypovolemia, and hemoconcentration. Depending on the site of the lesion, CDI can be permanent or transient.

Patients with severe TBI have a high risk for developing hypernatremia for a variety of reasons other than CDI; among these are inadequate water intake due to altered thirst or impaired sensorium and increased insensible water losses.[54] Even mild hypernatremia has been shown to be associated with increased risk of death in patients with severe TBI.[55]

Clinical Signs

Central diabetes insipidus is manifested by an abrupt onset of polyuria and polydipsia. The usual urine volume when this condition is present is 8 to 10 L/day. Conscious patients usually exhibit extreme thirst and will drink large volumes of fluid, if able to do so. Because of the sustained polyuria, sleep deprivation can be a problem. Failure to consume enough fluids to adequately match the large urine volume will produce profound volume depletion. Because the unconscious patient can neither experience thirst nor respond to it, fluids must be replaced by the parenteral route, titrated according to urine output and laboratory results. Classic laboratory findings include hypernatremia and serum hyperosmolality. Urine specific gravity is usually less than 1.005 and urine osmolality less than 200 mOsm/kg. Although the fluid deprivation test is sometimes used to establish a diagnosis of CDI, it must be done cautiously while observing the urine output and serum sodium level; regardless of fluid restriction, the patient with CDI will continue to excrete a large urine volume, perhaps leading to profound hypovolemia and hypernatremia.

In critically ill patients, CDI may follow a triphasic course. That is, it may occur transiently for a few days after surgery or trauma and then resolve for a few days, only to recur.

Management

Patients with large urinary losses from CDI need fluid replacement. If the patient is conscious, the fluid may be given orally. If the patient is not conscious, it may be given by the parenteral route in the form of lactated Ringer's solution or half-normal saline, depending on the patient's volume status and degree of water deficit. In addition to these IV fluids, magnesium and potassium supplementation may be needed to replace losses of these electrolytes through the excessive volume of urine.

Acute central diabetes insipidus after surgery or trauma may be treated with short-acting aqueous pitressin. After a period of time, this treatment may be temporarily discontinued to determine if the diabetes insipidus is transient or permanent. With the administration of an ADH analog, it is conceivable that the patient may become fluid overloaded if fluid intake (IV and oral) exceeds fluid output. Fluid overload may also result if third-space fluid accumulations from other injuries shift back into the vascular space when ADH is being administered. Excessive water retention may cause the patient's originally high serum sodium level to drop below normal. Such rapid vacillations in the serum sodium level can cause a worsened neurological status related to shifts in the brain water content. As a consequence, close monitoring assessment of neurological signs and laboratory data is required during treatment.

CASE STUDIES

Case Study 19-1

A 35-year-old man was involved in a multiple-vehicle accident and sustained a basilar skull fracture and multiple facial bruises. On admission to the emergency room, the patient was unconscious, with a Glasgow Coma Scale score of 7 and no focal neurologic abnormalities. A long bone fracture was discovered, and the patient received fluid resuscitation consisting of large amounts of lactated Ringer's solution. Mannitol was given to treat his head injury. Twelve hours after the injury, the patient's urine output was noted to exceed 1 L/hr and the following abnormal laboratory findings were observed: severe hypernatremia (Na = 175 mEq/L), hyperchloremia (Cl = 134 mEq/L), and a hyperosmolar serum (serum osmolality = 365 mOsm/L). The patient's urine was very dilute: urine osmolality = 80 mOsm/L and urine sodium = 10 mEq/L.

Commentary. The laboratory data were consistent with CDI. The serum sodium was markedly elevated, as was the serum osmolality. In contrast, the urine sodium and osmolality were low, reflecting large water loss in the urine. Basilar skull fracture is frequently associated with development of CDI. After treatment with vasopressin, the urine volume should diminish and the serum sodium level should decrease. Note that while a conscious patient with CDI would likely experience thirst and, therefore, drink extra fluid, an unconscious patient cannot make these responses. Thus continued loss of large volumes of urine without adequate fluid replacement could result in severe hypovolemia.

Case Study 19-2

A 30-year-old woman presented in the emergency room with complaints of severe headache, vertigo, and a stiff neck. She denied chest pain and had a normal electrocardiogram. Previously, she had been in good health and denied a history of hypertension or drug use. A head computed tomogram was performed in the emergency room and showed a subarachnoid hemorrhage.

On admission to the intensive care unit (ICU), the patient was lethargic, but opened her eyes when her name was called and responded appropriately to orientation questions before drifting back to sleep. Her pupils were 4/4 and brisk. She moved all extremities well; however, her left hand grasp was slightly weaker than her right hand grasp. A cerebral angiogram confirmed a right internal communicating artery aneurysm. The patient's heart rate ranged between 80 and 110 beats/min, mean blood pressure was between 90 and 118 mm Hg, respirations were 16 to 24 breaths/min, and her oxygen saturation was 94% to 98% on room air. She was started on oral doses of nimodipine, Decadron, Colace, Dilantin, Zantac, Apresoline, and morphine for pain.

Twenty-four hours after her initial subarachnoid hemorrhage, the patient underwent a craniotomy for aneurysm clipping. On return to the ICU, she was alert and oriented to her name and could follow simple commands using all four extremities; her speech was clear but occasionally inappropriate. A left radial arterial line was placed in the operating room to monitor her mean arterial blood pressure; orders were received to maintain the pressure at more than 100 mm Hg. In addition, a pulmonary artery catheter was placed in her right subclavian vein to monitor pulmonary artery wedge pressures every hour and cardiac output readings every 2 hours.

Twenty hours after surgery, the patient's level of consciousness changed; she became lethargic and did not follow commands. No other neurological deficits were apparent. Her mean arterial blood pressure was 70 mm Hg, while her central venous pressure and pulmonary wedge pressure were low. At this time, her serum sodium level was 130 mEq/L.

Commentary. This patient was experiencing a cerebral vasospasm, a potential complication from subarachnoid hemorrhage. Because healthcare providers failed to administer IV fluids in sufficient volume to match her urinary sodium loss, she developed fluid volume deficit with hyponatremia, which in turn contributed to the cerebral vasospasm. Hyponatremia can signal either SIADH or CSW. In this case, because the hyponatremia coexisted with clinical signs of fluid volume deficit, it was more likely a problem of CSW (true sodium loss in the urine). The patient required additional administration of 0.9% NaCl to reduce the adverse effects of the cerebral vasospasm and hyponatremia.

Case Study 19-3

A 48-year-old man sustained a fall and developed a headache thereafter; he sought care in a local hospital.[56] A brain CT showed no skull fracture or intracranial hemorrhage. When he developed vomiting, progressively severe headaches, and a deteriorating level of consciousness, the patient was sent to a different facility. There, a repeat CT scan showed a hematoma. Laboratory results were as follows: hyponatremia (Na = 122 mEq/L), low serum osmolality (263 mOsm/L), and high urine sodium (159 mEq/L). Renal function was normal (serum Cr = 0.7 mg/dL; BUN = 13 mg/dL). Urine osmolality was high at 710 mOsm/kg.

Surgery was not performed for the patient's small subdural hemorrhage; however, he received 3% sodium chloride and was placed on fluid restriction to treat his low serum sodium concentration (hyponatremia). A diagnosis of SIADH was made at this time. On day 10, his serum sodium concentration dropped again, to 110 mEq/L. The sodium concentration gradually returned to a level of 130 mEq/L over a period of several weeks. The patient was discharged at this time.

Another episode of hyponatremia occurred two months later, when the patient underwent surgery for a lumbar spine compression fraction. Prior to that surgery, the patient's serum sodium level was 131 mEq/L and he was symptom free. However, following the surgery, he experienced severe headaches and vomiting. At this time, a diagnosis of recurrent SIADH was made. Prior to the surgery, the serum sodium level was 131 mEq/L and no symptoms were present. The lowest serum sodium level reached during the hospitalization for spinal surgery was 108 mEq/L; it gradually resolved with water restriction to a level of 130 mEq/L.

A third episode of hyponatremia occurred 20 days after the second discharge when the patient was readmitted for a second spinal surgical procedure. Although the preoperative sodium level was near normal (133 mEq/L), the patient's sodium concentration dropped to 117 mEq/L following surgery. Again, the serum sodium level eventually normalized with conservative treatment. No subsequent hyponatremic events were reported.

Commentary. The authors of this case report emphasize that most TBI-associated hyponatremia occurs within 1 week after head injury, but that sodium levels tend to return to normal within 6 months.[57] Both of the repeat episodes of SIADH in this patient followed surgical procedures—a common precipitating event for SIADH. This case report highlights the clinical significance of recurrent trauma-related SIADH and the need for continual evaluation for hyponatremia for all patients with post-traumatic brain injury.

Case Study 19-4

A 39-year-old woman was admitted with a diagnosis of subarachnoid hemorrhage following a ruptured aneurysm. She subsequently underwent surgical clipping of the aneurysm without incident. In the postoperative period, the patient required therapeutic hypervolemia via the administration of isotonic saline to maintain her blood pressure and minimize risk for cerebral vasospasm. On the sixth postoperative day, her CVP dropped to 3 mm Hg and she became tachycardic. At this time, her blood pressure was 110/50 mm Hg and her skin was dry. During the previous 24 hours, her fluid intake was 3200 mL and her urine output was 4400 mL. Despite a relatively large IV fluid intake, her weight had decreased by 3 lb since her admission. The following laboratory values were reported: hyponatremia (Na = 126 mEq/L), normal serum potassium (K = 4.9 mEq/L), normal serum chloride (Cl = 100 mEq/L), low serum osmolality (270 mOsm/kg), and an elevated BUN:Cr ratio (22:1). The patient's serum glucose level was 115 mg/dL.

To treat the patient's low serum sodium concentration, a 3% solution of sodium chloride was given at a rate of 30 mL/hr over the next 12 hours, followed by isotonic saline at a rate of 120 mL/hr. It took two days for the serum sodium level to normalize. The serum sodium level remained in the normal range afterward and the patient made an uneventful recovery.

Commentary. This patient had developed cerebral salt wasting (hyponatremia) as a result of her neurological condition. The low serum osmolality was reflective of her low serum sodium concentration. Signs of volume depletion included tachycardia, drop in blood pressure, decreased weight, and a BUN:Cr ratio greater than 20:1.

See Case Study 4-14 for another case concerning a patient with a head injury.

Summary of Key Points

- Compensatory mechanisms for an expanding brain mass include: (1) shunting of cerebrospinal fluid (CSF) into the spinal dural sac, (2) increased absorption of CSF, and (3) vasoconstriction to decrease the volume of blood in the brain.

- Untreated cerebral edema, regardless of its etiology, leads to elevated intracranial pressure (ICP). An ICP value is most important in terms of its relationship with cerebral perfusion pressure (CPP).

- To assure adequate cerebral perfusion, attention must be given to both the patient's blood pressure and intracranial pressure: Cerebral perfusion pressure = mean arterial pressure minus intracranial pressure (CPP = MAP − ICP).

- It is important to maintain good ventilation in any patient with a head injury because decreased oxygenation (hypoxemia) and elevated levels of carbon dioxide (hypercarbia) are potent vasodilators that contribute to a high ICP.

- When ICP becomes dangerously high, hyperventilation may be employed to temporarily reduce the $PaCO_2$, thereby producing constriction of blood vessels with subsequent reduced brain volume. An undesirable effect of hyperventilation is reduced blood flow to brain tissues caused by vasoconstriction.

- Osmotic agents, such as mannitol or hypertonic saline, may be used to pull fluid from uninjured brain tissues to temporarily relieve elevated ICP.

- Barbiturate-induced coma can be associated with wide shifts in plasma potassium levels.

- Fluid management of patients with brain injury must provide sufficient volume to prevent hypotension while also considering intracranial hemodynamics and intracranial pressure.

- Hypotonic intravenous fluids should be avoided in patients with head injuries because they can induce brain swelling.

- Many clinicians agree that 0.9% sodium chloride solution is the best fluid to maintain normovolemia in brain-injured patients.

- The two conditions most commonly associated with hyponatremia in patients with brain injuries are syndrome of inappropriate antidiuretic hormone (SIADH) and cerebral salt wasting (CSW). Treatment for these two conditions is mutually exclusive: Fluid is restricted in SIADH patients, whereas fluid replacement is vital for CSW patients.

- The major cause of hypernatremia in patients with head injuries is central diabetes insipidus (CDI).

NOTES

1. Cohen, S. M., & Marin, D. W. (2005). Traumatic brain injury. In M. P. Fink et al. (Eds.), *Textbook of critical care* (5th ed.). Philadelphia. Elsevier Saunders, p. 384.

2. Sakowitz, O. W., Stover, J. F., Sarrafzadeh, A. S., Unterberg, A. W., & Kiening, K. L. (2007). Effects of mannitol bolus administration on intracranial pressure, cerebral extracellular metabolites, and tissue oxygenation in severely head-injured patients. *Journal of Trauma-Injury Infection & Critical Care, 62*(2), 292–298.

3. Kanter, M. J., & Narayan, R. K. (1991). Management of head injury. Intracranial monitoring. *Neurosurgery Clinics of North America, 2*(2), 257–265.

4. Kollef, M. H., Bedient, T. J., Isakow, W., & Witt, C. A. (Eds.). (2008). *The Washington manual of critical care.* Philadelphia: Wolters Kluwer/Lippincott Williams & Wilkins, p. 401.

5. Brain Trauma Foundation. (2007). Guidelines for the management of severe traumatic brain injury. IX. Cerebral perfusion thresholds. *Journal of Neurotrauma, 24*(suppl 1), S59–S64.

6. Brain Trauma Foundation. (2007). Guidelines for the management of severe traumatic brain injury. I. Blood pressure and oxygenation. *Journal of Neurotrauma, 24*(suppl 1), S7–S13.

7. Kollef et al., note 4, p. 402.

8. Kollef et al., note 4, p. 402.

9. Brain Trauma Foundation, note 5, p. 7.

10. Cohen & Marin, note 1, p. 384.

11. Kollef et al., note 4, p. 403.

12. Brain Trauma Foundation. (2007). Guidelines for the management of severe traumatic brain injury. XIV. Hyperventilation. *Journal of Neurotrauma, 24*(suppl 1), S87–S90.

13. Knapp, J. M. (2005). Hyperosmolar therapy in the treatment of severe head injury in children: Mannitol and hypertonic saline. *AACN Clinical Issues, 16*(2), 199–211.

14. Wakai, A., Roberts, I., & Schierhout, G. (2007). Mannitol for acute traumatic brain injury. *Cochrane Database of Systematic Reviews, 1,* CD001049.

15. Brain Trauma Foundation. (2007). Guidelines for the management of severe traumatic brain injury. II. Hyperosmolar therapy. *Journal of Neurotrauma, 24*(suppl 1), S14–S20.

16. Brain Trauma Foundation, note 15.

17. Cohen & Marin, note 1, p. 384.

18. Brain Trauma Foundation, note 15.

19. Cohen & Marin, note 1, p. 384.

20. Kollef et al., note 4, p. 403.

21. Brain Trauma Foundation, note 15.

22. Chang, C. H., Liao, J. J., Chuang, C. H., & Lee, C. T. (2008). Recurrent hyponatremia after traumatic brain injury. *American Journal of the Medical Sciences, 335*(5), 390–393.

23. Neil, M. J., & Dale, M. D. (2009). Hypokalaemia with severe rebound hyperkalaemia after therapeutic barbiturate coma. *Anesthesia & Analgesia, 108*(6), 1867–1868.

24. Bouchard, P. M., Frenette, A. J., Williamson, D. R., & Perreault, M. M. (2008). Thiopental-associated dyskalemia in severe head trauma. *Journal of Trauma-Injury Infection & Critical Care, 64*(3), 838–842.

25. Neil & Dale, note 23.

26. Neil & Dale, note 23.

27. Polderman, K. H., & Herold, I. (2009). Therapeutic hypothermia and controlled normothermia in the intensive care unit: Practical considerations, side effects, and cooling methods. *Critical Care Medicine, 37*(3), 1101–1120.

28. Jiang, J. Y. (2009). Clinical study of mild hypothermia treatment for severe traumatic brain injury. *Journal of Neurotrauma. 26*(3), 399–406.

29. Polderman, K. H., Peerderman, S. M., & Girbes, A. R. (2001). Hypophosphatemia and hypomagnesemia induced by cooling in patients with severe head injury. *Journal of Neurosurgery, 94*(5), 697–705.

30. Polderman, K. H. (2009). Mechanisms of action, physiological effects, and complications of hypothermia. *Critical Care Medicine, 37*(7 suppl), S186–S202.

31. Polderman, note 30.

32. Polderman, note 30.

33. Cohen & Marin, note 1, p. 384.

34. Garcia, A. (2006). Critical care issues in the early management of severe trauma. *Surgical Clinics of North America, 86*(6), 1359–1387.

35. Hahn, R. G., Prough, D. S., & Svensen, C. H. (2007). *Periperative fluid therapy.* London: Informa Healthcare, pp. 260–273.

36. Hahn et al., note 35, p. 260.

37. Cohen & Marin, note 1, p. 384.

38. Pascual, J. L., Maloney-Wilensky, E., Reilly, P. M., Sicoutris, C., Keutmann, M. K., Stein, S. C., et al. (2008). Resuscitation of hypotensive head-injured patients: Is hypertonic saline the answer? *American Surgeon, 74*(3), 253–259.

39. Froelich, M., Ni, Q., Wess, C., Ougorets, I., & Harti, R. (2009). Continuous hypertonic saline therapy and the occurrence of complications in neurocritically ill patients. *Critical Care Medicine, 37*(4), 1433–1441.

40. SAFE Study Investigators, Australian and New Zealand Intensive Care Society Clinical Trials Group, Australian Red Cross Blood Service, George Institute for International Health, Myburgh, J., Cooper, D. J., Finfer, S., et al. (2007). Saline or albumin for fluid resuscitation in patients with traumatic brain injury. *New England Journal of Medicine, 357*(9), 874–884.

41. Cohen & Marin, note 1, p. 385.

42. Diringer, M. N., & Zazulia, A. R. (2006). Hyponatremia in neurologic patients: Consequences and approaches to treatment. *Neurologist, 12*(3), 117–126.

43. Murphy, T., Dhar, R., & Diringer, M. (2009). Conivaptan bolus dosing for the correction of hyponatremia in the neurointensive care unit. *Neurocritical Care, 11*(1), 14–19.

44. Czosnyka, M., Radolovich, D., Balestreri, M., Lavinio, A., Hutchinson, P., Timofeev, I., et al. (2008). Gender-related differences in

intracranial hypertension and outcomes after traumatic brain injury. *Acta Neurochirurgica, 102*(suppl), 25–28.

45. Agha, A., Thornton, E., O'Kelly, P., Tormey, W., Phillips, J., & Thompson, C. J. (2004). Posterior pituitary dysfunction after traumatic brain injury. *Journal of Clinical Endocrinology & Metabolism, 89*(12), 5987–5992.

46. Chang et al., note 22.

47. Kumar, P. D., Nartsupha, C., & Koletsky, R. J. (2001). Delayed syndrome of inappropriate antidiuretic hormone secretion 1 year after a head injury. *Annals of Internal Medicine, 135*(10), 932–933.

48. Murphy et al., note 43.

49. Lu, D. C., Binder, D. K., Chien, B., Maisel, A., Manley, G. T. (2008). Cerebral salt wasting and elevated brain natriuretic peptide levels after traumatic brain injury: 2 case reports. *Surgical Neurology, 69*(3), 226–229.

50. Donati-Genet, P. C., Dubuis, J. M., Girardin, E., & Rimensberger, P. C. (2001). Acute symptomatic hyponatremia and cerebral salt-wasting head injury: An important clinical entity. *Journal of Pediatric Surgery, 36*(7), 1094–1097.

51. Steelman, R., Corbitt, B., & Pate, M. F. (2006). Early onset of cerebral salt wasting in a patient with head and facial injuries. *Journal of Oral and Maxillofacial Surgery, 64,* 746–747.

52. Cole, C. D., Gottfried, O. N., Liu, J. K., & Couldwell, W. T. (2004). Hyponatremia in the neurosurgical patient: Diagnosis and management. *Neurosurgical Focus, 16*(4), E9.

53. Frontera, J. A., Fernandez, A., Schmidt, J. M., Claassen, J., Wartenberg, K. E., Badjatia, N., et al. (2010). Clinical response to hypertensive hypervolemic therapy and outcome after subarachnoid hemorrhage. *Neurosurgery. 66*(1), 35–41.

54. Maggiore, U., Picetti, E., Antonucci, E., Parenti, E., Regolisti, G., Mergoni, M., et al. (2009). The relation between the incidence of hypernatremia and mortality in patients with severe traumatic brain injury. *Critical Care, 14*(4), R110.

55. Maggiore et al., note 54.

56. Chang et al., note 22.

57. Chang et al., note 22.

Chapter 20

Acute Pancreatitis

Approximately 2% of all patients admitted to U.S. hospitals are diagnosed with acute pancreatitis.[1] Further, approximately three-fourths of these cases are caused by either gallstones or alcoholism.[2] Less common causes of pancreatitis include hypertriglyceridemia, hypercalcemia, trauma, infection, neoplasms, and use of certain drugs (e.g., isoniazid, estrogens, thiazides, furosemide, sulfonamides, tetracycline, and corticosteroids).[3] In the United States, alcohol consumption accounts for approximately 40% of all cases of acute pancreatitis.[4] The clinical course of acute pancreatitis may range from mild local inflammation to multisystem organ failure secondary to a systemic inflammatory response.

When acute pancreatitis is limited to the mild form (roughly 75% to 85% of total cases), mortality is low. In these situations, the episode of pancreatitis is self-limited and is associated with mild symptoms that resolve within 3 to 5 days.[5] In contrast, a fatal outcome occurs in 10% to 24% of cases involving the acute hemorrhagic necrotizing form of pancreatitis.[6]

PATHOPHYSIOLOGY

In acute pancreatitis, trypsin is prematurely activated and leads to massive inflammation of the pancreas and systemic overproduction of pro-inflammatory products.[7] In severe acute pancreatitis, autodigestion of the organ occurs, with digestive enzymes then leaking into the circulation. Ultimately, remote organs (such as the kidneys and lungs) can be damaged through this process.

As a consequence of these changes, the pancreas becomes edematous and may pull enough fluid into itself to produce hypovolemia; swelling may be severe enough to compress the vascular bed and cause ischemia and necrosis. In addi-

tion, severe pancreatitis can lead to irritation of the peritoneal surface and cause the transudation of substantial volumes of protein-rich fluid. In this sense, an analogy can be made between the injury induced by severe pancreatitis and a chemical burn. Tissue changes are characterized by pancreatic and peri-pancreatic edema and by fat necrosis. A more severe form of the disease, referred to *hemorrhagic* or *necrotizing pancreatitis,* involves extensive pancreatic and peri-pancreatic fat necrosis and hemorrhage into and around the pancreas. Death in acute pancreatitis is most often related to multiple-organ failure.

Fluid and electrolyte status is an extremely important consideration during the care of patients with acute pancreatitis. Prognostic indicators for this disease include both fluid volume status and serum calcium concentrations.

Hypovolemia

The severity of the hypovolemia associated with acute pancreatitis depends on the extent of fluid and blood lost in the retroperitoneum and peritoneal cavity. Other factors influencing this imbalance include the volume of fluid sequestered in the bowel during adynamic ileus and the volume of vomitus or fluid lost through nasogastric (NG) suction. The hematocrit may be elevated in edematous pancreatitis because of plasma loss from the vascular space, which causes red blood cells to be suspended in a smaller blood volume. In contrast, a low hematocrit is likely in hemorrhagic pancreatitis as a result of blood loss. Mortality is increased in patients with acute pancreatitis who have hypovolemia (systolic blood pressure less than 100 mm Hg) at admission.[8]

The estimated amount of fluid sequestered in the abdomen after the onset of pancreatitis is one of the Ranson criteria for risk of complications (discussed later in this chapter). Another significant finding is the extent to which the hematocrit is decreased—a measure that reflects the amount of blood loss in hemorrhagic pancreatitis.

Hypocalcemia

Hypocalcemia in a patient with acute pancreatitis is suggestive of a poor outcome.[9–11] In part, the drop in the total serum calcium level (the sum of the ionized and bound fractions) is related to the concurrent hypoalbuminemia predictably associated with the leakage of protein-rich fluid into the peritoneal cavity. (Recall that when hypoalbuminemia is present, the total serum calcium appears deceptively low.) Nevertheless, true hypocalcemia can exist in patients with acute pancreatitis. Although the mechanisms responsible for the emergence of hypocalcemia in the setting of pancreatitis remain unclear, systemic endotoxin exposure appears to play a significant role in its development.[12] Another theory posits that calcium becomes trapped in necrotic tissue in and around the pancreas. For example, investigators found a markedly increased calcium content in necrotic tissues obtained from the peri-pancreatic areas of patients with severe pancreatitis.[13] Other investigators have suggested that a serum calcium less than 7.5 mg/dL is caused by widespread fatty necrosis; further, they hypothesize that a calcium level less than 7.5 mg/dL is indicative of disease severity and predictive of multisystem organ failure.[14] For some unknown reason, when a patient has pancreatitis, parathyroid hormone apparently does not increase as a compensatory method to raise the serum calcium concentration by pulling calcium from the bone.

Hypomagnesemia

Mild hypomagnesemia may occur during acute pancreatitis. As is the case with hypocalcemia, hypomagnesemia has been attributed to precipitation of magnesium ions in the inflamed tissues in and around the pancreas as insoluble magnesium "soaps." Also, as with hypocalcemia, hypomagnesemia is often at least partially related to hypoalbuminemia, meaning that much of the change may occur in bound magnesium rather than in ionized magnesium. Of course, one factor contributing to the development of hypomagnesemia in this population may be the direct loss of magnesium during vomiting, gastric suction, and diarrhea. If the pancreatitis is due to alcoholism, the hypomagnesemia is likely to be more severe because of the multiple magnesium-

lowering effects of alcohol. Patients with acute pancreatitis and hypocalcemia commonly have intracellular magnesium deficiency despite normal serum magnesium concentrations; therefore, magnesium deficiency may play a significant role in the pathogenesis of hypocalcemia.

In a study that compared 13 patients with chronic pancreatitis with 8 healthy control subjects, investigators found that 10 of the 13 patients with pancreatitis showed greater evidence of magnesium deficiency than did the control subjects.[15] The investigators concluded that routine evaluation of magnesium status could allow appropriate magnesium supplementation and possibly result in symptom improvement in patients with severe chronic pancreatitis.

Both serum calcium and magnesium levels should be monitored when patients with acute pancreatitis display symptoms of neuromuscular irritability, such as positive Chvostek's and Trousseau's signs.[16] Both of these signs are described in Chapter 2.

Hypophosphatemia

Hypophosphatemia in patients with acute pancreatitis may be caused by respiratory alkalosis—a condition that favors temporary shifting of phosphorus into the cells. Respiratory alkalosis is not uncommon in patients with acute pancreatitis because of the severe pain and anxiety associated with this disease. Other possible causes of hypophosphatemia in patients with acute pancreatitis may include shifting of phosphorus into the cells following insulin administration. Alcoholic patients are more likely to have low serum phosphorus levels than are non-alcoholic patients. Unfortunately, phosphate deficiency is often overlooked in patients with acute pancreatitis.[17] In fact, serum phosphate levels may need to be checked along with serum calcium levels in patients with acute pancreatitis, especially in those who are alcoholic.

Hyperglycemia

Several studies have shown that hyperglycemia that is present at the time of admission is associated with a worse prognosis in patients with acute pancreatitis.[18–20] That is, hyperglycemia (like hypocalcemia) is a marker for the severity of acute pancreatitis. Severe cases of acute pancreatitis result in destruction of pancreatic tissue and cause islet cell dysfunction, thereby interfering with the formation of insulin. In turn, the hyperglycemia can affect the patient's immune system and hinder the body's ability to combat infections.[21]

Acid–Base Imbalances

Acid–base disturbances may vary widely in patients with pancreatitis, depending on the clinical circumstances. On the one hand, metabolic alkalosis may result from the frequent vomiting associated with acute pancreatitis, as well as from the gastric suction used during treatment to alleviate adynamic ileus. On the other hand, a high anion gap (AG) metabolic acidosis is likely in the presence of poor tissue perfusion. Recall that multisystem organ failure is a complication of severe acute pancreatitis. The pulmonary complications to which patients with pancreatitis are predisposed—such as pneumonia, pleural effusions, pulmonary edema, pulmonary emboli, and atelectasis—may cause respiratory acid–base problems (either acidosis or alkalosis). As mentioned earlier, severe pain may stimulate hyperventilation, thereby causing respiratory alkalosis.

CLINICAL PRESENTATION

The patient with acute pancreatitis usually presents with constant midepigastric pain that radiates to the back, causing abdominal guarding. This pain is typically associated with nausea, vomiting, and abdominal distention. Bowel sounds may be absent if ileus is present. Lying in a supine position tends to exacerbate the pain, whereas sitting up and leaning forward tends to help. A low-grade fever with tachycardia and hypotension may be present. Weakness, sweating, and anxiety are often apparent during severe attacks of pancreatitis.

The presentation of acute pancreatitis may vary depending on its cause. For example, pain in biliary pancreatitis (caused by gallstones) often starts after a meal. In contrast, when pancreatitis develops in an alcoholic individual, it most often occurs 1 to 3 days after a heavy drinking binge.

A key finding used to make the diagnosis of acute pancreatitis is increased serum amylase activity coupled with abdominal pain. Total serum amylase activity level usually rises 2 to 12 hours after symptom onset and remains elevated for several days in most cases. Persistent elevations of serum amylase for longer than 10 days can indicate complications, such as pseudocyst formation.[22] While high serum amylase levels are frequently present in patients with non-alcoholic pancreatitis, as many as one-third of patients with alcoholic pancreatitis may have no or only moderately elevated elevations.[23] Serum lipase levels are also elevated in acute pancreatitis.

PROGNOSTIC INDICATORS

Because approximately 20% of all patients with acute pancreatitis will suffer severe illness, it is important to identify these individuals early. One set of markers commonly used to estimate the risk for major complications or death from acute pancreatitis are the Ranson criteria, which include age, white blood cell count, blood glucose level, liver enzymes, oxygenation, base deficit, estimated fluid sequestration, and the serum calcium concentration.[24] The Ranson criteria are evaluated over the initial 48 hours.

Other investigators have applied the APACHE II[25] criteria to patients with pancreatitis; an advantage of this set of criteria is that it can be used at any point in the patient's illness (not just the first 48 hours).[26] The APACHE II criteria incorporate a combination of physiological indicators, age, and chronic health to evaluate the status of critically ill patients. The range of scores varies from 0 to 71, with high scores being worse.

The Sequential Organ Failure Assessment Score, while not specific for pancreatitis, is helpful in identifying patients with increased morbidity and mortality.[27] Still other criteria include the serum C-reactive protein level to predict severity of pancreatitis; a level greater than 150 mg/L within the first 72 hours has been arbitrarily chosen as a marker for the occurrence of necrotizing pancreatitis.[28, 29] However, it is important to recognize that other factors may affect the C-reactive protein level (such as pneumonia or cholangitis) and must first be ruled out.[30]

A grading system based on a contrast-enhanced computed tomography (CT) scan includes scores for the level of inflammation as well as for the degree of tissue necrosis.[31] At the highest score (10 points), morbidity is estimated at 92% and mortality at 17%.[32] A more recently developed scoring system is the Pancreatitis Outcome Prediction (POP) score; this system emphasizes the effects of arterial pH, age, blood urea nitrogen, mean arterial pressure, oxygenation, and serum potassium on the course of pancreatitis.[33] A simple hematocrit value is helpful in distinguishing between edematous pancreatitis (elevated hematocrit) and hemorrhagic pancreatitis (decreased hematocrit).

COMPLICATIONS

Severe acute pancreatitis can be associated with both systemic and local complications. The two most common systemic complications are renal failure and respiratory failure. In a study of 267 consecutive patients admitted with acute pancreatitis, 63 (24%) developed multiple-system organ failure (defined as failure of two or more organ systems).[34] The most common complications noted in this patient population were renal, respiratory, and cardiovascular failure. Slightly more than half of the deaths in pancreatitis occur after the first week of illness, mostly associated with a combination of multiple-organ failure and sepsis.[35,36] Among the local complications are necrosis, pseudocysts, abscesses, fistulas, and gastrointestinal hemorrhage.

Acute Renal Failure

Severe intravascular volume depletion predisposes individuals to acute tubular necrosis and acute renal failure. Also, the systemic inflammatory response associated with severe acute pancreatitis can cause renal injury. For the most part, acute renal failure is explained on the basis of hypovolemia and hypotension. In fact, renal failure from inadequate fluid replacement is a frequent finding in patients who die from pancreatitis. The need for adequate fluid resuscitation to prevent this complication is obvious. Sufficient fluid replacement should be given to maintain adequate circulatory blood volume and urine output.

Respiratory Failure

Pulmonary complications occur in as many as 50% of patients with acute pancreatitis.[37] On admission, radiographic signs of lung injury are present in approximately 15% of patients with acute pancreatitis.[38] By the fifth day, radiographic evidence of abnormalities is evident in as many as 70% of patients.[39] The early acute lung injury observed in patients with severe acute pancreatitis is caused by inflammatory changes in the lung as well as by reduced chest wall expansion due to increased intra-abdominal pressure.[40] A chest x-ray may show left-sided or bilateral pleural effusions, elevation of the diaphragm, and basal atelectasis. Respiratory changes occurring later in the patient with severe acute pancreatitis are usually associated with pulmonary or extra-pulmonary infections. Factors contributing to respiratory complications may include immobility and retained secretions and overzealous fluid resuscitation.

The mortality rate for patients with acute pancreatitis who develop acute respiratory distress syndrome (ARDS) and require mechanical ventilation is high. In a laboratory study performed on rats with experimentally induced pancreatitis, the initial manifestations of pancreatitis-associated lung injury included a pronounced clustering of polymorphonuclear leukocytes in pulmonary microvessels, followed by severe damage of alveolar endothelial cells.[41] The increase in vascular permeability of the lung resulted in interstitial edema formation. Structural changes reached their maximal extent after 12 hours, but were reversed completely after 84 hours. The structural appearance of pulmonary injury in the laboratory animals was similar to that reported in the early stages of ARDS.

Abdominal Compartment Syndrome

Intra-abdominal hypertension can occur in patients with severe acute pancreatitis, in whom its development is related to the inflammatory process, retroperitoneal edema, fluid collections, ascites, and intestinal ileus.[42] The elevated intra-abdominal pressure is serious in that it can result in significant impairment of cardiac, pulmonary, renal, gastrointestinal, hepatic, and central nervous system function.[43] The critical intra-abdominal pressure in most patients appears to be 10 to 15 mm Hg; it is at this pressure that reduction in microcirculatory blood flow occurs and initial signs of organ dysfunction are seen.[44] Acute compartment syndrome (ACS) will develop if the intra-abdominal pressure is not corrected. Abdominal compartment syndrome may be defined as a sustained intra-abdominal pressure greater than 20 mm Hg, accompanied by new organ dysfunction.[45–47]

In patients with severe acute pancreatitis, it has been recommended that intra-abdominal pressure be measured every 4 hours or whenever evidence of clinical deterioration is noted.[48] In an intensive care unit, the drainage tubing of the patient's indwelling urinary catheter is clamped and connected to a pressure transducer and an electronic monitoring system to determine intra-abdominal pressure. Because this technology is not available outside ICU settings, a group of investigators described a simple, rapid screening method for bedside intra-abdominal pressure measurement using only the patient's indwelling urinary catheter and an intravenous tubing extension set.[49, 50]

Among possible signs of organ failure associated with ACS are hypercarbia (excessive CO_2), hypoxemia, oliguria that does not respond to volume administration, metabolic acidosis, and elevated intracranial pressure.[51] Gastric suction to decompress the gastrointestinal tract is helpful to prevent intra-abdominal hypertension. In some patients, decompressive laparotomy may be helpful in relieving this condition.[52–54] If intravenous fluid overload has occurred, continuous hemodiafiltration may be able to remove the excess fluid.[55] Loop diuretics are not helpful if acute kidney injury is concurrently present (and often it is).[56]

TREATMENT

The treatment of acute pancreatitis is primarily supportive. Monitoring of vital signs, oxygen saturation, and urine output is required every 4 hours for the first 24 to 48 hours after admission.[57] Patients with mild disease can be cared for on a general medical–surgical unit. In contrast, individuals with poor prognostic signs (such as hypotension, hypoxia, or tachypnea) are best cared for in an intensive care setting, where close monitoring of fluid and electrolyte status can be performed. Insulin therapy is indicated to control hyperglycemia, if present.

Fluid Replacement

The intravascular volume deficit may be 30% or greater; therefore, volume restoration should be rapid and efficient. Fluid losses through fluid pooling in the abdomen and retroperitoneal area, as well as from nasogastric suction, vomiting, and diaphoresis must be assessed and replaced. A practice guideline issued by the American College of Gastroenterology reads as follows: "Aggressive IV fluid replacement is of critical importance to counteract hypovolemia caused by third space losses, vomiting, diaphoresis, and greater vascular permeability caused by inflammatory mediators."[58] However, there is no clear agreement on how much fluid is needed.[59] One group of authors recommends a replenishment rate of 500 to 1000 mL/hr to treat severe volume depletion.[60] Others recommend at least 250 to 300 mL/hr for 48 hours.[61] In fact, the sickest patients may receive more than 10 to 15 L of fluid over the first 24 hours after diagnosis.[62] As a rule, crystalloid solutions (such as lactated Ringer's solution) will suffice for fluid replacement purposes because the fluid lost into the retroperitoneum has the same composition as extracellular fluid. When the serum albumin level is dangerously low, colloids may be needed. Some authors recommend considering blood transfusions when the hemoglobin concentration is less than 10 g/dL.[63]

Because it is difficult to gauge the needed volume of fluid replacement, a urinary catheter should be placed to monitor hourly urine output; an hourly output of more than 0.5 mL/kg body weight per hour is advocated.[64] Clinicians should recognize that a low urine output may signal either under-resuscitation (and thus a need for more fluid) or acute tubular necrosis (and thus a need for fluid restriction and possibly renal replacement therapy). To determine the appropriate treatment, serum creatinine and BUN levels should be closely monitored during fluid resuscitation.

Also, it is advisable to monitor the central venous pressure and blood gases at regular intervals. In seriously ill patients, a Swan-Ganz catheter may be needed to monitor central filling pressures and an indwelling arterial line to monitor arterial oxygen tension. Another method to assess the adequacy of fluid replacement is to observe the patient's response to a fluid bolus of 250 to 500 mL of a balanced salt solution.[65] If fluid resuscitation is successful, noticeable improvements should occur in urine output, arterial blood pressure, and peripheral perfusion (as evidenced by stronger peripheral pulses and increased limb temperature).[66]

Always of concern when massive amounts of fluid are administered is the potential for fluid overload. A particular concern in the patient with acute pancreatitis is the risk for abdominal compartment syndrome (described earlier in this chapter).

Electrolyte Replacement

Calcium gluconate, administered intravenously, is indicated if there is evidence of hypocalcemia with tetany.[67] Also, calcium supplementation may be indicated to prevent cardiac dysrhythmias. Serum magnesium and phosphate should be monitored in patients with pancreatitis—and especially in alcoholic patients—and both electrolytes replaced as needed.

Respiratory Support

Oxygen should be administered so as to maintain a pulse oximetry reading of 95% oxygen saturation.[68] Arterial blood gases should be measured every 12 hours for the first 3 days of an episode of acute pancreatitis to assess oxygenation and acid–base balance.[69] Patients with significant hypoxemia (such as those with a PaO_2 less than 60 mm Hg) despite a high inspired oxygen intake and patients with evidence of respiratory distress should be considered candidates for intubation and mechanical ventilation.[70] Other measures to improve cardiopulmonary performance may include sedation and pain management.

Gastrointestinal Decompression

If the patient has abdominal distention or is actively vomiting, a nasogastric tube may be inserted and connected to low suctioning to decompress the gastrointestinal tract. Although not supported by clinical studies, gastric suction is sometimes employed in an attempt to decrease neurohormonal stimulation of pancreatic secretions by emptying of gastric contents into the duodenum. In patients with intestinal ileus, low intermittent gastric suction is necessary.

Renal Support

Unfortunately, patients with severe acute pancreatitis are subject to impaired renal function, as evidenced by rising serum creatinine and blood urea nitrogen levels as well as decreased urinary output. In a recent report, an increase in serum creatinine within the first 48 hours of severe acute pancreatitis was strongly associated with pancreatic necrosis.[71] This relationship makes sense, given that necrotizing pancreatitis is associated with multiple-organ failure.

In some patients, low-dose dopamine may be needed to maintain renal function, in addition to adequate fluid resuscitation.[72] If necessary, temporary hemofiltration or hemodialysis may be started. In some patients, renal failure is self-limited. In others, it is part of the multiple-organ failure associated with severe pancreatitis.

Pain Management

Depending on the severity of acute pancreatitis, the pain associated with this disease can be quite strong. In the past, meperidine was widely used as analgesic agent in patients with pancreatitis. It has since fallen out of favor owing to the recognition that repeated doses of meperidine can cause the accumulation of normeperidine, a substance that can promote neuromuscular irritability (such as tremors and seizures). More acceptable pain-relieving agents may include hydromorphone (Dilaudid), morphine, and fentanyl. Epidural analgesia may be indicated for patients in whom intravenous analgesics are ineffective. For example, in a study of patients with severe acute pancreatitis admitted to a critical care unit, epidural anesthesia alone produced excellent analgesia on 1083 of 1496 observation days.[73]

Nutrition

Patients with pancreatitis are usually hypercatabolic and may require nutrition that fulfills as much as 140% of the usual caloric needs. This demand for extra calories is problematic when bowel rest is needed to minimize nausea and vomiting. After symptoms are relieved, small feedings of a low-fat diet may be started in patients with mild pancreatitis. Clear liquids are usually given first and gradually advanced to a low-fat diet, as determined by the patient's tolerance and absence of pain.

Some patients cannot tolerate oral feedings because of persistent pain or nausea and vomiting; the problem then becomes one of deciding how to supply nutrients in adequate amounts. Enteral nutrition is currently the preferred method for nutritional support because it is associated with a lower rate of infectious complications.[74] Compared to parenteral nutrition, when started within 48 hours, enteral nutrition may be more effective in reducing the risk of multiple-organ failure, pancreatic infectious complications, and mortality in patients with acute pancreatitis.[75] It has been recommended that enteral nutrition be started for patients with acute pancreatitis following the initial period of fluid resuscitation and control of pain and nausea. Nutrition support via nasojejunal feedings is favored by some clinicians.[76]

CASE STUDIES

Case Study 20-1

A 50-year-old intoxicated man with a long history of alcoholism was admitted to the hospital for evaluation of epigastric pain that radiated through to the midback. The only way he could find relief was to sit up in bed with his knees drawn to his chest. The patient stated that he was nauseated and had been vomiting intermittently since the abdominal pain started 2 days earlier. His vital signs were as follows: blood pressure = 108/64 mm Hg, pulse rate = 120/min, respiratory rate = 26/min, and temperature = 38.5°C.

On examination, the patient's abdomen was diffusely tender to palpation. A chest x-ray revealed a large effusion at the right lung base. Laboratory results from a venous blood sample were as follows:

Sodium = 143 mEq/L (normal, 135–145 mEq/L)
Potassium = 3.3 mEq/L (normal, 3.5 –5.0 mEq/L)
Chloride = 92 mEq/L (normal, 97–110 mEq/L)
CO_2 content = 22 mEq/L (normal, 21–31 mEq/L)
Total calcium = 8.2 mg/dL (normal, 8.9–10.3 mg/dL)
Magnesium = 1.2 mg/dL (normal, 1.6–2.5 mg/dL)
BUN = 48 mg/dL (normal, 8–25 mg/dL)
Creatinine = 1.2 mg/dL (normal, 0.6–1.5 mg/dL)
Amylase = 900 IU/L (normal, 60–180 IU/L)
Glucose = 200 mg/dL (normal, 65–110 mg/dL)
White blood cell count = 13,400 μL
    (normal, 4500–10,000 μL)

Laboratory results from an arterial sample for blood gases were as follows:

pH = 7.28 (normal, 7.35–7.45)
$PaCO_2$ = 41 mm Hg (normal, 35–45 mm Hg)
PaO_2 = 56 mm Hg (normal, 80–100 mm Hg)
HCO_3 = 19 mEq/L (normal, 22–26 mEq/L)

Laboratory results from a urinalysis were 3+ ketones (normal negative).

On the basis of these findings, a diagnosis of acute pancreatitis was made. The patient was treated with NG suction, IV fluid replacement, and parenteral analgesia. Within the next few days, his abdominal pain, fever, and nausea subsided.

Commentary. The patient's hypotension and tachycardia indicated a low blood volume, as did his elevated BUN (reflective of decreased renal perfusion). A number of potential problems were present in this patient:

- Hypoxemia (PaO_2 = 56 mm Hg) could cause lactic acidosis, a form of high AG metabolic acidosis.
- Inadequate food intake (common in alcoholics during heavy drinking spells) and ethanol intoxication could cause alcoholic ketoacidosis, a form of high AG metabolic acidosis (note that the patient had 3+ ketones in the urine).
- Loss of gastric acid by vomiting and NG suction could cause metabolic alkalosis and a lower than normal serum potassium (note that the patient's potassium was slightly lower than normal).

The lower than normal pH indicated *acidosis*. The lower than normal bicarbonate level (22 mEq/L) indicated *metabolic acidosis*; calculation of the AG indicates that this was a *high AG metabolic acidosis* due to excessive lactic acid production for hypoxemia (see Chapter 9). The bicarbonate level would have been even lower if vomiting has not been present to cause a predisposition to metabolic alkalosis (and thus an increase in bicarbonate concentration). *Respiratory acidosis* was also present. This imbalance can be determined by calculating the expected $PaCO_2$ and comparing that value to the actual reading. Using Winter's formula:

$$\text{Expected } PaCO_2 = 1.5 \, (HCO_3) + 8 \mp 2$$
$$1.5 \, (19) + 8 \mp 2 = 34.5\text{--}38.5 \text{ mm Hg}$$

Thus the $PaCO_2$ is expected to range between 34.5 and 38.5 mm Hg. Instead, it was 41 mm Hg in this case, indicating a slight degree of carbon dioxide retention in addition to the expected compensatory change. Note that the patient had a pleural effusion that could have interfered with ventilation, as could abdominal distention and splinting of the diaphragm. Release of pancreatic enzymes into the systemic circulation as a result of pancreatitis is also hypothesized to cause damage to pulmonary tissues.

A serum calcium level of less than 8 mg/dL is one indicator of poor outcome after the onset of pancreatitis. Although this patient's serum calcium level was not less than 8 mg/dL, it was below normal. In this case, calcium supplementation may have been indicated to prevent cardiac dysrhythmias. Because the patient was acidotic, a greater proportion of calcium existed in the ionized form, making the adverse effects of hypocalcemia less prominent.

Like hypocalcemia, hypomagnesemia has—at least in part—been attributed to precipitation of magnesium ions in the inflamed tissues in and around the pancreas as insoluble magnesium soaps. Losses from vomiting, gastric suction, and diarrhea intensify hypomagnesemia. Because this patient had a history of alcoholism, his hypomagnesemia may also have been related to the multiple magnesium-lowering effects of alcohol.

Case Study 20-2

A case was reported in which a 39-year-old man was admitted to the hospital with complaints of abdominal distention and cramps in his hands.[77] Four days earlier, he had experienced severe central abdominal pain accompanied by vomiting. His history revealed a daily intake of a large quantity of alcohol. Physical examination revealed positive Chvostek's and Trousseau's signs, along with absent bowel sounds. His vital signs were as follows: temperature 37.5°C, heart rate 120 beats/min, and respiratory rate 22/min. The following laboratory data were obtained upon admission:

- Serum Na = 133 mEq/L (normal, 135–145 mEq/L)
- Serum K = 3.8 mEq/L (normal, 3.5–5.0 mEq/L)
- Serum bicarbonate in venous blood = 23 mEq/L (normal, 22–31 mEq/L)
- Serum Ca = 4.3 mg/dL (normal, 8.9–10.3 mg/dL)
- Serum phosphate = 3.5 mg/dL (normal, 2.5–4.5 mg/dL)

The serum calcium levels on subsequent days were as follows:

Day 2: 3.8 mg/dL	Day 7: 7.2 mg/dL
Day 3: 3.8 mg/dL	Day 8: 7.4 mg/dL
Day 4: 7.2 mg/dL	Day 9: 7.8 mg/dL
Day 5: 6.3 mg/dL	Day 10: 8.1 mg/dL
Day 6: 6.7 mg/dL	Day 11: 9.2 mg/dL

Despite a normal serum amylase level, a CT scan showed acute pancreatitis; further, paracentesis revealed fluid with the appearance of "prune juice." The patient was treated with intravenous fluids, oxygen administration, intravenous calcium, broad-spectrum antibiotics, and a single peritoneal lavage. A persistent ileus developed, and the patient received intravenous nutrients for the next 10 days. Bowel function eventually returned to normal, and the patient was discharged from the hospital 3 weeks later.

Commentary. As pointed out earlier in this chapter, alcoholic pancreatitis may be present without elevated serum amylase levels. This patient's caregivers wisely followed through with assessment for pancreatitis because the patient's clinical picture and history made him a good candidate for this condition. The hand spasms were evidence of tetany secondary to the extremely low serum calcium concentration. The "prune juice"–colored fluid was evidence of hemorrhagic pancreatitis. As noted in the summary of laboratory results, the patient's serum calcium concentration was initially quite low, and it remained low for several days despite regular replacement of intravenous calcium gluconate. Finally, on day 11, the serum calcium level reached the normal range. The authors of the case report attributed the low serum calcium level to concurrent hypoalbuminemia, which occurred secondary to the large protein-rich exudates released from the inflamed pancreas and peripancreatic areas). The authors also speculated that a large amount of ionized calcium was deposited and sequestered into the areas of fat necrosis by saponification in the peripancreatic region.

Case Study 20-3

A case was reported in which a 42-year-old man was admitted to the hospital with epigastric pain, nausea, and vomiting.[78] A history revealed that he was an alcoholic and had experienced several previous admissions for pancreatitis. An enlarged, edematous pancreas was found by an abdominal sonogram. Although diminished, bowel sounds were

present. Vital signs were as follows: temperature 37.5°C, pulse rate 120/min, and respiratory rate 25/min. The table below summarizes the serum amylase and calcium and magnesium levels.

The elevated serum amylase levels on admission and again on days 2 and 3 demonstrated the presence of pancreatitis. Note that hypocalcemia was evident on all days except day 8; the most severe hypocalcemia was noted on days 2 and 3. Concurrently present with hypocalcemia was hypomagnesemia on admission and again on days 2 and 3. The hypomagnesemia on day 2 was especially of concern, as the serum magnesium was less than half of the lower limit of normal.

Commentary. The primary mechanism for the hypomagnesemia and hypocalcemia was presumed to be saponification of magnesium and calcium, respectively, in the necrotic fat tissue in and around the pancreas. The most significant of the electrolyte imbalances was the serum magnesium concentration of 0.8 mg/dL on day 2. The fact that the patient was an alcoholic likely partly explains the low serum magnesium levels. Recall that use of alcohol predisposes individuals to hypomagnesemia both by increasing urinary magnesium loss and by inhibiting magnesium absorption in the small bowel.

Case Study 20-4

A 37-year-old African American woman with type 2 diabetes presented to the emergency department with a two-day history of severe epigastric pain and vomiting that became bile stained on the second day. She reported that her pain started after she consumed a heavy meal on the evening preceding the acute onset of pain and vomiting. Her skin turgor was poor, and her tongue was dry and furry in appearance. At the time of admission, her blood pressure was 100/76 mm Hg and she was tachycardic (heart rate = 120 beats/min). Body weight was 205 lb. A low-grade temperature elevation (38° C) was found, along with the following abnormal laboratory values (see next page):

Laboratory Test	Admission	Day 2	Day 3	Day 4	Day 8
Serum calcium (normal, 8.5–10.5 mg/dL)	8.4 mg/dL	7.8 mg/dL	7.5 mg/dL	8.0 mg/dL	8.5 mg/dL
Serum magnesium (normal, 1.8–3.0 mg/dL)	1.4 mg/dL	0.8 mg/dL	1.5 mg/dL	2.3 mg/dL	1.8 mg/dL
Serum amylase (normal, 60–180 IU/L)	2800 IU/L	1200 IU/L	800 IU/L	?	95 IU/L

- Serum amylase = 1790 IU/L (normal, less than 180 IU/L)
- Total serum calcium = 7.7 mg/dL (normal, 8.9–10.2 mg/dL)
- Serum glucose = 338 mg/dL (normal, 65–110 mg/dL)
- WBC = 20,800 μL (normal, 4500–10,000 μL)

An abdominal sonogram revealed multiple gallstones, a dilated common bile duct, and an enlarged pancreas. The patient was admitted to the intensive care unit and treated with intravenous normal saline to restore her plasma volume, regular insulin to treat the hyperglycemia, and vancomycin to resolve a potential infectious process. Pain control was achieved with hydromorphone.

Three days later, an abdominal CT showed an enlarged and markedly hypoperfused pancreas; in addition, there was evidence of an extensive fluid collection in the peripancreatic area. A diagnosis of necrotizing pancreatitis was made at this time.

Following delivery of supportive care, the patient's serum amylase level returned to normal and she was discharged to home. She underwent a successful cholecystectomy two months later and was referred to a nutritional counselor and diabetic educator for assistance in controlling her diabetes.

Commentary. The elevated serum amylase and lower than normal serum calcium levels observed in this case are classically present in patients with acute pancreatitis. The serum amylase level typically becomes elevated within a few hours of the attack, but then gradually returns to normal. The reason for development of hypocalcemia remains a topic of debate, but is likely due to systemic endotoxins or trapping of calcium ions in necrotic tissue in and around the pancreas. Obesity is an established predictor of gallbladder disease and gallstones, which in turn are associated with increased risk for pancreatitis. Mortality from acute pancreatitis is higher in obese individuals as compared to persons of normal weight.[79] Also, mortality from acute pancreatitis is higher in blacks than in whites.[80] Thus the patient described in this case report was extremely fortunate in her recovery, given that she had two conditions that predisposed her to greater mortality. Cholecystectomy was needed to prevent future bouts of pancreatitis from occurring. To reduce the overall burden of pancreatitis, society should focus on preventable causes of pancreatitis (especially obesity and alcohol consumption).

Summary of Key Points

- Approximately three-fourths of all cases of pancreatitis are caused by either gallstones or alcoholism.
- In acute pancreatitis, trypsin becomes prematurely activated, which leads to massive inflammation of the pancreas and systemic overproduction of pro-inflammatory products.
- Factors associated with hypovolemia in patients with pancreatitis include fluid and blood lost in the retroperitoneum and peritoneal cavity, fluid sequestered in the bowel during adynamic ileus, and vomitus or fluid loss from nasogastric suction.
- An elevated hematocrit in a patient with pancreatitis is due to shifting of plasma from the vascular space into the retroperitoneum and peritoneal cavity, which causes the red blood cells to be suspended in a smaller blood volume.
- Low hematocrit is a likely finding in the patient with hemorrhagic pancreatitis.
- Hypocalcemia in a patient with acute pancreatitis is a marker for poor outcome. Although the mechanisms responsible for the emergence of hypocalcemia in pancreatitis remain unclear, systemic endotoxin exposure appears to play a significant role in its development in this population. Another theory is that calcium becomes trapped in necrotic tissue in and around the pancreas.
- In patients with severe acute pancreatitis, aggressive intravenous fluid replacement is needed to counteract the hypovolemia caused by third-space losses, vomiting, and diaphoresis.
- As a rule, crystalloid solutions (such as lactated Ringer's solution) suffice for fluid replacement in pancreatitis because the fluid lost into the retroperitoneum has the composition of the extracellular fluid. When the serum albumin level is dangerously low, colloids may be needed.
- Calcium gluconate, administered intravenously, is indicated if patients show evidence of hypocalcemia with tetany. Magnesium replacement may be needed in alcoholic patients.
- The two most common systemic complications associated with severe acute pancreatitis are renal failure and respiratory failure.
- Abdominal compartment syndrome may occur in patients with severe acute pancreatitis. For this reason, it has been recommended that intra-abdominal pressure be measured every 4 hours in inpatients or whenever there is evidence of clinical deterioration.

NOTES

1. Mayerle, J., Simon, P., & Lerch, M. M. (2004). Medical treatment of acute pancreatitis. *Gastroenterology Clinics of North America, 33*, 855–869.

2. Kollef, M. H., Bedient, T. J., Isakow, W., & Witt, C. A. (Eds.). (2008). *The Washington manual of critical care.* Philadelphia: Wolters Kluwer/Lippincott Williams & Wilkins, p. 344.

3. Klingensmith, M. E., Chen, L. I., Glasgow, S. C., & Goers, T. A. (2008). *The Washington manual of surgery* (5th ed.). Philadelphia: Wolters Kluwer/Lippincott Williams & Wilkins, p. 238.

4. Bongard, F. S., Sue, D. Y., & Vintch, J. R. (2008). *Current diagnosis and treatment, critical care* (3rd ed.). New York: McGraw-Hill/Lange, p. 47.

5. Klingensmith et al., note 3, p. 238.

6. Mayerle, J., Hlouschek, V., & Lerch, M. M. (2005). Current management of acute pancreatitis. *Nature Clinical Practice Gastroenterology & Hepatology, 2*(10), 472–483.

7. Hasibeder, W. R., Torgersen, C., Rieger, M., & Dunser, M. (2009). Critical care of the patient with acute pancreatitis. *Anaesthesia and Intensive Care, 37*(2), 190–206.

8. Eckerwall, G., Olin, H., Andersson, B., & Andersson, R. (2006). Fluid resuscitation and nutritional support during severe acute pancreatitis in the past: What have we learned and how can we do better? *Clinical Nutrition, 25*, 497–504.

9. Ranson, J. H., Rifkind, K. M., Roses, D. F., Fink, S. D., Eng, K., & Localio, S. A. (1974). Objective early identification of severe acute pancreatitis. *American Journal of Gastroenterology, 61*(6), 443–451.

10. Kawa, S., Mukawa, K., & Kiyosawa, K. (2000). Hypocalcemia < 7.5 mg/dL: Early predictive marker for multisystem organ failure in severe acute necrotizing pancreatitis, proposed by the study analyzing post-ERCP pancreatitis. *American Journal of Gastroenterology, 95*, 1096–1097.

11. Ammori, B. J., Barclay, G. R., Larvin, M., & McMahon, M. J. (2003). Hypocalcemia in patients with acute pancreatitis: A putative role for systemic endotoxin exposure. *Pancreas, 26*(3), 213–217.

12. Ammori et al., note 11.

13. Wills, M. R. (1966). Hypocalcaemia and hypomagnesaemia in acute pancreatitis. *British Journal of Surgery, 53*(3), 174–176.

14. Kawa et al., note 10.

15. Papazachariou, I. M., Martinez-Isla, A., Efthimiou, E., Williamson, R. C., & Girgis, S. I. (2000). Magnesium deficiency in patients with chronic pancreatitis identified by an intravenous loading test. *Clinica Chimica Acta, 302*(1–2), 145–154.

16. Wills, note 13.

17. Rizos, E., Alexandrides, G., & Elisaf, M. S. (2000). Severe hypophosphatemia in a patient with acute pancreatitis. *Journal of the Pancreas, 1*(4), 204–207.

18. Ranson et al., note 9.

19. Mentula, P., Kylanpaa, M. L., Kemppainen, E., & Puolakkainen, P. (2008). Obesity correlates with early hyperglycemia in patients with acute pancreatitis who developed organ failure. *Pancreas, 36*(1), e21–e25.

20. Dauphine, C., Kovar, J., Stabile, B. E., Haukoos, J. S., & de Virgilio, C. (2004). Identification of admission values predictive of complicated acute alcoholic pancreatitis. *Archives of Surgery, 139*, 978–982.

21. Turina, M., Fry, D. E., & Polk, H. C. (2005). Acute hyperglycemia and the innate immune system: Clinical, cellular, and molecular aspects. *Critical Care Medicine, 339*(7), 1624–1633.

22. Klingensmith et al., note 3, p. 239.

23. Lankisch, P. G., Burchard-Reckert, S., & Lehnick, D. (1999). Underestimation of acute pancreatitis: Patients with only small increase in amylase/lipase levels can also have or develop severe acute pancreatitis. *Gut, 44*, 542–544.

24. Ranson, J. H. (1982). Etiological and prognostic factors in human acute pancreatitis: A review. *American Journal of Gastroenterology, 77*(9), 633–638.

25. Knaus, W. A., Draper, E. A., Wagner, D. P., & Zimmerman, J. E. (1985). APACHE II: A severity of disease classification system. *Critical Care Medicine, 13*(10), 818–829.

26. Xin, M. J., Chen, H., Luo, B., & Sun, J. B. (2008). Severe acute pancreatitis in the elderly: Etiology and clinical characteristics. *World Journal of Gastroenterology, 14*(16), 2517–2521.

27. Vincent, J. L., Moreno, R., Takala, J., Willatts, S., De Mendonca, A., Bruining, H., et al. (1996). The SOFA (Sepsis-related Organ Failure Assessment) score to describe organ dysfunction/failure: On behalf of the Working Group on Sepsis-Related Problems of the European Society of Intensive Care Medicine. *Intensive Care Medicine, 22*, 707–716.

28. Robert, J. H., Frossard, J. L., Mermillod, B., Soravia, C., Mensi, N., Roth, M., et al. (2002). Early prediction of acute pancreatitis: Prospective study comparing computed tomography scan, Ranson, Glasgow, Acute Physiology, and Chronic Health Evaluation II scores, and various serum markers. *World Journal of Surgery, 26*, 612–619.

29. Yadav, D., Agarwal, N., & Pitchumoni, C. S. (2002). A critical evaluation of laboratory tests in acute pancreatitis. *American Journal of Gastroenterology, 97*, 1309–1318.

30. Mayerle et al., note 6.

31. Balthazar, E. J., Robinson, D. L., Megibow, A. J., & Ranson, J. H. (1990). Acute pancreatitis: Value of CT in establishing prognosis. *Radiology, 174*(2), 331–336.

32. Mayerle et al., note 6.

33. Harrison, D. A., D'Amico, G., & Singer, M. (2007). The Pancreatitis Outcome Prediction (POP) Score: a new prognostic index for patients with severe acute pancreatitis. *Critical Care Medicine, 35*, 1703–1708.

34. Tran, D. D., Cuesta, M. A., Schneider, A. J., & Wesdorp, R. I. (1993). Prevalence and prediction of multiple organ system failure and mortality in acute pancreatitis. *Journal of Critical Care, 8*(3), 145–153.

35. Andersson, R., Andersson, B., Haraldsen, P., Drewsen, G., & Eckerwall, G. (2004). Incidence, management and recurrence rate of acute pancreatitis. *Scandinavian Journal of Gastroenterology, 39*, 891–894.

36. Andersson, R., Sward, A., Tingstedt, B., & Akerberg, D. (2009). Treatment of acute pancreatitis: Focus on medical care. *Drugs, 69*(5), 506–514.

37. Klingensmith et al., note 3, p. 241.

38. Hasibeder et al., note 7.

39. Berry, A. R., Taylor, T. V., & Davies, G. C. (1981). Pulmonary function and fibrinogen metabolism in acute pancreatitis. *British Journal of Surgery, 68*, 870–873.

40. Gunther, A., Walmrath, D., Grimminger, F., & Seeger, W. (2001). Pathophysiology of acute lung injury. *Seminars in Respiratory & Critical Care Medicine, 22*, 247–258.

41. Willemer, S., Feddersen, C. O., Karges, W., & Adler, G. (1991). Lung injury in acute experimental pancreatitis in rats. *International Journal of Pancreatology, 8*, 305–321.

42. De Waele, J. J., & Leppaniemi, A. K. (2009). Intra-abdominal hypertension in acute pancreatitis. *World Journal of Surgery, 33*, 1128–1133.

43. Cheatham, M. L. (2009). Abdominal compartment syndrome: Pathophysiology and definitions. *Scandinavian Journal of Trauma, Resuscitation and Emergency Medicine, 17*(1), 10.

44. Cheatham, note 43.

45. Cheatham, note 43.

46. Keskinen, P., Leppaniemi, A., Pettila, V., Piilonen, A., Kemppainen, E., & Hynninen, M. (2007). Intra-abdominal pressure in severe acute pancreatitis. *World Journal of Emergency Surgery, 2*, 2.

47. Chen, H., Li, F., Sun, J. B., & Jia, J. G. (2008). Abdominal compartment syndrome in patients with severe acute pancreatitis in early stage. *World Journal of Gastroenterology, 14*(22), 3541–3548.

48. De Waele, J. J., De Laet, I., & Malbrain, M. L. (2007). Rational intraabdominal pressure monitoring: How to do it? *Acta Clinica Belgica-Supplementum, 1*, 16–25.

49. Cheatham, note 43.

50. Cheatham, M. L., & Fowler, J. (2008). Measuring intra-abdominal pressure outside the ICU: Validation of a simple bedside method. *American Surgeon, 74*(9), 806–808.

51. Cheatham, note 43.

52. Chen et al., note 47.

53. Al-Bahrani, A. Z., Abid, G. H., Holt, A., McCloy, R. F., Benson, J., Eddleston, J., et al. (2008). Clinical relevance of intra-abdominal hypertension in patients with severe acute pancreatitis. *Pancreas, 36*, 39–43.

54. De Waele, J. J., Hoste, E. A., & Malbrain, M. L. (2006). Decompressive laparotomy for abdominal compartment syndrome: A critical analysis. *Critical Care, 10*(2), R51.

55. Oda, S., Hirasawa, H., Shiga, H., Matsuda, K., Nakamura, M., Watanabe, E., et al. (2005). Management of intra-abdominal hypertension in patients with severe acute pancreatitis with continuous hemodiafiltration using a polymethyl methacrylate membrane hemofilter. *Therapeutic Apheresis and Dialysis, 9*(4), 355–361.

56. De Waele & Leppaniemi, note 42.

57. Muddana, V., Whitcomb, D. C., & Papachristou, G. I. (2009). Current management and novel insights in acute pancreatitis. *Expert Review of Gastroenterology and Hepatology, 3*(4), 435–444.

58. Banks, P. A., Freeman, M. L., & Practice Parameters Committee of the American College of Gastroenterology. (2006). Practice guidelines in acute pancreatitis. *American Journal of Gastroenterology, 101*(10), 2379–2400.

59. Gardner, T. B., Vege, S. S., Pearson, R. K., & Chari, S. T. (2008). Fluid resuscitation in acute pancreatitis. *Clinical Gastroenterology and Hepatology, 6*, 1070–1076.

60. Pandol, S. J., Saluja, A. K., Imrie, C. W., & Banks, P. A. (2007). Acute pancreatitis: Bench to the bedside. *Gastroenterology, 132*, 1127–1151.

61. Tenner, S. (2004). Initial management of acute pancreatitis: Critical issues during the first 72 hours. *American Journal of Gastroenterology, 99*, 2489–2492.

62. Parillo, J. E., & Dillinger, P. D. (2008). *Critical care medicine* (3rd ed.). Philadelphia: Mosby Elsevier, p. 1631

63. Bongard et al., note 4, p. 348.

64. Mayerle et al., note 6.

65. Bongard et al., note 4, p. 348.

66. Bongard et al., note 4, p. 348.

67. McPhee, S. J., & Papadakis, M. S. (2008). *2008 current medical diagnosis and treatment*. New York: McGraw Hill, p. 607.

68. Ma, J. O., Cline, D. M., Tintinalli, J. E., Kelen, G. D., & Stapczynski, J. S. (2004). *Emergency medical manual* (6th ed.). New York: McGraw-Hill, p. 251.

69. Klingensmith et al., note 3, p. 241.

70. Bongard et al., note 4, p. 349.

71. Muddana, V., Whitcomb, D. C., Khalid, A., Slivka, A., & Papachristou, G. I. (2009). Elevated serum creatinine as a marker of pancreatic necrosis in acute pancreatitis. *American Journal of Gastroenterology, 104*(1), 164–170.

72. Bongard et al., note 4, p. 349.

73. Bernhardt, A., Kortgen, B. A., Niesel, H. C., & Goertz, A. (2002). Using epidural anesthesia in patients with acute pancreatitis: Prospective study of 121 patients. *Anaesthesiologie und Reanimation, 27*(1), 16–22.

74. Parillo & Dillinger, note 62, p. 1632.

75. Petrov, M. S., Pylypchuk, R. D., & Uchugina, A. F. (2009). A systematic review on the timing of artificial nutrition in acute pancreatitis. *British Journal of Nutrition, 101*(6), 787–793.

76. Petrov, M. S., & Whelan, K. (2010). Comparison of complications attributable to enteral and parenteral nutrition in predicted severe acute pancreatitis: A systematic review and meta-analysis. *British Journal of Nutrition, 103*(9), 287–295.

77. Jones, P. A. (1985). Survival after profound hypocalcemia with tetany complicating severe haemorrhagtic acute pancreatitis. *Postgraduate Medical Journal, 61*(711), 43–45.

78. Liamis, G., Gianoutsos, C., & Elisaf, M. (2001). Acute pancreatitis-induced hypomagnesemia. *Pancreatology, 1*, 74–76.

79. De Waele et al., note 54.

80. Lowenfels, A. B., Maisonneuve, P., & Sullivan, T. (2009). The changing character of acute pancreatitis: Epidemiology, etiology, and prognosis. *Current Gastroenterology Reports, 11*(2), 97–103.

Chapter 21

Cirrhosis with Ascites

Cirrhosis is a consequence of most untreated chronic liver diseases and is characterized by the formation of fibrotic changes that replace normal liver cells. Among the conditions that can lead to cirrhosis are acute or chronic hepatitis, use of hepatotoxic drugs (such as acetaminophen), and alcoholic liver disease (which is the most common cause of cirrhosis in the United States). Acetaminophen toxicity accounts for as many as 50% of the cases of acute hepatic failure in the United States (approximately one-third of which are due to unintentional overdose).[1] Increased public education about safe dosing of acetaminophen is needed to reduce this risk for liver injury. Fortunately, acetaminophen toxicity has an antidote (N-acetylcysteine), which provides protection against hepatotoxicity if given within 12 hours of a nonstaggered ingestion.[2]

Symptoms vary according to the stage of cirrhosis; specifically, they are absent in the early phase and appear gradually or abruptly in a later phase. Among the early symptoms of cirrhosis are weakness, easy fatigability, and disturbed sleep. As the disease advances, anorexia is often present. It may be accompanied by nausea and vomiting, resulting in malnutrition. Although muscle wasting is common, it may be masked by fluid retention. Pain may result from enlargement of the liver. Hematemesis is the presenting symptom in 15% to 25% of patients.[3] Late findings include ascites and peripheral edema and perhaps a series of other complications described later in the chapter.

PATHOPHYSIOLOGY

Cirrhosis is the end result of hepatic injury that leads to fibrotic changes and nodular regeneration within the liver. As blood, lymph, and biliary channels become compressed, intrahepatic pressure increases, reducing the liver's capacity to fulfill its functions. At first the liver is enlarged with fatty tissue; later, it becomes small, hard, and nodular. Among the complications of cirrhosis are ascites, portal hypertension–related bleeding, hepatic encephalopathy, and spontaneous bacterial peritonitis. Cirrhosis has been reported to be the twelfth leading cause of death in the United States.[4]

Ascites Formation

More than half of all patients with cirrhosis will develop ascites.[5] Impeded venous outflow through the fibrotic liver results in an accumulation of serum-like fluid (ascites) within the peritoneal cavity. The two major factors involved in the pathogenesis of ascites are portal hypertension and renal retention of sodium and water.[6] Normally, less than 25 mL of fluid is located in the peritoneal cavity; in contrast, a patient with decompensated cirrhosis can accumulate more than 15 L of ascitic fluid, and accumulations of as much as 28 L have been reported.[7] Obviously, much discomfort—such as dyspnea, insomnia, and difficulty walking—is associated with the presence of a large quantity of fluid in the abdominal cavity. Ascites is a serious condition, associated with a 2-year mortality rate of 50%.[8]

When doubt arises regarding the origin of ascitic fluid, a laboratory test is performed on a sample of the fluid. If the ascites is due to portal hypertension, the serum-ascites albumin gradient will be greater than 1.1 g/dL (as opposed to a gradient less than 1.1 g/dL if the ascites originates from another source, such as inflammation or peritoneal malignancy).[9]

The ascitic patient with advanced liver disease has a distended abdomen; physical examination reveals a fluid wave, shifting dullness, and dullness to percussion. Measurement of abdominal girth with a millimeter tape is sometimes used to estimate the extent of ascites. Abdominal ultrasound can be used to detect small pools of ascitic fluid.

Decreased Effective Arterial Volume

"Decreased effective arterial volume" refers to a state in which the total extracellular fluid (ECF) volume is normal or even expanded, although the kidneys respond as if they were underperfused, resulting in renal retention of sodium. Presumably, this is what occurs in the patient with cirrhosis and ascites formation.

Hypoalbuminemia

Severe hypoalbuminemia may also contribute to ascites formation. Causes of low serum albumin levels in cirrhotic patients include decreased synthesis of protein by the diseased liver, dilution of serum protein (due to salt and water retention), and a shift of protein from the vascular space to the peritoneal cavity. However, hypoalbuminemia does not appear to be nearly as important in ascites formation as the increased pressure generated by the hepatic postsinusoidal obstruction. Relief from ascites occurs when portal hypertension is corrected by shunting procedures.

Edema

Edema formation in cirrhotic patients has several causes. For example, increased pressure in the vena cava—secondary to ascitic fluid and enlarged liver size—interferes with venous drainage of the lower extremities. Contributing to edema formation is the hypoalbuminemia that is frequently present in patients with advanced live disease. By lowering the plasma oncotic pressure, hypoalbuminemia promotes shifting of fluid from the intravascular space to the interstitial space. At first, edema appears in dependent areas; later, it spreads to nondependent areas, varying in severity with the degree of sodium intake. The edema associated with liver disease is of the "pitting" variety.

FLUID AND ELECTROLYTE DISTURBANCES

Common disorders of fluid, electrolyte, and acid–base metabolism observed in patients with hepatic cirrhosis include fluid volume excess with edema and ascites, hyponatremia, hypokalemia, respiratory alkalosis, and metabolic acidosis (**Table 21-1**).

Fluid Volume Excess

The patient with advanced cirrhotic disease has a complex fluid balance problem. Although such an individual has an excess of total body fluid with an accumulation in the peritoneal cavity (ascites) and in the interstitial space (edema), there is also a problem of decreased effective arterial blood volume. In response to this condition, the kidneys strive to build up the intravascular volume by retaining sodium and water (although the blood volume may actually be normal or even higher than normal). Plasma aldosterone levels are often higher than normal due to increased adrenal secretion and inability of the liver to deactivate this hormone. Nonsteroidal anti-inflammatory drugs (NSAIDs) should be avoided in such cases because they may cause deterioration in renal function, leading to further fluid retention.

Hyponatremia

Hyponatremia is common in patients with advanced hepatic cirrhosis and ascites. In these individuals, this imbalance is usually caused by intrarenal disturbances in water handling and excessive release of antidiuretic hormone (ADH).[10] This hyponatremia is superimposed on fluid volume excess. That is, although there is abnormal retention of both sodium and water, a relatively greater degree of water retention occurs. As such, the serum sodium level is diluted below normal even though the total body sodium is excessive. Other factors that can contribute to hyponatremia are sodium loss through frequent paracentesis or excessive diuretic use or too stringent sodium restriction. When the serum sodium concentration is less than 125 mEq/L, restriction of fluid intake to 800–1000 mL/day may be needed. Hyponatremia is associated with increased mortality in patients with liver failure; it is not known whether this condition actually increases mortality or whether it is merely a marker of poor hepatic function.

Hypokalemia

Hypokalemia is common in patients with chronic liver disease for a variety of reasons, such as increased renal losses of

Table 21-1 Possible Water and Electrolyte Disturbances in Patients with Advanced Cirrhosis and Ascites

Disturbance	Etiology
Increased total ECF volume but decreased effective arterial volume	• Enhanced renal tubular reabsorption of sodium. • Increased plasma aldosterone level due to increased adrenal secretion (in response to decreased effective arterial volume) and decreased degradation of this hormone by the diseased liver.
Increased water retention, causing dilutional hyponatremia	• Impaired renal water excretion related to excess ADH secretion (in response to decreased effective arterial volume).
Hypokalemia (This imbalance is especially harmful to patients with hepatic failure because it increases ammonia formation and can induce hepatic coma.)	• Excessive use of potassium-losing diuretics. • Decreased intake due to anorexia. • Direct loss in diarrhea or vomiting.
Hyperkalemia	• Excessive use of potassium-sparing diuretics, especially when renal insufficiency is present or potassium-containing salt substitutes are used to make the low-sodium diet more palatable.
Elevated serum ammonia level	• Under normal circumstances, the large amounts of ammonia formed in the intestines by bacterial action are absorbed into the bloodstream and carried to the liver to be converted to urea for renal excretion. In cirrhosis, the liver cannot convert the ammonia to urea; thus the blood ammonia level increases.
Hypomagnesemia	• Renal wasting of magnesium in patients with cirrhosis due to alcoholism. • Poor dietary intake. • Loss of magnesium in diarrhea.
Hypocalcemia	• Possibly a result of inadequate storage of vitamin D by diseased liver; also associated with hypoalbuminemia.
Respiratory alkalosis	• May be associated with high serum ammonia levels (which act as a respiratory stimulant).
Respiratory acidosis	• May occur if ascites is so severe that it interferes with movement of the diaphragm.
Metabolic alkalosis	• May occur in patients treated with potassium-losing diuretics; it is important to prevent metabolic alkalosis because of its association with hypokalemia.
Metabolic acidosis	• May occur in patients treated with spironolactone (Aldactone). • Associated with renal failure.

ADH = antidiuretic hormone; ECF = extracellular fluid.

potassium caused by diuretics and hyperaldosteronism, low dietary intake of potassium, and increased potassium losses from diarrhea or vomiting. In one study, almost two-thirds of the patients with cirrhosis developed a serum potassium level less than 3.1 mEq/L.[11]

In addition to increased risk for cardiac dysrhythmias, hypokalemia can contribute to the development of hepatic encephalopathy by increasing the serum ammonia level. Recall that ammonia is one of the toxins that can cause hepatic encephalopathy. Hypokalemia increases the formation of ammonia in the proximal tubules of the kidney (approximately half of which is returned to the systemic circulation by way of the renal veins).[12] The increased serum ammonia level may be sufficient to precipitate hepatic encephalopathy, or at least increase its severity if it already present. Additional adverse effects of hypokalemia include ileus, muscle weakness, and decreased renal concentrating ability.

Hyperkalemia

Hyperkalemia occasionally occurs in patients with chronic liver disease. Most often, it is associated with the use of potassium-sparing diuretics (such as spironolactone, amiloride, and triamterene). In a study of 150 patients who received spironolactone and were hospitalized for decompensated liver disease, investigators found that the best predictors of hyperkalemia were poor renal function (demonstrated by high serum creatinine and urea levels) and high doses of spironolactone.[13]

Acute hyperkalemia is also a frequent, potentially life-threatening complication in liver transplantation. Among the reasons for this association are the transplant recipients' high baseline preoperative potassium levels due to the use of potentially potassium-elevating medications (such as angiotensin-converting enzyme inhibitors, spironolactone, and heparin), the intraoperative administration of packed red blood cells, and release of potassium into the bloodstream from necrotic liver cells.[14]

Zinc Deficiency

Zinc, an essential trace element, is important in the regulation of protein and nitrogen metabolism. Thus zinc deficiency could conceivably disrupt protein metabolism and predispose individuals to increased risk for hepatic encephalopathy. Nevertheless, there is no clear evidence that zinc supplementation has beneficial effects in patients with hepatic encephalopathy.[15]

Acid–Base Imbalances

All four acid–base imbalances may be encountered in patients with liver disease, although the most frequently observed condition is respiratory alkalosis. As a rule, the degree of respiratory alkalosis increases as the severity of the hepatic disease increases. Although elevated blood ammonia levels may stimulate hyperventilation and respiratory alkalosis, it is unlikely that increased blood ammonia concentration is the sole factor driving the emergence of this imbalance. Another possible cause of hyperventilation is an elevated progesterone level; this hormone, which is normally degraded by the liver, is a respiratory stimulant.

Metabolic alkalosis occurs in many patients with hepatic disease and is usually associated with use of potassium-losing diuretics. It can also be caused by vomiting or nasogastric suction or by alkali loading from sources such as antacids or citrate from blood transfusions.

High anion gap metabolic acidosis can also occur in patients with chronic liver disease, especially as the severity of the disease increases. These patients may be more susceptible to lactic acidosis because their diseased livers are unable to remove lactic acid from the circulation. Also, they are more susceptible to increased lactic acid production, such as may occur with hypotension secondary to gastrointestinal hemorrhage.

Respiratory acidosis is possible when upward pressure on the diaphragm (from the distended abdomen) interferes with ventilation. Lung capacity may also be reduced due to hydrothorax when ascitic fluid leaks through the diaphragm into the pleural cavity.

GENERAL TREATMENT

Treatment of patients with advanced cirrhosis is, in part, directed at controlling the excess fluid in the peritoneal cavity (ascites) and the interstitial space (edema). Among the therapies for these problems are sodium restriction, diuretics, bedrest, water restriction (when hyponatremia is a problem), paracentesis, and various types of shunting procedures. Other interventions for patients with advanced hepatic disease are directed at preventing hepatic coma. These measures include dietary protein restriction and administration of lactulose and bowel-sterilizing antibiotics.

Sodium and Water Restriction

Patients with ascites are first treated with sodium-restricted diets (such as those allowing less than 2000 mg of sodium per day).[16] A more liberal sodium intake may be allowed after diuresis occurs. In some patients, sodium restriction is sufficient to induce diuresis, especially when combined with bedrest. Water restriction is not indicated for all patients. However, fluid restriction to 800–1000 mL/day may be required when dilutional hyponatremia (e.g., less than 125 mEq/L) occurs.[17] For more severe hyponatremia, fluid restriction to the amount necessary to replace only insensible loss plus urine output may be needed. If fluid restriction is indicated in tube-fed patients, a formula that is calorically dense can be selected (such as one that provides 1.5–2.0 cal/mL instead of one that provides 1.0 cal/mL).[18]

Diuretics

Spironolactone (an aldosterone-blocking agent) is usually the first diuretic prescribed when conservative measures (e.g., sodium restriction and bedrest) fail to induce an adequate diuresis. Patients with moderate to severe ascites may be prescribed a loop diuretic (such as furosemide) in conjunction with spironolactone. These diuretics act in different parts of the kidney, and combination therapy with both agents promotes greater diuresis than if either is used alone. Another benefit of their joint administration is the greater probability of a normal serum potassium concentration: Recall that spironolactone is a potassium-conserving diuretic, whereas furosemide is a potassium-losing diuretic. While both potassium imbalances (hyperkalemia and hypokalemia) are dangerous, an especially serious effect of hypokalemia is the increased probability of developing hepatic encephalopathy.

Only a limited amount of ascitic fluid (such as 750 mL) can be mobilized through the peritoneal capillaries each day; thus diuretic doses should be carefully calibrated to achieve a controlled weight loss. Over-vigorous use of diuretics may result in severe contraction of the intravascular fluid volume, producing azotemia and worsening of hepatic encephalopathy. Until ascites is controlled, the goal of diuretic therapy is a daily weight loss of not more than 1.0 kg in an edematous patient and approximately 0.5 kg is a patient without edema.[19] Of course, in edematous patients, diuretics promote fluid loss from the tissue space as well as from the pool of ascites.

Paracentesis

Eventually, patients with ascites may become unresponsive to diuretics and require paracentesis to relieve respiratory distress and symptoms of marked intra-abdominal pressure. Current guidelines support the performance of large volume paracenteses. As much as 4–5 L of fluid can be removed safely; in contrast, patients who undergo the removal of larger volumes of ascitic fluid may develop rapid contraction of the vascular fluid.[20]

There is controversy as to whether albumin administration is needed with large-volume paracentesis to prevent post-paracentesis circulatory dysfunction.[21] Post-paracentesis circulatory dysfunction is characterized by azotemia, increased plasma renin activity, and hyponatremia.[22] Fortunately, it is likely that the circulatory dysfunction can be prevented by the administration of plasma volume expanders, such as albumin. For example, in a clinical study reported in 1988, investigators randomly assigned 105 patients with severe ascites to large-volume paracentesis with and without concurrent albumin administration.[23] The 52 patients in the albumin infusion group had better

outcomes than the 53 patients who did not receive albumin during their paracentesis procedures. More specifically, there were no significant changes in standard renal function tests, plasma renin activity, and plasma aldosterone in the albumin-treated group. In contrast, the group who did not receive albumin had a significant increase in blood urea nitrogen, a marked elevation in plasma renin activity and plasma aldosterone concentration, and a significant reduction in serum sodium concentration.

In a more recent study, investigators found that albumin was more effective than isotonic saline in preventing paracentesis-induced circulatory dysfunction following the removal of more than 6 L of ascitic fluid.[24] Some clinicians favor administering intravenous albumin at a dosage of 10 g per liter of ascitic fluid removed to protect the vascular volume from effects of the rapid removal of fluid.[25] Until more studies are available, it is apparently reasonable (although not mandatory) to give albumin for paracenteses in which greater than 5 liters of ascitic fluid is removed.[26]

Dietary Protein Restriction

Impending hepatic coma is an indication that it is necessary to temporarily restrict dietary protein so as to decrease ammonia formation. In such a case, adequate non-protein calories (25–30 cal/kg) need to be supplied by the enteral or parenteral route. As the patient improves, more protein can be added in small increments every few days as tolerated. Protein supplements rich in branched-chain amino acids can be used with protein-restricted diets to help establish positive nitrogen balance without precipitating encephalopathy.[27] Specialized enteral and parenteral formulas are commercially available for malnourished patients with hepatic failure and probably are justified in only patients who have encephalopathy.[28]

Bowel-Sterilizing Antibiotics

An antibiotic (such as neomycin, rifaximin, or vancomycin) may be used to reduce the ammonia-producing flora in the intestinal tract. Neomycin can be given by mouth or as a retention enema.[29]

Transjugular Intrahepatic Portosystemic Shunt

Transjugular intrahepatic portosystemic shunt (TIPS) is a radiographic procedure that introduces an expandable stent between a branch of the hepatic vein and the portal vein.

The device is inserted via the internal jugular vein and provides portal decompression without altering the extrahepatic vascular anatomy—an important factor if the patient is to undergo a liver transplant. Complications associated with TIPS include increased risk for hepatic encephalopathy, infection, and shunt stenosis.

V$_2$-Receptor Antagonists

V$_2$-receptor antagonists are pharmacological agents that directly antagonize the effects of elevated plasma ADH levels, thereby inducing water diuresis. As such, they seem to be promising options for the treatment of patients with cirrhosis, ascites, and dilutional hyponatremia.[30] For example, in a double-blind study of 60 patients with cirrhosis and dilutional hyponatremia, half were assigned to a V$_2$-receptor antagonist (either 100 mg or 200 mg per day) and the remaining half was assigned to a placebo.[31] Fluid was restricted to 1000 mL/day until the serum sodium concentration normalized or for 7 days. The serum sodium concentration normalized in 27% of the patients who received 100 mg of the drug and in 50% of those who received 200 mg; none of the patients in the control group achieved normal sodium concentrations. The investigators concluded that an oral dose of a vasopressin-receptor antagonist can correct hyponatremia in patients with cirrhosis and ascites.

MANAGEMENT OF SPECIFIC COMPLICATIONS

Multiple complications are possible in the patient with end-stage liver disease and cirrhosis. This result is understandable when one considers the extent of tissue destruction and impeded circulation through the fibrotic liver.

Variceal Hemorrhage

Development of esophageal and gastric wall varices is a serious complication of hepatic failure and portal hypertension. Each episode of variceal hemorrhage is associated with a mortality rate of 20% to 40%.[32] Severity of bleeding from varices is intensified by coagulopathies associated with liver failure. When hemorrhage occurs from esophageal varices, protection of the airway takes precedence, followed by volume resuscitation in the form of packed red blood cells.

Attempts to treat coagulopathies may include the administration of fresh frozen plasma and platelets.[33] Upper endoscopy to perform band ligation or to sclerose the bleeding vessels is warranted. If endoscopy must be delayed for some reason, a balloon tamponade device (such as a Sengstaken-Blakemore tube) may be used to compress the bleeding vessels temporarily until endoscopy can be performed. A Sengstaken-Blakemore tube has both an esophageal and gastric balloon that can be inflated to compress bleeding varices. The lowest pressure needed to control bleeding is used to minimize local mucosal injury. The tube should be used for as short a time as possible (preferably less than 12 hours). Other possible complications associated with use of this tube include aspiration and esophageal rupture.

TIPS is an option for esophageal varices when endoscopy is not an option. This technique offers a rapid decompressive shunt that does not require surgery. Vasoconstrictors (such as terlipressin) suppress variceal bleeding by inhibiting splanchnic blood flow and thus reducing portal and variceal pressure.[34]

Hepatorenal Syndrome

Hepatorenal syndrome (HRS) is a type of renal failure that occurs in as many as 10% of patients with advanced cirrhosis and ascites.[35] It can be classified as a rapidly progressive type (type 1 HRS) or a slower-developing form (type 2 HRS). Dominant features of HRS include marked renal failure with oliguria, high serum creatinine and urea concentrations, a decreased glomerular filtration rate, and a low urinary sodium output. Although the cause of HRS is unknown, its pathogenesis involves intense renal vasoconstriction and reduced renal blood flow, perhaps because of impaired synthesis of renal vasodilators, such as prostaglandin E$_2$. This, in turn, causes reduced excretion of sodium by the kidney.

Typically, the kidneys are histologically normal and regain their function in the event of recovery of hepatic function. That is, when liver transplants are performed on patients with HRS, renal function may return to normal. Even though it is not associated with major histologic change in the kidneys, HRS is an ominous occurrence because this condition is usually progressive and fatal unless a liver transplant is performed. The decline in renal function often follows overzealous diuresis, large-volume paracentesis, or sepsis. Before a diagnosis of HRS is made, it is important to consider the possibility of other causes of renal deterioration, such as severe fluid volume depletion. To exclude the possibility of prerenal azotemia, it may be necessary to administer a fluid challenge (such as 1000 mL 0.9% NaCl).

Terlipressin (a vasopressin analogue) has been used to treat HRS. In a meta-analysis of five studies that involved

243 patients with HRS, researchers found that those who received terlipressin (versus those who received a placebo) had a significantly increased rate of HRS reversal.[36]

Because death from HRS is usually by caused liver failure (not renal failure), dialysis is generally not helpful. Conversely, if the liver disease is potentially reversible or the patient is a candidate for a liver transplant, dialysis may be considered. Following a liver transplant, patients experience a dramatic improvement in renal function and long-term survival is very good.[37]

Hepatic Encephalopathy

Hepatic encephalopathy is a condition associated with mental status changes and altered neuromuscular activity; in persons with cirrhosis, encephalopathy is partially due to the presence of excessive amounts of ammonia in the bloodstream. Recall that in the human body, ammonia is manufactured primarily from the metabolism of dietary protein products in the intestine. Normally, the ammonia that enters the portal system from the gut is converted to urea by the liver and excreted by the kidneys. Unfortunately, the diseased liver is incapable of converting ammonia to urea; thus it builds up in the bloodstream. Symptoms of hepatic encephalopathy may range from mild (such as sleep–wake disturbances and ataxia) to severe (such as coma and seizures).

Precipitating causes of episodes of hepatic encephalopathy include consumption of a high-protein diet, digestion of blood in the gastrointestinal tract, constipation, infection, fluid volume depletion from overzealous use of diuretics, progressive liver dysfunction, and hypokalemia with alkalosis. (Recall that hypokalemia increases ammonia production, while alkalosis promotes movement of ammonia and other toxins into the brain.)

Although ammonia is the most readily identified and measurable toxin associated with hepatic encephalopathy, others likely play a role in the development of this complication, such as increased brain glutamine levels and production of false neurotransmitters.[38] The exact biochemical trigger of encephalopathy is unknown; however, interference with cerebral metabolism and neurotransmission appears to be the basic underlying mechanism.

At present, the role of manganese in hepatic encephalopathy is poorly understood. Normally, manganese is cleared by the liver and excreted in bile; however, this process does not occur in patients with cirrhosis. Thus increased levels of manganese in the bloodstream could result in deposition of manganese in brain tissue. A study of brain tissue from alcoholic patients who died of hepatic encephalopathy showed manganese levels in the globus pallidus that were as much as 7 times higher than manganese levels in subjects without cirrhosis.[39]

Lactulose is a poorly absorbed substance that is used to promote more frequent stools and prevent or treat hepatic encephalopathy. The dose is typically titrated to a level that will produce 3 to 5 bowel movements per day. Almost all of the lactulose taken orally reaches the colon unabsorbed, where it is digested by bacteria and converted to short-chain fatty acids, resulting in acidification of the colon contents. Because the pH of the bowel vasculature is relatively higher than the contents of the colon under treatment with lactulose, ammonia (NH_3) is converted into ammonium (NH_4), preventing the absorption of ammonia. Lactulose can be administered rectally when it is not tolerated orally or when pulmonary aspiration is a great risk. The lactulose solution can be given through a rectal balloon catheter and retained for 30 to 60 minutes. If the solution is not retained, the treatment can be repeated immediately. This process is generally repeated every 4 to 6 hours until symptoms of encephalopathy begin to reverse and oral administration can be started.

Dietary protein should be restricted during acute episodes of hepatic encephalopathy. All narcotics, tranquilizers, and sedatives that are metabolized or excreted by the liver should be withheld from patients with hepatic encephalopathy.

Spontaneous Bacterial Peritonitis

Spontaneous bacterial peritonitis (SBP) is associated with an overall high mortality rate and is heralded by fever, abdominal pain, increasing ascites, and progressive encephalopathy.[40] SPB can also precipitate hepatorenal syndrome. The diagnosis is made by examining and culturing the ascitic fluid. The three most common bacteria present in SBP are *Escherichia coli*, *Klebsiella pneumoniae,* and *Streptococcus pneumoniae*.[41] To treat this form of peritonitis, antibiotics are administered and response to therapy is determined by examining the percentage of polymorphonuclear cells in ascitic fluid.

Hepatic Hydrothorax

Defects in the diaphragm may allow ascitic fluid to pass into the pleural space, resulting in hydrothorax. This condition can occur in as many as 13% of patients with ascites, typically presenting on the right side.[42] Placement of a TIPS may help to relieve this problem.

Infection

The patient with chronic hepatic failure has an increased risk for infection because the liver is no longer able to filter bacteria effectively from the blood. In addition, associated hypersplenism causes a decreased white blood cell count. Infection—particularly full-blown sepsis—places the patient at increased risk for fluid and electrolyte disturbances.

Anemia

Anemia may occur in hepatic failure because the hypersplenism caused by portal hypertension increases the rate of red blood cell destruction. Also, the malnutrition that commonly accompanies hepatic failure decreases the rate of red blood cell formation. Increased bleeding tendencies due to vitamin K deficiency and decreased prothrombin formation leave the patient at higher risk for excessive bleeding from menses, nosebleeds, gingivitis, GI mucosal changes, and even bruising. Recall that as bleeding in the GI tract increases, buildup of ammonia secondary to digestion of blood (a protein-containing substance) increases.

CASE STUDIES

Case Study 21-1

A 50-year-old woman with a long history of alcoholism and cirrhosis with ascites was admitted with complaints of difficulty breathing and a weight gain of 13 lb over the past 2 weeks. On questioning, she stated that she had skipped her diuretic medication (spironolactone) and had failed to adhere to her sodium-restricted dietary regimen over this same period. Physical examination revealed that her abdomen was largely distended with ascites. Her lower extremities were edematous, and she had jugular venous distention. Vital signs were as follows: temperature, 98.6°F; pulse rate, 100/min; respiratory rate, 20/min; blood pressure, 170/98 mm Hg. Laboratory results indicated that all serum electrolytes were within normal limits (serum sodium = 137 mEq/L).

Commentary. This patient's signs of excessive sodium and water retention included acute weight gain, lower extremity edema, ascites, hypertension, and jugular venous distention. Increasing ascitic fluid accumulation placed pressure on her diaphragm and made it difficult for her to breathe normally. Because she gained 13 lb over this relatively short period, it can be concluded that she retained approximately

6 L of fluid. (One liter of fluid weighs 2.2 lb.) The increased ascitic fluid accumulation that occurred over the 2-week period did not produce a deficit in the vascular space because it developed relatively slowly, allowing time for sodium and water to be retained by the kidneys so as to replace fluid shifted from the vascular space to the ascitic pool.

Treatment included diuretics and a sodium-restricted diet. Recall that the peritoneum limits the transfer of ascitic fluid into the vascular space to approximately 750 mL/day. Because this patient also had peripheral edema, she could be expected to diurese edema fluid in addition to the ascitic fluid (perhaps allowing her to excrete as much as 1 L of fluid per day initially without compromising her intravascular volume). Patients with ascites often are treated with spironolactone (a potassium-sparing diuretic) because it is an aldosterone antagonist that reduces sodium reabsorption by the kidney. This agent does not cause potassium depletion, which is an important consideration in cirrhotic patients because hypokalemia increases ammonia production and predisposes individuals to hepatic encephalopathy.

Case Study 21-2

A confused middle-aged man with cirrhosis of the liver was admitted for evaluation. His venous blood work yielded the following findings: mild hyponatremia (Na = 133 mEq/L), mild hypokalemia (K = 3.3 mEq/L), and mild hyperchloremia (Cl = 115 mEq/L). Arterial blood gas results included pH 7.44, $PaCO_2$ 20 mm Hg, and HCO_3 13 mEq/L (indicating chronic compensated respiratory alkalosis).

Commentary. Note that this patient's serum sodium and potassium levels were slightly below normal. Probably the slight hyponatremia was related to impaired renal water excretion and excessive release of ADH. The mild hypokalemia was likely due to use of potassium-losing diuretics. The most striking of these laboratory results was the low $PaCO_2$ level, which indicates primary respiratory alkalosis; the HCO_3 was also low due to a compensatory change. (In chronic respiratory alkalosis, the HCO_3 level is expected to decrease by about 5 mEq/L for every 10 mm Hg drop in the $PaCO_2$ level.) Because the $PaCO_2$ had dropped by 20 mm Hg (from a normal level of 40 mm Hg), the HCO_3 is expected to decrease by 10 mEq/L (from 24 to 14 mEq/L). Therefore, this patient had chronic compensated respiratory alkalosis. It has been postulated that elevated blood ammonia levels stimulate hyperventilation and result in respiratory alkalosis.

Case Study 21-3

A 50-year-old woman with long-term hepatitis C–related cirrhosis was admitted for treatment of ascites that failed to respond to a sodium-restricted diet (2 g/day) and large doses of diuretics (including spironolactone 200 mg/day and furosemide 160 mg/day). At the time of admission, her blood pressure was 88/68 mm Hg and her heart rate was 112 per minute. Lower extremity edema was prominent. Spider angiomas were noted, as was mild jaundice. The patient was unable to concentrate when being questioned about her recent activities; a mild hand tremor was noted. The following laboratory results were observed: hyponatremia (Na = 128 mEq/L), mild hyperkalemia (K = 5.4 mEq/L), elevated serum creatinine (Cr = 2.0 mg/dL), hypoalbuminemia (3.0 g/dL), and elevated liver enzymes.

Commentary. This patient had developed renal dysfunction, as manifested by increased retention of sodium and water with increasing ascites that was unresponsive to diuretics. Her retention of excessive amounts of water caused dilutional hyponatremia. The elevated serum creatinine demonstrated reduced renal function. A paracentesis was performed to remove 6 L of ascites; an infusion of 60 g of albumin was administered. Because of the patient's advanced liver disease, she was evaluated for a liver transplant.

Case Study 21-4

A case was reported in which a 4-day-old infant was admitted to the emergency department with signs of encepha-lopathy following an accidental overdose of acetaminophen to manage post-circumcision pain.[43] The child had markedly elevated liver enzymes, coagulopathy, and renal failure (necessitating extensive treatment in a neonatal ICU). Upon questioning, the parents revealed that they had given the infant acetaminophen every 4 hours since his circumcision on his second day of life. The parents administered the medication every 4 hours—not based on signs of pain, but instead in the belief that acetaminophen was safe and would cause no harm if given every 4 hours as instructed by hospital personnel. To manage the acetaminophen toxicity, the infant was treated with a 20-hour intravenous *N*-acetylcysteine infusion protocol without any side effects and eventually fully recovered.

Commentary. The authors of this case report made a series of important points for nurses to consider when providing education to parents of infants with circumcision. First, it is important to recognize that the average elimination half-life of acetaminophen is longer in infants than in older children and adults. Second, healthcare providers should use caution when suggesting repeated doses of acetaminophen for pain control after circumcision in newborns, emphasizing that acetaminophen not be used at all beyond 24 hours post-circumcision unless the infant is experiencing signs of pain.

Also see Case Study 17-9 for discussion of a patient with cirrhosis and a fluid balance problem that required renal replacement therapy.

Summary of Key Points

- Cirrhosis is the end result of hepatic injury that leads to fibrotic changes in the liver.
- Conditions that can lead to cirrhosis include acute or chronic hepatitis, hepatotoxic drugs (such as acetaminophen), and alcoholic liver disease. The last condition is the most common cause of cirrhosis in the United States.
- Educating patients about the safe use of acetaminophen is important to reduce risk for liver injury.
- Impeded venous outflow through a fibrotic liver results in an accumulation of serum-like fluid (ascites) within the peritoneal cavity. The impeded venous outflow through the liver also contributes to edema, as does hypoalbuminemia associated with poor protein synthesis in the diseased liver.
- Cirrhosis results in secondary hyperaldosteronism, in which the decreased effective arterial volume causes the kidneys to respond as if they were underperfused (by retaining sodium). In reality, the cirrhotic patient has a normal or over-expanded total extracellular fluid volume.
- Hypokalemia is common in patients with chronic liver disease for a variety of reasons, such as increased renal losses of potassium caused by diuretics and hyperaldosteronism, low dietary intake of potassium, and increased potassium losses from diarrhea or vomiting.

continues

- In addition to increased risk for cardiac dysrhythmias, hypokalemia can contribute to the development of hepatic encephalopathy by increasing the serum ammonia level.

- Hyponatremia is common in patients with advanced hepatic cirrhosis and is usually caused by intrarenal disturbances in water handling and excessive release of antidiuretic hormone.

- The most frequent acid–base imbalance in cirrhotic patients is respiratory alkalosis, which occurs secondary to high ammonia levels.

- Treatment for cirrhosis usually includes diuretics plus sodium and water restriction. When the disease becomes more severe, additional treatments may include paracentesis, protein restriction, and bowel-sterilizing antibiotics.

- The maximal volume of ascitic fluid that can be removed by diuretics is approximately 750 mL per day.

- To avoid circulatory collapse associated with the removal of large volumes (such as more than 5 L) of ascitic fluid by paracentesis, some clinicians favor administering intravenous albumin at a dosage of 10 g per liter of ascitic fluid.

- Hepatorenal syndrome (HRS) is a type of renal failure that occurs in as many as 10% of patients with advanced cirrhosis and ascites.

- Precipitating causes of hepatic encephalopathy episodes include fluid volume depletion from overzealous use of diuretics, consumption of a high-protein diet, digestion of blood in the gastrointestinal tract, constipation, infection, progressive liver dysfunction, and hypokalemia with alkalosis.

NOTES

1. Amar, P. J., & Schiff, E. R. (2007). Acetaminophen safety and hepatotoxicity: Where do we go from here? *Expert Opinion on Drug Safety, 6*(4), 341–355.

2. Parillo, J. E., & Dellinger, R. P. (2008). *Critical care medicine: Principles of diagnosis and management in the adult* (3rd ed.). Philadelphia: Mosby Elsevier, p. 1582.

3. McPhee, S. J., Papadakis, M. A., & Tierney, L. M. (2008). *2008 current medical diagnosis and treatment* (47th ed.). New York: McGraw-Hill Medical, p. 584.

4. McPhee et al., note 3, p. 548.

5. Bongard, F. S., Sue, D. Y., & Vintch, J. R. (2008). *Current diagnosis and treatment, critical care* (3rd ed.). New York: McGraw-Hill/Lange, p. 718.

6. Moore, K. P., & Aithal, G. P. (2006). Guidelines on the management of ascites in cirrhosis. *Gut, 55*(suppl 6), vi, 1–12.

7. Epstein, M. (1995, September 15). Renal sodium retention in liver disease. *Hospital Practice, 30*(9), 41–42.

8. Kolleff, M. H., Bedient, T. J., Isakow, W., & Witt, C. A. (Eds.). (2008). *The Washington manual of critical care*. Philadelphia: Wolters Kluwer/Lippincott Williams & Wilkins, p. 323.

9. Fink, M. P., Abraham, E., Vincent, J. L., & Kochanek, P. M. (2005). *Textbook of critical care* (5th ed.). Philadelphia: Elsevier Saunders, p. 967.

10. Akriviadis, E. A., Ervin, M. G., Cominelli, F., Fisher, D. A., & Reynolds, T. B. (1997). Hyponatremia of cirrhosis: Role of vasopressin and decreased "effective" plasma volume. *Scandinavian Journal of Gastroenterology, 32*(8), 829–834.

    Sherlock, S. (1970). Ascites formation and its management. *Scandinavian Journal of Gastroenterology, 7*(suppl), 9–15.

    Weiner, I. D., & Wingo, C. S. (1997). Hypokalemia: Consequences, causes and correction. *Journal of American Society of Nephrology, 8*(7), 1179–1188.

13. Abbas, Z., Mumtaz, K., Salam, A., & Jafri, W. (2003). Factors predicting hyperkalemia in patients with cirrhosis receiving spironolactone. *Journal of the College of Physicians & Surgeons—Pakistan, 13*(7), 382–384.

14. Kim, D. K., Chang, S. H., Yun, I. J., Kwon, W. K., & Woo, N. S. (2009). Salbutamol to facilitate management of acute hyperkalemia in liver transplantation: A case report. *Canadian Journal of Anaesthesia, 56*(2), 142–146.

15. Morgan, M. Y., Blei, A., Grungreiff, K., Jalan, R., Kircheis, G., Marchesini, G., et al. (2007). The treatment of hepatic encephalopathy. *Metabolic Brain Disease, 22*(3–4), 389–405.

16. McPhee et al., note 3, p. 586.

17. McPhee et al., note 3, p. 586.

18. Alpers, D. H., Stenson, W. F., Taylor, B. E., & Bier, D. M. (2008). *Manual of nutritional therapeutics* (5th ed.). Philadelphia: Wolters Kluwer/Lippincott Williams & Wilkins, p. 342.

19. Cooper, D. H., Krainik, A. J., Lubner, S. J., & Reno, H. E. (2007). *The Washington manual of medical therapeutics* (32nd ed.). Philadelphia: Wolters Kluwer/Lippincott Williams & Wilkins, p. 504.

20. Bongard et al., note 5, p. 719.

21. Cardenas, A., Gines, P., & Runyon, B. A. (2009). Is albumin infusion necessary after large volume paracentesis? *Liver International, 29*(5), 636–640; discussion 640–641.

22. Fink et al., note 9, p. 971.

23. Ginès, P., Tito, L., Arroyo, V., Planas, R., Panes, J., Viver, J., et al. (1988). Randomized comparative study of therapeutic paracentesis with and without intravenous albumin in cirrhosis. *Gastroenterology, 94*, 1493–1502.

24. Sola-Vera, J., Minana, J., Ricart, E., Planella, M., Gonzalez, B., Torras, X., et al. (2003). Randomized trial comparing albumin and saline in the prevention of paracentesis-induced circulatory dysfunction in cirrhotic patients with ascites. *Hepatology, 37*(5), 1147–1153.

25. Bongard et al., note 5, p. 719.

26. Runyon, B.A., & AASLD Practice Guidelines Committee. (2009). Management of adult patients with ascites due to cirrhosis: An update. *Hepatology, 49*(6), 2087–2107.

27. Alpers et al., note 18, p. 334.

28. Alpers et al., note 18, p. 343.

29. Cooper et al., note 19, p. 503.

30. Gines, P., & Cardenas, A. (2008). The management of ascites and hyponatremia in cirrhosis. *Seminars in Liver Disease, 28*(1), 43–58.

31. Gerbes, A. L., Gulberg, V., Gines, P., Decaux, G., Gross, P., Gandjini, H., et al. (2003). Therapy of hyponatremia in cirrhosis with a vasopressin receptor antagonist: A randomized double-blind multicenter trial. *Gastroenterology, 124*(4), 933–939.

32. Kolleff et al., note 8, p. 334.

33. Parillo & Dellinger, note 2, p. 1579.

34. Dohler, K. D., & Meyer, M. (2008). Vasopressin analogues in the treatment of hepatorenal syndrome and gastrointestinal haemorrhage. *Best Practice & Research: Clinical Anaesthesiology, 22*(2), 335–350.

35. McPhee et al., note 3, p. 587.

36. Fabrizi, F., Dixit, V., Messa, P., & Martin, P. (2009). Terlipressin for hepatorenal syndrome: A meta-analysis of randomized trials. *International Journal of Artificial Organs, 32*(3), 133–140.

37. Bongard et al., note 5, p. 720.

38. Sundaram, V., & Shaikh, O. S. (2009). Hepatic encephalopathy: Pathophysiology and emerging therapies. *Medical Clinics of North America, 93*(4), 819–836, vii.

39. Butterworth, R. F., Spahr, L., Fontaine, S., & Layrargues, G. P. (1995). Manganese toxicity, dopaminergic dysfunction and hepatic encephalopathy. *Metabolic Brain Disease, 10*(4), 259–267.

40. McPhee et al., note 3, p. 587.

41. Fink et al., note 9, p. 971.

42. Kolleff et al., note 8, p. 323.

43. Walls, L., Baker, C. F., & Sarkar, S. (2007). Acetaminophen-induced hepatic failure with encephalopathy in a newborn. *Journal of Perinatology, 27*, 133–135.

Chapter 22

Oncologic Conditions

Most oncology patients will experience a problem with fluid and electrolyte regulation at some point during the course of their illness. In some situations, fluid and electrolyte problems are the initial symptoms that cause the individual to seek medical attention. At other times, they are the result of aggressive anticancer therapy. Occasionally, fluid and electrolyte problems do not become evident until metastases occur. This chapter describes the mechanisms responsible for fluid and electrolyte imbalances in cancer patients.

Patients with cancer may also suffer from unrelated conditions that can cause fluid and electrolyte imbalances; among these are congestive heart failure, hypertension, renal disease, and gastrointestinal (GI) disorders. The complete picture of the cancer patient needs to be considered when evaluating fluid and electrolyte imbalances. These problems can be acute or chronic and vary significantly in the degree of severity.

HYPERCALCEMIA

Cancer-related hypercalcemia is the most frequent metabolic complication in patients with cancer.[1] Approximately 10% to 20% of all cancer patients will develop hypercalcemia.[2] This imbalance is most commonly observed in patients with carcinomas of the breast, lung, kidney, and head and neck; it is also associated with multiple myeloma and lymphoma.[3] Patients with breast cancer may develop a "flare" of hypercalcemia after the initiation of estrogen or antiestrogen therapy.[4] According to reports in the literature, these patients often achieve a good tumor response with continued therapy.[5]

Despite advances in treatment, overall survival is poor once hypercalcemia occurs. For example, in a retrospective study of 260 patients with cancer-associated hypercalcemia being treated with bisphosphonates, the median survival was 64 days.[6] In another study, the most common electrolyte imbalance associated with mortality in a group of palliative care patients was hypercalcemia.[7]

Laboratory Measurement

The total calcium level refers to a combination of albumin-bound calcium and freely ionized calcium; with minor variations, the normal range for total calcium is most laboratories in approximately 8.9 to 10.3 mg/dL. If the reporting laboratory measures total serum calcium instead of ionized calcium, it is important to consider the calcium value in relation to the serum albumin level. A lower than normal serum albumin concentration causes the total calcium value to appear lower than it actually is. That is, the reported serum calcium concentration is decreased by 0.8 mg/dL for every 1 g/dL the serum albumin concentration is below normal. An equation commonly used to identify the correct total calcium level is as follows:

Corrected calcium (mg/dL) = measured serum calcium + 0.8 × (4.0 − measured serum albumin g/dL)

For example, assume a patient's measured calcium level is 10.2 mg/dL and the measured albumin level is 1.0 g/dL:

Corrected Ca (mg/dL) = 10.2 + 0.8 × (4.0 − 1.0) = 12.6 mg/dL

Thus, although the reported calcium level is within the upper limit of normal, the patient's actual total calcium level is elevated above normal. Recognition of the effect of hypoalbuminemia on the measured serum calcium concentration is an especially important consideration in cancer patients because they frequently are hypoalbuminemic due to malnutrition.

Clinical Presentation

Symptoms of hypercalcemia generally develop when the total calcium level exceeds 12 mg/dL, although their emergence is partially dependent on the time over which the elevation occurred. That is, when the serum calcium concentration rises slowly, the patient may remain relatively asymptomatic for some time, despite a relatively high elevation of the calcium level. For example, a serum calcium concentration of 14 mg/dL or greater that developed over a period of days may make a patient unconscious; in contrast, the same degree of hypercalcemia, when it develops over a period of months, may not be accompanied with symptoms.[8]

The major presenting symptoms of hypercalcemia include the following:

- Anorexia, nausea, and vomiting
- Abdominal pain
- Constipation
- Weakness
- Changes in mental status
- Polyuria and polydipsia
- Dehydration

Hypercalcemia should be suspected if the patient displays any of these symptoms.

If this imbalance is allowed to progress untreated, it can lead to psychotic behavior, bradycardia, ventricular arrhythmias, seizures, coma, renal failure, and death. The muscle weakness and fatigue associated with hypercalcemia cause the patient to be less active, which only serves to worsen hypercalcemia. Recall that immobilization favors a shift of calcium from the bones to the extracellular fluid (ECF). Worsening renal function is manifested by elevated blood urea nitrogen (BUN) and creatinine levels. As indicated previously, hypercalcemia is life-threatening when it is severe, perhaps terminating in cardiac arrest or renal failure.

Although hypercalcemia is usually associated with a poor prognosis in patients with cancer, the aggressive management of this problem can bring about improvement in a patient's quality of life. For example, polyuria and nocturia caused by the kidneys' inability to concentrate urine interfere with the patient's rest and sleep. This excessive fluid loss is often accompanied by thirst; however, anorexia and vomiting may interfere with drinking and eating. At times, treatment of hypercalcemia can reverse the mental symptoms associated with hypercalcemia, allowing the patient more time to interact with family and friends. According to the literature, approximately 50% of delirium episodes associated with hypercalcemia are potentially reversible.[9]

Dehydration increases the probability of delirium at the end of life.[10] At this point in the patient's illness, there is uncertainty about the benefit of prolonging life with hydration in an effort to relieve unpleasant symptoms (such as thirst and delirium).

Management

Treatment of hypercalcemia is initiated when the total serum calcium exceeds 12 mg/dL.[11] In addition to addressing the underlying malignancy (to the extent possible), the aim of treatment is to increase renal calcium excretion and minimize release of calcium from the bone. The first line of treatment is rehydration with isotonic saline; however, this measure alone is likely not sufficient to manage severe hypercalcemia. Additional medications—such as a bisphosphonate, calcitonin, and corticosteroids—may be needed to produce a sustained decrease in the serum calcium concentration. Given that all anti-hypercalcemic agents have the potential to cause hypocalcemia, a careful watch on the serum calcium level is needed during treatment. The drugs are discontinued when the serum calcium concentration returns to normal or near normal.

Volume Expansion

Patients with hypercalcemia are often dehydrated and, therefore, have difficulty excreting the excess calcium load via the kidneys. The administration of isotonic saline (0.9% NaCl) expands the plasma volume and facilitates renal excretion of calcium by increasing the glomerular filtration rate. An aim of treatment is to increase the hourly urine output to 100 mL to 150 mL.[12] Before the initiation of any large fluid infusion, renal function should be evaluated. It is also advisable to monitor the central venous pressure when fluids are administered rapidly (such as at rates ranging from 250 to 500 mL/hr) because it is possible to overwhelm the patient's cardiovascular system and cause fluid overload. Among the signs of this condition are shortness of breath, rales (noted on auscultation of the lungs), peripheral edema, and distended neck veins. Furosemide may be added to the treatment regimen if signs of fluid overload are present. A potential additional benefit from administration of furosemide is increased renal excretion of calcium. A potential concern is that furosemide may worsen fluid volume deficit in patients who are not fully rehydrated.[13]

Bisphosphonates

The bisphosphonates (formerly called diphosphonates) have become the drugs of choice to treat malignancy-associated hypercalcemia; they are able to successfully control serum calcium in 80% to 90% of patients.[14] The bisphosphonates act by inhibiting calcium release from the bone. Among the drugs in this category are pamidronate and zoledronic acid, although zoledronic acid has largely replaced pamidronate because of its greater calcium-lowering effect. The serum calcium concentration will usually normalize 3 to 4 days after administration of one of these agents, and the effects may last from several weeks.

Calcitonin

Synthetic calcitonin promotes renal calcium excretion, even in patients with compromised renal function. The major advantages of calcitonin are its rapid onset of action (2 to 4 hours) and its comparatively low serious toxicity. A disadvantage is its relatively weak hypocalcemic effect. Another disadvantage is that its effect wanes after a period of several days.[15]

Owing to its rapid onset of action, calcitonin is sometimes used in conjunction with a bisphosphonate to treat acute hypercalcaemia.[16] The action of calcitonin starts quickly and helps lower the serum calcium level until the bisphosphonate activity is at peak effect. Potential side effects of calcitonin include nausea and flushing.

Glucocorticoids

Glucocorticoids can be helpful in the treatment of hypercalcemia associated with hematologic malignancies, including myeloma. Unfortunately, a glucocorticoid may take several days to lower the serum calcium level. Large doses of hydrocortisone may be required initially, followed by oral maintenance prednisone therapy.

Glucocorticoids lower the serum calcium level by increasing urinary calcium excretion and decreasing intestinal calcium absorption; they also inhibit cytokine release and have a direct cytolytic effect on some tumor cells.[17] Side effects of these agents can include hyperglycemia, gastrointestinal bleeding, osteoporosis, hypertension, and the development of opportunistic infections.

Gallium Nitrate

Gallium nitrate is effective in inhibiting bone resorption. However, a major adverse effect is nephrotoxicity; it is contraindicated if the patient's serum creatinine level is greater than 2.5 mg/dL.[18]

Diet and Hydration

Maintaining adequate hydration is important in preventing severe hypercalcemia. When possible, the patient's oral fluid intake should be at least 2 to 3 L per day to promote the excretion of calcium by the kidneys. Medications to treat nausea may be needed to facilitate fluid intake. Also, vomiting and diarrhea should be treated early to avoid dehydration.

A calcium-restricted diet in conjunction with an oral phosphate agent may be tried to inhibit intestinal calcium absorption (but only if the serum phosphorus level is < 3.0 mg/dL and kidney function is normal).[19] However, a calcium-restricted diet may have minimal effect in patients whose hypercalcemia is largely due to calcium resorption from the bones; further, dietary restriction of calcium-rich foods is unpleasant and may contribute to the chronic malnutrition often present in cancer patients.

Activity

Weight-bearing activities should be encouraged as much as possible in patients with cancer, because prolonged immobilization enhances bone resorption and is a contributing factor to the development of hypercalcemia. Given that ambulation is often associated with pain in cancer patients, it may be necessary to administer pain medication prior to exercise and to allow adequate periods of rest between activities.

Dialysis

Dialysis is helpful for patients with severe hypercalcemia (e.g., calcium concentrations greater than 16 mg/dL) in whom aggressive intravenous fluid replacement is contraindicated—for example, in patients with congestive heart failure or renal insufficiency.[20]

HYPONATREMIA

Hyponatremia is an important and common electrolyte disorder in cancer patients and is associated with a variety of primary diagnoses. The underlying pathophysiology in individual cases must be considered because it could affect the desired management strategy.[21]

Causes

Among possible causes for decreased serum sodium levels in this population are the following:

- Ectopic release of an antidiuretic hormone-like substance from certain tumors, especially small-cell lung cancer, leading to the syndrome of inappropriate antidiuretic hormone secretion (SIADH). Approximately 15% to 32% of patients with small-cell lung cancer experience hyponatremia caused by ectopic production of vasopressin by tumor cells.[22] Ectopic production of ADH is not controlled by any feedback mechanism; therefore, the serum sodium level continues to decrease because of sustained ADH production by the tumor site.
- SIADH secondary to administration of chemotherapeutic agents, such as cisplatin and cyclophosphamide.[23,24] For example, hyponatremia is a potentially disastrous consequence of cisplatin therapy and is rendered even more dangerous when a large volume of intravenous fluid is given to reduce the nephrotoxicity of cisplatin.[25]
- Loss of sodium through vomiting and diarrhea.
- Excessive use of hypotonic intravenous fluids, especially in the presence of SIADH.

Clinical Presentation

The clinical presentation of hyponatremia is discussed in Chapter 4. In some cases, symptoms of hyponatremia occur before a diagnosis of malignancy is recognized. The hyponatremia associated with malignancy usually develops gradually; therefore, patients may remain relatively free of symptoms until the serum sodium level falls quite low. (Recall that slowly developing imbalances do not produce symptoms nearly as often as imbalances that develop quickly.)

Management

Successful treatment of the tumor is the most direct treatment of hyponatremia associated with malignancy. Chemotherapy, radiation therapy, or surgery may be used, depending on the type of cancer involved. Close monitoring of serum sodium levels and serum osmolality is important when antineoplastic drugs known to induce hyponatremia are administered. In the case of drug-induced hyponatremia, discontinuation of the drug usually causes a resolution of the disorder.

Other standard measures to control water excess and restore normal serum sodium concentrations are described in Chapter 4. On a short-term basis, fluid intake is restricted to the extent that negative water balance is induced. If neurologic symptoms are present, hypertonic saline (3% or 5% NaCl) may need to be cautiously administered.

HYPOKALEMIA

Hypokalemia has been estimated to occur in as many as 75% of cancer patients at some point in their illness.

Causes

The poor dietary intake in an anorexic cancer patient, along with the potassium loss associated with nausea and vomiting, can lead to hypokalemia. Unfortunately, both poor intake and increased losses are common in cancer patients undergoing chemotherapy and radiotherapy. Although there is a direct loss of potassium in vomitus, the main cause of hypokalemia associated with vomiting is related to the presence of metabolic alkalosis.

Loss of intestinal fluid from diarrhea can lead to hypokalemia. A number of malignancies—for example, villous adenoma of the colon, pancreatic carcinoma, and carcinoma of the small or large intestinal cancers—have been associated with diarrhea. Diarrhea may also be present as a result of antibiotic therapy, infectious agents in the GI tract (such as *Clostridium difficile* and candidiasis), radiation therapy to the bowel, and certain antineoplastic drugs.

Both vomiting and diarrhea can also lead to a state of volume depletion. When this occurs, aldosterone production is increased, causing renal potassium loss. The administration of potassium-free IV fluids for treatment of dehydration simply exaggerates the potassium reduction.

Hypokalemia is frequently observed in patients with acute myeloid leukemia, apparently related to inappropriate renal potassium loss. Often patients are hypokalemic at the time they first present for treatment. In addition, excessive loss of potassium (due to renal tubular damage) occurs in many patients during induction therapy for acute non-lymphocytic leukemia. Renal tubular damage in this patient population is usually attributed to acute tubular necrosis caused by antineoplastic drugs, anti-infective therapy, or antifungal therapy with amphotericin B.

Certain malignancies release an adrenocorticotropic hormone (ACTH)-like substance that can cause increased renal loss of potassium, leading to hypokalemia. Among these malignancies are small-cell carcinoma of the lung, thymoma, tumors of the adrenal cortex, medullary carcinoma of the thyroid, and carcinoid tumors of the bronchus. ACTH stimulates the adrenal cortex to produce glucocorticoids and aldosterone (a mineralocorticoid). Aldosterone has a significant effect on the excretion of potassium and the retention of sodium, whereas glucocorticoids have a lesser effect on these electrolytes. The administration of large doses of prednisone and prednisolone—two drugs that have a mineralocorticoid effect—can result in hypokalemia. These steroids are sometimes used in the treatment of hematological malignancies, spinal cord compression, and sepsis.

Clinical Presentation

Clinical signs of hypokalemia are described in Chapter 5. The most significant problem associated with hypokalemia is the increased risk for cardiac arrhythmias.

Management

Therapy is directed at normalizing the serum potassium concentration to avoid the life-threatening complications (primarily cardiac dysrhythmias) associated with hypokalemia. Potassium losses can be replaced with oral supplements, although most often the emergent nature of hypokalemia necessitates intravenous potassium supplementation initially. For reasons that remain unclear, magnesium depletion affects potassium absorption. When hypokalemia is present, the magnesium level needs to be assessed; if decreased, it needs to be corrected before or concurrently with the correction of hypokalemia. Refer to Chapter 5 for a more detailed discussion of the treatment of hypokalemia.

HYPOPHOSPHATEMIA

Causes

Hypophosphatemia may be associated with some untreated rapidly proliferating malignancies (e.g., acute leukemia), presumably due to the consumption of phosphate by the tumor cells. However, hypophosphatemia associated with malignant disease usually occurs subsequent to nutritional deprivation and cachexia. Prolonged hyperalimentation without appropriate phosphate additives can lead to hypophosphatemia; further, respiratory alkalosis, which is associated with the septicemic episodes of neutropenic patients, may lower the serum phosphorus level by causing a shift of phosphorus from the extracellular space into the cells.

A phenomenon referred to as refeeding syndrome is commonly observed in malnourished cancer patients who are aggressively fed via the intravenous route or by tube feeding. Such feeding can produce a shift of phosphate, magnesium and potassium from the bloodstream into newly formed cells. Case Study 8-1 describes a case of hypophosphatemia associated with total parenteral nutrition in a cancer patient. Chapters 11 and 12 provide a more thorough discussion of refeeding syndrome.

Clinical Presentation

Clinical signs of hypophosphatemia are described in Chapter 8. When severe, hypophosphatemia can cause profound muscle weakness and pain. Weakness of chest wall muscles can interfere with ventilation. Hypophosphatemia may depress the chemotactic and phagocytic activity of granulocytes and thus may increase risk for infection.

Management

The treatment of hypophosphatemia is described in Chapter 8.

HYPOMAGNESEMIA

Causes

Hypomagnesemia may present as a single electrolyte imbalance or in combination with other disorders seen in cancer patients, such as hypokalemia, hypophosphatemia, and hypocalcemia. Hypomagnesemia can occur in this population for the same reasons as it occurs in any other population, including magnesium loss in chronic diarrhea or prolonged diuretic use, and inadequate magnesium supplementation during total parenteral nutrition or tube feedings. Although hypomagnesemia is a common clinical problem for cancer patients in general, this electrolyte imbalance is most prevalent in patients who are treated with certain pharmacological agents—specifically, cisplatin, cyclosporine, amphotericin B, and the aminoglycosides.

Cisplatin is a potentially nephrotoxic agent used to treat tumors occurring in a variety of sites; it has the potential to have a significant negative impact on total body magnesium due to renal wasting of this electrolyte.[26, 27] Hypomagnesemia reportedly occurs in as many as 90% of patients treated with cisplatin secondary to renal injury that impairs magnesium reabsorption.[28]

Amphotericin B—an agent commonly used in the treatment of fungal infections in immunocompromised patients—has been associated with both hypomagnesemia and hypokalemia. The aminoglycosides are associated with renal magnesium wasting. Cyclosporine causes increased magnesium excretion, although usually any associated hypomagnesemia is mild.[29]

Clinical Presentation

Clinical signs of hypomagnesemia are described in Chapter 7. The most serious problem associated with hypomagnesemia is its ability to increase myocardial electrical instability and dysrhythmias. An animal model study described an increased incidence of sudden death in hypomagnesemic rats, often following some triggering event.[30]

Management

The treatment of hypomagnesemia is described in Chapter 7.

THIRD-SPACE FLUID ACCUMULATION

Cancer patients frequently develop third-space fluid accumulations. These imbalances may be due to any of the following causes:

- *Malignant effusions into the peritoneal, pericardial, or pleural compartments.* Direct tumor involvement of the cavity's serous surface appears to be the most frequent cause of effusions in cancer patients. However, peritoneal effusions (also known as ascites) commonly occur with liver disease secondary to malignancy.
- *Edema.* Edema involves the trapping of excess fluid in the interstitial fluid space due to obstruction of lymphatic drainage or venous return secondary to tumor pressure. Protein seepage through the capillary bed in the edematous site pulls fluid with it, making the edema more severe. Low serum oncotic pressure (due to hypoalbuminemia), along with extremity dependence, contributes to ankle and leg swelling in oncology patients who sit for long periods.

Major shifts of water and electrolytes into potential fluid spaces result in extracellular fluid volume deficit (FVD). This condition is manifested by decreased urinary output, increased urinary specific gravity, and postural hypoten-sion. Body weight does not decrease (as it does with actual fluid loss) because fluid is trapped inside the body. In fact, weight may increase with parenteral fluid replacement; although given to correct the FVD, this treatment also allows an increase in the fluid volume trapped in the third space, which merely adds to the patient's discomfort.

In the case of peritoneal effusions, a paracentesis can be performed to drain the fluid for comfort measures. At the same time, replacement of the fluid, electrolytes, and albumin lost during this procedure must be considered. (Refer to Chapter 21 for a discussion of paracentesis for ascites.)

For a long-term resolution of third-space fluid accumulation, the cause of the fluid shift must be corrected. This can be accomplished only if the malignant process producing the third-space fluid accumulation responds to treatment.

TUMOR LYSIS SYNDROME

Tumor lysis syndrome (TLS) is a potentially life-threatening oncologic emergency that involves the massive necrosis of tumor cells following the administration of chemotherapy. The destroyed tumor cells release their cellular contents, resulting in hyperphosphatemia, hyperkalemia, and hyperuricemia. Hypocalcemia follows in the wake of the high serum phosphate concentration. Another potential problem with TLS is renal failure. While typically caused by chemotherapy, TLS may also result from radiotherapy.[31] Patients most at risk for TLS are those with acute and chronic leukemia, lymphomas, and (less often) bulky solid tumors.[32] Patients with underlying renal dysfunction or decreased urine output are at a higher risk of developing TLS because of their impaired ability to excrete the waste products generated by cell lysis.

TLS usually appears within 12 to 72 hours after the administration of cytotoxic thery and/or radiation.[33] The diagnosis is usually made on the basis of laboratory test results because symptoms of TLS may be nonspecific. Patients may present with a myriad of symptoms, including cardiac dysrhythmias, seizures, muscle cramps, confusion, delirium, nausea, vomiting, renal failure, and (potentially) sudden death.[34]

Treatment is directed toward correcting the hyperuricemia, hyperphosphatemia, and hyperkalemia; **Table 22-1** outlines treatment principles for TLS. As with most problems, the most important step in managing TLS is to prevent it from occurring. Fortunately, the renal failure caused by TLS may be reversible and patients can regain normal renal function as TLS resolves.

Table 22-1 Principles of Treatment for Tumor Lysis Syndrome (TLS)

Hydration	The goal of hydration is to preserve renal function and eliminate products of cellular breakdown during chemotherapy.
	When possible, hydration is recommended at least 48 hours before tumor-specific treatment is started.[35]
	An attempt is made to maintain the urine output at least at 100 ml/hr during chemotherapy.[36]
	To achieve diuresis, isotonic IV fluids may be infused at a rate of 200 to 300 ml/hr during the first 2 to 3 days of chemotherapy.[37]
	The ideal choice of an IV fluid to treat TLS is not clear. A solution of normal saline may be infused to maintain a high urine output (greater than 2.5 liters per day).[38] Sometimes used is the solution of 5% dextrose in 0.45% sodium chloride, with 50–100 mEq of sodium bicarbonate added per liter.[39]
Allopurinol or rasburicase	The goal is to lower the serum uric acid level with one of these agents, either prophylactically or as treatment for hyperuricemia.
	Allopurinol prevents further production of uric acid but does nothing to decrease existing pools of this substance.[40]
	Rasburicase rapidly catabolizes circulating uric acid into allantoin, a highly soluble by-product that is easily excreted by the kidneys. Rasburicine can reduce existing uric acid in the plasma as well as prevent further production of uric acid.[41]
Alkalinization of urine to increase solubility of urate	Alkalinization of the urine above a pH of 7 promotes solubility of uric acid and may prevent uric acid nephropathy.[42]
	When hyperphosphatemia accompanies a high blood urea concentration, urine alkalinization is avoided because calcium phosphate crystals may form in the renal tubules.[43]
	It has been recommended that bicarbonate therapy be stopped once uric acid levels normalize; and when the urine pH is greater than 8.0 and the serum bicarbonate concentration is greater than 30 mEq/L.[44]
Dialysis	Among the possible indications for initiation of renal replacement therapy are persistent hyperkalemia, hyperphosphatemia and severe metabolic acidosis.

Hyperuricemia

Rapid elevation of the serum uric acid level presents the danger of acute urate nephropathy caused by crystallization of uric acid in the kidney. Although hyperuricemia usually follows chemotherapy or radiation, it may also occur spontaneously in patients with rapidly proliferating tumors and in those with overproduction of uric acid precursors by the tumor (as in polycythemia vera and chronic granulocytic leukemia).

Diagnosis of hyperuricemia is established by measurement of uric acid in serum and urine. This imbalance is generally considered to be present if the serum uric acid concentration is more than 8 mg/dL or has increased more than 25% over baseline.[45]

Prevention of hyperuricemia is the cornerstone of management. Prophylactic treatment often consists of the following measures:

- Vigorous hydration
- Administration of allopurinol or rasburicase
- Alkalinization of the urine

Hyperuricemia should be viewed as a preventable complication rather than as an emergent condition. See Table 22-1.

Hyperkalemia

Lethal cardiac arrhythmias are the most serious consequence of hyperkalemia. When the hyperkalemia associated with TLS is mild, increased intravenous administration of

0.9% NaCl with a single dose of furosemide may be sufficient treatment. However, for those patients whose serum potassium level is between 5.5 and 6.0 mEq/L, it may be necessary to add an ion-exchange resin (such as Kayexalate) to the regimen. If the serum potassium level is greater than 6.0 mEq/L or the patient develops cardiac arrhythmias, it may be necessary to administer intravenous calcium gluconate first, and then follow this treatment with intravenous fluids, furosemide, and hypertonic dextrose and regular insulin.

Although hyperkalemia is most commonly associated with TLS, there are other possible causes of this electrolyte imbalance. An increased serum potassium level can result from acute renal failure, such as may occur in conjunction with untreated hyperuricemia, use of nephrotoxic or antineoplastic drugs, or renal malignancy. Also, a falsely high serum potassium level may be reported in the presence of a high white blood cell count, owing to increased leukocyte fragility and lysis that releases cellular potassium into the clotted serum sample. Validation of a supposed hyperkalemic state with the expected electrocardiographic changes and other clinical signs of hyperkalemia is needed to determine whether the serum potassium level is truly elevated in a patient with a high white blood cell count due to a leukemic process. Chapter 5 provides a more thorough discussion of the clinical manifestations and treatment of hyperkalemia.

Hyperphosphatemia

The elevated serum phosphate level associated with TLS may not occur until 1 or 2 days after treatment is initiated; levels as high as 20 mg/dL may persist for several days afterward. Hyperphosphatemia usually occurs along with hyperuricemia, hyperkalemia, and hypocalcemia. Renal damage—and perhaps even acute renal failure—may follow the precipitation of calcium phosphate in the kidneys. Thus reduction of the phosphate levels is critical to prevent or to correct renal damage. Treatment of TLS most often corrects hyperphosphatemia. Management of hyperphosphatemia associated with renal failure is described in Chapter 17.

Hypocalcemia

A reciprocal drop in the serum calcium level follows the elevated serum phosphate level described earlier. Other possible causes of hypocalcemia include production of calcitonin by medullary carcinomas, malabsorption due to extensive bowel resection or loss of small bowel absorptive surface secondary to tumor size, and magnesium depletion. As indicated earlier, a falsely low total serum calcium level may be present when the patient is hypoalbuminemic. However, a true deficit of calcium can result in muscle cramps and tetany. Symptomatic hypocalcemia can usually be corrected by the intravenous administration of calcium gluconate.

PATIENT/FAMILY EDUCATION

As indicated in this chapter, many fluid and electrolyte problems may occur in cancer patients. Thus frequent observation for these imbalances is important. When a patient is diagnosed with a malignancy, both the patient and the family should be taught about the fluid and electrolyte imbalances that pose the greatest risk in conjunction with oncologic diseases. They should be taught to recognize the signs and symptoms that need to be reported to caregivers and to follow up on routine laboratory evaluations to detect problems before they become severe. In some cases, the recurrence of a fluid and electrolyte disorder is the first sign of recurrence of the malignancy; therefore, it is essential that patients and family members understand the critical nature of reporting this information to the healthcare team. Chapter 2 reviews the process of assessment for fluid and electrolyte problems, and Chapters 3 through 9 offer information dealing with specific imbalances.

CASE STUDIES

Case Study 22-1

A 61-year-old woman, who had initially been diagnosed with lymphoma several years ago, was recently diagnosed with recurrent lymphoma. She had received cisplatin 3 days previously. Clinically, she displayed anxiety, decreased appetite, dehydration, and fatigue. Abnormal laboratory findings included the following data:

- Potassium = 3.0 mEq/L (usual laboratory normal = 3.5–5.0 mEq/L)
- Magnesium = 0.5 mEq/L (usual laboratory normal = 1.3–2.1 mEq/L)

Although she had decreased her fluid intake for several days, the patient had no symptoms of vomiting, diarrhea, or fistula drainage. She also had no obvious signs and symptoms of hypokalemia or hypomagnesemia.

To correct the imbalances, the patient was treated with intravenous potassium and magnesium followed by oral administration of these electrolytes for 3 days. On the day of discharge, her serum potassium and magnesium levels had returned to normal. Discharge medications included 40 mEq of oral potassium, three times daily, and 400 mg of magnesium oxide, three times daily. An appointment was set up to have the patient return to the clinic for laboratory evaluation of serum electrolytes in 3 days. A detailed instruction sheet was given to her regarding the administration of her medications. The patient also received a written list of signs of hyperkalemia/hypokalemia and hypermagnesemia/hypomagnesemia; she was instructed to report any signs described in the list to the clinic staff. In addition to being told of the importance of continuing the medications as prescribed, she was instructed to call the clinic staff if she had any difficulty taking the medications.

Commentary. This case involves a lymphoma patient 3 days after chemotherapy treatment. Instead of the expected tumor lysis syndrome, this patient's electrolyte problems were hypokalemia and hypomagnesemia. These imbalances were likely a side effect of cisplatin therapy. Both magnesium and potassium replacement were effective in restoring normal serum values of both electrolytes. However, long-term replacement was required because renal losses of these electrolytes were ongoing. Instructing the patient about the signs and symptoms of hypokalemia and hypomagnesemia is important in the event that this situation occurs again after the next chemotherapy treatment. Also, the patient needs to have detailed instructions about taking these medications and reinforcement that she should not discontinue them without direction from the clinic staff.

Case Study 22-2

A 68-year-old patient who was newly diagnosed with acute myelogenous leukemia was admitted to the hospital for induction therapy scheduled to begin the next day. Intravenous hydration was begun with 0.9% sodium chloride and added sodium bicarbonate at the rate of 150 mL/hr. Allopurinol was ordered to begin the day of admission and to continue daily. All admission blood work was within normal ranges (serum albumin = 4.0 g/dL). The next day, chemotherapy was begun with cytarabine (cytosine arabinoside) given by continuous infusion over 7 days and idamycin (idarubicin hydrochloride) given once daily for 3 days.

On the third day of treatment, abnormal laboratory results from venous blood were as follows:

- Potassium = 6.0 mEq/L (normal 3.5–5.0 mEq/L)
- Phosphorus = 14.9 mg/dL (normal 2.5–4.5 mg/dL)
- Uric acid = 10.3 mg/dL (normal < 8 mg/dL)
- Calcium = 7.5 mg/dL (normal 8.4–10.6 mg/dL)

Although all of these values were outside the normal range, the patient displayed no symptoms of electrolyte abnormalities. At this time, hydration with 0.9% sodium chloride (with added sodium bicarbonate) was increased to 300 mL/hr.

On the fourth day, the following abnormal serum values were reported by the laboratory:

- Phosphorus = 10.0 mg/dL (normal 2.5–4.5 mg/dL)
- Uric acid = 8.5 mg/dL (normal < 8 mg/dL)
- Calcium = 8.0 mg/dL (normal 8.4–10.6 mg/dL)

All laboratory results returned to within normal ranges on the final day of treatment (5 days after chemotherapy was begun).

Commentary. This patient experienced tumor lysis syndrome, a common occurrence in patients with a diagnosis of leukemia who are undergoing induction therapy. To prevent renal complications of hyperuricemia, large-volume intravenous hydration (along with sodium bicarbonate to keep the urine alkaline) was given. Allopurinol was given to reduce the production of uric acid (accomplished by inhibiting the chemical reactions that occur immediately preceding its formation). When the patient's laboratory results were abnormal (hyperkalemia, hyperphosphatemia, hyperuricemia, and hypocalcemia), treatment was initiated to correct these imbalances. The basic treatment consisted of increased hydration, preceded by assessment of renal function. The patient had no existing cardiac abnormality and had no symptoms from the hyperkalemia; therefore, no specific treatment of hyperkalemia was initiated. If the laboratory findings on the fourth day had failed to demonstrate any improvement in the tumor lysis syndrome, additional therapy to correct the hyperkalemia and the hypocalcemia likely would have been initiated. Although this syndrome can continue for several days after therapy has been completed, this patient had no further problems during this hospitalization.

Case Study 22-3

A case was reported in which a 64-year-old man with multiple myeloma was admitted with complaints of malaise, diffuse bone pain, and constipation.[46] Laboratory results confirmed the presence of anemia. A markedly elevated total serum calcium level was present (15.4 mg/dL).

Following treatment with 6 L of isotonic saline over a 48-hour period, the patient's serum calcium decreased to 14.4 mg/dL. Pamidronate (a bisphosphonate) was administered, and the patient was monitored for 2 weeks to assess renal function and electrolyte balance. Six days after treatment with pamidronate, the following abnormal laboratory values were observed:

- Calcium = 7.9 mg/dL (normal range 8.4–10.6 mg/dL)
- Phosphorus = 1.3 mg/dL (normal range 2.5–4.5 mg/dL)
- Magnesium = 0.7 mEq/L (normal range 1.3–2.2 mEq/L)

Commentary. The elevated serum calcium level responded to rehydration with isotonic saline and a single dose of pamidronate. However, a number of transient electrolyte imbalances occurred after the pamidronate was administered. The hypocalcemia was asymptomatic and did not require supplementation; this imbalance has been reported in other patients after high-dose pamidronate therapy (especially when in the presence of renal failure). Apparently, serum phosphorus levels tend to decrease after the administration of pamidronate, especially when the baseline phosphorus level is low (as it was in this patient). The most likely reason for the hypomagnesemia was magnesium wasting related to the hypophosphatemia. (Phosphate depletion is known to lead to an increase in the renal excretion of magnesium.)

Case Study 22-4

A case was reported in which a 26-year-old woman was admitted to the hospital with a history of six to eight episodes of diarrhea for a period of 3 days.[47] Her other symptoms included anorexia, nausea, abdominal cramping, and generalized fatigue. Mild abdominal tenderness was found, but the patient's vital signs were within normal limits. Her medical history revealed a diagnosis of osteosarcoma of the right tibia at the age of 16 that required an above-the-knee amputation and chemotherapy (consisting of bleomycin, cisplatin, cyclophosphamide, dactinomycin, doxorubicin, and methotrexate). Following the cisplatin therapy, the patient required treatment with oral electrolyte supplements for chronic hypomagnesemia and hypokalemia. Medications at home consisted of 1600 mg of magnesium sulfate daily, potassium supplements, and birth control pills. Although renal and liver function tests were within normal limits, the following abnormal laboratory data were found:

- Serum Mg = 0.5 mEq/L (normal 1.3–2.1 mEq/L)
- Serum K = 2.8 mEq/L (3.5–5.0 mEq/L)

A presumptive diagnosis of viral gastroenteritis was made, and the patient was treated with intravenous fluids and electrolyte replacement. A venipuncture performed 6 hours later resulted in sudden confusion and asystole that lasted for 15 to 20 seconds, after which a normal sinus rhythm returned spontaneously. Diarrhea persisted for the next 2 days, and a cardiology workup concluded that the asystolic episode originated in a vasovagal response to the venipuncture, which was exacerbated by the patient's chronic renal tubular disorder.

After two weeks, the patient was discharged with a normal serum magnesium level (1.5 mEq/L) and serum potassium level (3.7 mEq/L). Discharge medications consisted of magnesium oxide (2 g/day) and amiloride (10 mg/day). The patient's medical history revealed that her kidneys excreted magnesium excessively secondary to tubular damage caused by her previous cisplatin therapy. The patient's fractional excretion of magnesium ranged between 10% and 25% (normal is less than 2%).

Commentary. Cisplatin-related nephrotoxicity can result in excessive renal magnesium excretion even before renal function becomes affected. The patient's negative magnesium balance, which emerged while she was admitted with gastroenteritis, was likely exacerbated by large losses of magnesium in her diarrheal stools. The brief period of asystole that occurred during venipuncture was attributed to the effects of hypomagnesemia; no future periods of asystole were noted during venipunctures performed after the patient's serum magnesium level normalized. The authors of this case report emphasize the need to avoid hypomagnesemia in patients with cisplatin-induced tubular dysfunction.[48]

Also see Case Studies 4-2, 6-8, 6-9, 6-10, 7-4, 12-3, and 17-8 for a discussion of other oncology patients with fluid and electrolyte problems.

Summary of Key Points

- Symptoms from fluid and electrolyte problems may cause the cancer patient to seek medication attention for the first time.
- Hypercalcemia is the most frequently noted metabolic complication in patients with cancer. It is most commonly observed in patients with carcinomas of the breast, lung, kidney, and head and neck; it is also associated with multiple myeloma and lymphoma.
- A lower than normal serum albumin concentration causes the total calcium value to appear lower than it actually is. The following equation is used to identify the correct total calcium level: Corrected calcium (mg/dL) = measured serum calcium + 0.8 × (4.0 − measured serum albumin g/dL).
- Symptoms of hypercalcemia generally develop when the total calcium level exceeds 12 mg/dL, although they are partially dependent on the time over which the elevation occurred. Major presenting symptoms include anorexia, nausea, vomiting, abdominal pain, constipation, weakness, changes in mental status, polyuria and polydipsia, and fluid volume deficit.
- Although hypercalcemia is usually associated with a poor prognosis in patients with cancer, the aggressive management of this problem can bring about significant improvements in patients' quality of life.
- Treatment of hypercalcemia includes attacking the underlying malignancy (to the extent possible), aggressively treating volume depletion with intravenous isotonic saline, and using medications (such as bisphosphonates, calcitonin, and corticosteroids).
- Hyponatremia is a common electrolyte disorder in patients with cancer; it is associated tumors that produce antidiuretic-hormone like substances (such as small-cell lung cancer), chemotherapeutic agents that cause syndrome of inappropriate antidiuretic hormone (SIADH), and loss of sodium through vomiting and diarrhea.
- Hypokalemia has been estimated to occur in as many as 75% of cancer patients at some point in their illness. Causes include poor dietary intake due to anorexia, and potassium losses with nausea and vomiting during chemotherapy.
- Hypophosphatemia may be associated with some untreated rapidly proliferating malignancies (e.g., acute leukemia), presumably due to the consumption of phosphate by the tumor cells. Significant hypophosphatemia may be observed when the severely malnourished cancer patient is fed aggressively, a phenomenon known as refeeding syndrome.
- Although hypomagnesemia is a common clinical problem in cancer patients in general, it is most prevalent in patients who are treated with certain pharmacological agents—namely, cisplatin, cyclosporine, amphotericin B, and the aminoglycosides.
- Tumor lysis syndrome (TLS) is a potentially life-threatening oncologic emergency that involves the massive necrosis of tumor cells following the administration of chemotherapy. The destroyed tumor cells release their cellular contents, resulting in hyperphosphatemia, hyperkalemia, and hyperuricemia.

NOTES

1. Penel, N., Dewas, S,, Doutrelant, P., Clisant, S., Yazdanpanah, Y., & Adenis, A. (2008). Cancer-associated hypercalcemia treated with intravenous diphosphonates: A survival and prognostic factor analysis. *Supportive Care in Cancer, 16,* 387–392.

2. McPhee, S. J., Papadakis, M. A., & Tierney, L. M. (2008). *2008 current medical diagnosis and treatment* (47th ed.). New York: McGraw-Hill/Lange, p. 1450.

3. McPhee et al., note 2, p. 1450.

4. McPhee et al., note 2, p. 1451.

5. McPhee et al., note 2, p. 1451.

6. Penel et al., note 1.

7. Alsirafy, S. A., Sroor, M. Y., & Al-Shahri, M. Z. (2009). Predictive impact of electrolyte abnormalities on the admission outcome and survival of palliative care cancer referrals. *Journal of Palliative Medicine, 12*(2), 177–180.

8. Govindan, R. (Ed.). (2008). *The Washington manual of oncology* (2nd ed.). Philadelphia: Wolters Kluwer/Lippincott Williams & Wilkins, p. 404.

9. Delgado-Guay, M. O., Yennurajalingam, S., & Bruera, E. (2008). Delirium with severe symptom expression related to hypercalcemia in a patient with advanced cancer: An interdisciplinary approach to treatment. *Journal of Pain & Symptom Management, 36*(4), 442–449.

10. Lawlor, P. G. (2002). Delirium and dehydration: Some fluid for thought? *Supportive Care in Cancer, 10*(6), 445–454.

11. Cooper, D. H., Kranik, A. J., Lubner, S. J., & Reno, H. E. (2007). *The Washington manual of medical therapeutics* (32nd ed.). Philadelphia: Wolters Kluwer/ Lippincott Wilkins & Wilkins, p. 80.

12. Govindan, note 8, p. 404.

13. LeGrand, S. B., Leskuski, D., & Zama, I. (2008). Narrative review: Furosemide for hypercalcemia: An unproved yet common practice. *Annals of Internal Medicine, 149,* 259–263.

14. Govindan, note 8, p. 405.

15. Cooper et al., note 11, p. 81.

16. Sekine, M. & Takami, H. (1998). Combination of calcitonin and pamidronate for emergency treatment of malignant hypercalcemia. *Oncology Reports, 5,* 197–199.

17. Cooper et al., note 11, p. 81.

18. Cooper et al., note 11, p. 81.

19. Cooper et al., note 11, p. 81.

20. Cooper et al., note 11, p. 81.

21. Onitilo, A. A., Kio, E., & Doi, S. A. (2007). Tumor-related hyponatremia. *Clinical Medicine & Research, 5*(4), 228–237.

22. Lin, M., Liu, S. J., & Lim, I. T. (2005). Disorders of water imbalance. *Emergency Medicine Clinics of North America, 23*(3), 749–770.

23. Webberley, M. J., & Murray, J. A. (1989). Life-threatening acute hyponatraemia induced by low dose cyclophosphamide and indomethacin. *Postgraduate Medical Journal, 65*(770), 950–952.

24. Bissett, D., Cornford, E. J., & Sokal, M. (1989). Hyponatraemia following cisplatin chemotherapy. *Acta Oncologica, 28*(6), 823.

25. Bissett et al., note 24.

26. Hunter, R. J., Pace, M. B., Burns, K. A., Burke, C. C., Gonzales, D. A., Webb, N. F., et al. (2009). Evaluation of intervention to prevent hypomagnesemia in cervical cancer patients receiving combination cisplatin and radiation treatment. *Supportive Care in Cancer, 17*(9), 1195–1201.

27. Kramer, J. H., Spurney, C., Iantorno, M., Tziros, C., Mak, I. T., Tejero-Taldo, M. I., et al. (2009). Neurogenic inflammation and cardiac dysfunction due to hypomagnesemia. *American Journal of the Medical Sciences, 338*(1), 22–27.

28. Bashir, H., Crom, D., Metzger, M., Mulcahey, J., Jones, D., & Hudson, M. M. (2007). Cisplatin-induced hypomagnesemia and cardiac dysrhythmia. *Pediatric Blood & Cancer, 49,* 867–869.

29. Saif, M. W. (2008). Management of hypomagnesemia in cancer patients receiving chemotherapy. *Journal of Supportive Oncology, 6*(5), 243–248.

30. Fiset, C., Kargacin, M. E., Kondo, C. S., Lester, W. M., & Duff, H. J. (1996). Hypomagnesemia: Characterization of a model of sudden cardiac death. *Journal of the American College of Cardiology, 27,* 1771–1776.

31. Noh, G. Y., Choe. D. H., Kim, C. H., & Lee, J. C. (2008). Fatal tumor lysis syndrome during radiotherapy for non–small-cell lung cancer. *Journal of Clinical Oncology, 26*(36), 6005–6006.

32. Cheson, B. D. (2009). Etiology and management of tumor lysis syndrome in patients with chronic lymphocytic leukemia. *Clinical Advances in Hematology and Oncology, 7*(4), 263–271.

33. Govindan, note 8, p 405.

34. Govindan, note 8, p 405.

35. Tosi, P., Barosi, G., Lazzaro, C., Liso, V., Marchetti, M., Morra, E., et al. (2008). Consensus conference on the management of tumor lysis syndrome. *Haematologica, 93*(12), 1877–1885.

36. Tosi, note 35.

37. Kollef, M. H., Bedient, T. J., Isakow, W., & Witt, C. A. (2008). *The Washington manual of critical care.* Philadelphia: Wolters Kluwer/Lippincott Williams & Wilkins, p. 219.

38. Govindan, note 8, p 406.

39. Bongard, F. S., Sue, D. Y., & Vinch, J. R. (2008). *Current diagnosis and treatment* (3rd ed.). New York: McGraw-Hill/Lange, p. 462.

40. Givens, M. L., & Wethern, J. (2009). Renal complications in oncologic patients. *Emergency Medicine Clinics of North America, 27*(2), 283–291.

41. Givens & Wethren, note 40.

42. Cooper et al., note 11, p. 592.

43. Cooper et al., note 11, p. 592.

44. Givens & Wethren, note 40.

45. Govindan, note 8, p. 406.

46. Elisaf, M., Kalaitizidis, R., & Siamopoulos, K. (1998). Multiple electrolyte abnormalities after pamidronate administration. *Nephron, 79,* 337–339.

47. Bashir et al, note 28.

48. Bashir, et al. note 28.

Chapter 23

Pregnancy

Normal changes in fluid and electrolyte balance occur during pregnancy to support fetal growth. Unfortunately, harmful changes may occur in pathologic conditions associated with pregnancy, such as hyperemesis gravidarum and eclampsia. Before discussing the latter conditions, it is helpful to briefly review the normal fluid and electrolyte status in pregnancy.

NORMAL PHYSIOLOGICAL WATER AND ELECTROLYTE CHANGES IN PREGNANCY

Retained Sodium and Water

Increased production of progesterone and aldosterone occurs during pregnancy. These hormones, in turn, contribute to expansion of maternal plasma volume by promoting sodium and water retention.[1] During pregnancy, a 30% to 45% gain in blood volume may be expected.[2,3] Because of the increased plasma volume, hemoglobin and hematocrit levels decrease slightly, resulting in decreased blood viscosity.

During a normal pregnancy, the average weight gain is approximately 24 pounds, most of which is accrued during the second and third trimesters.[4] Approximately 6 of these 24 pounds result from extra fluid in the extracellular compartment (plasma and interstitial space).[5] The extra sodium and water retained during pregnancy are excreted in the mother's urine during the first few postpartum days.[6]

Edema

Approximately three-fourths of pregnant women experience edema at some time during their pregnancy. Redistribution of fluid between the intracellular and extracellular compartments, secondary to sodium retention, is associated with the "physiological" edema of many normal pregnancies. Most common is the *dependent edema* observed when the pregnant woman assumes an upright position. Impingement of blood flow through the inferior vena cava by the pregnant uterus causes stagnation of blood in the lower extremities. When the pregnant woman elevates her legs or lies on her side, the hydrostatic pressure is partially overcome and interstitial fluid is returned to the general circulation. *Generalized edema* is manifested by rapid weight gain and edema of the hands and upper half of the body. This type of edema can also occur in normal pregnancy. When generalized edema is accompanied by a rise in blood pressure and proteinuria, however, it is considered a disease process.

Serum Electrolyte Concentrations

Although a pregnant woman retains approximately 1000 mEq of sodium during pregnancy, the serum sodium concentration is decreased slightly because of her expanded plasma volume.[7] The serum sodium concentration may decrease by 5 mEq/L during late pregnancy and the plasma osmolality may decrease by 10 mOsm/kg.[8] These responses are partly due to increased levels of antidiuretic hormone (ADH), which in turn cause water retention.

Approximately 300 mEq of potassium is retained during pregnancy (two-thirds of which is present in the products of conception); however, the maternal serum potassium level decreases slightly because of dilution by the expanded plasma volume.[9] Both the total and ionized magnesium fractions decline during pregnancy; however, the serum phosphate level remains within the nonpregnant range.[10] The maternal total serum calcium concentration begins to decrease during the second or third month of pregnancy and reaches its lowest point during the third trimester. Contributing to the lowered total serum calcium concentration is a reduced albumin concentration. Despite the lowered total serum calcium level, the ionized calcium concentration remains within normal range.[11]

Calcium Balance

Enlargement of the maternal parathyroid glands with subsequent increased production of parathyroid hormone (PTH) occurs during pregnancy and serves to increase calcium absorption from the mother's bones as the fetal bones are developing. Also, maternal absorption of calcium from the small bowel doubles during pregnancy.[12] After the baby's birth, the PTH secretion intensifies during lactation because the growing baby requires even more calcium than does a fetus.[13]

The amount of calcium required by the fetus during pregnancy is small in relation to the total maternal store of calcium. Given this fact, the recommendation for adequate intake of calcium in pregnant women is the same as in non-pregnant women: 1000 mg per day in women 19 years or older, and 1300 mg for adolescents 18 years or younger.[14]

Acid–Base Changes

Progesterone has a potent stimulating effect on the medullary respiratory center. The resulting hyperventilation causes the partial pressure of arterial carbon dioxide ($PaCO_2$) to decrease by several millimeters of mercury and the arterial pH to become elevated (mild respiratory alkalosis). To compensate for these changes, the serum bicarbonate concentration also decreases slightly. Therefore, if the serum bicarbonate concentration is normal or elevated in late pregnancy, the possibility of a second imbalance—specifically, metabolic alkalosis—should be investigated. Possible causes of the latter could be persistent vomiting or excessive use of potassium-losing diuretics.

ABNORMAL CONDITIONS IN PREGNANCY ASSOCIATED WITH FLUID AND ELECTROLYTE IMBALANCES

Hyperemesis Gravidarum

Hyperemesis gravidarum (HG) apparently represents the extreme end of the spectrum of nausea and vomiting of

pregnancy.[15] While most pregnant women experience mild to moderate nausea and vomiting during the first 14 to 16 weeks of gestation, only a small percentage develop HG. In an attempt to quantify nausea and vomiting, a group of investigators developed a scale named the Pregnancy-Unique Quantification of Emesis and Nausea Index (PUQE).[16] The three components of the scale, measured over a 12-hour period, are frequency of nausea, frequency of emesis, and frequency of retching without vomiting. In a more recent publication, the investigators expanded the scale to cover a 24-hour period.[17] See **Table 23-1**.

Risk factors for HG include multiple gestations, family history (genetics), a history of HG during previous pregnancies, and motion sickness.[18] Serious problems associated with HG include weight loss, dehydration, metabolic alkalosis, and hypokalemia (secondary to prolonged vomiting and loss of gastric acid). In a retrospective study of 166 women hospitalized with HG, hypokalemia was found to be associated with adverse pregnancy outcome.[19] If caloric intake is severely decreased, starvational ketoacidosis—a form of metabolic acidosis—can also complicate the situation. HG is the second most common reason for hospitalization of pregnant women.[20]

The incidence of HG is reported to range from 0.5% to 2% of pregnancies.[21] Two recent studies suggest that the incidence of HG is less than 1%. For example, a study of 520,739 births in California found that HG complicated 0.47% (2466) of the births.[22] Similarly, a study of 156,091 singleton pregnancies in Nova Scotia found that hospital admission for HG occurred in 0.81% (1270) women.[23] As mentioned earlier, a genetic component has been suggested for HG because of the high prevalence of severe nausea and vomiting/hyperemesis gravidarum among relatives of women with HG.[24]

Infants of HG women are more likely to have a low birth weight compared to infants of women without HG.[25] Because poor maternal weight gain is generally associated with adverse outcomes, it is not surprising that obese women who develop HG are less likely to require hospitalization.[26]

Use of vitamin B_6, or vitamin B_6 plus doxylamine, has been recommended as a first-line form of pharmacotherapy.[27] A recent survey of more than 1000 obstetrician-gynecologists found that the most frequently recommended treatments for pregnant women with moderate to severe nausea with occasional vomiting were "eat frequent, small meals" (93%), "snack on soda crackers" (68.5%), and "take vitamin B_6 plus doxylamine" (67.1%).[28] It has also been

Table 23-1 Motherisk PUQE-24 Scoring System

In the last 24 hours, for how long have you felt nauseated or sick to your stomach?	Not at all (1)	1 hour or less (2)	2–3 hours (3)	4–6 hours (4)	More than 6 hours (5)
In the last 24 hours, have you vomited or thrown up?	7 or more times (5)	5–6 times (4)	3–4 times (3)	1–2 times (2)	I did not throw up (1)
In the last 24 hours, how many times have you had retching or dry heaves without bringing anything up?	No time (1)	1–2 times (2)	3–4 times (3)	5–6 times (4)	7 or more times (5)

PUQE-24 score: Mild ≤ 6; Moderate = 7–12; Severe = 13–15

How many hours have you slept out of 24 hours? Why?
On a scale of 0 to 10, how would you rate your well-being?
0 (worst possible); 10 (the best you felt before pregnancy)
Can you tell me what causes you to feel that way?

Source: Reprinted from Ebrahimi, N., Maltepe, C., Bournissen, F. G., & Koren, G. (2009). Nausea and vomiting of pregnancy: Using the 24-hour Pregnancy-Unique Quantification of Emesis (PUQE-24) Scale. *Journal of Obstetrics & Gynaecology Canada, 31*(9), 803–807. Permission to reprint has been provided courtesy of the Society of Obstetricians and Gynaecologists of Canada.

suggested that ginger, an herbal remedy, may be effective (although more research has been advocated).[29] Fortunately, in most women, the nausea and vomiting eventually subside as the pregnancy progresses.

A variety of treatments have been used for women with HG. For those whose vomiting is so severe that fluids cannot be retained, intravenous fluid replacement is required. It is important to prevent dehydration, as prolonged dehydration can lead to acute renal failure.[30] Among the types of parenteral fluids described in the treatment of HG are lactated Ringer's solution and isotonic saline, with added dextrose and multivitamins.[31] Of course, fluid replacement needs will vary according to the individual patient.

A protocol of drug therapy found to be effective in a cohort of 130 pregnant women with HG consisted of a combination of metoclopramide and diphenhydramine.[32] In a study of 92 women with HG, a placebo-controlled trial of oral pyridoxine, in conjunction with metoclopramide, did not improve the vomiting frequency or the nausea score; however, the investigators recommended a larger trial before completely ruling out the efficacy of these medications.[33] Alternative therapies, such as herbal teas and P6 accupoint stimulation, have been considered. However, in a randomized controlled trial that involved 80 patients with nausea and vomiting (plus ketonuria) before 14 weeks of gestation, acupressure at the P6 point did not reduce the amount antiemetic medication or fluid required between treatments.[34]

Prolonged starvation in the pregnant woman has adverse effects on both the mother and the fetus. For example, thiamine deficiency associated with malnutrition in the pregnant woman with HG can lead to Wernicke's encephalopathy. For this reason, prophylactic thiamine supplementation is recommended, along with a method to improve nutrient intake.[35] Inability to consume adequate calories may necessitate the use of a feeding tube[36, 37] or a central line for parenteral nutrition. Some authors caution against the routine use of a peripherally inserted central venous catheter in women with HG because of the possibility of complications such as infection and thrombophlebitis.[38] In rare instances,

HG may lead to termination of the pregnancy. Among the reasons reported by women with HG who chose to terminate their pregnancies were inability to care for their family or self, fear that the baby could die, or fear that the baby would be abnormal.[39]

Preeclampsia/Eclampsia

Preeclampsia is a multiorgan disease of unknown etiology that occurs in as many as 6% to 8% of all pregnancies, usually after 20 weeks gestation.[40] It is characterized by hypertension with proteinuria (greater than 1.0 g/L in a random urine specimen or 0.3 g/L in a 24-hour urine specimen).[41] In women with severe preeclampsia, edema is usually much greater than the edema found in normal pregnant women.[42] In addition to generalized edema and proteinuria, there is a decreased plasma oncotic pressure, which adds to the probability of movement of fluid from the vascular space into the interstitium.[43] Electrolyte concentrations are not appreciably different in women with preeclampsia when compared to those of normal pregnant women, unless sodium has been restricted or vigorous diuresis has been achieved.[44] Arterial spasms occur in multiple parts of the mother's body (especially the kidneys, brain, and liver).[45] A systolic blood pressure of 140 mm Hg or greater or a diastolic pressure of 90 mm Hg or greater observed after 20 weeks of gestation raises the suspicion for preeclampsia. A more severe form of preeclampsia is characterized by a systolic pressure of 160 mm Hg or greater or a diastolic pressure of 110 mm Hg or greater, plus proteinuria of 5 g/L or more in 24 hours.[46]

Eclampsia is a more severe condition in which seizures occur in addition to vascular spasms throughout the mother's body. Following seizures, lactic acidosis—a form of metabolic acidosis—may occur. The severity of the lactic acidosis depends on the amount of lactic acid produced during the seizure activity. In addition to seizures, eclampsia may be accompanied by coma, extreme hypertension, and impaired urine output.[47] Without treatment, eclampsia is associated with a high mortality.[48] Eclamptic women do not develop the expected plasma volume expansion seen in normal pregnant women.[49] Although plasma levels of aldosterone in eclamptic women are higher than the nonpregnant values, they do not approach the levels found in normal pregnancy.[50]

Management

Hospitalization is considered for pregnant women with new-onset hypertension, especially if this condition is accompanied by proteinuria. Important clinical findings to consider include headache, visual disturbances, worsening hypertension, and elevated serum creatinine levels. Several studies support the benefit of restricted activity.[51, 52] However, "complete bedrest" predisposes pregnant women to thromboembolism.[53] Termination of pregnancy is the only cure for preeclampsia.[54]

Magnesium Sulfate as an Anticonvulsant. Magnesium sulfate is widely used to prevent and treat eclamptic seizures. By acting as a vasodilator, it may decrease peripheral vascular resistance or relieve vasoconstriction.[55] Magnesium sulfate most likely exerts an anticonvulsant action on the cerebral cortex while avoiding central nervous system depression in both mother and infant.[56] Although it can be given intramuscularly, it is almost always administered intravenously.

Magnesium sulfate has been found to be superior to a variety of other drugs for managing eclampsia, including phenytoin,[57] nimodipine,[58] and diazepam.[59] Protocols for magnesium sulfate administration begin with a loading dose followed by a maintenance dose for as long as needed. Because magnesium sulfate is primarily cleared through the kidneys, it is important to monitor renal function during its administration. An adequate urine output (such as 25 mL/hr or more) is often used as an indicator that it is safe to administer magnesium sulfate. However, the best way to assess renal function is to monitor the serum creatinine level.[60] When the serum creatinine level is greater than 1.0 mg/dL, the magnesium infusion rate is adjusted according to serum magnesium levels.[61] The therapeutic serum magnesium level during treatment for preeclampsia/eclampsia is between 4 and 7 mEq/L (4.8 and 8.4 mg/dL).[62] **Table 23-2** identifies approximate total serum magnesium levels to consider in the management of preeclampsia/eclampsia.

A serum magnesium level should be requested if any of the following conditions is present:

- Respiratory rate < 12 breaths per minute
- Urine output < 100 mL in 4 hours
- Patellar reflex absent

Calcium gluconate or calcium chloride should be readily available as an antidote during the administration of magnesium sulfate. When respiratory depression is severe, tracheal intubation and mechanical ventilation may be needed to support ventilation.

Other Therapies. If severe hypertension is present, cerebrovascular hemorrhage, hypertensive encephalopathy, and

Table 23-2 Approximate Total Serum Magnesium Levels to Consider in Treatment of Eclampsia

Total Serum Magnesium Concentration	mEq/L	mg/dL	mmol/L
Normal range	1.3 to 2.1	1.6 to 2.5	0.65 to 1.10
Therapeutic range to prevent convulsions	4 to 7	4.8 to 8.4	2.0 to 3.5
Patellar reflex is lost	7 to 10	8.4 to 12	3.5 to 5.0
Respiratory depression	10	12	5.0
Respiratory paralysis	10 to 15	12 to 18	5.0 to 7.5
Cardiac arrest	15 to 20	18 to 24	7.5 to 10

eclamptic convulsions may occur. Thus treatments are initiated to lower systolic pressures to 160 mm Hg or less, using agents such as hydralazine, labetalol, and nifedipine.[63]

Healthcare providers must be aware that women with severe preeclampsia have a diminished intravascular volume compared to women with normal pregnancy. Thus aggressive fluid replacement in women with severe preeclampsia increases risk for pulmonary edema, cerebral edema, and pharyngolaryngeal edema.[64] An example of a reasonable fluid rate might be 60 mL to no more than 125 mL per hour of lactated Ringer's solution in a preeclamptic woman;[65] however, individual patient characteristics will dictate actual fluid orders in specific patients.

Hyponatremia and Oxytocin Administration

Oxytocin is used in a majority of births in the United States.[66, 67] As with any medication, it has the potential for adverse effects. The possible adverse effects associated with electrolyte balance are discussed in this section.

The hyponatremia associated with water overload is often called "water intoxication" or "dilutional hyponatremia." Symptoms associated with this condition include lethargy, headache, blurred vision, twitching, seizures, and coma. A case was reported in 2009 in which a 26-year-old woman with postpartum bleeding was given 7500 mL of 5% dextrose in water that contained oxytocin (100 IU/L) over a 15-hour period.[68] Roughly 24 hours later, the patient's serum sodium concentration decreased to 113 mEq/L; 3 hours afterward, she suffered generalized convulsions and lost consciousness. Fortunately, following treatment with hypertonic saline and mannitol, she regained consciousness; her serum sodium concentration normalized after 48 hours and a full recovery was eventually made. (The treatment for hyponatremia is discussed in depth in Chapter 4.) Without treatment, hyponatremia can lead to permanent neurologi-

cal sequelae or even death of the mother. Moreover, the newborn infant of a hyponatremic mother is at high risk for developing hyponatremia because of the close correlation between maternal and cord blood.[69, 70]

In the United States, virtually all facilities routinely administer oxytocin in an isotonic electrolyte solution (such as lactated Ringer's or isotonic saline). For example, a study reported in 2002 showed that only 2% of randomly selected obstetrical units in the United States used 5% dextrose in water to administer oxytocin or for the mainline intravenous solution.[71]

Hydration During Labor

In most labor units, oral fluids are restricted because of the risk for aspiration if an unanticipated general anesthetic is required.[72] Typical fluid orders call for 125 mL of IV fluid per hour in laboring nulliparous women with limited oral intake.[73] In women who receive an epidural block, it is common practice to administer a fluid bolus prior to placement of the epidural catheter.[74, 75] This fluid bolus is given because sympathetic blockage from an analgesic that is injected epidurally may cause hypotension and decreased cardiac output.[76]

Hydration with 500 to 1000 mL of lactated Ringer's solution may be recommended for this purpose. After the fluid bolus, IV fluids are typically provided continuously.[77] In a study reported in 1997, researchers found that 31% of 243 women who received a epidural block experienced hypotension.[78] In the same study, intravenous fluids were given to treat hypotension (defined as a systolic blood pressure less than 25% of the baseline or a systolic blood pressure less than 100 mm Hg). If hypotension was persistent, it was treated with ephedrine as needed.

Finally, although extremely rare, cases have been reported in which laboring women drank large quantities of water and lowered their serum sodium concentrations to dangerous levels.[79,80] In one case report, a woman had consumed approximately 8 L of water within a 13.5-hour period during labor; her infant's serum sodium level was found to be 121 mEq/L.[81] This issue is important because maternal hyponatremia can be transferred to the infant via the placenta.

Fluid and Electrolyte Disturbances Associated with Tocolytic Therapy

Nearly half of the more than 500,000 preterm births each year are the result of preterm labor; further, the focus of treatment for these women is tocolytic therapy.[82] Administration of tocolytic agents may delay delivery for at least 48 hours in some women.[83, 84] Among the drugs used for this purpose are magnesium sulfate, beta-adrenergic receptor agonists, prostaglandin inhibitors, and calcium-channel blockers.

Pharmacologic doses of magnesium are frequently used to inhibit labor. However, because of this drug's potential for toxicity, women receiving magnesium sulfate must be monitored closely for signs of hypermagnesemia (see Table 7-4). Hypocalcemia may be associated with magnesium sulfate tocolytic therapy, possibly because it leads to decreased parathyroid hormone secretion or increased renal excretion of calcium; however, only rarely does symptomatic hypocalcemia occur.[85, 86] The risk for symptomatic hypocalcemia may potentially be greater when magnesium sulfate and nifedipine are used together as tocolytic agents.[87] The overall efficacy of magnesium sulfate as a tocolytic agent has been questioned by some authors.[88] While toxic maternal magnesium levels can injure the fetus,[89] some evidence suggests that maternal magnesium sulfate therapy has a fetal neuroprotective effect.[90]

Ritodrine and terbutaline are beta-adrenergic receptor agonists used in the United States to inhibit preterm labor.[91,92] These drugs may cause hypokalemia by stimulating cellular uptake of potassium in women treated for preterm labor. For this reason, it is recommended that electrolytes be monitored during tocolytic therapy with ritodrine and terbutaline.[93] Beta-adrenergic receptor agonists also cause retention of sodium and water, and their administration can lead to volume overload.[94] As such, tocolytic therapy with beta-adrenergic agonists is a risk factor for pulmonary edema in pregnant women; another risk factor is the infusion of large volumes of crystalloids intravenously.[95]

Although calcium-channel blockers were developed to treat hypertension, they are also used as tocolytics. Several studies have suggested that these agents—such as nifedipine—are safer and more effective than the beta-adrenergic agonists for the latter indication.[96, 97] For example, in a study that compared metabolic changes after ritodrine and nifedipine tocolysis, researchers found that mean serum potassium levels were lower in the ritodrine-treated group 48 hours after starting tocolysis; for this reason, the investigators preferred nifedipine for the treatment of preterm labor.[98]

Pica

Pica is an eating disorder defined as the compulsive ingestion of a nonfood substance.[99]

It is most commonly reported in areas of low socioeconomic status and in women, especially those who are pregnant.[100] The cause of pica remains unclear.

In a study reported in 2003, more than one-third (38%) of 128 women receiving prenatal care in two rural communities reported practicing pica.[101] The practice was more frequent among African American women than in other ethnic groups. Among the substances ingested by these women were clay dirt, baked clay dirt, laundry starch, cornstarch, and freezer frost. The women who reported pica were significantly more likely to have been underweight and have low hematocrit concentrations prior to pregnancy, as compared to women who did not practice pica. The authors of the study recommended that nurses query patients in a nonjudgmental manner about pica practices, because the practices may have cultural implications unknown to the nurse. Clay (sometimes referred to as "white dirt") can be readily purchased in some southern states.

Other nonfood substances reportedly consumed by individuals practicing pica include ashes, chalk, crayons, and detergent.[102] Depending on the ingested substance, pica can lead to electrolyte disorders. Case Study 5-3 describes a pregnant woman who ate large quantities of baking soda and subsequently developed metabolic alkalosis and hypokalemia.[103] In yet another case, a 44-year-old pregnant woman at 31 weeks gestation was admitted to the emergency department with progressive fatigue and muscle weakness for 1 month and leg pain for 3 days.[104] Her serum potassium level at admission was 1.5 mEq/L; despite intravenous and oral potassium replacement, the serum potassium concentration did not normalize over the next 4 days. On the fourth day, a family member pointed out that the patient regularly ingested clay (a large bag of which was found in the patient's purse). The patient was advised to stop eating clay. Over the next 2 days, her weakness and myalgia resolved as her serum potassium level normalized. Ingested clay likely binds to potassium in the bowel and, therefore, can lead to hypokalemia.[105]

CASE STUDIES

Case Study 23-1

A case was reported in which a 21-year-old multiparous woman at 16 weeks gestation was admitted to the emergency department with an altered mental status.[106] According to the patient's family, she had experienced nausea and vomiting for the previous 6 weeks. A previous pregnancy was complicated by severe hyperemesis gravidarum and required multiple hospital admissions for intravenous therapy. At the end of the previous pregnancy, the patient had delivered a normal term infant.

Upon admission to the emergency department for her current illness, the patient had a heart rate of 130 beats per minute, a temperature of 37.4°C, and a blood pressure of 89/43 mm Hg. Although there was no history of prior renal disease, her blood urea nitrogen (BUN) was 171 mg/dL and her serum creatinine level was 10.7 mg/dL. Following insertion of a Foley catheter, her hourly urine output was 10 mL. Several liters of intravenous fluid were administered and hemodialysis was started within 5 hours of admission. The hemodialysis was continued for 5 consecutive days, during which serial measurements of serum creatinine and BUN showed improvements.

A psychological consult was obtained on the third hospital day and revealed no element of disorder. An abdominal ultrasound revealed a 16-week gestation with ventriculomegaly and a Dandy-Walker malformation. On the fifth hospital day, the patient elected to terminate her pregnancy. A renal biopsy on day 6 demonstrated acute tubular necrosis. By the twelfth hospital day, the patient's BUN and serum creatinine were significantly improved— 15 mg/dL and 2.2 mg/dL, respectively. Two weeks after discharge, her serum creatinine was 0.5 mg/dL and her BUN was 6 mg/dL.

Commentary. This case demonstrates that the dehydration associated with hyperemesis gravidarum can lead to renal hypoperfusion and acute tubular necrosis. Fortunately, following appropriate management, the patient's renal function eventually returned to normal.

Case Study 23-2

A case was reported in which a one-day-old male infant was admitted to the ICU of a children's hospital because of episodes of slight cyanosis, paleness, and oxygen desaturation (pulse oximetry = 74%).[107] The neonate's breathing was shallow and periodic (20 breaths per minute), with normal symmetrical sounds. Venous blood sampling demonstrated hypochloremic metabolic alkalosis (pH = 7.48), elevated bicarbonate concentration (38.5 mEq/L), and decreased chloride concentration (82 mEq/L). The infant's serum potassium level was also low (2.4 mEq/L). A serum potassium level from the infant's mother just prior to delivery (a routine measurement) was 1.5 mEq/L; at the same time, a venous blood gas analysis revealed that the mother also had hypochloremic metabolic alkalosis (pH = 7.63, serum bicarbonate = 34.6 mEq/L, and serum chloride = 84 mEq/L).

Because of the similar electrolyte and blood gas disturbances in the infant and the mother, the authors reviewed the mother's pregnancy history and found that she had eaten poorly during the first 3 to 5 months of pregnancy due to nausea and vomiting. Following resolution of the nausea and vomiting, she deliberately continued to eat poorly. As a result, she apparently gained only 2 kg during the pregnancy. A possible explanation for the maternal hypochloremic metabolic alkalosis was self-induced vomiting, although this behavior was denied by the mother. Therefore, the cause of the mother's metabolic alkalosis was deemed inconclusive. It was presumed that the infant's shallow slow breathing was compensatory for metabolic alkalosis and led to the lowered oxygenation status. Fortunately, the infant's metabolic abnormalities resolved.

Commentary. The authors of the case study pointed out that an electrolyte/acid–base disturbance of the mother can be transplacentally transferred to the infant.[108] Further, a transplacentally transferred metabolic alkalosis can cause compensatory hypoventilation with oxygen desaturation on the newborn.

Case Study 23-3

A case was reported in which a 31-year-old primigravida at 32 weeks gestation with twins experienced spontaneous rupture of her membranes.[109] Tocolytic therapy with magnesium sulfate ($MgSO_4$) was administered, along with betamethasone and prophylactic antibiotics. (A loading dose of 4 g $MgSO_4$ was followed by $MgSO_4$ infusion at a rate of approximately 2.5 g/hr.) After almost a day of tocolytic therapy, a routine blood test revealed a serum magnesium level of 9.0 mg/dL. (According to the case report, the upper limit desired for this patient was 7 mg/dL.) As a result of the elevated serum magnesium level, tocolysis was stopped immediately. Although the mother stated she was sleepy, she could be aroused and was oriented. Her deep tendon reflexes were present, although depressed. External fetal monitoring showed normal heart rates, decreased beat-to-beat variability, and no periodic decelerations. Approximately 42 hours after the mother's admission, a cesarean delivery was performed and twins were delivered. The first twin died 30 minutes after delivery, despite vigorous resuscitation attempts; no abnormalities were noted on autopsy. The second twin required intubation at the time of delivery. On the day of delivery, the second twin had a serum magnesium level of 3.9 mg/dL (the upper limit of normal in the reporting laboratory was 2.5 mg/dL). On the sixth day after delivery, an ECG revealed nonspecific S-T wave abnormalities; by day 13, the infant's ECG was normal.

Commentary. The authors of this case report concluded that the death of the first infant was probably attributable to maternal magnesium toxicity.[110] While the mother's serum magnesium level was 9.0 mg/dL, the fetal magnesium level may have been even higher. The day after delivery, the surviving twin's serum magnesium level was still 56% above normal. The authors recommended that neonatologists who attend deliveries be aware that unexpected death may occur in infants who were exposed to high doses of tocolytic $MgSO_4$.

Case Study 23-4

A case was reported in 2006 in which an 18-year-old woman who was 7 months pregnant died from an overdose of magnesium sulfate administered to slow her early labor.[111] Instead of administering 4 g of magnesium sulfate, a nurse inadvertently administered 16 g of the drug. Shortly after receiving this dose, the patient experienced difficulty breathing. When the condition was recognized, caregivers administered calcium but were unsuccessful in resuscitating the patient.

Commentary. Errors in administering magnesium sulfate are facilitated by the availability of the drug in various strengths and containers. Extreme caution is warranted to prevent errors. (See Table 7-3.) Excellent recommendations to prevent errors in the administration of magnesium sulfate in an obstetric setting are provided by Simpson.[112]

Summary of Key Points

- Although a pregnant woman retains approximately 1000 mEq of sodium, her serum sodium concentration will be decreased slightly because of her expanded plasma volume. The serum sodium concentration may decrease by 5 mEq/L during late pregnancy.

- Approximately 300 mEq of potassium is retained during pregnancy (two-thirds of which is present in the products of conception); however, the serum potassium level decreases slightly owing to dilution by the expanded plasma volume.

- Progesterone has a potent stimulating effect on the medullary respiratory center. The resulting hyperventilation causes the partial pressure of arterial carbon dioxide ($PaCO_2$) to decrease by several millimeters of mercury and the arterial pH to become elevated (mild respiratory alkalosis).

- Maternal absorption of calcium from the small bowel doubles during pregnancy to support the developing fetus.

- Serious problems associated with hyperemesis gravidarum include fluid volume deficit, metabolic alkalosis, and hypokalemia (secondary to prolonged vomiting and loss of gastric acid).

- Magnesium sulfate is widely used as a tocolytic agent and to prevent and treat eclamptic seizures in pregnant women. If used incorrectly, it can lead to life-threatening hypermagnesemia.

- Because the pharmacological action of oxytocin includes a potent antidiuretic effect, this agent can lead to severe hyponatremia if it is administered in a high dose in a large volume of electrolyte-free aqueous dextrose solution.

- Depending on the ingested substance, pica—the compulsive ingestion of a nonfood substance—can lead to electrolyte disorders.

Also see Case Studies 3-3, 5-3, and 6-11 regarding fluid and electrolyte problems that have occurred in pregnant women.

NOTES

1. Escher, G. (2009). Hyperaldosteronism in pregnancy. *Therapeutic Advances in Cardiovascular Disease, 3*(2), 123–132.

2. Guyton, A. C., & Hall, J. E. (2006). *Textbook of medical physiology* (11th ed.). Philadelphia: Saunders Elsevier, p. 1034.

3. Whittaker, P. G., Macphail, S., & Lind, T. (1996). Serial hematologic changes and pregnancy outcome. *Obstetrics & Gynecology, 88,* 33–39.

4. Guyton & Hall, note 2, p. 1034.

5. Guyton & Hall, note 2, p. 1034.

6. Guyton & Hall, note 2, p. 1034.

7. Cunningham, F. G., Leveno, K. J., Bloom, S. L., Hauth, J. C., Rouse, D. J., & Spong, C. Y. (2010). *Williams obstetrics* (23rd ed.). New York: McGraw-Hill Medical, p. 114.

8. Paller, M., & Ferris, T. (1994). Fluid and electrolyte metabolism during pregnancy. In: G. Narins (Ed.), *Maxwell and Kleeman's clinical disorders of fluid and electrolyte metabolism* (5th ed.). New York: McGraw-Hill, p. 1128.

9. Lindheimer, M. D., Richardson, D. A., Ehrlich, E. N., & Katz, A. I. (1987). Potassium homeostasis in pregnancy. *Journal of Reproductive Medicine, 32*(7), 517–522.

10. Cunningham et al., note 7, p. 113.

11. Cunningham et al., note 7, p. 114.

12. Cunningham et al., note 7, p. 114.

13. Guyton & Hall, note 2, p. 1034.

14. Alpers, D. H., Stenson, W. F., Taylor, B. E., & Bier, D. M. (2008). *Manual of nutritional therapeutics* (5th ed.). Philadelphia: Wolters Kluwer/Lippincott Williams & Wilkins, p. 66.

15. Klebanoff, M. A., Koslowe, P. A., Kaslow, R., & Rhoads, G. G. (1985). Epidemiology of vomiting in early pregnancy. *Obstetrics & Gynecology, 66,* 612–616.

16. Koren, G., Boskovic, R., Hard, M., Maltepe, C., Navioz, Y., & Einarson, A. (2002). Motherisk-PUQE (Pregnancy-Unique Quantification of Emesis and Nausea) scoring system for nausea and vomiting of pregnancy. *American Journal of Obstetrics & Gynecology, 186*(5 Suppl), S228–S231.

17. Ebrahimi, N., Maltepe, C., Bournissen, F. G., & Koren, G. (2009). Nausea and vomiting of pregnancy: Using the 24-hour Pregnancy-Unique Quantification of Emesis (PUQE-24) scale. *Journal of Obstetrics & Gynaecology Canada, 31*(9), 803–807.

18. ACOG (American College of Obstetrics and Gynecology) Practice Bulletin 52: Nausea and vomiting of pregnancy. (2004). *Obstetrics & Gynecology. 103*(4), 803–814.

19. Tan, P. C., Jacob, R., Quek, K. F., & Omar, S. Z. (2007). Pregnancy outcome in hyperemesis gravidarum and the effect of laboratory clinical indicators of hyperemesis severity. *Journal of Obstetrics & Gynecology Research, 33*(4), 457–464.

20. Lacasse, A., Lagoutte, A., Ferreira, E., & Berard, A. (2009). Metoclopropamide and diphenhydramine in the treatment of hyperemesis gravidarum: Effectiveness and predictors of rehospitalisation. *European Journal of Obstetrics, Gynecology & Reproductive Biology, 143*(1), 43–49.

21. ACOG Practice Bulletin 52, note 18.

22. Bailit, J. L. (2005). Hyperemesis gravidarum: Epidemiologic findings from a large cohort. *Obstetrics & Gynecology, 193*(3 Part 1), 811–814.

23. Dodds, L., Fell, D. B., Joseph, K. S., Allen, V. M., & Butler, B. (2006). Outcomes of pregnancies complicated by hyperemesis gravidarum. *Obstetrics & Gynecology, 107*(2 Part 1), 285–292.

24. Fejzo, M. S., Ingles, S. A., Wilson, M., Wang, W., MacGibbon, K., Romero, R., et al. (2008). High prevalence of severe nausea and vomiting of pregnancy and hyperemesis gravidarum among relatives of affected individuals. *European Journal of Obstetrics, Gynecology, and Reproductive Biology, 141*(1), 13–17.

25. Bailit, note 22.

26. Cedergren, M., Brynhildsen, J., Josefsson, A., Sydsjo, A., & Sydsjo, G. (2008). Hyperemesis gravidarum that requires hospitalization and the use of antiemetic drugs in relation to maternal body composition. *American Journal of Obstetrics & Gynecology, 198,* 412.

27. ACOG Practice Bulletin 52, note 18.

28. Power, M. L., Milligan, L. A., & Schulkin, J. (2007). Managing nausea and vomiting of pregnancy: A survey of obstetrician-gynecologists. *Journal of Reproductive Medicine, 52*(10), 922–928.

29. Borrelli, F., Capasso, R., Aviello, G., Pittler, M. H., & Izzo, A. A. (2005). Effectiveness and safety of ginger in the treatment of pregnancy-induced nausea and vomiting. *Obstetrics & Gynecology, 105*(4), 849–856.

30. Hill, J. B., Yost, N. P., & Wendel, G. D. (2002). Acute renal failure in association with severe hyperemesis gravidarum. *Obstetrics & Gynecology, 100*(5 Part 2), 1119–1121.

31. Tasci, Y., Demir, B., Dilbaz, S., & Haberal, A. (2009). Use of diazepam for hyperemesis gravidarum. *Journal of Maternal–Fetal and Neonatal Medicine, 22*(4), 353–356.

32. Lacasse et al., note 20.

33. Tan, P. C., Yow, C. M., & Omar, S. Z. (2009). A placebo-controlled trial of oral pyridoxine in hyperemesis gravidarum. *Gynecologic & Obstetric Investigation, 67*(3), 151–157.

34. Heazell, A., Thorneycroft, J., Walton, V., & Etherington, I. (2006). Acupressure for the in-patient treatment of nausea and vomiting in early pregnancy: A randomized control trial. *American Journal of Obstetrics & Gynecology, 194*(3), 815–820.

35. Selitsky, T., Chandra, P., & Schiavello, H. J. (2006). Wernicke's encephalopathy with hyperemesis and ketoacidosis. *Obstetrics & Gynecology, 107*(2 Part 2), 486–489.

36. Saha, S., Loranger, D., Pricolo, V., & Degli-Esposti, S. (2009). Feeding jejunostomy for the treatment of severe hyperemesis gravidarum: A case series. *Journal of Parenteral & Enteral Nutrition, 33*(5), 529–534.

37. Vaisman, N., Kaidar, R., Levin, I., & Lessing, J. B. (2004). Nasojejunal feeding in hyperemesis gravidarum: A preliminary study. *Clinical Nutrition, 23*(1), 53–57.

38. Holmgren, C., Aagaard-Tillery, K. M., Silver, R. M., Porter, T. F., & Varner, M. (2008). Hyperemesis in pregnancy: An evaluation of

treatment strategies with maternal and neonatal outcomes. *American Journal of Obstetrics & Gynecology, 198*(1), 56.

39. Poursharif, B., Korst, L. M., Macgibbon, K. W., Fejzo, M. S., Romero, R., & Goodwin, T. M. (2007). Elective pregnancy termination in a large cohort of women with hyperemesis gravidarum. *Contraception, 76(6),* 451–455.

40. Turner, J. A. (2009). Severe preeclampsia: Anesthetic implications of the disease and its management. *American Journal of Therapeutics, 16,* 284–288.

41. McPherson, R. A., & Pincus, M. R. (2007). *Henry's clinical diagnosis and management by laboratory methods* (21st ed.). Philadelphia: Saunders Elsevier, p. 376.

42. Cunningham et al., note 7, p. 718.

43. Cunningham et al., note 7, p. 718.

44. Cunningham et al., note 7, p. 718.

45. Guyton & Hall, note 2, p. 1035.

46. McPhee, S. J., Papadakis, M. A., & Tierney, L. M. (2008). *2008 current medical diagnosis & treatment.* New York: McGraw-Hill/Lange, p. 672.

47. Guyton & Hall, note 2, p. 1035.

48. Guyton & Hall, note 2, p. 1035.

49. Cunningham et al., note 7, p. 117.

50. Cunningham et al., note 7, p. 118.

51. Abenhaim, H. A., Bujold, E., Benjamin, A., & Kinch, R. A. (2008). Evaluating the role of bedrest on the prevention of hypertensive disease of pregnancy and grown restriction. *Hypertension in Pregnancy, 27*(2), 197–205.

52. Meher, S., & Duley, L. (2006). Rest during pregnancy for preventing preeclampsia and its complications in women with normal blood pressure. *Cochrane Database of Systematic Reviews, 19,* CD005939.

53. Knight, M., on behalf of UKOSS. (2007). Eclampsia in the United Kingdom 2005. *British Journal of Obstetrics and Gynecology, 114(9),* 1072–1078.

54. Cunningham et al., note 7, p. 729.

55. Euser, A. G., & Cipolla, M. J. (2009). Magnesium sulfate for the treatment of eclampsia: A brief review. *Stroke, 40,* 1169–1175.

56. Cunningham et al., note 7, p. 737.

57. Duley, L., & Henderson-Smart, D. (2003). Magnesium sulphate versus phenytoin for eclampsia. *Cochrane Database of Systematic Reviews, (4)CD000128.*

58. Belfort, M. A., Anthony, J., Saade, G. R., & Allen, J. C., for the Nimodipine Study Group. (2003). A comparison of magnesium sulfate and nimodipine for the prevention of eclampsia. *New England Journal of Medicine, 348,* 304–411.

59. Duley, L., & Henderson-Smart, D. (2003). Magnesium sulphate versus diazepam for eclampsia. *Cochrane Database of Systematic Reviews, (4)CD000127.*

60. Cunningham et al., note 7, p. 738.

61. Cunningham et al., note 7, p. 738.

62. Cunningham et al., note 7, p. 738.

63. Cunningham et al., note 7, p. 740.

64. Cunningham et al., note 7, p. 458.

65. Cunningham et al., note 7, p. 741.

66. McCoy, S., & Baldwin, K. (2009). Pharmacotherapeutic options for the treatment of preeclampsia. *American Journal of Health-System Pharmacy, 66,* 337–344.

67. Clark, S. L., Simpson, K. R., Know, E., & Garite, T. J. (2009). Oxytocin: New perspectives on an old drug. *American Journal of Obstetrics & Gynecology, 200(1),* 35.

68. Bergum, D., Lonnee, H., & Hakli, T. F. (2009). Oxytocin infusion: Acute hyponatremia, seizures and coma. *Acta Anesthesiologica Scandinavica, 53,* 826–827.

69. Ophir, E., Solt, I., Odeh, M., & Bornstein, J. (2007). Water intoxication: A dangerous condition in labor and delivery rooms. *Obstetrical and Gynecological Survey, 62*(11), 731–738.

70. Johannson, N., Lindow, S., Kapadia, H., & Norman, M. (2002). Perinatal water intoxication due to excessive oral intake during labour. *Acta Paediatrica, 91,* 811–814.

71. Ruchala, P., Metheny, N., Essenpreis, H., & Borcherding, K. (2002). Current practice in oxytocin dilution and fluid administration for induction of labor. *Journal of Obstetric and Gynecological Nursing, 31,* 545–550.

72. Garite, T. J., Weeks, J., Peters-Phair, K., Pattillo, C., & Brewster, W. R. (2000). A randomized controlled trial of the effect of increased intravenous hydration on the course of labor in nulliparous women. *American Journal of Obstetrics & Gynecology, 183*(6), 1544–1548.

73. Garite et al., note 72.

74. Lowdermilk, D. L., & Perry, S. E. (2007). *Maternity and women's health care* (9th ed.). St. Louis, Mo: Mosby Elsevier, p. 486.

75. Davidson, M., London, M., & Ladewig, P. (2008). *Olds' maternal–newborn nursing & women's health across the lifespan* (8th ed.). Upper Saddle River, NJ: Pearson Prentice Hall. p. 696.

76. Cunningham et al., note 7, p. 455.

77. Davidson et al., note 75, p. 697.

78. Sharma, S. K., Sidawi, J. E., Ramin, S. M., Lucas, M. J., Leveno, K. J., & Cunningham, F. G. (1997). Cesarean delivery: A randomized trial of epidural versus patient-controlled meperidine analgesia during labor. *Anesthesiology, 87*(3), 487–494.

79. Graham, K., & Palmer, J. (2004). Severe hyponatraemia as a result of primary polydipsia in labour. *Australian & New Zealand Journal of Obstetrics & Gynaecology, 44*(6), 586–587.

80. Johannson et al., note 70.

81. Johannson et al., note 70.

82. Mercer, B. M., & Merlino, A. A. Society for Maternal-Fetal Medicine. (2009). Magnesium sulfate for preterm labor and preterm birth. *Obstetrics & Gynecology, 114*(3), 650–668.

83. ACOG (American College of Obstetrics and Gynecology) Practice Bulletin 80: Premature rupture of membranes. (2007). *Obstetrics & Gynecology, 109*(4), 1007–1009.

84. Cunningham et al., note 7, p. 822.

85. Nassar, A. H., Salti, I., Makarem, N. N., & Usta, I. M. (2007). Marked hypocalcemia after tocolytic magnesium sulphate therapy. *American Journal of Perinatology, 24*(8), 481–482.

86. Koontz, S. L., Friedman, S. A., & Schwartz, M. L. (2004). Symptomatic hypocalcemia after tocolytic therapy with magnesium sulfate and nifedipine. *American Journal of Obstetrics & Gynecology, 190(6)*, 1773–1776.

87. Koontz et al., note 86.

88. Grimes, D. A., & Nanda, K. (2006). Magnesium sulfate tocolysis: Time to quit. *Obstetrics & Gynecology, 108(4)*, 986–989.

89. Herschel, M., & Mittendorf, R. (2001). Tocolytic magnesium sulfate toxicity and unexpected neonatal death. *Journal of Perinatology, 21(4)*, 261–262.

90. Grether, J. K., Hoogstrate, J., Walsh-Greene, E., & Nelson, K. B. (2000). Magnesium sulfate for tocolysis and risk of spastic cerebral palsy in premature children born to women without preeclampsia. *American Journal of Obstetrics & Gynecology, 183(3)*, 717–725.

91. Braden, G. L., von Oeyen, P. T., Germain, M. J., Watson, D. J., & Haag, B. L. (1997). Ritodrine- and terbutaline-induced hypokalemia in preterm labor: Mechanisms and consequences. *Kidney International, 51*, 1867–1875.

92. Cunningham et al., note 7, p. 823.

93. Braden et al., note 91.

94. Cunningham et al., note 7, p. 823.

95. Cunningham et al., note 7, p. 823.

96. King, J. F., Flenady, V., Papatsonis, D., Dekker, G., & Carbonne, B. (2003). Calcium channel blockers for inhibiting preterm labour: A systematic review of the evidence and a protocol for administration of nifedipine. *Australian & New Zealand Journal of Obstetrics & Gynaecology, 43(3)*, 192–198.

97. Papatsonis, D. N., van Geijn, H. P., Bleker, O. P., Ader, H. J., & Dekker, G. A. (2003). Hemodynamic and metabolic effects after nifedipine and ritodrine tocolysis. *International Journal of Gynaecology & Obstetrics, 82(1)*, 5–10.

98. Papatsonis et al., note 97.

99. Mills, M. E. (2007). Craving more than food: The implications of pica in pregnancy. *Nursing for Women's Health, 11(3)*, 266–273.

100. Rose, E. A., Porcerelli, J. H., & Neale, A. V. (2000). Pica: Common but commonly missed. *Journal of the American Board of Family Practice, 14(1)*, 353–358.

101. Corbett, R. W., Ryan, C., & Weinrich, S. P. (2003). Pica in pregnancy: Does it affect pregnancy outcomes? *American Journal of Maternal–Child Nursing, 28(3)*, 183–189; quiz 190–191.

102. Ukaonu, C., Hill, D. A., & Christensen, F. (2003). Hypokalemic myopathy in pregnancy caused by clay ingestion. *Obstetrics & Gynecology, 102(5 Pt 2)*, 1169–1171.

103. Grotegut, C. A., Dandolu, V., Katari, S., Whiteman, V. E., Geifman-Holtzman, O., & Teitelman, M. (2006). Baking soda pica: A case of hypokalemic metabolic alkalosis and rhabdomyolysis in pregnancy. *Obstetrics & Gynecology, 107(2 Pt 2)*, 484–486.

104. Ukaonu et al., note 102.

105. Mengel, C. E., Carter, W. A., & Horton, E. S. (1964). Geophagia with iron deficiency and hypokalemia. *Archives of Internal Medicine, 114*, 470–474.

106. Hill et al., note 30.

107. Schimert, P., Bernet-Buettiker, V., Rutishauser, C., Schams, M., & Frey, B. (2007). Transplacental metabolic alkalosis. *Journal of Paediatrics and Child Health, 43*, 851–853.

108. Schimert et al., note 107.

109. Herschel, M., & Mittendorf, R. (2001). Tocolytic magnesium sulfate toxicity and unexpected neonatal death. *Journal of Perinatology, 21(4)*, 261–262.

110. Herschel & Mittendorf, note 109.

111. Greene, L. (2006, June 8). Hospital says error killed woman. *St. Petersburg Times*. Retrieved March 6, 2010, from http://www.sptimes.com/2006/06/08/Tampabay/Hospital_says_error_k.shtml.

112. Simpson, K. R. (2006, September–October). Minimizing risk of magnesium sulfate overdose in obstetrics. *American Journal of Maternal–Child Nursing, 31(5)*, 340.

UNIT V

Special Considerations in Children and the Elderly

Chapter 24

Fluid and Electrolyte Balance in Children

Linda L. Haycraft, RN, MSN(R), CPNP

INTRODUCTION

While children and adults share many similarities in fluid and electrolyte balance, some distinct differences exist between these populations. For example, body fluids are distributed differently in young children than in adults, and children have a higher metabolic rate and a proportionately larger body surface area. All of these conditions place the child at greater risk for developing fluid and electrolyte problems. Although adults may be able to tolerate fluid imbalances for days, infants may tolerate similar disturbances for only hours before the situation becomes acute.

Serum Electrolyte Concentrations

Most serum electrolyte concentrations do not vary strikingly among infants, small children, and adults. However, there are differences in phosphorus, calcium, and potassium values (**Table 24-1**). Phosphorus levels are normally higher in young children than in adults because the bones of youths are actively growing. Serum calcium levels are known to correlate with gestational age, being lower in premature infants.

Body Water Content and Distribution

The percentage and distribution of body water are significantly different in young children than in adults. Whereas the total body water of an adult usually does not exceed 60% of body weight, it reaches much higher percentages in children. For example, 90% of a premature infant's body weight may be water when the infant's gestational age is 23 to 27 weeks; approximately 75% of a full-term infant's body weight is water. Further, distribution of fluid in the extra-

Table 24-1 Variations in Electrolyte Concentrations and Creatinine Levels According to Age

	Phosphorus (Inorganic)
Child, 1 year	3.6–6.0 mg/dL (serum)
Adult	2.3–4.7 mg/dL (serum)
	Calcium
Premature infant, first week	6.0–10.0 mg/dL (serum)
Full-term newborn, first week	7.0–12.0 mg/dL (serum)
Adult	9.2–11.0 mg/dL (serum)
	Potassium
Child, 3 months–1 year	3.7–5.6 mEq/L (serum)
Adult	3.8–5.0 mEq/L (plasma)
	Creatinine
Child younger than age 2 years	0.3–0.6 mg/dL (serum or plasma)
Adult	0.6–1.2 mg/dL (serum or plasma)

Source: Information from McPherson, R. A., & Pincus, M. R. (2007). *Henry's clinical diagnosis and management by laboratory methods* (21st ed.). Philadelphia: Saunders Elsevier, pp. 1405, 1406, 1408, 1416, 1418.

cellular and intracellular spaces is different in young children and adults. The percentage of body fluid in the extracellular space is almost twice as high in a full-term newborn as in an adult (40% versus 15–20%, respectively). An even higher percentage (60%) is located outside the cells of a neonate with a gestational age of 23 to 27 weeks. After one year of age, the child's total body water content begins to decrease toward the average adult value. The adult body fluid percentage and distribution are reached near the time of puberty.

Factors That Increase Risk for Fluid Loss in Children

Fluid is lost more easily from the extracellular space than from the cellular space. As a consequence, the young child's higher proportion of extracellular fluid is a significant factor in predicting fluid loss during times of illness. Another factor that increases risk for fluid loss is the child's proportionately greater body surface area. For example, compared with older children and adults, the premature infant has five times as much body surface area in relation to weight, and the newborn, three times. This factor is important because the skin represents a major route of insensible fluid loss. (Recall that insensible fluid loss refers to "invisible" losses of fluid via radiation from the skin and via exhalation from the lungs.) Infants who must undergo phototherapy for hyperbilirubinemia have increased insensible water loss, as do those who require radiant warmers to maintain body temperature. In addition, compared to adults, healthy infants and children have greater insensible water losses from the respiratory tract because of higher respiratory rates. Insensible respiratory water losses are even more significant in children who require mechanical ventilation, especially when inadequate humidification is provided. Children with birth defects, such as myelomeningocele and extrophy of the bladder, are also at increased risk for insensible water loss.

The young infant has a relatively greater gastrointestinal membrane surface area than does an older child or adult. Hence, relatively greater losses occur from the gastrointestinal tract in the sick infant than in the older child and adult.

Infants exchange approximately half of their extracellular fluid each day; by comparison, adults exchange only one-sixth of their extracellular fluid. The daily fluid exchange is relatively greater in infants in part because their metabolic rate is roughly two times higher per unit of weight than the corresponding metabolic rate for adults. The high metabolic rate increases the amount of metabolic wastes that must be excreted by the kidneys. Because water is needed by the kidneys to excrete these wastes, a large urinary volume is formed each day.

It is unclear precisely when a child's kidneys mature, although this phase of development is thought to occur by the end of the second year of life. An infant's kidneys have a limited concentrating ability and require more water to excrete a given amount of solute. Further, the infant has difficulty conserving body water when it is needed.

DEHYDRATION DUE TO GASTROENTERITIS

In pediatric patients, it is common to refer to "isotonic dehydration," "hyponatremic dehydration," and "hypernatremic dehydration." Any of these conditions may occur in the child with gastroenteritis. Gastroenteritis—an inflammation or infection of the gastrointestinal tract—is the most common cause of dehydration in children and can be caused by a multitude of bacterial, viral, or parasitic agents. The World Health Organization estimates that each year more than 525,000 children younger than the age of five years die from gastroenteritis due to the rotavirus.[1] Attempts to develop a vaccine for this virus have been plagued with problems.

Regardless of the origin of gastroenteritis, clinical manifestations of this condition may include nausea and vomiting, diarrhea, abdominal cramping, and fever. Left untreated, children can quickly become severely dehydrated.

Electrolyte and Acid–Base Problems Associated with Vomiting and Diarrhea

Chapter 13 provides an in-depth description of the fluid and electrolyte problems associated with vomiting and diarrhea. As noted in that chapter, vomiting results in a loss of acidic gastric secretions and may lead to metabolic alkalosis. In contrast, loss of bicarbonate-rich intestinal fluid from diarrhea may lead to metabolic acidosis. If the child with gastroenteritis is unable to eat for a prolonged period (and nutrients are not provided by another route), ketosis of starvation—another form of metabolic acidosis—may occur.

Assessment for Dehydration

Assessment of a dehydrated child involves both objective and subjective information and requires clinical judgment. Unfortunately, no single clinical manifestation is diagnostic of this condition. Roland et al. developed a standardized scoring system to aid physicians in assessing dehydration in children; however, use of this scoring system did not decrease variability among their diagnoses.[2]

History

The assessment should begin with a thorough history, obtained from the child's caregivers. The information should include the following items:

- Pre-illness weight (if known)
- Number of occurrences of emesis and/or diarrhea

- Changes in tear production
- Changes in fluid intake
- Changes in urine output

This information is often estimated because caregivers do not keep a written log of events. The caregivers may report a change in the child's behavior, however, and it is important to pay attention to their descriptions of subtle changes. Examples of behavior changes include a decrease in activity, increased sleepiness, and increased crankiness.

Physical Assessment

The physical examination should begin with an assessment of the child's general appearance and activity level. During the examination, the child should be in a comfortable position, such as sitting on a caregiver's lap. The respiratory status should be assessed while the child is relaxed; note both the respiratory rate and pattern. **Table 24-2** describes the clinical manifestations of dehydration in pediatric patients.

Weight. A sudden change in body weight is usually reflective of a change in body water content. Comparison of the child's pre-illness and illness weights provides an excellent measure of the degree of dehydration. The following formula is commonly used to calculate the percentage of dehydration:[3]

$$\% \text{ Dehydration} = \frac{(\text{pre-illness weight} - \text{illness weight})}{\text{pre-illness weight}} \times 100$$

Another method for estimating the extent of dehydration is to simply subtract the child's illness weight from the pre-illness weight. For example, a loss of 500 g of body weight is equivalent to a loss of 500 mL of body fluid (1 milliliter of fluid weighs 1 gram).

The problem with the previously described methods for calculating the extent of dehydration is that most caregivers rarely know the child's precise pre-illness weight. For this reason, other parameters for physical assessments take on added importance in determining the extent of fluid loss.

Appearance of Fontanel. The posterior fontanel closes by the time the infant is 6 weeks old and is not useful in assessing hydration status. In contrast, the anterior fontanel usually does not close until the child is approximately 18 months old; thus its appearance can be used to assess for dehydration in children younger than this age. In normal conditions, the anterior fontanel feels soft and flat. In the presence of moderate dehydration, it appears slightly depressed. When severe dehydration is present, the fontanel has a sunken appearance. Assessment of the fontanel should occur when the child is quiet (because crying increases intracranial pressure and may result in a faulty assessment.) If meningitis is present, the fontanel will feel full and tense.

Eyes and Tearing. A healthy child's eyes are shiny and bright; in contrast, a dehydrated child's eyes will appear

Table 24-2 Clinical Manifestations of Stages of Dehydration in Infants and Children

Clinical Manifestation	Mild Dehydration	Moderate Dehydration	Severe Dehydration
Weight loss (from pre-illness weight)	3% loss	5% loss	10% loss
Fontanel (infants only)	Flat	Soft	Sunken
Eyes	Normal	Slightly sunken	Sunken
Tears	Normal	Slightly decreased	Absent
Mucous membranes	Moist	Tacky	Dry
Skin turgor	Normal	Delayed	Tenting
Skin color	Normal	Pale	Mottled
Capillary refill	Brisk	2–3 seconds	> 3 seconds
Urine output	Normal	Oliguric	Anuric
Pulses	Strong	Weak	Thready
Heart rate	Normal	Slightly ↑	Tachycardic
Blood pressure	Normotensive	Normotensive	Hypotensive

sunken with surrounding dark circles. A normally hydrated child who is at least 1 to 3 months of age will produce tears when crying. In contrast, the volume of tears decreases as a child becomes dehydrated. A severely dehydrated child may produce no tears when crying.

Mucous Membranes. Infants and children normally have very moist mucous membranes. A pacifier removed from an infant's mouth is usually wet with saliva. As dehydration progresses, however, the pacifier will be less moist. The dehydrated child will have tacky mucous membranes; in the presence of severe dehydration, the child's lips will be dry and cracked. Bubbles of saliva, which are normally present under the tongue of a well-hydrated child, are absent when dehydration is present.

Skin Turgor. In a healthy person, pinched skin will immediately fall back to its normal position when released; in contrast, pinched skin will remain briefly elevated when dehydration is present. A dehydrated adult will display poor skin turgor more readily than will a dehydrated child, because infants and children have greater skin elasticity that can withstand changes in fluid volume. As a consequence, skin turgor is not an especially sensitive indicator of dehydration in infants and children. Generally, skin turgor begins to diminish after 3% to 5% of the body weight is lost. In the presence of severe dehydration, the child's skin may remain tented for several seconds when pinched, indicating a deficit of interstitial fluid. The skin of a child with hypernatremia may feel thick and "doughy." An obese child may have a deceptively normal skin turgor in the presence of dehydration.

Skin Color. Because skin color is highly subjective, the healthcare provider should ask the child's caregiver if the child's skin color has changed in any way. Children with moderate dehydration may appear pale; however, the paleness could also reflect lack of sun exposure. Mottling—an uneven discoloration of the skin—may occur in a child who is hypovolemic.[4]

Capillary Refill Time. Capillary refill time is a noninvasive method for measuring tissue perfusion. Although this test is frequently used as a quick method to assess circulation, there is considerable variability in how it is performed and how the results are interpreted.[5]

The usual method consists of applying pressure on the nail beds of the upper extremities until blanching occurs. Alternatively, a capillary refill test can be performed over the sternum if the digits are cool. The Pediatric Advanced Life Support Manual recommends that the extremity be elevated slightly above the level of the heart while performing a test for capillary refill time.[6] A capillary refill time of 2 seconds or less is regarded as normal, while a capillary refill time longer than 2 seconds is regarded as indicative of dehydration.[7, 8]

Because visual inspective of capillary refill is subjective, a group of investigators compared visual assessments of capillary refill time with assessments obtained by digital videography.[9] These researchers found that digitally measured capillary refill time was more accurate than visually assessed capillary refill time in predicting significant dehydration in a group of 83 young children with gastroenteritis.

Urine Output. A dehydrated child produces less urine. For example, a caregiver may report that an infant has fewer wet diapers. However, a decrease in urine output may be difficult for a caregiver to detect if the infant is having frequent episodes of diarrhea, because it is difficult to determine if the wet diaper is due to urine or liquid stool.

Once a child is hospitalized, various methods can be used to measure urine output. The simplest, and less invasive, is measurement of diaper weights. With this technique, the diaper is weighed before use, and then again after use. The weight of the dry diaper is then subtracted from the weight of the wet diaper. The end value will reflect urine volume (with approximately 1 milliliter of urine representing 1 gram of body weight). Another method consists of applying a temporary urine bag to the child's perineum. Unfortunately, these bags tend to leak and may cause skin excoriation; thus they are primarily used to obtain a single urine specimen as opposed to measuring urinary output.

Although an indwelling urinary catheter provides the most accurate measure of urine output, use of these catheters is limited to situations in which they are absolutely necessary (e.g., when a child with a head injury is receiving an osmotic diuretic). Risk for urinary tract infection is significantly increased in children with indwelling catheters. For example, a 5-year prospective study revealed that 92% of children between the ages of 4 days and 15 years who developed a hospital-acquired urinary tract infection had an indwelling urinary catheter.[10]

Pulses. Central and peripheral pulses should be assessed in children when dehydration is suspected. The central pulses are normally stronger than the peripheral pulses. As hypovolemia worsens, peripheral pulses become weaker. When a child's central pulses become weak, the healthcare provider must intervene quickly to prevent cardiac arrest.[11]

Heart Rate. Tachycardia is common in the dehydrated child. It arises because beta receptors in the myocardium sense the decreased intravascular volume and respond by increasing the heart rate. The extent of tachycardia increases as the dehydration worsens.

Blood Pressure. Blood pressure is a less sensitive indicator of volume status in children than in adults. Even when moderately dehydrated, children usually remain normotensive. Infants and children do not generally become hypotensive until their fluid loss is severe and their physiologic compensatory mechanisms have failed.[12]

As in adults, correct measurement of blood pressure requires the use of a cuff appropriate to the individual's size. The cuff bladder should cover approximately 40% of the mid-upper arm circumference.[13]

Management

A variety of routes are available for fluid replacement in dehydrated children. While mild to moderate dehydration may be treated by oral rehydration or parenteral fluids (either intravenous or subcutaneous), severe dehydration mandates use of either the intravenous or intraosseous route.

A review of treatment outcomes in 1811 children with acute gastroenteritis found no clinically significant differences when oral rehydration was used, as opposed to intravenous therapy.[14] However, the group who received oral rehydration did have a greater risk for paralytic ileus, and the group who received intravenous therapy was exposed to the risks associated with IV therapy. The authors reported that for every 25 children treated with oral replacement therapy, one would fail to respond to this treatment and require intravenous fluid replacement.

Oral Rehydration Therapy

Oral rehydration fluids were first developed in the 1960s.[15] For children with mild to moderate dehydration, oral rehydration therapy (ORT) is recommended as the first-line treatment by the American Academy of Pediatrics and the Centers for Disease Control and Prevention.[16, 17] These solutions are inexpensive and are less difficult to administer than are intravenous fluids (which, of course, require the insertion of an intravenous device). However, some children cannot drink the oral solutions because of uncontrollable vomiting or a low level of consciousness.

A typical oral rehydration solution contains dextrose as well as electrolytes. For example, the rehydration solution used by the World Health Organization (WHO) contains sodium (75 mEq/L), potassium (20 mEq/L), chloride (65 mEq/L), and citrate (10 mEq/L), in addition to glucose. Commercial sources also provide oral rehydration solutions with varying concentrations of electrolytes and glucose. Compared to the WHO solution, oral rehydrating solutions used in the United States are generally lower in sodium content and, therefore, are less likely to cause hypernatremia if used in excess.

Mildly to moderately dehydrated children typically receive 50 to 100 mL/kg of oral rehydration solution within a 3- to 4-hour period.[18] The fluid may be administered via a teaspoon or syringe every 1 to 2 minutes. Extra fluid may be prescribed for each watery stool and each emesis.

Although ORT is the recommended treatment for children with mild to moderate dehydration from gastroenteritis, evidence suggests that this regimen is underused, primarily because clinicians believe it requires more time to administer than does intravenous fluid replacement.[19] Countering this belief, some studies have found that patients who receive ORT have shorter emergency department stays than do those who receive intravenous therapy.[20]

Intravenous Fluids

While many children can tolerate oral rehydrating solutions, others (such as those with severe dehydration) will require intravenous fluid therapy.[21] The evidence indicates that normal saline (0.9% sodium chloride) is superior to half-strength saline (0.45% sodium chloride) in the treatment of children with gastroenteritis.[22] Children who receive isotonic saline are less likely to experience dilutional hyponatremia than are those who receive half-strength saline. A bolus of normal saline (20 mL/kg) over 20 minutes may be prescribed and repeated as necessary to restore tissue perfusion. The adequacy of fluid replacement is gauged by the child's response, evidenced by improved urine output, reduced heart rate, increased blood pressure, improved capillary refill time, and a more alert affect. It is critical to maintain accurate intake and output records in such cases and to observe the child's electrolyte values and vital signs while assessing response to fluid replacement.

Several methods have been developed to calculate maintenance fluid needs in children. One method is based on the child's body weight:

- 100 mL/kg for the first 10 kg of body weight
- 50 mL/kg for the next 10 kg
- 20 mL/kg for each kilogram above 20 kg

For example, a 17-kg child will require

1000 mL + (7 × 50)/24 hr
1000 mL + 350 mL/24 hr
1350 mL/24 hr = 56.25 mL/hr

In children with vomiting, it is common practice to use normal saline (0.9% sodium chloride) to replace the gastric fluid losses; potassium chloride may be added to the solution in a concentration of 10 mEq/L.[23] In children with diarrhea, a replacement solution may contain sodium chloride, potassium chloride, and sodium bicarbonate; for example, a solution of 0.2% sodium chloride plus 20 mEq/L of sodium bicarbonate plus 20 mEq/L of potassium chloride may be used.[24]

During treatment for gastroenteritis, special attention must be paid to the child's serum sodium concentration. That is, the child may have "isotonic dehydration" (dehydration with a near normal serum sodium concentration), "hyponatremic dehydration" (dehydration with a low serum sodium concentration), or "hypernatremic dehydration" (dehydration with a high serum sodium concentration). If the child has hyponatremic dehydration, care must be taken to correct the serum sodium concentration slowly, so as to avoid causing central pontine myelinolysis (CPM; discussed in Chapter 4). Hypernatremic dehydration is an especially dangerous form of dehydration, and care must be taken to avoid correcting the serum sodium concentration too quickly and subsequently producing cerebral edema. (See Chapter 4 for a discussion of the treatment of hypernatremia.)

Intravenous Route for Infusion. Obtaining peripheral vascular access in the child who is already fluid compromised poses a challenge for healthcare providers. If time permits, a topical anesthetic may be applied to the insertion site. Once vascular access has been achieved, the device must be secured to prevent its inadvertent removal. If the device has been placed in an arm or leg, the extremity may need to be secured to an armboard. Central venous access is also a possibility, but is more invasive and requires advanced skills for insertion.

Subcutaneous Route for Infusion. Because of the difficulty associated with inserting peripheral intravenous devices, the subcutaneous route for administering fluids is an option for the mildly or moderately dehydrated child. Potential injection sites in the child include the subcutaneous space on the anterior thigh or between the scapulae. Usually, a drug called hyaluronidase is first injected at the infusion site to decrease the subcutaneous tissue's resistance to fluid; then a small-gauge device is inserted into the site.

To date, relatively few studies have examined the efficacy and safety of subcutaneous fluids in dehydrated children. A pilot study was recently reported that involved 51 mildly to moderately dehydrated children who sought care at nine emergency departments in the United States where they received subcutaneous fluids.[25] The children ranged in age from 2 months to 10 years; among the exclusion criteria were severe dehydration, shock, life-threatening conditions, a serum sodium concentration less than 130 mEq/L, a serum sodium concentration greater than 155 mEq/L, a serum potassium concentration less than 3.0 mEq/L, and hypersensitivity to hyaluronidase. The children had a 24-gauge catheter or needle placed in the mid-anterior thigh or interscapular area. Hyaluronidase was injected subcutaneously through the infusion device, followed by the subcutaneous infusion of 20 mL/kg of isotonic fluid over 1 hour. Additional fluids were continued for up to 72 hours as needed. Of the 51 children, 48 were deemed clinically rehydrated primarily through subcutaneous therapy. Of these 48 children, 43 were rehydrated in the emergency department; the others had continuing subcutaneous infusions following hospitalization. Infusion site reactions were experienced by all of the children, and the severity of pain reported by the children varied widely. Cellulitis (a serious adverse event) occurred in one child. The authors of this report recommended further study to compare the efficacy of subcutaneous fluid replacement in mildly to moderately dehydrated children with that of other routes.

Among the suitable fluids for subcutaneous administration are isotonic saline (0.9% sodium chloride) or half-strength saline (0.45% sodium chloride), with or without added small concentrations of dextrose. Most medications and nutrient additives are not suitable for subcutaneous administration. Irritating additives (such as potassium chloride) produce pain at the infusion site and, therefore, can be administered via this route only in low concentrations.

Intraosseous Route for Infusion. The intraosseous route provides a noncollapsible access to the systemic venous circulation via the marrow or medullary cavity of the bone.[26] Use of the intraosseous route is reserved for emergent, life-saving situations when vascular access cannot be readily achieved. While in the past this technique was used only in children younger than 6 years of age, intraosseous infusions are currently used for children of all ages (as well as for adults).

A variety of intraosseous devices are available. The EZ10 (Vidacare Corporation, Shawana Park, Texas), a battery-powered intraosseous insertion device, has made the procedure less complicated and faster to perform than was possible with previously used manual devices (**Figure 24-1**). For infants and children younger than 6 to 8 years of age, the preferred access site is the anteromedial surface of the tibia, approximately 1 to 2 cm below the tibial tuberosity.[27] Other sites may include the distal tibia, distal femur, and sternum. Prior to insertion, the site is cleansed thoroughly. The needle is then inserted into the bone at a 90-degree angle. As the needle passes into the bone matrix, a sudden release of pressure will be felt and the needle will stand up without support. Once correct placement is confirmed, the stylet may be removed (a flash of blood may be observed in the catheter when the stylet is removed). Further confirmation of correct placement of the catheter may be achieved by attaching a syringe to the needle and withdrawing bone marrow. It should be possi-

ble to easily instill fluid via the catheter. Any fluid (including crystalloids, colloids, and blood) and medications that can be given via the blood vessels can also be administered into the bone matrix and rapidly dispersed into the vascular system.

As with any invasive procedure, complications may occur during the intraosseus infusion process. Failure to achieve access may occur due to bending of the needle or failure to use appropriate landmarks for needle insertion. Further, there is potential for bone fracture. Other complications may include extravasation of fluids (perhaps resulting in compartment syndrome), skin infection, and osteomyelotis. The likelihood of osteomyelitis may be increased by the infusion of hypertonic solutions via the intraosseous device—thus suggesting that hypertonic solutions should be diluted before intraosseous administration.[28] To minimize risk for infection, the intraosseous device should be removed as soon as the child is stable and a peripheral intravenous site can be established.

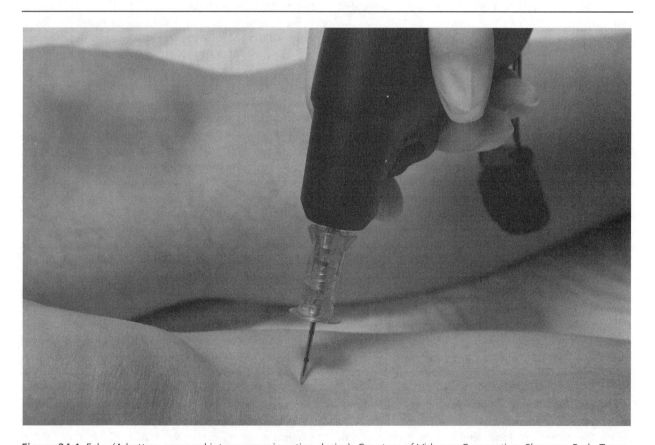

Figure 24-1 Ezlo. (A battery powered intraosseous insertion device). Courtesy of Vidacare Corporation, Shawana Park, Texas.

OTHER CONDITIONS AFFECTING FLUID AND ELECTROLYTE STATUS IN CHILDREN

Hypertrophic Pyloric Stenosis

Hypertrophic pyloric stenosis is a condition in which the pyloric sphincter muscle becomes enlarged. As a result of this abnormality, the pyloric canal is narrowed and causes delayed emptying of gastric contents into the duodenum. Pyloric stenosis usually occurs in children around 3 weeks of age, but may occur in infants as old as 5 months. In such a case, the infant will develop non-bilious vomiting immediately after feeding. After vomiting, the infant will want to eat, resulting in a cycle of eating followed by projectile vomiting, until the child quickly becomes dehydrated. Repeated loss of gastric juice (which typically has a low pH and high hydrochloric acid content) will result in metabolic alkalosis. Because metabolic alkalosis is associated with hypokalemia, the child with severe vomiting will develop a condition referred to as hypokalemic, hypochloremic metabolic alkalosis. (Chapter 13 reviews the various imbalances associated with vomiting.)

Diagnosis of pyloric stenosis begins with a thorough history. The clinician may be able to palpate an "olive-shaped" mass in the right upper quadrant of the abdomen, indicating enlargement of the sphincter. Visible peristaltic waves may be observed in the abdomen, moving from left to right, after the infants eats. An abdominal ultrasound will show an enlarged pyloric sphincter. An abdominal radiograph will likely reveal a distended stomach. An upper gastrointestinal series with contrast may demonstrate delayed gastric emptying—a phenomenon known as the "string sign," because the contrast media looks like a string as it exits the stomach via the narrowed pyloric sphincter.

The infant with pyloric stenosis will be hospitalized and oral intake will be stopped. Intravenous fluids, such as isotonic saline (0.9% sodium chloride) or half-strength saline (0.45% sodium chloride), will be administered until the child is rehydrated and the serum bicarbonate level is normalized. Potassium chloride is added to the intravenous fluids as soon as an adequate urine volume has been verified. As indicated in Chapter 13, the high chloride content of isotonic saline is ideal for replacing lost hydrochloric acid–rich gastric fluid, thereby correcting the metabolic alkalosis associated with gastric fluid loss.

Following stabilization, the infant is taken to the operating room, where a pyloromyotomy will be performed to relieve the stenosis. (Pyloric stenosis is the most common reason for surgery during the first 6 months of life.) Postoperatively, the infant will be offered an oral electrolyte solution. Caregivers should be aware that half of all infants with this condition will continue to vomit after surgery secondary to gastric irritation and pyloric edema. After tolerance of the oral electrolyte solution has been established, the child is offered half-strength formula. The concentration of the formula is gradually increased to full strength. The infant is discharged after multiple, full-strength formula feedings are tolerated—an achievement usually accomplished within 48 hours after surgery.[29]

Dilutional Hyponatremia from Excessive Water Intake

Children may develop hyponatremia for the same reasons as adults, such as gastrointestinal fluid losses, head injuries, diuretics, malignancies, and heart failure. Hyponatremia is a common electrolyte imbalance in both age groups. Chapter 4 provides a thorough discussion of the causes and management of hyponatremia. Only conditions directly related to hyponatremia in children are discussed in this section.

Dilution of formula with water by an infant's caregiver may lead to hyponatremia. The children most at risk from this cause are infants of parents who are living in poverty and are unaware of the risks associated with feeding excess water to their infants. In one report, 25 cases of hyponatremic seizures in infants were found to be related to excess water intake; 17 infants were fed straight tap water, 4 were given sugar water (prepared at home), and 4 were fed tea, soda, or Kool-Aid.[30] In some of the cases, parents reported feeding their infants dilute formula to save money or because they ran out of formula. A case reported by Bruce and Kliegman involved a 55-day-old African American infant who was admitted to the emergency department with "eye twitching" and generalized tonic–clinic seizures.[31] Laboratory analysis revealed a serum sodium concentration of 116 mEq/L; a review of the infant's history showed that the 22-year-old mother had been buying cow's milk and supplementing feedings with bottled drinking water for several days. The infant's mother and grandmother related to the clinicians that the bottled water product they administered to the infant was inexpensive and labeled in such a way that it seemed to contain nutrients adequate for use as an infant feeding supplement. Following treatment and hospitalization for 5 days, the infant was sent home in good condition on formula feedings.

Hospital-acquired hyponatremia can result from the administration of excessive volumes of hypotonic intravenous fluid, especially in children. This condition occurs most commonly in previously healthy children for whom maintenance intravenous fluids have been prescribed in the form of hypotonic saline, such as 0.2% or 0.3% sodium chloride.[32] Children are at especially high risk for developing neurological symptoms of hyponatremia because they have a large brain-to-skull ratio.[33]

Abuse is another cause for hyponatremia in children. For example, some reports have described the deaths of children who were forced to drink large quantities of water.[34, 35]

Hypernatremia from Breastfeeding

Despite the recognized benefits of breastfeeding, a serious potential complication of insufficient breastfeeding is severe hypernatremic dehydration, especially during the infant's first week of life.[36] This condition can be so severe that it results in death.[37–39]

In a report of 21 cases of breastfeeding-related hypernatremia, researchers found that the infants' weight loss ranged between 8% and 30% of their birth weight, and that their serum sodium levels ranged between 146 mEq/L and 207 mEq/L.[40] Common conditions identified in these cases were poor breastfeeding technique and problems with infant suckling. The incidence of breastfeeding-associated hypernatremia is unclear, however. In a study conducted at the University of Pittsburgh, the incidence was found to be 1.9%; researchers identified 70 cases in 3718 consecutive term and near-term hospitalized neonates over a 5-year period.[41]

The cause of breastfeeding-associated hypernatremia is multifaceted. Obviously, the infant is not consuming sufficient fluid to match the obligatory large fluid losses of infancy. Also, a high sodium concentration in the mother's milk may be a factor in promoting this electrolyte imbalance. For example, a case report of an 11-day-old exclusively breastfed infant with dehydration and hypernatremia (sodium = 170 mEq/L) revealed that the sodium content in the mother's milk was three times higher than that found in breast milk from other women.[42]

Prevention of breastfeeding-related hypernatremia can be promoted through family education—specifically, by providing appropriate lactation support for new mothers and emphasizing the importance of monitoring the infant's weight and urine output.[43]

Hypernatremia from Administration of Baking Soda

Several reports have described cases in which children were given baking soda (sodium bicarbonate) to relieve indigestion. For example, a 6-week-old infant developed life-threatening complications following the administration of sodium bicarbonate, which was given to help the child "burp."[44] The child's serum sodium level increased to 180 mEq/L and the bicarbonate concentration increased to 47 mEq/L (about twice the normal level). The authors recommended that parents be educated to guard against the use of harmful home remedies, such as this one. It is disturbing that an informal survey conducted at Johns Hopkins Hospital revealed that 11% of this facility's clinic population had heard of using baking soda as a home remedy, and 4% had actually added baking soda to their infants' formulas.[45]

Hypocalcemia of Infancy

The infants at greatest risk for developing hypocalcemia are those with very low birth weight, those born to diabetic mothers, and those who were subjected to difficult deliveries. Often this condition is asymptomatic and resolves spontaneously. When clinical manifestations require treatment, it usually consists of the slow intravenous injection of a 10% solution of calcium gluconate. It is important to give the solution slowly while monitoring the cardiac rate for bradycardia. Severe tissue necrosis may occur if the solution is allowed to extravasate into the tissue space.

Enemas

Undesirable effects of enemas for the treatment of constipation in infants and children are discussed in Chapters 8 and 13. The risk for electrolyte problems—hypernatremia, hyperphosphatemia, and hypocalcemia—is high when guidelines for the safe administration of hypertonic sodium phosphate enemas are not followed (see Table 8-3). Caregivers should be instructed to consult a healthcare provider before administering an enema to an infant or small child.

Burns

Burns are the second leading cause of unintentional death in children. Among common causes for burn injury in children is contact with hot surfaces or flames, scalding with hot liquids, and exposure to electricity or fireworks. Unfortunately, burns are also a common form of child abuse, such as forced immersion in hot water or burning with cigarettes. Clinicians must assess the burn injury to assure that the pattern of the burn correlates with the history provided by the child's caregiver.

Numerous physiological changes occur during the first 48 to 72 hours following burn injury. An increase in capillary permeability allows protein-rich plasma to leak out of the capillaries into the interstitial space at the burn site (referred to as "third-spacing"). This fluid is nonfunctional because it is no longer available in the vascular space. The associated fluid and electrolyte shifts must be treated immediately to prevent burn shock. While mildly burned children (such as those who are 2 years or older with burns that cover less than 10% of their total body surface area) may be treated with oral electrolyte solutions, those with more severe burns require intravenous fluid replacement. Severe hypovolemia—manifested by tachycardia, hypotension, and low urine output—may develop quickly, accompanied by an elevated serum hematocrit and osmolality. Prompt fluid replacement with an isotonic sodium solution, such as lactated Ringer's solution or 0.9% sodium chloride, is mandated to prevent shock and its associated metabolic acidosis (due to poor tissue perfusion). Adequate fluid resuscitation will perfuse the kidneys so that a minimum of 1 mL of urine per 1 kg of body weight will be produced hourly.

The extensive tissue trauma associated with burns results in a release of cellular potassium into the vascular space. For this reason, to minimize risk for hyperkalemia, potassium is not added to intravenous fluids until adequate urine output is established and serum potassium levels are normal. At times, a colloid (such as plasma) may also be indicated to maintain an adequate vascular volume. A patient who has lost red blood cells secondary to the burn injury may develop anemia and require blood transfusion. Ionized calcium levels are more accurate in assessing calcium status in the burned patient than are total calcium levels. (Recall that the total calcium measurement consists of both ionized calcium and calcium bound to albumin; because albumin is lost into the burned tissues, the total calcium level will be falsely low.)

Numerous formulas are available to guide fluid resuscitation in burn patients. For example, the Parkland formula calls for the administration of crystalloids at a volume of 2 to 4 mL/kg of body weight for each 1% of total burn surface area; half of this volume is infused in the first 8 hours and the remainder over the next 16 hours.[46] The 24-hour time frame is based on the time when the burn injury occurred—not the time of arrival at the hospital. Children who are hypotensive or who are not producing the minimal volume of urine should receive additional fluid boluses (such as 20 mL/kg) of either 0.9% sodium chloride or lactated Ringer's solution. Because the response to fluid resuscitation is unpredictable, every child must be closely monitored. Chil-

dren with burn injuries may experience seizures; while the cause of this complication is unknown, it is hypothesized to be related to rapid fluid and electrolyte shifts, hypoxemia, and medications required for pain relief.

Approximately 48 to 72 hours after the burn injury is incurred, the capillaries heal sufficiently to allow fluid to shift back from the interstitial space into the bloodstream. During this period, the child must be observed for signs of fluid overload if intravenous fluids are continued at a high rate.

Burned patients are instructed to avoid exposure to sunlight to prevent hyperpigmentation of any areas that were scarred from the burn. This lack of exposure to sunlight offer leads to a vitamin D deficiency. Children with burns covering more than 40% of their total body surface area have reduced bone mineral density, placing them at risk for fractures. They may also develop post-burn osteopenia.[47]

CASE STUDIES

Case Study 24-1

An 8-month-old child with nasal congestion, diffuse wheezing, and diminished breath sounds was brought to the emergency department. The past medical history revealed a premature birth (26 weeks) with a birth weight of 672 g (1 lb, 8 oz). Also noted on the history were closure of a patent ductus arteriosus, pulmonary hypertension, adrenal suppression, and bronchi pulmonary dysplasia. Home medications included hydrochlorothiazide, furosemide, spironolactone, potassium chloride, ammonium chloride, famotidine, hydrocortisone, and albuterol. Blood work revealed the following: sodium = 153 mEq/L (normal range, 137–145 mEq/L), potassium = 11.9 mEq/L (normal range, 3.5–5.1 mEq/L), chloride = 123 mEq/L (normal range, 98–107 mEq/L), carbon dioxide content = 23.8 mEq/L (normal range, 18–27 mEq/L), BUN = 74.9 mg/dL (normal range, 5–17 mg/dL), serum creatinine = 0.8 mg/dL (normal range, 0.1–0.7 mg/dL), and serum glucose = 127 mg/dL (normal range, 70–106 mg/dL).

The child was intubated and an intraosseous line was established. Ventricular fibrillation developed with evidence of inadequate perfusion; electrocardiography revealed persistent wide-complex tachycardia. Chest compressions were started and electrical cardioversion was attempted. A calcium gluconate drip was initiated, along with an infusion of insulin and dextrose. Approximately 90 minutes following the initial blood work, additional blood was drawn for analysis. Findings at this time included sodium = 153 mEq/L, potassium = 9.8 mEq/L, chloride =

122 mEq/L, carbon dioxide content = 19.4 mEq/L, BUN = 72.3 mg/dL, creatinine = 1 mg/dL, and serum glucose = 152 mg/dL.

Additional insulin and glucose were administered, and a sodium polystyrene sulfonate (Kayexalate) enema was started. Four hours later, blood work revealed the following: sodium = 153 mEq/L, potassium = 8.1 mEq/L, chloride = 121 mEq/L, carbon dioxide content = 27.5 mEq/L, BUN = 75 mg/dL, creatinine = 0.8 mg/dL, and serum glucose = 46 mg/dL. On day 4, the following laboratory values were noted: sodium = 144 mEq/L, potassium = 3.3 mEq/L, chloride = 100 mEq/L, carbon dioxide content = 39 mEq/L, BUN = 16.2 mg/dL, and creatinine = 0.8 mg/dL.

Eventually the child was extubated and recovered sufficiently to be discharged to a pediatric extended care facility. Unfortunately, several months after the initial admission, the child developed respiratory failure and required mechanical ventilation (from which she could not be weaned).

Commentary. The child was admitted with severe hyperkalemia (potassium = 11.9 mEq/L). The cause of this profound imbalance was never discovered. As noted in her home medications, she received two medications that could account for a higher than normal serum potassium concentration, if used improperly: spironolactone (a potassium-conserving agent) and potassium chloride. Clinicians who cared for the child suspected that she may have been given too much potassium chloride at home. It is interesting to note that the child also received several drugs than could reduce her serum potassium concentration—namely, hydrochlorothiazide and furosemide (both potassium-losing diuretics). In addition, albuterol can decrease the serum potassium concentration. Use of multiple electrolyte-altering drugs, especially in the home setting, can lead to serious electrolyte abnormalities.

Case Study 24-2

A 4-month-old child with active seizures was brought to the emergency department. The child's initial serum sodium concentration was 103 mEq/L (normal range, 135–145 mEq/L). The parents reported that they had run out of formula and had fed the baby water for 3 days. Treatment consisted of 10 mL/kg of 3% sodium chloride given over a 60-minute period. Serum sodium levels were monitored at 15, 30, and 60 minutes during the infusion. The child was admitted to a pediatric intensive care unit, where the serum sodium concentration eventually increased 135 mEq/L.

Commentary. The neurologic sign (seizures) displayed by this infant was a result of cerebral edema caused by the extremely low serum sodium concentration. (See Figure 4-1 in Chapter 4.) Fortunately, the child recovered fully and a social service consultation was obtained to help ensure that the child would have an adequate supply of formula. Hyponatremia due to excessive water intake (such as occurred in this case) is not an uncommon problem, especially in poverty situations.

Case Study 24-3

A 10-month-old child was brought to the emergency department with multiple linear burns on her back. The child's mother reported that the child rolled over on a hot curling iron that had been placed on the bed. The burn area was less than 10% of the child's total body surface area. A plastic surgeon was consulted and the following fluid orders were given: D5 in 0.45% NaCl with 2 mEq of KCl/100 mL at a rate of 25 mL/hr. Morphine was prescribed every 3 hours as needed for pain.

Commentary. An experienced nurse questioned the inappropriate fluid order and was able to get it changed to lactated Ringer's solution at 40 mL/hr without added potassium. Twelve hours after the burn injury, the child's serum potassium level was 6.8 mEq/L.

Case Study 24-4

Kaplan et al.,[48] reported a case in which an infant was born to a 35-year-old primigravida at term by vaginal delivery. Normal Apgar scores were noted, and the baby and mother were discharged 24 hours after delivery. The mother chose to breastfeed the baby exclusively. At 4 days of age, the infant was brought in for an unscheduled visit because the mother was concerned that the baby was not breastfeeding effectively. A greater than 10% weight loss was considered by the pediatrician to be within acceptable limits for a breastfed baby. The infant was released to home with advice to supplement breastfeeding as needed. When the infant was 9 days old, the mother returned with the child to the pediatrician's office. At this time, the infant was lethargic, had poor skin turgor and dry mucous membranes, and apparently had not urinated in the past 24 hours. A serum sodium concentration of 191 mEq/L was found, confirming hypernatremic dehydration. The infant developed uncontrollable seizures and subsequently died from a massive intraventricular hemorrhage. (Hypernatremia causes the brain to contract as water is pulled from the cells by the hypertonic extracellular fluid; this contraction can produce tearing of cerebral blood vessels.)

Commentary. Maternal breastfeeding failure leading to dehydration of newborn infants has been recognized as a possibility for many years. A clinical profile often includes a well-motivated, intelligent primipara of older maternal age who is determined to breastfeed. It is extremely unfortunate that this mother was released from the hospital without the benefit of specific instructions regarding breastfeeding and that the pediatrician did not follow through with the infant following the initial visit.

Case Study 24-5

Helkison et al.[49] reported a case in which a 3-year-old child developed severe hyperphosphatemia and hypocalcemia after the administration of three adult-size hypertonic phosphate (Fleet) enemas. The child's serum phosphate level rose to 74.7 mg/dL (normal range, 2.6–5.0 mg/dL) and her ionized serum calcium level fell markedly below normal. The child also developed metabolic acidosis (pH = 7.15). With early intervention and treatment, the child survived without sequelae.

Commentary. The authors of this report point out the need to be aware of possible adverse effects of improperly administered hypertonic sodium phosphate enemas. They further emphasize that the commonly held notion that these enemas are not absorbed is incorrect. Use of adult-size sodium phosphate enemas for constipation or bowel cleansing before surgery or diagnostic procedures in children can produce disastrous results. Recommendations from the manufacturer of hypertonic sodium phosphate enemas are provided in Table 8-3; it is important that clinicians be familiar with these recommendations.

Case Study 24-6

A case was reported a case in which a 2-week-old infant was brought to an emergency department with a 2-day history of episodes of rapid eye blinking, trembling, and jerking of all four extremities.[50] The episodes occurred several times each day and lasted about 1 minute, followed by a brief period of sleep. No history of trauma, fever, or other illness was present. The infant had not received a formula with high-phosphorus content. (A high phosphorus intake is expected to cause a reciprocal drop in the serum calcium concentration.) A review of the infant's history revealed that the mother's pregnancy was complicated by gestational diabetes and hypertension and that the father had a family history of seizure disorder. During examination, the infant cried incessantly and had severe episodes of seizure activity. Otherwise, the physical examination was normal. Blood work revealed a serum calcium level of 5.2 mg/dL (the lower limit of normal for a 1-week infant is approximately 7 mg/dL).

The infant was admitted to the hospital for treatment of hypocalcemia and received oral calcium replacement over the next 3 days. On correction of the low serum calcium level, the infant's symptoms resolved. At the time of discharge from the hospital, the infant was seizure-free, was less irritable, and had a serum calcium level of 9.9 mg/dL. Calcium supplementation was continued and no further difficulties occurred.

Commentary. Neonatal seizures are common, with an overall incidence of 1 per 200 live births.[51] A specific cause can be determined in only 70% of these cases. Early-onset hypocalcemia is commonly seen in association with infants of diabetic mothers. The seizures are usually brief because the infant's immature neurons are unable to sustain repetitive activity for a prolonged period. Fortunately, the seizures in this infant did not compromise the airway; also, the cardiovascular status was normal. It was concluded that the infant probably had transient idiopathic hypocalcemia.

NOTES

1. World Health Organization. (2008). Global networks for surveillance of rotavirus gastroenteritis. *Weekly Epidemiological Record*, 47(83), 421.

2. Roland, D., Clarke, C., Borland, M. L., & Pascoe, E. M. (2010). Does a standardized scoring system of clinical signs reduce variability between doctor's assessments of the potentially dehydrated child? *Journal of Paediatrics and Child Health*, 46(3), 103–107.

3. Custer, J. W., & Rau, R. E. (Eds.). (2009). *The Harriet Lane handbook* (18th ed.). Philadelphia: Elsevier/Mosby, p. 303.

4. Ralston, M., Hazinski, M. F., Zaritsky, A. L., et al. (Eds.). (2006). *Pediatric life support provider manual.* American Heart Association. Dallas, Texas. p. 20.

5. Labos, A.T., & Menon, K. (2008). A multidisciplinary survey on capillary refill time: Inconsistent performance and interpretation of a common clinical test. *Pediatric Critical Care Medicine*, 9(4), 386–391.

6. Ralston et al., note 4.

7. Ralston et al., note 4.

8. Gray, K., Briseno, M. R., & Otsuka, N. Y. (2008). The association between capillary refill time and arterial flow in the pediatric upper extremity. *Journal of Pediatric Orthopaedics Part B, 17*(5), 257–260.

9. Shavit, I., Braunt, R., Nisjssen-Jordan, C., Galbraith, R., & Johnson, D. W. (2006). A novel imaging technique to measure capillary-refill time: Improving diagnostic accuracy for dehydration in young children with gastroenteritis. *Pediatrics, 118*(6), 2402–2408.

10. Lohr, J. A. (1999). Urinary tract infections: from pathogenesis to outcome. *Pediatric Annals, 28*(10), 637.

11. Ralston et al., note 4.

12. Ralston et al., note 4.

13. National High Blood Pressure Education Program Working Group on High Blood Pressure in Children and Adolescents. (2004). The fourth report on the diagnosis, evaluation, and treatment of high blood pressures in children and adolescents. *Pediatrics, 114*(2 suppl 4th Report), 555–576.

14. Hartling, L., Bellemare, S., Wiebe, N., Russell, K. F., Klassen, T. P., Craig, W., et al. (2006). Oral versus intravenous hydration for treating dehydration due to gastroenteritis in children. *Cochrane Database of Systematic Reviews, 3*, CD004390.

15. Dale, J. (2004). Oral rehydration solutions in the management of acute gastroenteritis among children. *Journal of Pediatric Health, 18*(4), 211–212.

16. King, C. K., Glass, R., Bresee, J. S., Duggan, C., & Centers for Disease Control and Prevention. (2003). Managing acute gastroenteritis among children: Oral rehydration, maintenance, and nutritional therapy. *Morbidity and Mortality Weekly Report, Recommendations and Reports. 52*(RR-16), 1–16.

17. American Academy of Pediatrics, Provisional Committee on Quality Improvement, Subcommittee on Acute Gastroenteritis. (1996). Practice parameter: The management of acute gastroenteritis in young children. *Pediatrics, 97*(3), 424–435.

18. Reid, S. R., & Losek, J. D. (2009). Rehydration: Role for early use of intravenous dextrose. *Pediatric Emergency Care, 25*(1), 49–52.

19. Ozuah, P. O., Avner, J. R., & Stein, R. E. (2002). Oral rehydration, emergency physicians, and practice parameters: A national survey. *Pediatrics, 109*(2), 259–261.

20. Atherly-John, Y. C., Cunningham, S. J., & Crain, E. F. (2002). A randomized trial of oral vs. intravenous rehydration in a pediatric emergency department. *Archives of Pediatric and Adolescent Medicine, 156*, 1240–1243.

21. Bass, D. M. (2009). Rotaviruses, caliciviruses, and astroviruses. In R. M. Kliegman, R. E. Behrman, H. G. Jenson, & B. F. Stanton (Eds.), *Nelson textbook of pediatrics* (18th ed.). Philadelphia: Saunders/Elsevier, p. 1401.

22. Neville, K. A., Verge, C. F., Rosenberg, A. R., O'Meara, M. W., & Walker, J. L. (2006). Isotonic is better than hypotonic saline for intravenous rehydration of children with gastroenteritis: A prospective randomized study. *Archives of Disease in Childhood, 91*, 226–232.

23. Greenbaum, L. A. (2009). Pathophysiology of body fluids and fluid therapy. In R. M. Kliegman, R. E. Behrman, H. G. Jenson, & B. F. Stanton (Eds.), *Nelson textbook of pediatrics* (18th ed.). Philadelphia: Saunders/Elsevier, p. 312.

24. Greenbaum, note 23.

25. Allen, C. H., Etzwiler, L. S., Miller, M. K., Maher, G., Mace, S., Hostetler, M. A., et al. (2009). Recombinant human hyaluronidase-enabled subcutaneous pediatric rehydration. *Pediatrics, 124*(5), e858–e867.

26. Tobias, J. D., & Ross, A. K. (2010). Intraosseous infusions: A review for the anesthesiologist with a focus on pediatric use. *Anesthesia & Analgesia, 110*(2), 391–401.

27. Tobias & Ross, note 26.

28. Tobias & Ross, note 26.

29. Wyllie, R. (2009). Pyloric stenosis and congenital anomalies of the stomach. In R. M. Kliegman, R. E. Behrman, H. G. Jenson, & B. F. Stanton (Eds.), *Nelson textbook of pediatrics* (18th ed.). Philadelphia: Saunders/Elsevier, p. 1557.

30. Bruce, R. C., & Kliegman, R. M. (1997). Hyponatremic seizures secondary to oral water intoxication in infancy: Association with commercial bottled drinking water. *Pediatrics, 100*(6), E4.

31. Bruce & Kliegman, note 30.

32. Hurdowar, A., Urmson, L., Bohn, D., Geary, D., Laxer, R., & Stevens, P. (2009). Compliance with a pediatric clinical guidelines for intravenous fluid and electrolyte administration. *Healthcare Quarterly, 12*, 129–134.

33. Moritz, M. L., & Ayus, J. C. (2003). Prevention of hospital-acquired hyponatremia: A case for using isotonic saline. *Pediatrics, 111*(2), 227–230.

34. Arieff, A. I., & Kronlund, B. A. (1999). Fatal child abuse by forced water intoxication. *Pediatrics, 103*(6 Pt 1), 1292–1295.

35. Lin, C. Y., & Tsau, Y. K. (2005). Child abuse: Acute water intoxication in a hyperactive child. *Acta Paediatrica Taiwanica, 46*(1), 39–41.

36. Uras, N., Karadag, A., Dogan, G., Tonbul, A., & Tatli, M. M. (2007). Moderate hypernatremic dehydration in newborn infants: Retrospective evaluation of 64 cases. *Journal of Maternal–Fetal and Neonatal Medicine, 20*(6), 449–452.

37. Yldzdas, H. Y., Satar, M., Tutak, E., Narl, N., Buyukcelik, M., & Ozlu, F. (2005). May the best friend be an enemy if not recognized early: Hypernatremic dehydration due to breastfeeding. *Pediatric Emergency Care, 21*(7), 445–448.

38. Jaramillo, I., Lopez, G., & Hernandez, H. (2003). Hypernatremic dehydration and death in an infant. *Pediatric Emergency Care, 19*(1), 62–63.

39. van Amerongen, R. H., Moretta, A. C., & Gaeta, T. J. (2001). Severe hypernatremic dehydration and death in a breast-fed infant. *Pediatric Emergency Care, 17*(3), 175–180.

40. Livingstone, V. H., Willis, C. E., Abdel-Wareth, L. O., Thiessen, P., & Lockitch, G. (2000). Neonatal hypernatremic dehydration associated with breast-feeding malnutrition: A retrospective survey. *Canadian Medical Association Journal, 162*(5), 647–652.

41. Moritz, M. L., Manole, M. D., Bogen, D. L., & Ayus, J. C. (2005). Breastfeeding-associated hypernatremia: Are we missing the diagnosis? *Pediatrics, 116*, e343–e347.

42. Marzouk, M., Neffati, F., Khelifa, H., Douki, W., Monastiri, K., Gueddiche, M. N., et al. (2008). A case of hypernatremic dehydration due to breast-feeding (French). *Annales de Biologie Clinique, 66*(4), 471–474.

43. Iyer, N. P., Srinivasan, R., Evans, K., Ward, L., Cheung, W. Y., & Matthes, J. W. (2008). Impact of an early weighing policy on neonatal hypernatraemic dehydration and breast feeding. *Archives of Disease in Childhood, 93*(4), 297–299.

44. Nichols, M. H., Wason, S., Gonzales del Rey, J., & Benfield, M. (1995). Baking soda: A potentially fatal home remedy. *Pediatric Emergency Care, 11*(2), 109–111.

45. Nichols et al., note 44.

46. Baxter, C. R., & Shires, T. (1968). Physiological response to crystalloid resuscitation of severe burns. *Annals of the New York Academy of Sciences, 150,* 874–894.

47. Klein, G. L., Langman, C. B., & Herndon, D. N. (2002). Vitamin D depletion following burn injury in children: A possible factor in postburn osteopenia. *Journal of Trauma Injury, Infection and Critical Care, 52*(2), 346–350.

48. Kaplan, J. A., Siegler, R. W., & Schmunk, G. A. (1998). Fatal hypernatremic dehydration in exclusively breast-fed newborn infants due to maternal lactation failure. *American Journal of Forensic Medicine and Pathology, 19*(1), 19–22.

49. Helikson, M. A, Parham, W. A, & Tobias, J. D. (1997). Hypocalcemia and hyperphosphatemia after phosphate enema use in a child. *Journal of Pediatric Surgery, 32*(8), 1244–1246.

50. Sheth, D. P. (1997). Hypocalcemic seizures in neonates. *American Journal of Emergency Medicine, 15*(7), 638–641.

51. Sheth, note 49.

Chapter 25

Fluid and Electrolyte Balance in the Aged

INTRODUCTION

Risk for fluid and electrolyte imbalances is greater in the elderly than in younger adults. This is largely because aged persons have less total body water (TBW), a decreased thirst sensation, and impaired renal ability to conserve water when needed. These three mechanisms work together to increase their risk for fluid volume deficit (FVD) and hypernatremia (dehydration). Further, the elderly are likely to have one or more disease conditions that predispose to fluid balance problems.

Changes in Body Composition

Normal aging is associated with a decrease in muscle mass and a gain in fat (a water-poor tissue); thus, TBW declines with aging. For example, a 75-year-old man with a 70-kg body weight may have as much as 7 to 8 L less TBW than a 35-year-old man of the same weight.[1] The percent of body fluid is even lower in elderly women because they have proportionately more fat tissue than elderly men.[2] The age-related change in TBW increases the elderly person's susceptibility to stresses on fluid balance.

Decreased Thirst

When challenged by fluid deprivation, elderly persons exhibit less thirst and consume less fluid than younger adults.[3] This difference reflects an intrinsic defect in the thirst mechanism associated with aging. Recall that the major stimulus to thirst is an elevated serum osmolality; it appears that the point at which an elevated osmolality stimulates thirst is higher in the aged (as compared to younger adults).[4]

Changes in Renal Function

Structural changes in the kidney occur with aging. For example, the thickness of the renal cortex decreases approximately 10% per decade of life after the age of 30.[5, 6] Moreover, the number of glomeruli decreases by roughly one-third with increasing age.[7] Renal blood flow declines 10% per decade of life after young adulthood.[8]

Glomerular Filtration Rate and Serum Creatinine Concentration

On average, the glomerular filtration rate (GFR) decreases approximately 1 mL/min per year after the age of 50 years.[9] Despite this change, the serum creatinine level tends to remain in the normal range because of a concurrent reduction in creatine formation due to reduced muscle mass. An increased serum creatinine level in an elderly person implies a GFR low enough to result in symptoms of uremia if even a small physiological stress occurs.[10] Chapter 17 provides a more in-depth discussion of GFR and serum creatinine concentration.

Renal Concentrating Ability

Maximal urinary concentration is significantly less—relative to the same degree of dehydration—in aged persons than in younger persons.[11] As such, the elderly are less able to adapt to fluid losses by conserving urine. The decreased ability to concentrate urine partially explains the nocturia of aging.

Hormonal Changes

Although some controversy persists regarding changes in antidiuretic hormone (ADH) levels with aging, reports indicate that basal ADH levels are elevated in healthy elderly adults as compared to younger individuals.[12] Because of their relatively increased ADH level, the elderly are less able to purge excess water, which in turn increases their susceptibility to hyponatremia.[13,14]

Reduced aldosterone production in the elderly causes the kidneys to excrete sodium even in the presence of hypovolemia when sodium conservation is needed.[15] This inability to conserve sodium when needed predisposes older individuals to FVD. Another effect of reduced aldosterone production is a less vigorous response to hyperkalemia. Recall that in a young person, hyperkalemia stimulates aldosterone release to facilitate renal excretion of excess potassium.

Cardiopulmonary Changes

Cardiovascular and vasomotor responses to an acute drop in blood volume may decline in elderly individuals.[16] As a result, the aged are more susceptible to hypovolemic shock. Other cardiovascular changes associated with aging include stiffening of the large vessels and decreased beta-adrenergic responsiveness of the heart, which limits the maximum achievable heart rate.[17] Changes in the respiratory system in the aged include increased rigidity of the chest wall, decreased respiratory muscle strength, and a decreased forced expiratory volume. In addition, the arterial partial pressure of oxygen (PaO_2) decreases progressively with age.[18] Structural changes in the respiratory system interfere with the elderly patients' ability to respond to hypoxia (oxygen lack) and hypercapnea (carbon dioxide excess).

Fluid and Electrolyte Imbalances in the Elderly

Terminology for Salt and Water Imbalances

Authors may use different terms when referring to salt and water imbalances. In the following discussion, *fluid volume deficit* is defined as an isotonic loss of both water and sodium, yielding a decreased fluid volume with an essentially normal serum sodium concentration. In contrast, *dehydration* is defined as primarily a loss of water, yielding an increased serum sodium concentration (hypernatremia). Either hyponatremia or hypernatremia can be superimposed on fluid volume deficit. For example, when more water is lost than sodium, the condition is called "fluid vol-

ume deficit with hypernatremia," although some authors refer to this condition as "hypertonic dehydration."[19] When more sodium is lost than water, the condition is called "fluid volume deficit with hyponatremia"; some authors call this condition "hypotonic dehydration." **Table 25-1** compares isotonic fluid volume deficit and fluid volume deficit with hypernatremia.

Isotonic Fluid Volume Deficit

As described above, isotonic FVD results when water and electrolytes are lost in an isotonic fashion (see Figure 3-1). Unless concurrent electrolyte imbalances are present, serum electrolyte levels remain essentially unchanged in isotonic FVD. Causes of FVD in the elderly are similar to those observed in younger adults—for example, loss of gastrointestinal fluids, polyuria related to hyperglycemia, excessive use of diuretics, fever, sweating, and third-spacing of fluids in a bowel obstruction (see Table 3-1). However, elderly persons are less well equipped to adapt to FVD and, therefore, are at greater risk for adverse outcomes when excessive fluid losses occur. This imbalance is almost always due to loss of body fluids but is intensified when fluid intake is low.

Hypernatremia

Hypernatremia in the elderly is typically due to decreased water intake along with increased water losses, such as occurs in acute illnesses associated with fever, hyperventilation, or watery diarrhea. For example, in a study in which 264 nursing home residents required hospitalization for an acute illness, more than one-third became markedly hypernatremic.[20]

Hypernatremia significantly increases the risk for mortality among elderly persons. For example, in a study involving more than 15,000 hospitalized patients who were 60 years of age or older, investigators found that those with hypernatremia had a 7 times higher mortality rate than did other age-matched, hospitalized patients.[21] The elderly person is at increased risk for fluid volume deficit, often with accompanying hypernatremia, for a multitude of reasons (**Table 25-2**).

Dehydration in the elderly may be viewed as an indicator of neglect, especially in those persons who are cared for in nursing homes.[22] For example, in a study of 56 records of hypernatremic patients at two public hospitals, investigators found that the average serum sodium concentration of patients transferred from nursing homes was significantly higher than that of patients who developed hypernatremic

Table 25-1 Summary of Fluid Volume Deficit/Hypernatremia Associated with Aging

Imbalance	Precipitating Causes	Clinical Indicators
Isotonic fluid volume deficit	Physiologic changes associated with aging: • Decreased total body water content due to loss of muscle (a water-rich tissue) and gain of fat (a water-poor tissue) increases stress on water balance. • Decreased renal concentration ability interferes with fluid conservation by the kidneys, even in the presence of water deprivation. • Decreased thirst associated with aging prevents the elderly from consuming extra fluid during times of need. • Reduced aldosterone production causes the kidneys to excrete sodium even in the presence of hypovolemia, when sodium conservation is needed. Clinical events: • Loss of gastrointestinal fluids (vomiting and diarrhea). • Fever. • Diuresis (as in excessive use of diuretics or hyperglycemia).	• Dry oral mucous membranes. • Decreased salivation. • Decreased tissue turgor. • Sunken eyes. • Decreased urine volume. • Dark, concentrated urine. • Weight loss over a short period of time (indicating fluid loss; see Chapter 3). • Postural hypotension (increased risk for falls). • BUN elevated out of proportion to serum creatinine level (see Chapter 3). • Elevated hematocrit level. • Body temperature that is slightly lower than normal in a cool room (related to reduced basal metabolic rate associated with FVD).
Fluid volume deficit with hypernatremia	Same as above, plus: • Greater loss of water than of sodium. • Central nervous symptoms of hypernatremia are likely due to cellular dehydration of neurons.	Same as above, plus: • Serum sodium > 145 mEq/L. An elevated serum Na concentration is a more reliable marker of hypernatremia than other clinical indicators. • Thirst (while commonly present in younger individuals) is blunted or absent in the elderly person with hypernatremia. • Dry, sticky mucous membranes. • Possibly a mild temperature elevation. • Disorientation, delusions, and hallucinations in severe hypernatremia. Alternatively, the patient may be lethargic when undisturbed and irritable and hyper-reactive when stimulated. • Lethargy, stupor, or coma. The level of consciousness depends not only on actual sodium levels, but also on the rate of development of hypernatremia. For example, a patient may have a serum sodium level of 170 mEq/L and remain conscious if the imbalance developed slowly.

Table 25-2 Summary of Factors Associated with Poor Fluid Intake in the Elderly

- Impaired thirst due to changes in the thirst center (interfering with the older person's ability drink extra fluid in times of need).
- Impaired cognition, as in dementia and delirium. A direct correlation exists between the Mini-Mental Status Examination score and impairment of water intake.
- Impaired ability to gain access to fluids due to physical disabilities (e.g., poor mobility, arthritis, stroke).
- Impaired swallowing.
- Failure of caregivers to provide adequate fluids for debilitated patients (either by mouth, feeding tube, intravenously, or subcutaneously).

dehydration at home or in an acute care hospital.[23] An in-depth discussion of the recognition and treatment of hyper-natremia is provided in Chapter 4; also see Case Study 4-1. (See the sections on oral hydration, enteral hydration, and parenteral hydration later in this chapter as well.)

Hyponatremia

During normal aging, the serum sodium concentration may decrease by approximately 1 mEq/L for each decade of life after adulthood.[24] In a study of 5000 sets of plasma electrolytes taken from a population of hospitalized individuals (mean age = 54 years), the mean serum sodium concentration was found to be 134 ± 6 mEq/L, with a tendency toward the hyponatremic end of the distribution.[25] Hyponatremia is estimated to occur in 7% of healthy elderly persons,[26] and it may be present in 15% to 18% of elderly patients living in long-term care facilities.[27]

Hyponatremia is a complex imbalance with many causes. Nevertheless, the major classifications for causes are excessive water gain (dilutional hyponatremia) or excessive sodium loss (depletional hyponatremia). See **Table 25-3**.

Dilutional hyponatremia may be caused by too much water and is commonly observed when patients are given excessive amounts of hypotonic intravenous fluids (such as

Table 25-3 Summary of Differences Between Hyponatremia Due to Gain of Water Versus Hyponatremia Due to Loss of Sodium (Usually Accompanied by Fluid Volume Deficit)

Gain of Water	Loss of Sodium
- Excessive administration of D_5W or other hypotonic IV fluids - Excessive water administration with isotonic or hypotonic tube feedings - Psychogenic polydipsia **Disease Conditions** - Oat-cell carcinoma of lung - Carcinoma of duodenum or pancreas - Head trauma - Stroke - Pulmonary disorders (tuberculosis, pneumonia, asthma, respiratory failure) **Drugs** - Tricyclic antidepressants - Selective serotonin reuptake inhibitors - Desmopressin acetate (DDAVP) - Antineoplastic agents (cyclophosphamide, vincristine, cisplatin) **Hydrational Status** - Normal volume or perhaps edema **Laboratory Findings** - Normal or decreased hematocrit - Normal or decreased blood urea nitrogen - Urine sodium > 20 mEq/L - Serum sodium < 135 mEq/L - Serum sodium concentration often much lower when hyponatremia is due to water overload (as compared to when it is due to sodium loss)	- Diuretics - Vomiting - Gastric suction - Diarrhea - Adrenal insufficiency - Osmotic diuresis - Salt-losing nephritis **Hydrational Status** - Hypotension - Tachycardia - Dry mucous membranes - Decreased skin turgor **Laboratory Findings** - Elevated hematocrit - Elevated blood urea nitrogen - Urine sodium < 15 mEq/L - Serum sodium < 135 mEq/L

See Table 4-3 for a list of clinical characteristics of hyponatremia.
Neurological symptoms tend to be more pronounced when hyponatremia is due to water overload.

5% dextrose in water) or too much water with tube feedings. Another cause of dilutional hyponatremia is a condition referred to as syndrome of inappropriate ADH secretion (SIADH; see Chapter 4). Patients with stroke and malignancies (such as small-cell carcinoma of the lung) are at increased risk for SIADH. Use of certain antidepressants—such as the selective serotonin reuptake inhibitors (SSRIs)—is associated with hyponatremia in the elderly (see the discussion of this topic later in the chapter). The elderly person is at especially high risk for dilutional hyponatremia because of decreased ability to purge excess water via the kidneys (due to ADH production changes associated with aging).[28]

Another form of hyponatremia results from decreased sodium intake (as occurs with a low-sodium diet or low-sodium tube feedings) or increased sodium loss (as may occur in vomiting, diarrhea, gastric suctioning, or cerebral salt wasting). Recall that the sodium content of gastrointestinal fluids is relatively high (see Table 13-1). Cerebral salt wasting is associated with neurologic conditions—such as stroke or a brain tumor—that signal the kidneys to excrete more sodium; this condition is described in detail in Chapter 19.

An in-depth discussion of the causes, clinical signs, and treatment of hyponatremia is provided in Chapter 4. As a rule, the hyponatremia caused by sodium loss is associated with less severe neurologic symptoms than is that due to excessive water gain.

Hyperkalemia

Sluggish control of potassium concentration by the aged kidney plus lower aldosterone production makes hyperkalemia a common imbalance in the elderly.[29,30] Although baseline serum potassium levels are not typically elevated in elderly patients, these levels may rise quickly when potassium homeostatic mechanisms are threatened—such as occurs in the presence of volume depletion, change in cardiac function, or therapy with certain medications.[31] A variety of drugs that predispose individuals to hyperkalemia, such as spironolactone and angiotensin-converting enzyme (ACE) inhibitors, may be prescribed for elderly patients with congestive heart failure (a prevalent condition in this population).[32] Because elderly patients with congestive heart failure are also often prescribed a salt-poor diet, they may choose to use salt substitutes, most of which contain potassium chloride. Use of nonsteroidal anti-inflammatory drugs (NSAIDs) can predispose individuals to hyperkalemia as well as sodium and water retention; as such, elderly patients should be cautioned to use these agents judiciously, especially if they are taking other agents with potassium-elevating capacity. Potassium levels should be monitored at regular intervals when geriatric patients are prescribed potassium-altering medications. An in-depth discussion of the recognition and treatment of hyperkalemia is provided in Chapter 5.

Calcium Imbalances

Hypercalcemia occurs in 2% to 3% of institutionalized elderly patients.[33] Causes of this imbalance in the elderly are the same as those in younger adults, including malignant tumors, hyperparathyroidism, immobilization, and thiazide diuretic use. Hypocalcemia is observed less frequently than hypercalcemia in the elderly; the causes of hypocalcemia in this population are also similar to those in younger adults, such as chronic renal failure and chronic malabsorption.[34]

Magnesium Imbalances

Hypomagnesemia may be present in as many as 7% to 10% of hospitalized elderly patients, most commonly due to malnutrition as well as loss of magnesium from use of laxatives or diuretics.[35] Hypermagnesemia is less common and is typically found in patients with renal insufficiency who take magnesium-containing laxatives and antacids. See Chapter 7 for an in-depth discussion of magnesium imbalances.

Phosphorus Imbalances

The most common cause of hypophosphatemia in the elderly is the refeeding syndrome, a condition that occurs when malnourished patients are fed too aggressively—usually via tube feedings or total parenteral nutrition, although it can also be precipitated by oral feedings. (See Chapters 11 and 12.) The most common cause of hyperphosphatemia in the elderly is improper use of phosphate-containing laxatives and enemas. Chapter 8 provides an in-depth discussion of phosphorus imbalances; also see Case Studies 12-1 and 12-3.

Metabolic Acidosis

Reduced ability of the aged kidney to excrete excessive hydrogen ions predisposes elderly persons to metabolic acidosis.[36] Pulmonary changes associated with aging—such as reduced respiratory muscle strength and increased rigidity of the chest wall—may interfere with respiratory compensation for metabolic acidosis via hyperventilation. An in-depth discussion of acid–base imbalances is provided in Chapter 9.

Assessment for Fluid Volume Deficit/Dehydration

Ongoing assessment for fluid volume deficit, and for fluid volume deficit associated with hypernatremia (referred to as dehydration), is important to facilitate early detection and treatment of these imbalances. Dehydration is one of the most frequent reasons why an elderly person is transferred from a nursing home to an acute care hospital.[37] According to one report, approximately one-fourth of the nursing home patients admitted to a hospital are dehydrated.[38]

Intake and Output/Body Weight

A negative fluid balance—as detected on an intake and output (I & O) record—should raise concern and cause the caregiver to initiate a fluid replacement regimen. Of course, an I & O record is useful only if the measurements are properly and reliably obtained. It behooves healthcare institutions to provide proper training on this procedure to ensure the highest degree of accuracy. For example, I & O forms placed at the bedside should list the volume of fluid containers (e.g., glasses, cups). Bouts of incontinence should be recorded and the volume estimated.

Because it is difficult to obtain accurate I & O records, especially when patients are incontinent, it is important to weigh elderly individuals on a regular basis to detect fluid losses. As with I & O records, attention to accuracy is crucial. Scales used to weigh patients should be calibrated at regular intervals, and the patient should be weighed at the same time of day while wearing the same amount of clothing. A loss or gain of 1 kg of body weight in a short period of time is equivalent to the loss of or gain of 1 L of fluid. Decline in food intake has been correlated with a decline in fluid intake (recall that solid foods also contain fluid).

Urine Color

Nurse investigators evaluated the efficacy of a urine color chart to assess hydration status in a group of 98 elderly nursing home residents.[39] A significant correlation was found between colors on the chart and average urine specific gravity readings; the investigators concluded that urine color can be used as an indicator of hydration status. Because nurse assistants spend more time with institutionalized elderly patients than do registered nurses, it is important to teach these individuals about the need to observe for signs of fluid deficit, including the color of urine and frequency of urination.

Skin and Tongue Turgor

Although the purpose of the skin turgor test is to measure only interstitial fluid volume, it also measures skin elasticity. This dual nature of the test presents a problem in the elderly because of age-related decreases in skin elasticity (commonly noted in persons older than 55 to 60 years of age). Thus reduced skin turgor is not diagnostic in the absence of other signs of FVD. Probably the best site to assess skin turgor in elderly people is over the forehead or sternum, where reduced skin elasticity is minimal.

In a person with FVD, the tongue is smaller and has additional longitudinal furrows, again reflecting loss of interstitial fluid. Fortunately, tongue turgor is not affected appreciably by age and, therefore, is a useful assessment in all age groups.

Body Temperature

An elevated body temperature may be observed in a hypernatremic (dehydrated) patient, presumably related to a direct effect on the heat-regulating portion of the hypothalamus and reduced availability of fluid for sweating. In contrast, a patient with an isotonic fluid deficit may be slightly hypothermic in a cool room, a condition probably related to the decreased basal metabolic rate associated with FVD. After partial correction of the FVD, the patient's temperature generally increases to an appropriate level.

Changes in body temperature do not merely reflect fluid balance problems. Fever *causes* fluid balance problems if not promptly recognized and treated. An elevated body temperature causes an increased formation of metabolic wastes that require additional urine production. Fever also causes an increased breathing rate, which is associated with extra water vapor loss. Because fever increases loss of body fluids, temperature elevations must be detected early and appropriate interventions taken. A10% increase in need for water may be needed for every degree of body temperature above 37° C.[40]

Behavior

One of the major causes of acute confusion in frail elders is dehydration. An independent risk factor for delirium is a BUN/Cr ratio greater than 18:1.[41] Hyperosmolality for any reason—such as hypernatremia, hypercalcemia, or uremia—can lead to delirium. Signs of delirium include decreased ability to focus, perceptual disturbances, and drowsiness. The Confusion Assessment Method (CAM) is widely used in a variety of settings to assess for delirium.[42–44]

Blood Pressure

Monitoring for positional changes in blood pressure is helpful in assessing hydration status. For example, one nursing study indicated that a drop of at least 15 mm Hg in the systolic pressure and 10 mm Hg in the diastolic pressure occurred when volume-depleted patients were quickly shifted from a lying to a standing position.[45]

Ability to Obtain Fluids

Functional assessment of an aged patient's ability to obtain fluids is essential. For example, visual impairment may make it difficult for the patient to locate a water glass and pitcher. Tremors or stiffness of hands and fingers may make it difficult for the patient to grasp a pitcher or glass. Alterations in mental status may significantly interfere with the patient's ability to verbalize fluid preferences.

For healthcare providers, it is important to recognize that merely delivering a drink or a food tray to a debilitated elderly person is not sufficient. The food and drink must be placed within the patient's reach, and plastic-wrapped utensils and containers (such as milk and juice cartons) must be opened so they can be accessed by the patient. Sadly, it is not uncommon to see trays removed from an elderly person's bedside, virtually untouched, because these simple rules were ignored.

Ability to Swallow

When an elderly patient coughs or gags when eating or drinking, it likely indicates aspiration (secondary to dysphagia). Another sign of frequent small aspirations of fluid and food is chronic hoarseness. If simple maneuvers to reduce aspiration during feeding are not effective, a swallowing study performed by a speech pathologist may be indicated.[46]

Providing Oral Hydration

When possible, it is always best to administer fluids by mouth to elderly patients. **Table 25-4** summarizes factors to consider when encouraging fluid intake by elderly patients.

In normal circumstances, the requirement for daily fluid intake is approximately 30 mL per kilogram of body weight.

Table 25-4 Suggestions to Increase Fluid Intake in Elderly Individuals

Institutionalized Patients	Elderly Individuals Living at Home
• Place fluids within reach.	• Encourage the individual to drink between 1500 mL and 2000 mL of fluid daily, unless otherwise instructed by physician (e.g., when fluid restriction is ordered in case of congestive heart failure).
• Keep water pitchers filled with fresh, cool water.	
• Provide glasses and cups that are easy to grasp.	
• Have straws available at the bedside.	
• Open milk cartons and other packaged drinks and utensils for the patient if he or she is a self-feeder.	• Encourage the individual to drink extra fluids during hot weather and exercise.
• Offer small volumes of fluid frequently throughout the day; a large container of fluid may discourage the elderly person from drinking.	• Instruct the individual how to self-monitor urine color and report changes to the caregiver.
• Identify several types of fluids that the patient likes and offer them frequently.	• Instruct the patient not to restrict fluid intake in an attempt to reduce episodes of incontinence.
• Offer frozen items (such as frozen juice bars).	• Encourage the individual to follow recommendations from caregivers for fluid intake when disease conditions (such as congestive heart failure) are present.
• Encourage family involvement in increasing fluid intake.	
• Elevate the patient during a sitting position (preferably 90 degrees) to facilitate swallowing.	
• When feeding patients, alternate solids and liquids to increase ease of swallowing.	
• Avoid rushing patients during meals.	
• For dysphagic patients, thickened liquids may be easier to swallow than thin liquids.	
• In some types of dysphagia, a "chin-down" position during feeding may improve swallowing.	

The need is even greater in the presence of fever, increased gastrointestinal fluid losses, and high environmental temperatures. Researchers suggest that at least 1500 to 2000 mL of fluid is necessary to keep long-term care residents sufficiently hydrated.[47] Evidence suggests that adequate fluid intake in the elderly decreases the risk for falls, decreases the need for laxatives to relieve constipation, and perhaps even decreases the risk for more serious conditions (such as heart disease). For example, findings from a study of more than 20,000 men and women between the ages of 38 and 100 years suggested that drinking five or more 8-ounce glasses of water per day is associated with lower rates of fatal coronary heart disease in older adults, as compared to drinking two or fewer glasses of water.[48]

Elderly persons who receive suboptimal fluid intake are more susceptible to confusion and disorientation, urinary tract infections, respiratory infections, renal failure, and pressure ulcers. Those who primarily have water loss (resulting in hypernatremia) are at greater risk for delirium. Unfortunately, proper hydration of the institutionalized elderly is frequently overlooked in practice.[49] A quote from Florence Nightingale is pertinent here: "Every careful observer of the sick will agree in this, that thousands of patients are annually starved in the midst of plenty, from want of attention to the ways which alone make it possible for them to take food."[50] While Nightingale was referring to food, it is important to remember that solid foods also contain water.

The following factors should be considered when analyzing risk for fluid volume deficit ("dehydration") in an elderly patient:

- Amount of fluid consumed (including water consumed with medications and estimates of solid food consumed)
- Comparison of fluid gained versus fluid lost (for example, does fluid output exceed fluid intake?)
- Ability to swallow
- Ability to feed self
- Cognitive ability
- Ability to communicate with caregivers

Providing Hydration/Nutrients by Feeding Tubes

Patients with severe dysphagia are unable to consume adequate fluid by the oral route. In this situation, it is relatively easy to hydrate patients with a feeding tube. For example, in a study that compared hydration status in 28 long-term, swallowing-impaired patients who received oral feedings to that of 67 long-term care patients with nasogastric tube feedings, a higher percentage of dehydration was observed in the orally fed group (75% versus 18%, respectively).[51] Among the markers for dehydration used in the study were low urine output (less than 800 mL/day), elevated values of blood urea nitrogen/serum creatinine, and elevated urine osmolality.

Although tube feedings are sometimes necessary, it is important to recognize the need to provide oral feedings whenever possible. While it takes considerably more time and effort to hand-feed cognitively impaired patients, this approach is the preferred route if they are able to swallow and enjoy food. A recent study compared two nursing homes in which patients with advanced dementia received care.[52] One nursing home had a high tube-feeding rate (41.8%), while the other had a much lower rate (10.7%). The investigators concluded that the nursing home with the lower tube-feeding rate had greater administrative support to empower the staff to hand-feed patients; further, it included a physical environment that promoted the enjoyment of food.

Chapter 12 discusses fluid and electrolyte problems associated with tube feedings. One of the more prominent problems associated with this method in severely malnourished patients is refeeding syndrome (described in Chapters 11 and 12). The most common imbalance associated with refeeding syndrome is hypophosphatemia. For example, in a group of 40 elderly patients who had feeding problems for at least 72 hours prior to the start of nasogastric tube feedings, significant electrolyte changes (including hypophosphatemia) were observed in the first 2 to 3 days following refeeding.[53]

Ethical concerns regarding the use of feeding tubes in elderly patients are beyond the scope of this textbook. Note, however, that it is important to involve the patient (when possible) as well as the patient's family in making this decision.

Providing Parenteral Hydration

When adequate fluid cannot be administered orally or by feeding tube, it is necessary to use the intravenous or subcutaneous route. There are pros and cons for each site, depending on individual patient characteristics.

Intravenous Route

The intravenous route is usually reserved for patients with advanced fluid volume depletion/dehydration. Elderly patients often have poor-quality veins, making it difficult to use peripheral veins for feeding purposes over a prolonged period. Chapter 10 describes commonly used intravenous fluids and their applications. Intravenous management of fluid volume deficit is described in Chapter 3, and intravenous management of hypernatremia is described in Chapter 4.

Subcutaneous Route (Hypodermoclysis)

Hypodermoclysis is the infusion of fluids into the subcutaneous tissue with an intravenous needle or catheter. For elderly debilitated patients who need short-term hydration to treat mild or moderate fluid volume deficit/dehydration, the subcutaneous route may be considered. Although the thigh area is the most commonly used site for parenteral hydration in the elderly, other sites may include the upper back and abdominal wall. The hypodermoclysis injection site should be changed when signs of poor absorption, swelling, or redness appear.

Among the suitable fluids for subcutaneous administration are isotonic saline (0.9% sodium chloride) or half-strength saline (0.45% sodium chloride); both of these solutions may be used with or without added small concentrations of dextrose. Flow rates used in clinical practice are highly variable. Some clinicians will administer a bolus of 500 mL over a period of 2 to 6 hours.[54] Others may administer the fluid continuously at a rate of 75 mL or more per hour.[55] Tolerance at the infusion site is the major determinant of flow rate. Rarely is more than 3000 mL administered in a 24-hour period (using two sites concurrently).[56]

Major advantages of the subcutaneous route for fluid administration include the following points:

- This method is easy to set up for use in long-term care facilities, acute care settings, or even the patient's home.
- Insertion of devices into the subcutaneous tissues is far easier than insertion of devices into the venous system (so a relatively low skill level is required for hypodermoclysis).
- Subcutaneous delivery has a low cost (compared to the skill level needed for intravenous administration of fluids).
- This method is valuable for short-term use during brief periods when the patient is unable to consume adequate oral fluid or is experiencing increased fluid losses.
- Subcutaneous infusions may reduce the transfer of mildly volume-depleted nursing home patients to acute care settings for hydration.

Major disadvantages include the following issues:

- Less fluid can be administered via the subcutaneous route than by the intravenous route.
- Limited types of fluids can be administered subcutaneously (for example, hypertonic solutions are not suitable for subcutaneous administration).
- Most medications and nutrient additives are not suitable for subcutaneous administration.
- Irritating additives (such as potassium chloride) produce pain at the infusion site and, therefore, can be infused at only low concentrations.
- Edema at the infusion site is common and necessitates moving the insertion sites if subcutaneous infusions are used for more than a limited time.
- Cellulitis may occur if aseptic technique is not observed.
- Bleeding is possible, especially in patients with coagulopathy.[57]
- Although rare, it is possible to puncture the bowel when the abdominal site is used in a very thin patient. (See Case Study 25-3.)

Hypodermoclysis is used more frequently in Europe, Asia, and Canada than in the United States.[58] However, it is gaining favor in the United States, especially in non-acute settings.

Special Problems in Elderly Patients

Discussed in this section are conditions that place elderly patients at increased risk for fluid and electrolyte problems.

Hyponatremia Associated with Antidepressants

Because depression in common in elderly patients, antidepressants are often prescribed for members of this population. Investigators have reported that users of selective serotonin receptor inhibitors (SSRIs) have approximately a four times higher risk for hyponatremia (as compared to patients who use other antidepressant drugs).[59] Elderly patients who take SSRIs while also taking diuretics fall into the highest risk category.[60] Examples of SSRIs include citalopram (Celexa), escitalopram (Lexapro), fluoxetine (Prozac), fluvoxamine (Luvox), paroxetine (Paxil), and sertraline (Zoloft).[61] An estimated 12% of older adults taking SSRIs may develop clinical symptoms.[62] Additional risk factors for antidepressant-induced hyponatremia include low body weight, female sex, use of other medications that can cause hyponatremia (such as diuretics), and a previous history of hyponatremia.

Hyponatremia associated with antidepressant use usually occurs within the first few weeks of treatment.[63] Changes in mental status, including confusion and lethargy, should be investigated immediately.[64] Because symptoms of hyponatremia can mimic depression or psychosis, it is important to be aware of the possibility of this imbalance and to periodically monitor serum sodium levels. Some authors recommend checking serum sodium levels in older adults at least once during the first month of use of antidepressants.[65] If hyponatremia is found, the medication should be discontinued until the imbalance is corrected.[66] (See Case Study 25-1.)

Nephropathy Associated with Use of Contrast Dyes for Diagnostic Tests

Contrast-induced nephropathy (CIN) is a common cause of acute renal failure in hospitalized patients. Elderly patients are at increased risk for CIN because of age-related renal changes, especially if their baseline serum creatinine level is elevated. The cornerstone of care for preventing CIN is the administration of intravenous fluids beginning 12 to 24 hours before the contrast study and ending 12 hours after the study.[67] The fluids most often recommended for this purpose are isotonic saline and half-strength saline.[68–70] A drug sometimes administered prior to use of the contrast medium is N-acetylcysteine, an agent that improves renal vasodilation (see Chapter 17).

Nocturia

Nocturnal urination is a common problem in many older adults and is frequently overlooked as a cause of sleep disturbance. For example, in a survey of 1424 individuals between the ages of 55 and 84 years, 53% reported that nocturia was a self-perceived cause for sleep disturbance; this condition was identified more than four times as frequently as the next most cited cause of poor sleep, pain (12%).[71]

In elderly individuals, the diurnal pattern of ADH secretion may be disrupted. Recall that in younger adults there is increased production of ADH during the night to reduce urine formation; for example, the night-time urine volume in these individuals represents 25% or less of their total urine volume.[72] However, due to renal changes associated with aging, the elderly person's night-time urine volume might actually exceed the daytime urine output. Adding to the likelihood of nocturnal voiding is reduced bladder capacity and detrussor muscle instability (common conditions in the elderly). Sometimes used to treat nocturnal polyuria is the vasopressin analogue, desmopressin acetate (DDAVP), which is given in the evening. This drug causes the kidneys to retain water, however, its use is associated with an increased risk for developing dilutional hyponatremia.

The risk–benefit ratio for the use of DDAVP to reduce nocturia in an elderly population should be considered before this agent is prescribed. The key question is this: Does the potential benefit for reduced nocturia exceed the potential risk for hyponatremia? A study of 10 carefully screened nursing home patients, 65 years of age and older, with night-time urinary incontinence did not find a significant improvement in night-time nocturia.[73] In an attempt to reduce night-time incontinence, 6 patients were given oral DDAVP in a dose of 0.1 mg; the other 4 patients were given oral DDAVP in a dose of 0.2 mg. Both DDAVP dosages yielded a mean reduction of 0.7 night-time events of incontinence. One patient in each group developed hyponatremia; in both instances, the hyponatremia resolved when the DDAVP was discontinued. The investigators concluded that the modest average reduction in nighttime urination was of little clinical significance.

From personal experience, Miller has observed that as many as 20% of older adults treated with oral DDAVP experience hyponatremia.[74] A meta-analysis of 7 studies led to the conclusion that hyponatremia is relatively common in older adults taking DDAVP for the treatment of nocturia.[75] Because of the risk of hyponatremia, individuals who are given DDAVP should have their serum sodium levels monitored within 3 to 7 days after initiation of the treatment and periodically thereafter.[76] Some authors have recommended that patients with a baseline serum sodium concentration below the normal range should not be treated with DDAVP.[77]

Imbalances Associated with Diuretics

Diuretics are among the most frequently prescribed drugs for hypertension and congestive heart failure in the elderly. Potassium-losing diuretics (such as the thiazides and furosemide) have a greater tendency to induce hypokalemia in the aged than in the younger adult population. Hypokalemia potentiates the action of digitalis and can precipitate toxic symptoms. Use of a potassium-sparing diuretic, such as spironolactone (Aldactone) or triamterene (Dyrenium), may produce a higher incidence of hyperkalemia in elderly patients.[78]

Hyponatremia has been attributed to thiazide diuretic use in the elderly; at greatest risk are persons with a small body mass, low fluid intake, or excessive intake of low-sodium nutritional supplements.[79] Because of the orthostatic hypotension associated with diuretic-induced FVD, an older patient taking such a medication may become dizzy upon position change and experience a fall. Indeed, the use of diuretics has been identified as a characteristic of patients at risk for falls.

Patients on diuretic therapy should be weighed daily. Serum electrolyte levels should be determined at regular intervals. In addition, older patients should be monitored closely for signs of weakness, lethargy, and postural hypotension.

Imbalances Associated with Laxatives and Enemas

In the elderly, reduced motility of the intestinal tract and a lessened sense of the need to eliminate can lead to chronic constipation and dependence on laxatives and enemas. In addition to decreased gastrointestinal motility with aging, certain drugs—such as anticholinergics and antacids containing calcium carbonate or aluminum hydroxide—predispose patients to constipation. Persons older than age 70 take laxatives far more frequently than do younger adults. Prolonged use of strong laxatives predisposes individuals to large losses of intestinal fluid with resultant hypokalemia and FVD (see Chapter 13). Unfortunately, use of laxatives in the aged often becomes a habit, requiring larger and more frequent doses to achieve results.

Hypermagnesemia. Magnesium-containing laxatives (such as milk of magnesia and citrate of magnesia) and antacids are readily available as over-the-counter products and are frequently used by the aged. Even usual doses of magnesium laxatives or antacids are sufficient to cause toxic serum levels in patients with impaired renal function—which is not an unusual finding in the elderly. (See Case Studies 13-7 and 13-8.) Recall that the kidneys are the major route for excretion of magnesium from the body.

Hyperphosphatemia. Hyperphosphatemia and even phosphate nephropathy may result from the improper use of phosphate-containing laxatives. Individuals at increased risk for acute phosphate nephropathy include those of advanced age, those with kidney disease or decreased intravascular volume, and those using medicines that affect renal perfusion or function (e.g., diuretics, ACE inhibitors, angiotensin-receptor blockers, and possibly NSAIDs). Hyperphosphatemia may also result from the improper use of phosphate-containing enemas, especially in patients with slowed colonic motility or megacolon. (See Case Studies 8-4 and 13-4.)

Fluid Volume Deficit. Standard colon-cleansing techniques for diagnostic studies constitute a threat to the fluid status of elderly persons who are only marginally hydrated when these measures are implemented. Most gastrointestinal studies are now performed in outpatient settings, making it impossible to observe the elderly person undergoing rigorous bowel preparation for adverse events. Isotonic sodium-containing intravenous fluids may be needed to maintain an adequate fluid status during and immediately after the procedure. Patients should be encouraged to increase their fluid intake when they return home until their fluid status returns to normal.

Hyperglycemic Hyperosmolar Syndrome

Diabetes mellitus is common among the elderly, especially those residing in nursing homes. With advancing age, there is a decrease in the insulin secretory reserve and in insulin sensitivity.[80] Further, elderly individuals do not experience normal thirst urges and typically tend to drink too little fluid. Thus elderly individuals are especially vulnerable to hyperglycemia and dehydration, usually in the form of hyperglycemic hyperosmolar syndrome (HHS).[81]

The major characteristics of HHS are severe hyperglycemia, hyperosmolality, and dehydration (without ketoacidosis). Most elderly patients who develop HHS have relatively mild (perhaps undetected) diabetes mellitus, which may initially become manifest during a sudden acute illness. Precipitating factors in the elderly person with diabetes may include infections (often pneumonia), hyperosmolar tube feedings, high carbohydrate administration (as in total parenteral nutrition), and certain medications (such as osmotic diuretics or steroids).

Recall that normal aging reduces the kidneys' ability to retain needed fluid. As such, the elderly patient may continue to excrete relatively large volumes of urine even when little fluid is being consumed. Monitoring the adequacy of fluid intake in the elderly diabetic patient is an important assessment that can lead to early detection of HHS.

Diabetic ketoacidosis (DKA) is relatively uncommon in older adults, unless they have type 1 diabetes mellitus. The mortality rate for HHS is much higher than in DKA, primarily because HHS is more likely to occur in elderly patients with significant comorbidities. Chapter 18 provides an in-depth discussion of HHS and DKA.

Perioperative Period

Elderly persons tolerate major surgery and its complications less well than younger adults; therefore, it is important to identify conditions that can adversely affect fluid balance in older patients who are undergoing surgical procedures. For example, a recent report of increased mortality in elderly patients who experienced hip fractures and had elevated blood urea nitrogen (BUN) and abnormal electrolyte values prior to surgery emphasizes the need to correct imbalances prior to surgery whenever possible.[82] Moderate FVD and decreased circulating blood volume are not uncommon in the elderly *before* surgery. Giving intravenous fluids (such as isotonic saline or lactated Ringer's solution) may be necessary prior to anesthesia induction to assure an adequate urine output. Hypotension is poorly tolerated by the aged and, unless corrected quickly, is frequently complicated by renal damage, stroke, or myocardial infarction. Shock also becomes irreversible earlier than this population in young patients.

Aged patients develop sodium deficit faster than younger adults; thus it is important to be alert for this imbalance when a patient is losing sodium-rich fluids. The risk for hyponatremia is intensified by the use of hypotonic intravenous fluids. Recall that all postoperative patients (regardless of age) are at increased risk for hyponatremia owing to increased release of ADH associated with stress, pain, and nausea.

Control of pH balance is less efficient in elderly patients undergoing surgery, so pH disturbances are more likely to occur in this group than in younger adults. Further, changes in pH are less well tolerated by the elderly. These individuals have a tendency toward metabolic acidosis, as the kidneys have an (age-related) impaired ability to excrete excess acids. Diminished respiratory function interferes with carbon dioxide elimination; thus the elderly patient is at risk for respiratory acidosis. In addition to decreased renal and pulmonary reserves, the presence of anemia, with its decreased hemoglobin, depletes one of the major buffer systems. Emphysema is not uncommon in the aged and also disrupts pH control. Measures to improve pulmonary function should be used both preoperatively and postoperatively in older patients, such as frequent turning, encouraging maximal physical activity, avoiding restrictive clothing, and keeping the respiratory tract free of excess secretions.

For patients who are diabetic, oral hypoglycemic agents are usually held the night before surgery to reduce risk for operative hypoglycemia. For insulin-requiring diabetics, the typical practice is to administer half of the usual dose of intermediate-acting insulin on the morning of surgery and to administer appropriate amounts of a 5% glucose solution intravenously, based on blood glucose monitoring.[83]

Malnutrition is more common in aged individuals than in younger adults and contributes to the increased incidence of postoperative complications in the elderly population. Preoperative dietary management is particularly important. Optimal nutrition helps the aged patient withstand the electrolyte deficits and pH changes occurring with surgery. If the patient is unable to eat, tube feedings or parenteral nutrients are indicated to meet nutritional needs and build up reserves. (Tube feedings are discussed in Chapter 12 and parenteral nutrition is discussed in Chapters 10 and 11.)

CASE STUDIES

Case Study 25-1

A case was reported in which a 90-year-old woman with depression was treated with citalopram 10 mg (an SSRI).[84] Following use of the medication, the patient reported an improved mood. Other medications concurrently used by the patient included an ACE inhibitor, hydrochlorothiazide, and atorvastatin. Later, the patient experienced a fall and sustained a hip fracture that required placement of a prosthetic femoral head. While in the hospital, the patient appeared desponded and thus her dose of citalopram was increased to 20 mg. The surgery was tolerated well and the patient was eventually discharged to an assisted living facility.

Two days following discharge from the hospital, the patient was found disoriented and confused on the floor in her room. A serum sodium level at that time was 112 mEq/L. She was again admitted to the hospital, this time for treatment of hyponatremia. Both the SSRI and diuretic were discontinued. Following treatment, the serum sodium level normalized and she was discharged on a fluid restriction of 1000 mL per day. After several weeks, the fluid restriction was lifted and the patient's serum sodium concentration remained within a normal range. The patient's mild symptoms of depression persisted and no additional antidepressant was prescribed.

Commentary. Multiple risk factors for antidepressant-induced hyponatremia were present in this patient. First, a review of her history revealed several notations over the past few years of mild hyponatremia found on routine blood tests.[85] Second, she received other medications that predisposed her to developing hyponatremia, such as hydrochlorothiazide and an ACE inhibitor. Yet another risk factor for antidepressant-induced hyponatremia was her female gender. The risk for hyponatremia was further increased when the patient's dosage of the SSRI was doubled while she was hospitalized. Her serum sodium concentration was quite low (112 mEq/L) and accounted for the neurologic symptoms of confusion and disorientation. Recall that hyponatremia causes cellular swelling throughout the body, including the brain. It is likely that the patient experienced more subtle symptoms earlier.

Case Study 25-2

A case was reported in which a 70-year-old man had a medical history of chronic alcoholism, congestive heart failure with swollen legs, diabetes mellitus, and hypertension.[86] At the time of his admission to a long-term care facility, he had significant hypokalemia (serum K = 2.5 mEq/L) and mild hypomagnesemia (serum Mg = 1.2 mg/dL). To help correct these imbalances, the patient was given 40 mEq of potassium chloride once daily as well as 500 mg of magnesium oxide once daily. In addition, he was given spironolactone 50 mg twice daily, propranolol 40 mg once daily, thiamine 100 mg daily, and folic acid 1 mg daily.

A few weeks later, when admitted to an acute care facility, the patient was confused and combative and appeared cachetic. The fluid overload present at the time of his admission to the long-term care facility was no longer evident; in fact, the patient had poor skin turgor. Although he had been able to ambulate when first admitted to the long-term care facility, he was unable to walk—due to profound muscle weakness—when admitted to the acute care facility. Prominent among his laboratory data upon admission to the acute care facility were profound hyperkalemia (K = 9.7 mEq/L), hyperglycemia (glucose = 418 mg/dL), mild hyponatremia (Na = 131 mEq/L), and a high BUN/Cr ratio (65 mg/dL:2.1 mg/dL). An ECG showed evidence of peaked T waves, a finding consistent with hyperkalemia. Treatment for the profound hyperkalemia included intravenous calcium, dextrose and insulin, sodium bicarbonate, and oral sodium polystyrene sulfonate. The potassium-elevating drugs (spironolactone and potassium chloride) the patient had been prescribed at the long-term care facility were discontinued.

The patient's serum potassium level normalized within the first 24 hours. As his potassium level normalized, the patient regained strength and generally improved. Fortunately for this patient, he was transferred to a facility where clinicians quickly identified the potentially fatal serum potassium concentration and administered correct treatment.

Commentary. The hypokalemia present at the time of this patient's admission to the long-term care facility was caused by poor nutritional intake and chronic alcoholism. The drug regimen instituted at the long term care facility consisted of a potassium-conserving agent (spironolactone) and potassium chloride. Spironolactone, as a potassium-sparing diuretic, can significantly elevate the serum potassium concentration, especially when used in a large dose for several weeks in combination with potassium supplementation (40 mEq of KCl each day) and in the presence of chronic renal disease (indicated by the serum creatinine level of 2.1 mg/dL). Recall that the elderly are at higher risk for developing hyperkalemia than younger adults because of age-related changes in the kidney. The authors of this case study recommend that serum potassium levels be carefully monitored when nursing home patients receive drugs that can elevate the serum potassium concentration—for example, potassium-sparing diuretics, potassium supplements, and ACE inhibitors.

Case Study 25-3

A case was reported in which an 86-year-old woman with advanced dementia experienced a complication of hypodermoclysis while being cared for in a long-term care facility.[87] The patient was very thin (99 pounds) and developed difficulty in eating and drinking. To administer a solution of 0.9% sodium chloride (isotonic saline), her caregivers inserted a 26-gauge short needle in the right inferior quadrant of her abdomen. No immediate complication was observed during the insertion of the needle; however, 2 hours later, the patient experienced increased confusion. The next day, the patient experienced bilious vomiting. At that time, the patient was transferred to an acute care facility. Her temperature was 36.4°C. Pain and diffuse tenderness were evident during an abdominal examination. Inspection of the abdominal wall noted a needle puncture hole in the right iliac fossa. An abdominal computed tomography (CT) scan showed subcutaneous emphysema, pneumoperitoneum, and global intestinal distention. During surgery, a cecal puncture was observed close to the puncture site of the hypodermoclysis. A cecal resection was performed with ileostomy and colostomy. Antibiotics were administered to treat the patient's generalized peritonitis. After 2 weeks, the patient recovered and was returned to the long-term care facility.

Commentary. The authors of this case report commented on the difficulties encountered in long-term care facilities when trying to provide fluids to patients who are unable to eat and drink. As compared to the intravenous route or insertion of a nasogastric tube, the subcutaneous route for fluid administration is perceived to be less invasive and easier to perform. In this patient, the abdominal site was selected over sites in the leg or arm. Unfortunately, the needle perforated the cecum when it was inserted in the right iliac fossa of this very thin woman.

The authors of the case report recommend that, when the abdomen is selected for hypodermoclysis, it is best to use the left iliac fossa because at that point there is a maximal distance between the colon and the abdominal wall.

They also suggest that careful aspiration from the needle should be the rule to so as to detect blood vessel injury or air aspiration. Despite the unfortunate occurrence in this patient, the authors of the case report believe that hypodermoclysis seems to be a reasonable alternative to intravenous rehydration in the elderly, provided safety rules are respected.

Also see Case Studies 4-5, 4-7, 4-10, 4-11, 5-4, 5-11, 5-12, 5-13, 8-4, 8-6, and 13-2 for a discussion of other geriatric patients with fluid and electrolyte problems.

Summary of Key Points

- Reduction in total body water in the aged increases elderly patients' susceptibility to stresses on fluid balance.
- The glomerular filtration rate (GFR) decreases approximately 1 mL/min per year after the age of 50 years. However, the serum creatinine level tends to remain in the normal range because of a concurrent reduction in creatine formation due to reduced muscle mass in older persons.
- An intrinsic defect in the thirst mechanism is associated with aging. As a result, when elderly persons are challenged by fluid deprivation, they exhibit less thirst and consume less fluid than younger adults.
- During normal aging, the serum sodium concentration decreases by approximately 1 mEq/L for each decade of life after adulthood.
- Causes of hyponatremia in the elderly vary widely. Use of SSRIs as a treatment for depression is an especially common cause of this electrolyte imbalance in older patients.
- Elderly persons experience fluid volume deficit, or fluid volume deficit with hypernatremia, more frequently than younger adults.
- Dehydration is one of the most frequent reasons that an elderly person is transferred from a nursing home to an acute care hospital.
- Hypernatremia significantly increases risk for mortality in the elderly.
- Sluggish control of potassium concentration by the aged kidney plus lower aldosterone production makes hyperkalemia a common electrolyte imbalance observed in the elderly.
- Potassium imbalances associated with diuretic use are more common in the elderly than in younger adults.
- Nocturnal urination is a common problem in many older adults and is frequently overlooked as a cause of sleep disturbance. It is apparently caused by renal changes associated with aging and possibly a disruption in the diurnal pattern of ADH production.
- Elderly individuals use laxatives and enemas more often than do younger adults. Because of their reduced renal function, older individuals are at greater risk for hypermagnesemia, hyperphosphatemia, and other electrolyte imbalances from excessive use of laxatives and enemas.

NOTES

1. Beck, L. H., & Lavizzo-Mourey, R. (1987). Geriatric hypernatremia. *Annals of Internal Medicine, 107,* 768–769.

2. Fulop, T., Worum, I., Csongor, J., Foris, G., & Leovey, A. (1985). Body composition in elderly people: Determination of body composition by multiisotope method and the elimination kinetics of these isotopes in healthy elderly subjects. *Gerontology, 31,* 6–14.

3. Phillips, P. A., Rolls, B. J., Ledingham, J. G., Forsling, M. L., Morton, J. J., Crowe, M. J., et al. (1984). Reduced thirst after water deprivation in healthy elderly men. *New England Journal of Medicine, 311,* 753–759.

4. Kenney, W. L., & Chiu, P. (2001). Influence of age on thirst and fluid intake. *Medicine and Science in Sports and Exercise, 33,* 1524–1532.

5. Tedla, F. M., & Friedman, E. A. (2008). The trend toward geriatric nephrology. *Primary Care Clinics in Office Practice, 35,* 515–530.

6. Epstein, M. (1996). Aging and the kidney. *Journal of the American Society of Nephrology, 7,* 1106–1122.

7. Miller, M. (2009). Disorders of fluid balance. In J. B. Halter et al., *Hazzard's geriatric medicine and gerontology* (6th ed.). New York: McGraw-Hill Medical, p. 1047.

8. Miller, note 7, p. 1048.

9. Epstein, note 6.

10. Beck, L. H. (1990). Perioperative renal, fluid, and electrolyte management. *Clinics in Geriatric Medicine, 6,* 557–569.

11. Beck & Lavizzo-Mourey, note 1.

12. Miller, note 7, p. 1050.

13. Luckey, A. E., & Parsa, C. J. (2003). Fluid and electrolytes in the aged. *Archives of Surgery, 138,* 1055–1060.

14. Miller, M. (1995). Hormonal aspects of fluid and sodium balance in the elderly. *Endocrinology Metabolism Metabolic Clinics of North America, 24,* 233–253.

15. Beck, L. H. (2000). The aging kidney: Defending a delicate balance of fluid and electrolytes. *Geriatrics, 55,* 26–28, 31–32.

16. Allison, S. P., & Lobo, D. N. (2004). Fluid and electrolytes in the elderly. *Current Opinion in Clinical Nutrition and Metabolic Care, 7,* 27–33.

17. Aalami, O. O., Fang, T. D., Song, H. M., & Nacamuli, R. P. (2003). Physiological features of aging persons. *Archives of Surgery, 138,* 1068–1076.

18. Aalami et al., note 17.

19. Allison & Lobo, note 16.

20. Miller, note 7, p. 1055.

21. Snyder, N. A., Feigal, D. W., & Arieff, A. I. (1987). Hypernatremia in elderly patients: A heterogeneous, morbid, and iatrogenic entity. *Annals of Internal Medicine, 107*(3), 309–319.

22. Himmelstein, D. U., Jones, A. A., & Woolhandler, S. (1983). Hypernatremic dehydration in nursing home patients: An indicator of neglect. *Journal of the American Geriatrics Society, 31*(8), 466–471.

23. Himmelstein et al., note 22.

24. Luckey & Parsa, note 13.

25. Miller, note 7, p. 1052.

26. Caird, F. I. (1973). Problems of interpretation of laboratory findings in the old. *British Medical Journal, 4,* 348–351.

27. Beck, L. H. (1998). Changes in renal function with aging [abstract]. *Clinical Geriatric Medicine, 14,* 199–200.

28. Kugler, J. P., & Hustead, T. (2000). Hyponatremia and hypernatremia in the elderly. *American Family Physician, 61,* 3623–3630.

29. Beck, note 15.

30. Lerma, E. V. (2009). Anatomic and physiologic changes of the aging kidney. *Clinics in Geriatric Medicine, 25*(3), 325–329.

31. Perazella, M. A., & Mahnensmith, R. L. (1997). Hyperkalemia in the elderly: Drugs exacerbate impaired potassium homeostasis. *Journal of General Internal Medicine, 12,* 646–656.

32. Vanpee, D., & Swine, C. H. (2000).Elderly heart failure patients with drug-induced serious hyperkalemia. *Aging & Clinical and Experimental Research, 12,* 315–319.

33. Lerma, note 30.

34. Lerma, note 30.

35. Lerma, note 30.

36. Luckey & Parsa, note 13.

37. Schols, J., De Groot, C. P., Van der Cammen, T. J, Olde Rikkert, M. G. (2009). Preventing and treating dehydration in the elderly during periods of illness and warm weather. *Journal of Nutrition, Health & Aging, 13,* 150–157.

38. Lavizzo-Mourey, R., Johnson, J., & Stolley, P. (1988). Risk factors for dehydration among elderly nursing home residents. *Journal of the American Geriatrics Society, 36,* 213–218.

39. Mentes, J. C., Wakefield, B., & Culp, K. (2006). Use of a urine color chart to monitor hydration status in nursing home residents. *Biological Research for Nursing, 7*(3), 197–203.

40. Pestana, C. (2000). *Fluids and electrolytes in the surgical patient* (5th ed.). Philadephia: Lippincott Williams & Wilkins, p. 26.

41. Inouye, S. K. (2000). Prevention of delirium in hospitalized older patients: Risk factors and targeted intervention strategies. *Annals of Medicine, 32*(4), 257–263.

42. Inouye, S. K., vanDyck, C., Alessi, C. A., Balkin, S., Siegal, A. P., & Horwitz, R. I. (1990). Clarifying confusion: The confusion assessment method. *Annals of Internal Medicine, 113,* 941–948.

43. Wei, L. A., Fearing, M. A., Sternberg, E. J., & Inouye, S. K. (2008). The Confusion Assessment Method: A systematic review of current usage. *Journal of the American Geriatrics Society, 56*(5), 823–830.

44. Adamis, D., Treloar, A., MacDonald, A. J., & Martin, F. C. (2005). Concurrent validity of two instruments (the Confusion Assessment Method and the Delirium Rating Scale) in the detection of delirium among older medical inpatients. *Age & Ageing, 34*(1), 72–75.

45. Robinson, S. B., & Demuth, P. L. (1985). Diagnostic studies for the aged: What are the dangers? *Journal of Gerontologic Nursing, 11*(6), 6–9.

46. Metheny, N. A., & Hartford Institute for Geriatric Nursing. Preventing aspiration in older adults with dysphagia. (2007). *MEDSURG Nursing, 16*(4), 271–272.

47. Chidester, J. C., & Spangler, A. A. (1997). Fluid intake in the institutionalized elderly. *Journal of the American Dietary Association, 97,* 23–28.

48. Chan, J., Knutsen, S. F., Blix, G. G., Lee, J. W., & Fraser, G. E. (2002). Water, other fluids, and fatal coronary heart disease: The Adventist Health Study. *American Journal of Epidemiology, 155,* 827–833.

49. Chidester & Spangler, note 47.

50. Nightingale, F. (1859/1946). *Notes on nursing: What it is and what it is not.* Philadelphia: Edward Stern & Company, p. 36.

51. Leibovitz, A., Baumoehl, Y., Lubart, E., Yaina, A., Platinovitz, N., & Segal, R. (2007). Dehydration among long-term care elderly patients with oropharyngeal dysphagia. *Gerontology, 53*(4), 179–183.

52. Lopez, R. P., Amella, E. J., Strumpf, N. E., Teno, J. M., & Mitchell, S. L. (2010). The influence of nursing home culture on the use of feeding tubes. *Archives of Internal Medicine, 170*(1), 83–28.

53. Lubart, E., Leibovitz, A., Dror, Y., Katz, E., & Segal, R. (2009). Mortality after nasogastric tube feeding initiation in long-term care elderly with oropharyngeal dysphagia: The contribution of refeeding syndrome. *Gerontology, 55,* 393–397.

54. Slesak, G., Schnürle, J. W., Kinzel, E., Jakob, J., & Dietz, P. K. (2003). Comparison of subcutaneous and intravenous rehydration in geriatric patients: A randomized trial. *Journal of the American Geriatrics Society, 51,* 155–160.

55. Frisoli, A. Jr., de Paula, A. P., Feldman, D., & Nasri, F. (2000). Subcutaneous hydration by hypodermoclysis: A practical and low

cost treatment for elderly patients. *Drugs & Aging, 16*(4), 313–319.

56. Dasgupta, M., Binns, M. A., & Rochon, P. A. (2000). Subcutaneous fluid infusion in a long-term care setting. *Journal of the American Geriatrics Society, 48,* 795–799.

57. O'Hanlon, S., Sheahan, P., & McEneaney, R. (2009). Severe hemorrhage from a hypodermoclysis site. *American Journal of Hospice and Palliative Care, 26,* 135–136.

58. Remington, R., & Hultman, T. (2007). Hypodermoclysis to treat dehydration: A review of the evidence. *Journal of the American Geriatrics Society, 55,* 2051–2055.

59. Movig, K. L., Leufkens, H. G., Lenderink, A. W., & Egberts, A. C. (2002). Association between antidepressant drug use and hyponatremia: A case-control study. *British Journal of Clinical Pharmacology, 53,* 363–369.

60. Movig et al., note 59.

61. Bowen, P. D. (2009). Use of selective serotonin reuptake inhibitors in the treatment of depression in older adults: Identifying and managing potential risk for hyponatremia. *Geriatric Nursing, 30*(2), 85–89.

62. Fabian, T. J., Amico, T. A., Kroboth, P. D., Mulsant, B. H., Corey, S. E., Begley, A. E., et al. (2004). Paroxetine-induced hyponatremia in older adults: A 12-week prospective study. *Archives of Internal Medicine, 164,* 327–332.

63. Mago, R., Mahajan, R., & Thase, M. E. (2008). Medically serious adverse effects of newer antidepressants. *Current Psychiatry Reports, 10*(3), 249–257.

64. Mentes, J. (2006). Oral hydration in older adults: Greater awareness is needed in preventing, recognizing, and treating dehydration. *American Journal of Nursing, 106,* 40–49.

65. Mago et al., note 63.

66. Sharma, H., & Pompei, P. (1996). Antidepressant-induced hyponatremia in the aged: Avoidance and management strategies. *Drugs and Aging, 8*(6), 430–435.

67. Cooper, D. H., Kranik, A. J., Lubner, S. J., & Reno, H. E. (Eds.). (2007). *The Washington manual of medical therapeutics* (32nd ed.). Philadelphia: Wolters Kluwer/Lippincott Williams & Wilkins, p. 320.

68. Marenzi, G., & Bartorelli, A. L. (2004). Recent advances in the prevention of radiocontrast-induced nephropathy. *Current Opinion in Critical Care, 10*(6), 505–509.

69. Asif, A., Garces, G., Preston, R. A., & Roth, D. (2005). Current trials of interventions to prevent radiocontrast-induced nephropathy. *American Journal of Therapeutics, 12*(2), 127–132.

70. Chen, S. L., Zhang, J., Yei, F., Zhu, Z., Liu, Z., Lin, S., et al. (2008). Clinical outcomes of contrast-induced nephropathy in patients undergoing percutaneous coronary intervention: A prospective, multicenter, randomized study to analyze the effect of hydration and acetylcysteine. *International Journal of Cardiology, 126*(3), 407–413.

71. Bliwise, D. L., Foley, D. J., Vitiello, M. V., Ansari, F. P., Ancoli-Israel, S., & Walsh, J. K. (2009). Nocturia and disturbed sleep in the elderly. *Sleep Medicine, 10*(5), 540–548.

72. Miller, note 7, p. 1056.

73. Johnson, T. M. 2nd, Miller, M., Tang, T., Pillion, D. J., & Ouslander, J. G. (2006). Oral ddAVP for nighttime urinary incontinence in characterized nursing home residents: A pilot study. *Journal of the American Medical Directors Association, 7*(1), 6–11.

74. Miller, note 7, p. 1057.

75. Weatherall, M. (2004). The risk of hyponatremia in older adults using desmopressin for nocturia: A systematic review and meta-analysis. *Neurourology & Urodynamics, 23*(4), 302–305.

76. Miller, note 7, p. 1057.

77. Rembratt, A., Riis, A., & Norgaard, J. P. (2006). Desmopressin treatment in nocturia: An analysis of risk factors for hyponatremia. *Neurourology & Urodynamics, 25*(2), 105–109.

78. Todd, B. (1989). Oral potassium supplements. *Geriatric Nursing, 9*(2), 121–122.

79. Sonnenblick, J., Friedlander, Y., & Rosin, A. (1993). Diuretic-induced severe hyponatremia: Review and analysis of 129 reported patients. *Chest, 103,* 601–606.

80. Gaglia, J. L., Wyckoff, J., & Abrahamson, M. J. (2004). Acute hyperglycemic crisis in the elderly. *Medical Clinics of North America, 88*(4), 1063–1084.

81. MacIsaac, R. J., Lee, L. Y., McNeil, K. J., Tsalamandris, C., & Jerums, G. (2002). Influence of age on the presentation and outcome of acidotic and hyperosmolar diabetic emergencies. *Internal Medicine Journal, 32*(8), 379–385.

82. Lewis, J. R., Hassan, S. K., Wenn, R. T., & Moran, C. G. (2006). Mortality and serum urea and electrolytes on admission for hip fracture patients. *Injury, 37,* 698–704.

83. Malani, P. N., Vaitkevicius, P. V., & Orringer, M. B. (2009). Perioperative evaluation and management. In J. B. Halter et al., *Hazzard's geriatric medicine and gerontology* (6th ed.). New York: McGraw-Hill Medical, p. 410.

84. Wright, S. K., & Schroeter, S. (2008). Hyponatremia as a complication of selective serotonin reuptake inhibitors. *Journal of the Academy of Nurse Practitioners, 20,* 47–51.

85. Wright & Schroeter, note 84.

86. Dharmarajan, T. S., Nguyen, T., & Russell, R. O. (2005). Life-threatening, preventable hyperkalemia in a nursing home resident: Case report and literature review. *Journal of the American Medical Directors Association, 6,* 400–405.

87. Mongardon, N., Le Manach, Y., Tresallet, C., Lescot, T., & Langeron, O. (2008). Subcutaneous hydration: A potentially hazardous route. *European Journal of Anaesthesiology, 25*(9), 771–772.

Index